Spoken Discourse Impairments in the Neurogenic Populations

Anthony Pak-Hin Kong
Editor

Spoken Discourse Impairments in the Neurogenic Populations

A State-of-the-Art, Contemporary Approach

Springer

Editor
Anthony Pak-Hin Kong
Academic Unit of Human Communication, Learning, and Development
The University of Hong Kong
Pokfulam, Hong Kong SAR

ISBN 978-3-031-45189-8   ISBN 978-3-031-45190-4 (eBook)
https://doi.org/10.1007/978-3-031-45190-4

This Springer imprint is published by the registered company Springer Nature Switzerland AG
The registered company address is: Gewerbestrasse 11, 6330 Cham, Switzerland

Paper in this product is recyclable.

To my parents, Imalda and Simon

To my niece, Meredith, and nephew, Anakin

and

To my grandma, PorPor

Foreword

Discourse refers to spoken or written communication between people, i.e., conversation. For linguists, discourse refers to a unit of language longer than a single sentence. However, this notion can be extended to any form of communication, e.g., email, gesture, sign, and texting. Spoken discourse impairments are difficulties in communication that can arise as a result of neurological damage including brain injuries, strokes, degenerative diseases, e.g., Alzheimer's disease, Parkinson's disease, or neurological conditions such as primary progressive aphasia (PPA) (see Chaps. 1–6). Such impairments can affect functional communication, making it challenging for individuals to engage in conversations and convey their thoughts effectively. These include aphasia defined as a difficulty finding words and constructing grammatically correct sentences (see Chaps. 10–18), but also dysarthria, e.g., slurred speech and reduced articulation; apraxia of speech, e.g., poor planning and coordination of speech movements; cognitive communication disorders, e.g., deficits to attention, memory, and problem solving; and social communication disorders, e.g., difficulty using cues such as gestures and facial expressions in conversations. Studies of these impairments range from qualitative analyses of pragmatics, e.g., adjusting spoken language to social expectations to quantitative analyses of fluency, e.g., hesitations and interruptions (see Chaps. 7, 12–17) to executive functions, e.g., control over language in conversation (see Chap. 18). Management and rehabilitation strategies for spoken discourse impairments include cognitive neuropsychological methods (see Chaps. 8, 9, 20); speech and language therapy, cognitive rehabilitation, interlocutor (partner) training, and teaching communication strategies (see Chaps. 19–26).

This collection is written by world experts in topics ranging from conversation and discourse analysis (e.g., Chap. 7) to AI technology (e.g., Chaps. 16, 17). One conclusion to emerge from this important collection is that there is now a network of international collaborators in place who are well equipped to build capacity in this important field (see Chaps. 1 and 21).

How can this collection be translated to clinical work in order to maximize impact? Discourse plays a significant role in psychotherapy as well as speech therapy, as it is through language and communication that therapists and clients engage in the therapeutic process. Therapy relies on verbal discourse as clients communicate their thoughts, feelings, and experiences. Through these communication channels, clients can express their concerns, anxieties, and emotions, which are central to healing. Loss of communication abilities means that patients are likely to develop mental health difficulties if early intervention is not provided. Indeed, some therapeutic approaches, such as narrative therapy, place an emphasis on the stories people tell about themselves and their lives. Therapists typically work with clients to explore and reshape these narratives, helping them to learn different perspectives to make positive changes to their thinking. Critically, these narratives need not be conveyed via the medium of speech only. Signs, symbols, and semiotics can play a part, as well as the use of electronic media that require no speech at all to enhance comprehension. For all therapists, language serves as a mirror reflecting cognitive processes that lead to problematic behavior. Specific discourse techniques facilitate emotional healing, behavioral and cognitive change by using active listening, paraphrasing, and vocalizing. These techniques also improve awareness of differences in communication genre and, in an increasingly multilingual world, can empower excluded groups in society, e.g., migrants, refugees, and seniors via enhancing their self-esteem. Several nonverbal therapeutic approaches specifically utilize metaphorical language and semiotics to help clients explore and express unique feelings and experiences. For example, within art, dance, music, and play therapies, clients use symbols and metaphors to represent their emotions and thoughts. These techniques could also have an important role in therapy when nonverbal communication is impaired. Research testing this hypothesis is nascent (1).

In summary, spoken discourse is a fundamental aspect of well-being. However, discourse is a broader concept and includes use of language in any communication, including the structure and organization of the meaning of signs, symbols, and writing (2). Similarly, discourse in sign language requires the same processes as spoken or written language, but conveyed through gestures, facial expressions, and body movements not via sound or text. Symbols provide an abstract representation of meaning but can be used to converse nevertheless. Text is a form of discourse and can be impaired in neurogenic populations, i.e., acquired reading and writing impairments (3, 4). Given the recent developments in AI, rehabilitation of acquired dyslexia and dysgraphia could take advantage of "transliterating" between speech and text to improve conversation, discourse, and well-being in a wide range of individuals, especially clients who do not speak the dominant language in their linguistic environment (5). In just the past three years alone, the capacity to transliterate text into speech and vice versa has accelerated to the standard whereby any client who has a smartphone or access to a camera can use "ChatGPT" or Zoom to participate in virtual discourse online, thus making "impairments" obsolete. AI and discourse processing should be considered *related* fields that focus on understanding, generation, and analysis of language and communication. Natural Language Processing (NLP) is a subfield of AI that deals with the interaction between computers and human language. It encompasses various techniques and algorithms for understanding and processing language. Discourse processing is actually a component of NLP, as it involves the interpretation of text or speech in context, taking into account the structure, meaning, and flow of a conversation. This opens up the possibility of developing

NLP for therapeutic purposes in speech therapy (see Chaps. 7, 16, 17, 18 for examples). AI systems can be designed to identify discourse markers, speech acts, and rhetorical structures. AI-powered chatbots and virtual assistants are applications that require discourse processing and therefore could be applied clinically.

As with human language, AI requires techniques to understand user input, generate relevant responses, and maintain coherence and context awareness in conversations. For clients with communication difficulties, their carers, and their therapists, these same cognitive processes are needed to generate a sense of meaning in any therapeutic context. AI systems also rely on dialogue management techniques to keep track of ongoing discourse, as do all therapists. AI translation systems exploit deep learning to translate text from one language to another as do multilingual speakers. However, they lack linguistic nuances in their current form as do some clients with multilingual aphasia. AI requires discourse processing to maintain flow and coherence in translated texts. Similar to the therapist who is working with spoken discourse impairments in neurogenic populations, specific techniques developed for discourse therapy could be applied as a learning criterion in AI to enable the software to understand, generate, and analyze language in a coherent and context-aware manner. As AI tools become smarter, with more data it may be possible to transfer deep learning algorithms to discourse therapy.

Discourse Analysis is a major topic in a wide range of nontherapeutic research fields such as critical justice, literature, and social theory, with work spanning fields including anthropology, art, education, law, music, poetry, philosophy, psychotherapy, religion, semiotics, sociology, and philosophy. In all of these fields, consideration of historical background, social, linguistic, psychological, visual, gestural, ritual, and technological processes requires an understanding of the cultural diversity within populations for theoretical developments to emerge. Speech therapists could scaffold their work with excluded clients by applying conceptual frameworks to understand communication styles chosen by their clients. For example, critical race theory can be used to assess, research, and treat spoken discourse impairments in excluded groups by understanding education, healthcare, and science within their socio-political context (6).

References

1. Pieri M, Foote H, Grealy MA, Lawrence M, Lowit A, Pearl G. Mind-body and creative arts therapies for people with aphasia: a mixed-method systematic review. Aphasiology 2022;37(3):504–62. doi: 10.1080/02687038.2022.2031862
2. Weekes BS. Literacy in contact and context. Letrônica 2020;13(4):e37538.
3. Weekes BS. Acquired disorders of reading and writing: cross-script comparisons. Behav Neurol 2005;16(2–3):51–7.
4. Weekes BS. Acquired dyslexia and dysgraphia across scripts. Behav Neurol 2012;25(3);159–63.

5. Weekes BS. Transliterating in space and time. 2022. Recorded keynote presentation for the association of reading and writing. https://www.youtube.com/watch?v=w2DoxKOQi9M
6. Horton R. Critical race theory for speech-language pathology: how race-conscious practice mitigates disparities. In Horton R, editor. Critical perspectives on social justice in speech-language pathology; 2021, pp. 84–104. doi: 10.4018/978-1-7998-7134-7.ch005

The University of Hong Kong
Pokfulam, Hong Kong SAR

Melbourne School of Psychological Sciences at the University of Melbourne
Melbourne, Australia

Brendan Stuart Weekes

Preface

The focus of this book is on the research and clinical aspects of discourse deficits in various neurological conditions such as aphasia, dementia, traumatic brain injury, and right hemisphere damage. It explores a wide range of topics such as historical reviews of discourse deficits research, discourse characteristics in different conditions, the neural correlates of spoken discourse, assessment methods, treatment approaches, and communication training. The scope of the book encompasses examining discourse deficits, understanding their neural basis, assessing impairment, and implementing interventions to improve discourse production in individuals with various neurological disorders.

Discourse impairment can have a significant impact on one's ability to communicate effectively, and can lead to social isolation and decreased quality of life. Engaging in research on discourse impairment can provide valuable insights in several areas: uncovering the neural mechanisms that underlie these deficits, enhancing the development of improved diagnostic tools and assessments, and facilitating the design of more effective intervention approaches and treatment strategies. As the need for research and theory around neurogenic discourse impairments (along with its clinical applications) has increased, it is my aim to draw together a group of expert researchers and clinicians to contribute articles within their specific areas of expertise to (i) share findings of their recent investigations to help understand spoken discourse analysis in various disorder populations, (ii) discuss principles of evaluating spoken discourse in adult patients with a variety of neurogenic communication disorders, and (iii) summarize and document their experiences with discourse intervention of different restorative approaches and explain their philosophies behind specific rehabilitation programs.

Compared with the recent text I wrote in 2016 *Analysis of Neurogenic Disordered Discourse Production: From Theory to Practice* and its second edition published in 2022 *Analysis of Neurogenic Disordered Discourse Production: Theories, Assessment and Treatment*, this volume is more comprehensive and holistic in its coverage of topics. The volume also addresses more specific and contemporary topics on spoken discourse impairments and allows contributing authors to discuss and highlight clinically relevant and important details in each chapter.

The chapters within this volume delve into the intricacies of discourse use, deficits, and language research and have implications for both research and clinical settings. As a result, they are relevant to individuals in different fields including researchers, clinicians, and students. I sincerely hope that users of this volume will enjoy the curated content. Constructive input, feedback, and comments are welcomed. More importantly, suggestions on additional relevant information and/or updates will allow potential creation of a better edition in the near future.

Hong Kong, Hong Kong SAR Anthony Pak-Hin Kong

Acknowledgments

I would like to express my gratitude to all the chapter authors for their tremendous efforts to produce these excellent contributions. Thank you for sharing your wisdom, knowledge, expertise, and outstanding work. I am also grateful to the Springer team for believing in this exciting book project and the support offered along the way.

Introduction

Discourse broadly refers to a unit of language longer than a single sentence, typically used in a spoken or written format to express ideas, feelings, and opinions or to interact with others. As the field of research in aphasia and related neurogenic disorders (particularly in terms of clinical decision making to evaluate and manage neurogenic communication impairments) is rapidly expanding, there has been an increased focus on spoken discourse analysis and therapy. Various user groups and people with lived experience, such as those with aphasia, dementia, traumatic brain injury, right hemisphere damage, etc., are also increasingly focused on the impact of neurogenic impairments on domains of conversation and changes in language skills beyond the smaller linguistic components of single words and sentences that are traditionally supported by speech-language therapy.

This comprehensive volume, *Spoken Discourse Impairments in the Neurogenic Populations: A State-of-the-Art, Contemporary Approach*, is an attempt to provide general overviews, state-of-the-art information and discussions, updated contents and resources, as well as evidence-based recommendations on the areas that are most crucial to the understanding of neurogenic discourse impairments. The volume contains 26 chapters, authored by a target international group of experts based in Asia, Australia, Europe, North and South America, and United Kingdom that provide a balanced and easily readable text of contemporary topics around discourse production. There are three general sections in this volume:

- Part I—Basic principles, historical perspectives, neural basis, and recent advancements of neurogenic disordered discourse analysis
- Part II—Current methods and technology in neurogenic disordered discourse elicitation, processing, and analysis
- Part III—Evidenced-based training strategies, interventions, and innovative technology to improve neurogenic disordered discourse

Collectively, these chapters highlight the international appeal and relevance to researchers, clinicians, and students in the field of communication sciences and disorders, speech and language therapy, gerontology, (neuro-) linguistics, psychology, and related fields in medical or social care. More importantly, these chapters pertain to research of language and capture the complexities of discourse use with implications for both the research and applied clinical settings.

The first part of this volume is oriented toward several issues that are germane to the overall theme of neurogenic discourse impairments. Topics summarized here include the historical perspectives (i.e., history and developmental milestones) and basic principles of discourse analysis, evolutions of and recent advancement in analyzing discourse production in acquired communication disorders, as well as discussion of the neural basis of impaired discourse. In the first chapter, Stark establishes the definition of discourse production and provides a historical overview of studying discourse in four neurogenic populations—aphasia, primary progressive aphasia, right hemisphere disorder, and traumatic brain injury. Recent advances in discourse databases and technology-based strategies to enhance examination of discourse in neurogenic populations are also discussed. In Chap. 2, Kintz focuses on the genres, tasks, and measures of discourse analysis among adults with aphasia. After describing the different levels (i.e., microlinguistic and macrolinguistic) of discourse performance in aphasia, together with the corresponding linguistic and cognitive systems used for both levels, the author provides a thorough discussion to compare and contrast the discourse characteristics between fluent and non-fluent aphasia.

Speech, language, and communication deficits are early symptoms in people living with dementia. Recent studies have suggested that spoken discourse may act as an early linguistic biomarker for diagnosing dementia and predicting its prognosis. In Chap. 3, Themistocleous discusses the language and communication biomarkers elicited through Clinical Discourse Analysis for dementia assessment and treatment efficacy evaluation. This is followed by details relative to the impact of dementia on microstructure and macrostructure of spoken discourse, as well as its cognitive representations. In Chap. 4, Mueller presents the current knowledge about cutting-edge biomarker detection and progression in Alzheimer's disease. In particular, the temporal relationships between development of the pathology, biomarker positivity, and co-occurrence of cognitive and discourse impairment are described.

Chapters 5 and 6 provide coverage for traumatic brain injury (TBI) and right hemisphere damage (RHD), respectively. More specifically, Chap. 5 (Lê and Coelho) contains a comprehensive description of the major characteristics of impaired spoken discourse comprehension and production, and written discourse deficits in TBI, together with their widespread functional impacts on major life domains. Apart from outlining the cognitive bases of discourse impairments secondary to brain injury, Lê and Coelho explain the application of Structure Building Framework (SBF) as a cognitive model for TBI discourse and the relationships between discourse and mental health factors among Veterans with TBI. In Chap. 6, Cornwell and Hewetson remind us that the RHD population are known to be heterogeneous in terms of their communication domains of discourse, prosody, semantics, and pragmatics. The authors summarize how discourse after RHD may differ across genres with reference to the meaning, appropriateness, cohesion, and efficiency of spoken output.

At present, the TalkBank system is the largest open-access, multimedia repository for studying spoken language data. In Chap. 7 (MacWhinney and

Fromm), the basic principles of this database (e.g., its adoption of international standards, use of the CHAT transcription format and CHAT-consistent software for analysis) are introduced. Apart from reviewing the establishment and research utilization of specific adult language databases, including the AphasiaBank, TBIBank, RHDBank, and DementiaBank, the authors illustrate how new and existing TalkBank tools can facilitate Language Sample Analysis (LSA) for adult neurogenic language disorders.

Chapters 8 and 9 approach discourse production and impairments from a neuroscience perspective. In Chap. 8, Alyahya outlines the neuroimaging methods for studying language and cognitive processing, with a highlight on the mechanisms associated with spoken discourse production. She focuses on how the structural neuroimaging literature on the neural correlates of spoken discourse can be synthesized, and discusses challenges we need to consider when conducting and interpreting findings of experiments that investigate the neural underpinnings of oral discourse. Chapter 9 (Schnur, Brown, and Guess), on the other hand, focuses on the use of functional neuroimaging methodologies to examine macrolinguistic properties of overt, unrehearsed multi-utterance speech. The authors nicely summarize existing contemporary work that informs a bilateral network of brain regions to support linguistic and cognitive processes involved during the production of coherent discourse. Multiple research avenues that will allow a better understanding of the functional relationships between brain regions and these cognitive and linguistic processes are also discussed.

In Chap. 10, Chick, Garrard, Buxbaum, and Vigliocco focus on co-speech gesture production at the discourse level. More specifically, while gestures are used naturally in human communication, how they are impaired in different populations with neurogenic communication disorders is still poorly understood. The authors review existing classification schemes and key features of co-speech gestures in unimpaired speakers as well as those impacted by acute (e.g., stroke) and chronic (e.g., dementia and Parkinson's disease) neurological conditions. To account for the characteristics of gesture production in neurogenic populations, two cognitive models to explain how speech and gestures interact during language production are also discussed.

At present, the number of multilingual speakers worldwide has exceeded those who are monolingual; this phenomenon is also reflected in various clinical populations. In Chap. 11, Goral starts by explaining the clinical characteristics of discourse production in multilingual people with aphasia. The importance of using discourse to examine the strengths and weaknesses of their multiple languages, as well as the need to pay attention to language mixing behaviors and the specific challenges associated with these analyses are also discussed. Both Chaps. 10 and 11 conclude nicely with avenues for future study.

When it comes to clinical evaluation of language skills in individuals with neurological conditions, discourse analysis is still, at present, an underutilized tool, despite its important and valuable benefits for informing diagnosis and subsequent remediation. **The second part of this volume outlines and illustrates current methods for discourse elicitation and analysis across different clinical populations. How assessment of discourse, when**

properly conducted, can help improve quantification of one's communication strengths and weaknesses is discussed. Recent leaps forward in technology that can assist in the recording, processing, and analysis of discourse are also highlighted.

Chapter 12 (Dalton and Richardson) summarizes a range of clinically feasible analyses of spoken discourse. More specifically, the discussion of these assessment options is first divided into the transcription-less and transcription-based options. For the latter approach, details on various word-level (e.g., correct information units) and proposition-level (e.g., Main Concept Analysis, Main Event Analysis) measures are given. The authors also direct readers to some web-based scoring tools that are currently available for analysis in English and conclude that more research is needed to confirm the accuracy and reliability of non-transcription-based implementation of these clinical measures.

In Chap. 13, Richardson, Dalton, and Greenslade focus on macrostructural analysis of discourse in aphasia and present several measures based on picture description and story (re)telling tasks that have been reported in aphasia research. Note, these measures are carefully selected for discussion because they have clear instructions on how to elicit and code spoken samples clinically, have relevant norms for references, and demonstrate promise for quantifying the degree of impairments as well as estimating changes in discourse performance, such as tracking recovery or monitoring treatment outcomes.

Concerning the TBI population, in Chap. 14, Mozeiko, Suting, and Lindsey first compare and contrast discourse assessment and other traditional options of evaluations (e.g., standardized assessments). They then detail different approaches (conventional paper-based vs. and technology-enhanced methods) to record, transcribe, and conduct analysis of TBI discourse. A summary of various relevant discourse elicitation tasks and quantification measures is also given.

Chapter 15 (Johnson and Preston) provides an overview of assessment of discourse in people with right hemisphere brain damage (RHD). The authors highlight the apragmatic deficits associated with RHD and explain how apragmatism (in terms of linguistic, paralinguistic, and/or extralinguistic problems) can be evaluated. There is also a nice summary of the RHDBank assessment protocol that clinicians can modify for use to assess discourse clinically.

Rather than focusing on the aforementioned qualitative and/or quantitative discourse measures alone, Chap. 16 (Qin and Lee) points out that automatic speech assessment, i.e., the computational process of deriving and analyzing symptoms-related speech features from acoustic signals, is gaining increasing attention in the fields of speech engineering. The authors explain that many methods and systems of automatic speech and language assessment in speech-language pathology are empowered by digital signal processing, machine learning (ML), and natural language processing (NLP). Apart from summarizing the principles of two mainstream approaches to automatic assessment (i.e., the two-step and end-to-end approaches), their challenges, pros, and cons are also discussed. Chapter 17 (Clarke and Garrard) follows on this topic and details how machine readable text has revolutionized discourse analysis. In particular, the authors present the core concepts of ML algorithms and pitfalls when training prediction models. Apart from reviewing how NLP is used to model natural human language, how features of different linguistic domains (e.g., lexical, syntactic, entropic, and word-embedding features) are automatically computed is described. This is followed by a discussion on how different computational approaches to speech analysis are operationalized in both the clinical and research contexts.

Chapter 18 (Choy, Dai, Kong, and Wong) is slightly different from other chapters in this part in that it focuses on remote assessment of discourse production and cognition. The authors first provide an overview of the latest developments in tele-assessments of people living with dementia (PWD) and survivors of stroke. Some experiences implementing tele-assessment of cognition and virtual discourse evaluation amid the COVID-19 pandemic, along with specific practical guidelines, are shared by the authors.

The final part of this volume deals with various approaches of recognized interventions or evidence-based treatment programs and training strategies to improve neurogenic disordered discourse. Reviews and summaries of key developments in rehabilitation across various clinical groups are provided, and utilization of innovative technology to clinically improve discourse impairments is discussed. To set the stage for discussion, the first chapter of this part—Chap. 19 (Dipper, Carragher, and Whitworth)—provides an overview of developments in discourse interventions in the aphasiology literature, highlighting the historical and theoretical frameworks of discourse examinations. Various approaches, genres, and discourse therapy contexts that clinicians should consider are discussed. In addition, with reference to the Rehabilitation Treatment Specification System (RTSS) that was previously devised for a more systematic characterization of individualized rehabilitation, the authors illustrate how the planning and implementation of three multi-level intervention programs of aphasic discourse (including interactive storytelling therapy, NARNIA, and LUNA) can be mapped against the RTSS components. The importance of integrating suitable cognitive processes and meta-linguistic/meta-cognitive strategies into discourse therapies is also discussed.

Chapter 20 (Bakhtiar, Carthery-Goulart, and Kong) discusses the neuromodulation methods to improve spoken discourse in two clinical populations—aphasia and primary progressive aphasia (PPA). Traditionally, this approach of neurorehabilitation has a primary focus on decontextualized word production, with much less attention toward its potential benefits to functional communication such as discourse production. The authors provide a state-of-the-art overview of investigations that applied neuromodulation accompanied with discourse production therapy and highlight some directions of future research that will consider, for example, individualized neuromodulation and bilateral versus unilateral brain stimulation protocols.

In Chap. 21, Dutta, Murray, Stark, and Bryant introduce an international working group of FOQUSAphasia that aims to address current issues and to improve the state of research regarding the assessment and treatment of spoken discourse. The authors illustrate how various FOQUSAphasia task forces initiatives and deliverables have successfully translated into improved evidence-based practice for managing spoken discourse in aphasia and related acquired language disorders.

Chapter 22 (Volkmer and Beeke) describes the Better Conversations (BC) approach to Communication Partner Training that focuses on individualized strategies to help people with communication difficulties and their communication partners. Apart from explaining the principles of this treatment approach, the authors present and summarize two case studies on its application to aphasia and PPA—i.e., the Better Conversation with Aphasia (BCA) and PPA (BCPPA) programs, respectively. Readers will find the given examples and details of intervention useful.

Chapter 23 (Brandão, de Lira, and Freitas) focuses on a socio-cognitive approach of improving discourse production in dementia, which is coherent with the person-centered perspectives on facilitating communication involving PWD. The intervention methods and protocols summarized here emphasize not only the functional aspects of communication, but also the importance for PWD and communication partners to make joint decisions regarding the planning of communication interventions.

In Chap. 24, Togher, Elbourn, and Steel address the heterogeneity of the population of TBI and, therefore, the need of a diverse range of intervention options to improve spoken discourse. These intervention methods include communication partner training, group-based social skills-based treatments, narrative-based interventions, social cognition treatments, project-based treatments, and vocational rehabilitation. The important theory behind these intervention approaches and corresponding clinical guidelines are provided.

As for Chap. 25, Hubner, Carthery-Goulart, and Rodrigues concentrate their efforts on telepractice on spoken discourse by first providing an overview of the recent research advances in stimulation, training, and rehabilitation of language and communication. The summary of different existing, published language-based telepractice interventions in healthy older adults and multiple clinical groups (including stroke, mild cognitive impairment, Alzheimer's disease, and primary progressive aphasia) as well as the recommendations on methodological considerations for these telepractice options are of interests to both researchers and healthcare professionals.

Finally, in Chap. 26 (Pais and Jagoe), the application of Communication Partner Training (CPT) in discourse intervention focusing on aphasia and its roles in addressing communication, conversation, and mental health or well-being is discussed. To broaden the cultural-linguistic and geographic representation in CPT research, the authors present clinical evidence of CPT generated in the Indian context and analyze the positive outcomes using the framework of Communication Accommodation Theory (CAT). Also contained in this chapter is the authors' illustration on how CAT can support rigorous and rich analysis of conversation and the psychosocial process underlying interaction.

Final Notes

As the need for research and theory around neurogenic discourse impairments (along with its clinical applications) has increased, it is my aim to draw together a group of expert researchers and clinicians to contribute articles within their specific areas of expertise to (i) share findings of their recent investigations to help understand spoken discourse analysis in various disorder populations, (ii) discuss principles of evaluating spoken discourse in adult patients with a variety of neurogenic communication disorders, and (iii) summarize and document their experiences with discourse intervention of different restorative approaches and explain their philosophies behind specific rehabilitation programs.

Compared with the recent text I wrote in 2016 *Analysis of Neurogenic Disordered Discourse Production: From Theory to Practice* and its second edition published in 2022 *Analysis of Neurogenic Disordered Discourse Production: Theories, Assessment and Treatment*, this volume is more comprehensive and holistic in the topics it covers. The volume also addresses more specific and contemporary topics on spoken discourse impairments and allows contributing authors to discuss and highlight clinically relevant and important details in each chapter.

I sincerely hope that users of this volume will enjoy the curated content. Constructive input, feedback, and comments are welcomed. More importantly, suggestions on additional relevant information and/or updates will allow potential creation of a better edition in the near future.

Contents

About the Editor

Anthony Pak-Hin Kong holds a Ph.D. in Speech and Hearing Sciences and is a professor and research scientist specialized in aphasiology a The University of Hong Kong. He is a Fellow of the American Speech-Language-Hearing Association (ASHA) and Academy of Aphasia. In 2013, he received the ASHA Recognition for Outstanding Contribution in International Achievement. Dr. Kong is the former Unit Head of *Academic Unit of Human Communication, Development, and Information Sciences* at The University of Hong Kong. He currently serves as the Founding Unit Head of Academic *Unit of Human Communication, Learning, and Development* and Director of *Aphasia Research and Therapy (ART) Laboratory* at The University of Hong Kong.Trained as a speech-language pathologist, Dr. Kong's research interests include stroke-induced aphasia, discourse analyses, neurogenic communication disorders in multilingual speakers, gesture production and multimodal communication in aphasia, acoustic analysis and automatic speech assessment for disordered speech, neuromodulation and technology-based training for acquired communication disorders, and community support to people with aphasia and their caregivers. His research has received continuous funding from the National Institutes of Health, the Hong Kong Government, the Government of the People's Republic of China, and multiple national and international universities and private foundations.Over the years, Dr. Kong has developed several important language and cognitive tools/batteries for clinical evaluation of Chinese speakers, such as the *Main Concept Analysis (MCA)* for oral discourse production, the Hong Kong version of the *Oxford Cognitive Screen*, and the Cantonese version of *Birmingham Cognitive Screen*. He is also the organizer of the Cantonese AphasiaBank (https://speech.edu.hku.hk/caphbank/search/), the first data-sharing corpus of multimodal discourse production by Chinese-speaking people with aphasia and healthy individuals. His most recent authored book is *Analysis of neurogenic disordered discourse production: Theories, assessment and treatment* (2nd edition) (Routledge).Dr. Kong is the Founding Editor-in-Chief of *Cogent Gerontology* (Taylor & Francis) and was elected as Vice Chairperson of the Hong Kong Association of Speech Therapists (2004-07). As a world-renowned scholar in communication sciences and disorders, Dr. Kong serves and served as Consultant/Advisor to provide research, clinical, and/or professional consultations to many national and international agencies, such as Aphasia United, Voices of Hope for Aphasia, Project BRIDGE (Building

Research Initiatives by Developing Group Effort, USA), the Self-help Group for the Brain Damaged, National Clinical Research Center for Aging and Medicine at Fudan University (China), Hong Kong Hospital Authority, and Hong Kong Society for Rehabilitation.

Contributors

Reem S. W. Alyahya Department of Language and Communication Sciences, School of Health and Psychological Sciences, City, University of London, London, UK

Department of Communication and Swallowing Disorders, King Fahad Medical City, Riyadh, Saudi Arabia

Mehdi Bakhtiar Speech and Neuromodulation Laboratory, Faculty of Education, The University of Hong Kong, Hong Kong, Hong Kong SAR

Academic Unit of Human Communication, Learning, and Development, The University of Hong Kong, Pokfulam, Hong Kong SAR

Suzanne Beeke Division of Psychology and Language Sciences, University College London, London, UK

Lenisa Brandão Department of Speech, Language and Hearing Sciences, Federal University of Santa Maria, Santa Maria, Brazil

Danielle A. Brown Department of Physical Medicine and Rehabilitation, University of Texas Health Science Center at Houston McGovern Medical School, Houston, TX, USA

Lucy Bryant Graduate School of Health, University of Technology Sydney, Sydney, Australia

Laurel J. Buxbaum Moss Rehabilitation Research Institute, Thomas Jefferson University, Philadelphia, PA, USA

Marcella Carragher Aphasia Centre of Research Excellence, La Trobe University, Melbourne, VIC, Australia

Maria Teresa Carthery-Goulart Center for Mathematics, Cognition and Computing, Federal University of ABC, Santo André, Brazil

Cognitive and Behavioral Neurology Unit (GNCC), University of São Paulo, São Paulo, Brazil

Academic Unit of Human Communication, Learning, and Development Faculty of Education, Unit of Human Communication, Learning, and Development, The University of Hong Kong, Pokfulam, Hong Kong SAR

Isobel Chick Language and Cognition Lab, University College London, London, UK

Jacky Chak Pui Choy Department of Social Work and Social Administration, The University of Hong Kong, Pok Fu Lam, Hong Kong SAR

Natasha Clarke Centre de recherche de l'Institut universitaire de gériatrie de Montréal, Montreal, Canada

Carl Coelho Department of Speech, Language, and Hearing Sciences, University of Connecticut, Storrs, CT, USA

Petrea Cornwell School of Health Sciences and Social Work, Griffith University, Gold Coast, QLD, Australia

Maria Isabel d'Ávila Freitas Department of Speech, Language and Hearing Sciences, Federal University of Santa Catarina, Florianópolis, Brazil

Ruizhi Dai Department of Psychology, Guangzhou University, Guangzhou, China

Center for Brain and Cognitive Sciences, Guangzhou University, Guangzhou, China

Sarah Grace H. Dalton Department of Speech Pathology and Audiology, Marquette University, Milwaukee, MI, USA

Juliana Onofre de Lira Faculty of Ceilândia, University of Brasília, Brasília, Brazil

Lucy Dipper Department of Language and Communication Science, School of Health and Psychological Sciences, City University of London, London, UK

Erica dos Santos Rodrigues Departament of Letters, Center for Theology and Human Sciences, Pontifical Catholic University of Rio de Janeiro (PUC-Rio), Rio de Janeiro, Brazil

Manaswita Dutta Department of Speech and Hearing Sciences, Portland State University, Portland, OR, USA

Elise Elbourn Department of Speech Pathology, The University of Sydney, Sydney, Australia

Davida Fromm Department of Psychology, Carnegie Mellon University, Pittsburgh, PA, USA

Peter Garrard Molecular and Clinical Sciences Research Institute, St George's University of London, London, UK

Mira Goral Department of Speech-Language-Hearing Sciences, Lehman College, The City University of New York, Bronx, New York, USA

Kathryn J. Greenslade Department of Communication Sciences and Disorders, University of New Hampshire, Durham, NH, USA

Kennedy K. Guess Department of Physical Medicine and Rehabilitation, University of Texas Health Science Center at Houston McGovern Medical School, Houston, TX, USA

Ronelle Hewetson School of Health Sciences and Social Work, Griffith University, Gold Coast, QLD, Australia

Lilian Cristine Hübner School of Humanities in the Graduate Course of Linguistics, Pontifical Catholic University of Rio Grande do School (PUCRS), Porto Alegre, Brazil

Caroline Jagoe Department of Clinical Speech and Language Studies, Trinity College Dublin, The University of Dublin, Dublin, Ireland

Human & Community Development, University of the Witwatersrand, Johannesburg, South Africa

Melissa Johnson Communication Sciences and Disorders Department, Nazareth University, Rochester, NY, USA

Stephen Kintz Department of Speech Language Pathology, University of Arkansas at Little Rock, Little Rock, AR, USA

Anthony Pak-Hin Kong Aphasia Research and Therapy (ART) Laboratory, The University of Hong Kong, Pok Fu Lam, Hong Kong SAR

Academic Unit of Human Communication, Learning, and Development, The University of Hong Kong, Pokfulam, Hong Kong SAR

Tan Lee Department of Electronic Engineering, The Chinese University of Hong Kong, Hong Kong, Hong Kong SAR

Karen Lê Audiology and Speech Pathology Service, VA Connecticut Healthcare System, West Haven, CT, USA

André Lindsey School of Education, Nevada State University, Henderson, NV, USA

Brian MacWhinney Department of Psychology, Carnegie Mellon University, Pittsburgh, PA, USA

Jennifer Mozeiko Department of Speech, Language and Hearing Sciences, University of Connecticut, Storrs, CT, USA

Kimberly D. Mueller Department of Communication Sciences and Disorders, University of Wisconsin, Madison, WI, USA

Division of Geriatrics in School of Medicine and Public Health, University of Wisconsin, Madison, WI, USA

Laura L. Murray School of Communication Sciences and Disorders, Western University, London, ON, Canada

Analisa Pais School of Health and Social Care, University of Essex, Colchester, UK

Jessie Preston Communication Sciences and Disorders Department, Nazareth University, Rochester, NY, USA

Ying Qin Institute of Information Science in School of Computer and Information Technology, Beijing Jiaotong University, Beijing, People's Republic of China

Jessica D. Richardson Department of Speech and Hearing Sciences, University of New Mexico, Albuquerque, NM, USA

Tatiana T. Schnur Department of Physical Medicine and Rehabilitation, University of Texas Health Science Center at Houston McGovern Medical School, Houston, TX, USA

Brielle C. Stark Department of Speech, Language and Hearing Sciences, Indiana University Bloomington, Bloomington, IN, USA

Joanne Steel School of Health Sciences (Speech Pathology), The University of Newcastle, Callaghan, Australia

Louisa Suting Department of Speech, Language and Hearing Sciences, University of Connecticut, Storrs, CT, USA

Charalambos Themistocleous Department of Special Needs Education, University of Oslo, Oslo, Norway

Leanne Togher Department of Speech Pathology, The University of Sydney, Sydney, Australia

Gabriella Vigliocco Language and Cognition Lab, University College London, London, UK

Anna Volkmer Division of Psychology and Language Sciences, University College London, London, UK

Anne Whitworth School of Health Sciences, University of Tasmania, Hobart, TAS, Australia

Gloria H. Y. Wong Department of Social Work and Social Administration, The University of Hong Kong, Pok Fu Lam, Hong Kong SAR

List of Figures

List of Tables

Part I

Basic Principles, Historical Perspectives, Neural Basis, and Recent Advancements of Neurogenic Disordered Discourse Analysis

Historical Review of Research in Discourse Deficits and Its Recent Advancement

1

Brielle C. Stark

Preview of What Is Currently Known

Individuals with aphasia cite improving their ability to converse—a type of discourse—as a top priority [1]. Further, researchers and clinicians agree that assessing and analyzing discourse in aphasia enable comprehensive characterization of language and its use [2, 3]. It is therefore unsurprising that discourse has a long history of study in the field of communication sciences and disorders, and discourse analysis has helped to characterize the communication strengths and weaknesses of individuals with neurogenic communication disorders. There are constant improvements to the ways in which we assess and analyze discourse as it relates to neurogenic communication, improving our ability to comprehensively understand (and treat) discourse in this population.

Objectives

(a) To introduce and define discourse analysis
(b) To provide a historical overview of interest in studying discourse in neurogenic communication disorders
(c) To discuss approaches to discourse analysis specific to neurogenic communication populations
(d) To provide an overview of advances for better understanding the preservation, breakdown, and treatment of discourse in neurogenic populations

Introduction

Discourse drives human communication as the means by which we express our feelings, thoughts, ideas, and emotions using words. We tell stories about our lives, we teach others how to do tasks, we have conversations, we give academic presentations, and we write fictional stories. People with neurogenic communication disorders often find engaging in discourse difficult and may demonstrate discourse impairments, which can lead to frustration, lower quality of life, psychosocial stress, and social isolation.

It is important to establish the definition by which this chapter approaches discourse. This chapter aligns itself with three commonly used definitions of discourse in the communication sciences and disorders field:

> *Any language that is "beyond the boundaries of isolated sentences" (Ulatowska & Olness, 2004, p. 300)* [4]

> *A set of utterances aimed at conveying a message among interlocutors ... [it] may be the most elaborative linguistic activity (Ska, Duong, & Joanette, 2004, p. 302)* [5]

B. C. Stark (✉)
Department of Speech, Language and Hearing Sciences, Indiana University Bloomington, Bloomington, IN, USA
e-mail: bcstark@iu.edu

A. P.-H. Kong (ed.), *Spoken Discourse Impairments in the Neurogenic Populations*,
https://doi.org/10.1007/978-3-031-45190-4_1

Language beyond a single simple clause used for a specific purpose (Armstrong 2000, Halliday 2004) [6, 7]

Discourse can be spoken or written and is typically accompanied by multimodal communicative elements such as gesture, eye gaze, and facial expression. Further, discourse can be monologic or dialogic/conversational. This chapter focuses on spoken discourse.

Given that discourse is more than just the production of a single word and reflects the type of natural communication we engage in on a daily basis, many researchers and clinicians in the field of communication sciences and disorders are interested in analyzing it. *Analyzing* discourse is to closely inspect components within the discourse, so that we may better understand them (e.g., understand how brain injury impacts this component), as well as accurately measure them. Accurate measurement enables researchers and clinicians to use these components as diagnostic markers, to quantify recovery, and as targets of treatment.

Discourse can be assessed by employing a variety of instructions, usually grouped into genres and tasks. Genre includes the general variety of discourse, such as a narrative, and task includes the specific instructions that guide the discourse, such as "tell me a story about …." Genres/tasks employ different cognitive components (e.g., telling a personal story requires access to episodic long-term memory and executive function to organize its components in addition to verbal language). As such, anything extracted from discourse, regardless of which component it represents, may be specific to type (monologic/dialogic), genre, and task. It is, therefore, often best practice to acquire discourse samples across genres/tasks. Indeed, Armstrong [6] highlights that some of the measures extracted from a single task are not generalizable beyond that task, and researchers/clinicians are thus cautioned about broader interpretation related to treatment effectiveness and recovery.

The benefits of acquiring and analyzing discourse are many. One can evaluate aspects of language structure (e.g., phonology, semantics) as well as use/function (e.g., topic management, context appropriateness), thus providing a holistic means of assessing a person's language capabilities. Discourse appears to have good face and ecological validity, seeming more like everyday language than language typically assessed in standardized batteries. Further, discourse analysis may be more sensitive to picking up language issues in mildest aphasia, which in turn enables clinicians to continue to advocate for services for that population [8, 9]. Discourse has a tendency to elicit manual gesture (which has been shown to be produced by individuals with aphasia at a much higher rate and used to supplement speech [10–18]), enabling one to assess the use and quality of multimodal communication in addition to verbal communication. Analysis of discourse may help predict severity of dementia [19], being a sensitive means of detecting early disease and potentially improving quality of life by engaging in earlier remediation strategies. Because there are so many diverse aspects of discourse to evaluate, both qualitative and quantitative analyses have been used to better understand its breakdown (and its preservation) in the neurogenic communication populations.

A recent review by Dipper and colleagues [20] proposes a theoretical framework which conceptualizes the building blocks, or components, of discourse. The goal of conceptualizing discourse in this way is to aid in developing discourse-specified treatments, measuring discourse change during recovery, and conceptualizing the relationship between discourse levels to better understand complex recovery patterns often demonstrated in those with neurogenic communication disorders. Specifically, Dipper and colleagues divide discourse into four components: linguistic, propositional, macrostructural/planning, and pragmatic (Fig. 1.1). These components are derived from several other influential

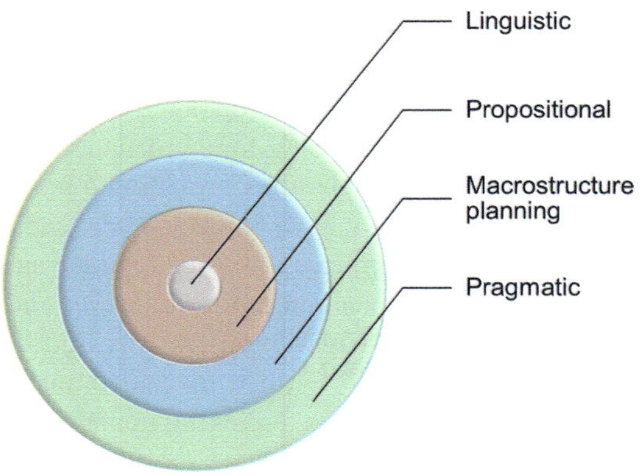

Fig. 1.1 My interpretation of Dipper et al.'s [20] unified theoretical framework of discourse

theories [7, 21–23] and form a unified framework for interpretation of discourse in the context of neurogenic populations. Within each component of discourse, researchers and clinicians measure variables that are thought to be representative of the core function of that level. Dipper et al. [20] give several examples as follows:

- Linguistic: measuring language variables like syntax, lexical semantics, lemma and lexemes, and phonology
- Propositional: measuring sequencing, sentence semantics, cohesion, and semantic content
- Macrostructural/planning: measuring structure, gist, story content, framing, and coherence
- Pragmatic: evaluating context, interpersonal factors, interactional factors, and influences on discourse from situational and external influences

Whilst pragmatics has been described in a variety of ways, it is largely concerned with the social appropriateness of language [24]. Examples of actual outcome measures seen in the aphasia literature from each of these levels include percentage paraphasias and correct information units [25] (linguistic level), main concept analysis [26, 27] and sequencing [9] (propositional level), story grammar [28] (macrostructural/planning), and evaluation of the context's influence on discourse, e.g., how discourse is molded across different tasks or in monologic vs. dialogic settings [29–33] (pragmatic). Conversation analysis [34] contains elements that can fit into each of these levels, as well. Therefore, researchers and clinicians are able to quantify preservation, or deficit, in variables within each component.

A Historical Overview of Studying Discourse in Neurogenic Populations

Discourse has been a topic of interest in the field of communication sciences and disorders since at least the mid-1900s, with a steep increase in publications related to discourse, especially in aphasia, occurring from the 1970s and 1980s [2]. As eloquently summarized by Ulatowska and Bond Chapman in 1989 [35], observations of communicative competence [via discourse analysis] reveal a discrepancy between performance on standardized language tests and functional communication (i.e., communicating in everyday life), making discourse analysis an especially sensitive means of fully comprehending the communication ability of individuals with aphasia [35]. In the following sections, historical approaches to spoken discourse assessment and analysis are discussed (non-exhaustively). A summary of select findings, divided by neurogenic population, is also given in Fig. 1.2.

Aphasia

Aphasia is characterized by an impairment of language, which can affect speaking, listening, reading, and writing. Aphasia occurs most commonly after a left hemisphere stroke but can be due to other etiologies such as head injury, tumor (and resection), and viruses/bacterial infections. Aphasia is acutely present in approximately one-third of strokes and, in a further one-third of cases [36], can persist into the chronic stage (i.e., present 6 months after the injury). Aphasia is

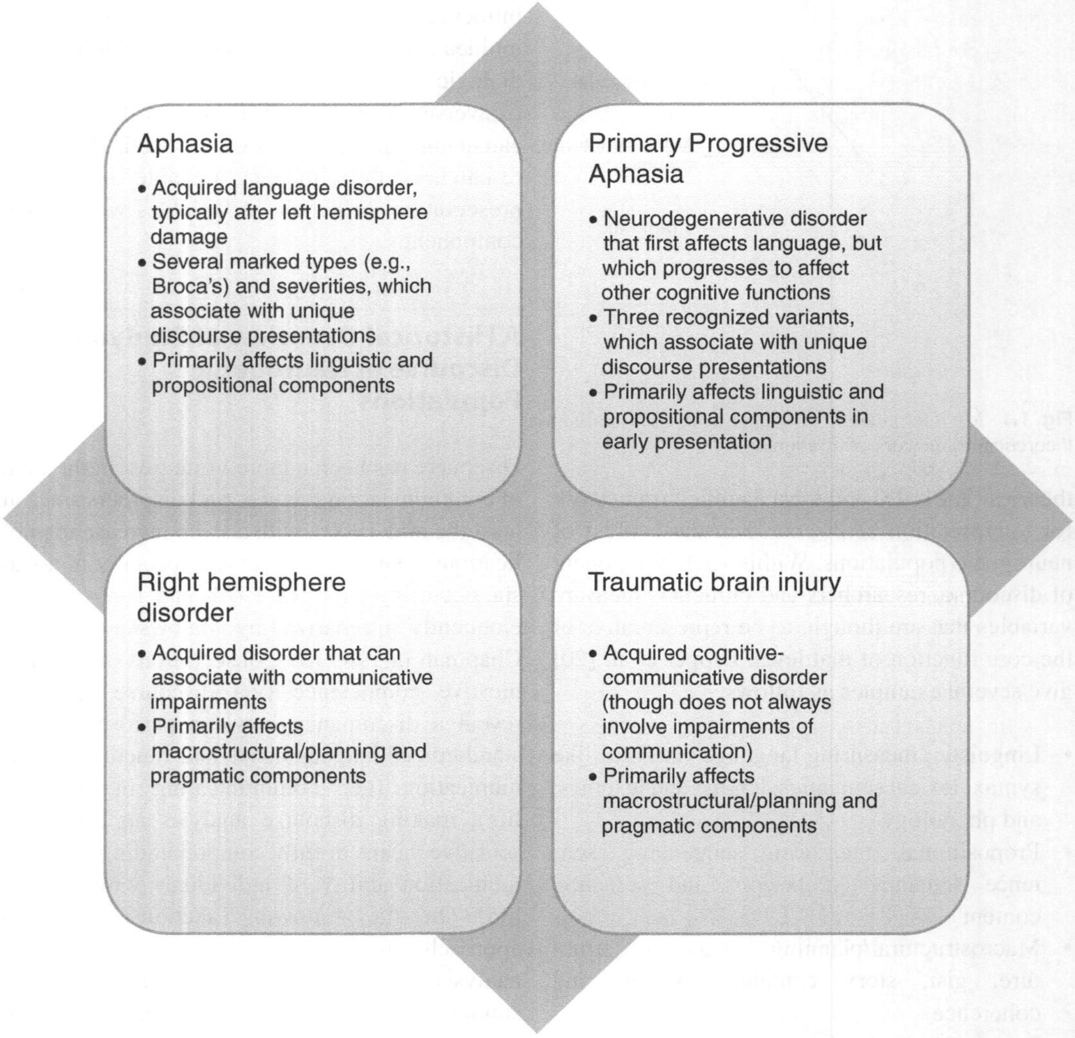

Fig. 1.2 Four neurogenic communication disorders and the components of discourse that are most affected

characterized as predominantly affecting production (often called "non-fluent" or "expressive" type of aphasia) or comprehension (often called "fluent" or "receptive" type of aphasia). Some standardized tests, such as the Western Aphasia Battery-Revised [37], further delineate aphasia into specific subtypes, e.g., Broca's aphasia.

A review by Bryant et al. [2] demonstrated the sharp increase in discourse studies in aphasia since the 1980s, which emphasizes growing research and clinical interest in this area. In Armstrong's [6] review of discourse studies in aphasia, she points out that the bulk of early research in aphasia involved analysis of "microstructure," which, for our purposes, largely contains the linguistic and propositional components discussed earlier. A recent review by Linnik et al. [38] emphasizes that much work still takes place at those levels, with increasing amounts of research at the macrostructural/planning and pragmatic levels. Typically, focus has been on characterizing impairments at the linguistic level, given that aphasia impacts lexical, syntactic, phonological, and semantic processes. We refer readers to each of these comprehensive reviews for extended information about discourse production in aphasia.

Linguistically, individuals with aphasia produce a variety of paraphasias (word errors) in discourse [39, 40] and demonstrate various word retrieval issues, such as elongated or filled pauses, false starts, and word fragments, as well as repetitions and retracings (for a review, see Linnik et al. [38]). Syntax can also be impaired, being either impoverished (agrammatic) [41–43] or misused (paragrammatic) [44, 45]. As mentioned in the introduction, context and task have an impact on discourse production. For example, increased syntactic complexity within narratives may result in a higher proportion of syntactic errors in narrative as opposed to procedural discourse [35]. Individuals with aphasia may also have difficulty with producing core vocabulary that individuals without aphasia typically produce (core lexicon [46]) and producing informative and efficient information [25, 47]. The linguistic weaknesses demonstrated by individuals with aphasia also vary by aphasia type and severity; for example, individuals with Broca's aphasia (a non-fluent type of aphasia, typically severe to moderate in severity) tend to produce more nouns than verbs, as well as simpler syntax due to the prevalence of agrammatism [48].

At the propositional level, individuals with aphasia have been shown to have difficulties with cohesion, which refers to the semantic connectedness between propositional elements [49]. The reason for impaired cohesion may be due to impairments in coreference [30, 50], where individuals with aphasia may omit antecedents of pronouns, thus introducing ambiguity [6, 51]. When comparing dialogues and monologues in two individuals with aphasia, it has been found that cohesion may be facilitated in dialogues [52]. Cohesion also involves the ability to time reference (i.e., shift between past and present), a concept with which individuals with syntactic impairments may have difficulty [53, 54]. For example, individuals with Broca's aphasia and agrammatism tend to be selectively impaired in the use of grammatical morphology associated with reference to the past (e.g., by producing a verb that is unmarked for tense, like "peel the potato" rather than "peeled the potato") [53]. Other studies have shown that tense accuracy is likely mediated by task, whereas more challenging tasks (like discourse compared to sentence completion) had a tendency to reveal a past tense disadvantage, suggesting that verb tense impairment is exacerbated in the more complex environment of discourse in agrammatic aphasia [55]. Another impairment commonly found at the propositional level is the production of accurate and complete main concepts [27, 56]. Main concept analysis [27] evaluates the extent to which utterances provide the gist of the task and extends into evaluating the utterance's accuracy and completeness [57]. As with linguistic impairments, propositional level impairments vary by aphasia type and severity [8, 26].

Within the macrostructural/planning component, coherence [58–61] and story grammar/sequencing [9] may be impaired in the aphasia population. Coherence refers to the semantic connectedness across several propositions or the entire discourse, whilst story grammar/sequencing is the logical organization of the discourse into parts (e.g., beginning, middle, end). In a sample of native Russian speakers with ($N = 10$) and without ($N = 10$) aphasia, it was found that coherence (as rated on a 4-point scale) was lower for those with aphasia, and when investigating further, it was found that different combinations of linguistic (e.g., syntactic and word-level errors) and macrostructural variables (e.g., discourse structure) likely combined to support (or impair) coherence [62]. Research using conversation analysis has also explored macrostructural/planning components, with evidence indicating that individuals with aphasia may have issues with topic maintenance and switching [63, 64]. Some research suggests that discourse organization may be intact independent of aphasia severity (except in most severe cases) [50, 65]. Olness and Ulatowska [50] suggest that, in many cases, aspects of macrostructure and pragmatics can be preserved due to multiple factors that contribute to the overall coherence of a narrative. For example, leveraging a small number of agents in the story (thus limiting the need to constantly refer to different agents), shared cultural knowledge of the story's gist or main events, and the knowledge that past tense tends to be explicitly marked in personal narratives. The following example is originally from Olness and Ulatowska:

> *Man it's stroke. It's comin'. Yes okay. After it's seure [seizure]. "Uh:"! [sound of having a seizure] Oh Lord, oh Lord. Talking. And now, "Woo:"! [ambulance sound] An(d) then, "Why?" "I can't talking." It's and for, for long, not long time. Man it's angry! It angry boy. Oh. But it's okay. It's praise God.*

The authors rated this story as relatively coherent overall, given that the topic (stroke) has been established and is contextually appropriate (the prompt was to discuss a frightening experience). The authors also cited that there is temporal-causal order which is explicit (i.e., "and now"). Therefore, even with impaired lexical retrieval or morphosyntax, oftentimes macrostructure and/or pragmatics can be preserved due to these implicit factors.

Pragmatics are generally thought to be intact in this population [66]. However, context and different interlocutors (e.g., at home with familiar conversation partners vs. in research settings with an experimenter) can affect aphasic discourse. As noted by Ulatowska and Olness, a complete understanding of communicative competence must outline limitations or boundaries and the contexts by which these boundaries manifest [50]. A recent study investigated whether individuals with aphasia's discourse benefitted when completing a collaborative communication task with a partner that they were familiar with; their performance was also compared to a group of neurologically healthy controls [67]. It was concluded that individuals with aphasia showed faster communication (though similar accuracy) when a familiar conversation partner was present.

Whilst I have thus far focused on impairments, it should be noted that, despite language impairments, individuals with aphasia can be very good communicators [68]. Indeed, individuals with aphasia have been shown to use multimodal communication effectively, including manual gestures that supplement speech [13, 14], and to use strategies that aid in word retrieval issues, such as circumlocution, singing, and onomatopoeia [69]. This has sometimes been termed as successful "codification of ideas" [70], referring to the ability to convey a message with available linguistic and nonlinguistic cognitive resources. Given sufficient time and space to think [71, 72], many individuals with aphasia will successfully convey their intended message.

Primary Progressive Aphasia (PPA)

Primary progressive aphasia (PPA) is a progressive type of aphasia caused by a neurological disease, most commonly Alzheimer's disease and frontotemporal dementia (a group of related disorders affecting the frontal and temporal lobes of the brain) [73]. Like acquired aphasia, PPA can affect speaking, listening, reading, and writing. As of 2023, there are three acknowledged variants: logopenic, agrammatic/non-fluent, and semantic (sometimes called semantic dementia) [74].

Because PPA is a relatively new diagnosis (first described by Mesulam in 1982 [73, 75]), analyzing the linguistic and propositional components of discourse has played a role in characterizing the speech of PPA, usually by subgroup or across subgroups [76–81]. Wilson et al. (2010), evaluated discourse samples in patients with non-fluent variant of PPA and found that they were characterized by slow rate, distortions, syntactic errors, and reduced syntactic complexity [76]. Patients with the semantic variant of PPA, in contrast, demonstrated a typical rate and few speech or syntactic errors but instead showed higher proportions of closed class words, pronouns, verbs and higher frequency nouns. The authors attributed this to reduced lexical retrieval typical of this variant. Finally, in the logopenic variant of PPA, speech rate was intermediate (between semantic and non-fluent variants), and this was also the case for distortions and syntactic errors (less common than the non-fluent variant) and lexical access (less common than the semantic variant). This early study in PPA demonstrates the benefits of using discourse to differentiate the variants of PPA. Similar to aphasia types and severities differing in the types of discourse weaknesses (and strengths) that they demonstrate, PPA variants and severities similarly differ. Early [82] and more recent research [43, 83] suggest that, in order to understand how language degrades over time in PPA, the most sensitive means may be investigating measures from discourse rather than standard batteries (e.g., naming batteries).

In the macrostructural/planning domain, individuals with PPA may have trouble with gist and, in the propositional domain, with main concept production [84]. Forty individuals with PPA (20 with semantic PPA, 20 with non-fluent/agrammatic PPA) described a picture and produced fewer main concepts than a group of matched controls [85]. Individuals with semantic PPA may also have issues with coherence, as individuals with semantic PPA may produce ambiguous or inaccurate semantic information, which degrades the coherence of the discourse. This is due to their selective impairment in semantics and the role of semantic connectedness in coherence [86]. Individuals with semantic PPA may substitute superordinate terms (like "animal" instead of the more appropriate "horse") and increasingly vague words (like "that" and "thing") as time progresses "horse" or "animal" [81], reflecting increased difficulty with accessing more specific semantic information (a linguistic impairment). Even superordinate terms become difficult for these patients over time, and as the disease progresses, the meaningfulness of words becomes increasingly vague and ultimately consists of terms like "that" and "thing" [81]. There is some evidence that individuals with PPA can omit episodes in a narrative (like the Cinderella story) and narrate other episodes incompletely, perhaps suggesting an impairment of story grammar [87].

In the pragmatic component, early research (in 14 individuals with frontal lobe dementia without PPA [$N = 3$] and those with PPA [$N = 5$ with non-fluent PPA and $N = 6$ with fluent PPA], which today likely means semantic and logopenic variants together) suggested that individuals with PPA produced fewer on-topic phrases than those with frontotemporal lobe dementia without PPA [88]. Moreover, the non-fluent PPA group produced the most off-topic utterances and the highest percentage of perseverative and intrusive utterances (e.g., stereotypies and automatic language) [88]. The use of coined or automatic phrases that lack meaning (e.g., "you know") can reflect word-finding difficulty. More recent research on dyadic conversations between individuals with PPA and their partners suggested that individuals with PPA have a reduced mean length of turn but maintained their turn-taking abilities, that conversation partners often bore a greater burden of highlighting issues in conversation and initiating their repair, and that each dyad (pair) demonstrated unique patterns of language during conversation [89].

The syndrome of PPA highlights the interaction of cognition and language by task, with many individuals with PPA having more difficulty in more complex tasks (e.g., narratives [87]). This suggests that complex tasks, in particular, may be more sensitive to exploring discourse production and/or deficits in this population.

Right Hemisphere Disorders (RHDs)

Right hemisphere disorder (RHD) is an acquired brain injury (e.g., stroke, traumatic brain injury) that causes impairments in language and cognition. Historically, differences in discourse following RHD are thought to be "less obvious" when compared to left hemisphere brain damage. RHD rarely leads to aphasia (typically called "crossed aphasia" when this occurs). In general, it is thought that linguistic levels are generally most intact in RHD, with issues arising primarily at propositional, macrostructural, and pragmatic levels.

An early study evaluated narrative and procedural samples from individuals with RHD, demonstrating group differences in informativeness, efficiency, total main concepts, and number of absent main concepts, compared with age-similar controls [90]. Individuals with RHD produced similar language and main concepts as a control group during the procedural tasks, but varied significantly from controls on the narrative task. Notably, the RHD group did not differ from the control group on several cognitive measures, suggesting that it was the interaction of language and complexity in the narrative that likely produced the between-group difference. Minga [91] in a review published in 2016 makes it clear that discourse weaknesses seem to be more prominent in narratives than in other types of tasks, probably because of the wide-reaching cognitive components involved in producing narratives (e.g., executive function, episodic memory) [91].

Individuals with RHD are thought to produce less informative narratives (as perceptually rated by listeners) [92], which may be due to exclusion or oversimplifying of core propositions, reflecting an impairment at the propositional level [93]. This is despite narratives of individuals with RHD having just as many words [94] or more words [95] compared to controls. In one study of those with right hemisphere brain damage and control participants, the numbers of words and T units (a way of delineating an utterance) were equal, though the narratives produced by the right hemisphere brain damage group contained significantly less information, in terms of fewer complex propositions (which contain more than one piece of information or link two pieces of information) and number of core propositions (those expected to be produced in the narrative) [93]. Cohesion may be impaired following right hemisphere injury, including impairments in referential cohesion, logical coherence, and accuracy of narration (and again, more obvious with more complex narrative tasks) [96]. Coherence and story grammar, too, may be impacted [94].

At the pragmatic level, researchers have found that participants with RHD were more tangential in their narratives, with some tending to terminate their script productions prematurely [97]. In two case studies, the individuals had to be prompted to return to task, because their scripts were being taken over by tangential remarks (e.g., off topic) or excessive script detail. The authors hypothesized that in these two cases, the individuals were led away from the topic by an inability to prevent their intrusive (e.g., tangential remark) behavior [97]. Conversationally, there are issues with macrostructure and pragmatics, including issues with topic choice or maintenance, as well as failure to adhere to turn-taking rules [98–101]. Individuals with RHD may also request for additional information less often, may assert more facts or opinions, and may ask fewer questions [102].

Traumatic Brain Injury (TBI)

Adulthood traumatic brain injury (TBI) is an acquired disorder that has several etiologies (i.e., closed or open head injury), brain injury presentations (e.g., diffuse axonal injury), and severities. Because TBI can affect a variety of brain structures, and be relatively diffuse, the discourse impairments vary across the TBI population. A historically difficult thing with interpreting discourse impairments in the TBI population is that many early papers did not discuss whether the included individuals with TBI also had concomitant aphasia or other motor speech impairments, such as apraxia of speech. Some studies on discourse including individuals with TBI purposively exclude individuals with concomitant aphasia.

Carl Coelho has a large body of work in this area, with an early review of 17 studies suggesting that impairment at the linguistic level of discourse was difficult to conclusively identify, due to unclear presence of aphasia and dysarthria, but that generally word retrieval issues are common in TBI [103]. In some cases, total word production was found to be similar in individuals with severe TBI, mild or moderate TBI, and controls, yet differed when evaluating syntax (specifically, percentages of complete sentences), where the individuals with severe TBI performed significantly worse than the control group (but note that they did not perform significantly different from the mild-to-moderate group) [104]. Individuals with TBI (who typically do not demonstrate significant deficits based on traditional clinical language tests, i.e., do not have aphasia) may have difficulty at the propositional level, producing fewer propositions per T-unit [105]. A more recent study in 14 individuals with severe (though not aphasic) TBI also demonstrated issues with cohesion and coherence, producing narratives with frequent interruption of ongoing utterances, derailments, and extraneous utterances that rendered their discourse vague and ambiguous [104, 106]. However, some other studies have not reported issues with cohesion), though this may be due, once again, to the complexity of the elicitation task [103, 107–109]. Propositional level issues in TBI may be related to deficient organization and monitoring of language representations in working memory [110, 111]. Global coherence during narrative production may be impacted in TBI [104]. Errors of global coherence include production of tangential utterances, utterances that are incongruent with the narrative, propositional repetitions, or simple fillers. The authors gave the example of the following: /It is a picnic/I like picnics/I have made several picnics in my life/[104], where the second and third utterances are tangential, as they provide information that is irrelevant for the task and is simply triggered by a specific idea depicted in the stimulus. Individuals with severe TBI may produce fewer thematic units (i.e., missing more of the story content) than controls [104]. Further research suggests errors of global coherence, and less informative speech, can even be present in mild TBI [112]. Pragmatically, the production of social norms is thought to be impaired in TBI discourse [113, 114], and individuals with TBI may have difficulty with topic maintenance in both monologic and dialogic tasks [113, 115, 116].

In general, it is recognized that analyzing discourse is fruitful during TBI assessment, as the sufficiently challenging narrative genre (in particular, when the narrative involves recall of events, thus drawing on declarative memory) enables sensitive assessment of language and discourse [117, 118].

Recent Advances in Studying Discourse in Neurogenic Populations

Advances in Databases, Technology, and Analyses

A huge advance in the analysis of discourse has been the growth of publicly available databases, like those curated by the TalkBank project [119–121]. AphasiaBank [122], TBIBank [123], RHDBank [124], and DementiaBank all contain discourse from those respective populations, as well as detailed demographic and neuropsychological information. There are several languages represented in these corpuses. As of the writing of this chapter, AphasiaBank contains speech samples from over 350 individuals with aphasia and over 200 individuals without aphasia. The databases contain audio and/or video eliciting discourse using their standard protocol (which includes a free speech sample, autobiographical narratives, a fictional narrative, several picture sequence descriptions, a single-picture description, and a procedural "how to" narrative) as well as contributed audio and/or video files that are "off protocol" and comprise things like group therapy sessions, other non-protocol discourse tasks, and standardized test batteries. Many of these projects also contain curated Grand Rounds, which use several samples from the discourse protocol to educate learners about discourse components and how they are impacted by the disorders. Because there is finally a critical mass of data available (something inherently hard to do in clinical populations), researchers have been able to mine data using innovative approaches like natural language processing and artificial intelligence. CLAN [121], which is the software curated by the TalkBank team for analysis of the speech transcripts, has been advancing since its advent in the early 2000s and is now capable of producing a variety of automatic analyses such as moving average type-token ratio (a measure of lexical diversity) and core lexicon analysis (a measure of core vocabulary produced for a given sample).

With a growing understanding of the many levels of discourse (i.e., linguistic through pragmatic) has come an increased emphasis on measuring language across those levels. Multilevel analysis has become increasingly more common [58, 125, 126], and so has analysis focused on higher levels of discourse, e.g., macrostructure [9]. Multilevel analysis in individuals with anomic aphasia demonstrated that, despite a more mild type of aphasia, these individuals tended to make linguistic, propositional, and macrostructural errors, such as more semantic paraphasias (linguistic), cohesion errors (propositional), and global coherence errors (macrostructural) but demonstrated preserved thematic selection (another aspect of macrostructure) [51]. Recent research in multilevel analysis has evaluated main concept analysis, sequencing, and story grammar in aphasia, demonstrating that individuals with aphasia differ across all of these areas when compared to a matched, non-brain-damaged group, and that this was true across each aphasia subtype and even for individuals with aphasia who had a very mild impairment (i.e., scoring higher than the aphasia cutoff on a standard aphasia battery) [9]. Continued work in streamlining multilevel analysis will provide more comprehensive and sensitive understanding of discourse.

A survey that my team recently completed [3] coupled with other surveys [127, 128] demonstrates that a major barrier in discourse analysis is time, principally time to analyze and interpret the samples, and a lack of training and/or availability of tools to analyze discourse. To combat this, we and others have urged for the creation and validation of tools which would streamline discourse analysis. Core lexicon analysis has been one such way of achieving this goal [46, 56, 129, 130] (recently, an automated version available in CLAN [131]). Core lexicon checklists were developed by analyzing a variety of discourse genres and tasks in speakers without brain damage, representative of the core vocabulary (inclusive of nouns, verbs, adjectives, adverbs) produced during these samples. The resultant lexemes then become a checklist by which samples from speakers with neurogenic communication disorders can be compared, e.g., by demonstrating that a person with aphasia produces 40% of possible core lexicon items for a given sample. A perceptual rating scale, the Auditory-Perceptual Rating of Connected Speech in Aphasia (APROCSA), was recently developed to rate acoustic-phonological characteristics of discourse [132]. This tool rates across several discourse elements (e.g., anomia, empty speech, paraphasias, paragrammatism, retracings), using 5-point rating scales (0, not present; 1, mild [detectable from infrequent]; 2, moderate [frequently evident but not pervasive]; 3, marked [moderately severe, pervasive]; 4, severe [nearly always evident]) and has demonstrated good inter-rater reliability and validity. More research is needed to evaluate utility of these tools in clinical settings, but they represent a promising future direction to streamline analysis.

Another critical feature that large sample sizes have made possible is the improvement of speech recognition and automatic transcription software. Automatic speech recognition (ASR) has also proven to be a fruitful endeavor in aphasic speech, given that transcription is arguably the most time-consuming part of and a major barrier to discourse analysis [3, 127]. Research leveraging AphasiaBank's large database suggests that ASR for aphasic speech is possible [133–135], and future work in this area will be a critical step for cutting down analysis time.

A Focus on Best Practices for Discourse Analysis and Collaboration

A critical issue in synthesizing discourse literature has been a lack of consistency and standardization of what is reported in published articles [136, 137]. A good example of this is the inconsistency with which the literature uses the terms "microlinguistic" vs. "microstructural" (which do not necessarily mean the same thing—microlinguistic likely means linguistic component, and microstructural may be both linguistic and propositional components), as well as the terms "macrolinguistic" vs. "macrostructural." To address this, my colleagues and I conducted a three-round e-Delphi survey methodology, which drew upon expert opinion to establish a set of best practice guidelines for reporting information about discourse [138]. The results of this e-Delphi survey encouraged reporting of 13 necessary and 7 recommended items in all research evaluating spoken discourse in persons with adult neurogenic language disorders. Some examples of necessary items include describing the discourse elicitation stimulus/task, providing inter-rater reliability metrics for primary outcome measures, and including detailed descriptions of any perceptual rating scale used, accompanied with a copy of the scale if not previously published. Evidencing how these guidelines are specialized for the aphasic population, two necessary items relate to characterizing the persons eliciting the discourse. Similar to encouraging the use of the EQUATOR network for accurate and consistent reporting of human subject research, scientific investigations evaluating discourse in aphasia can be improved by using these types of guidelines, thereby improving the ability to synthesize across studies.

Another core future direction in this area is the creation of working groups where people can network and share information about discourse in aphasia, which is further discussed in Chap. 21 of this book, describing the FOQUSAphasia working group.

Improving Quality of Psychometric Data Available for Discourse

Psychometric properties, like reliability and validity, are important components of assessments, because they provide insights into the assessment's appropriateness (a type of validity) and stability (a type of reliability). A long-standing issue in the discourse literature is sparse availability and low quality of psychometric data on measures [139]. Of interest, because we evaluate discourse usually at multiple time points (e.g., pre- and post-therapy), test–retest reliability is critical. Test-retest reliability is the consistency (or absolute similarity) of a measure when evaluated across a short interval during a time when no intervention takes place. If a measure is not reliable across this short duration of testing, i.e., there is a lot of variation or inherent error in the measure when retested, then the measure is unlikely to sensitively reflect treatment-induced changes. Discourse changes from day to day and context to context (as discussed above in relation to tasks, for example), and we therefore must be confident that any alternations in a measure after therapy are reflective of intervention-related change and not this variability. Establishing this reliability directly improves our ability to detect intervention-related change in spoken discourse, thereby demonstrating which therapies instill the most improvements to this real-life communication ability. A few studies have explored test–retest reliability of linguistic measures of aphasia, finding that, in general, some metrics (e.g., correct information units) are reliable over multiple testing sessions [140–142]. Research in primary progressive aphasia and Alzheimer's disease found excellent test-retest reliability of measures across lexical content, fluency, and informativeness measures, with variability across discourse tasks [143]. Recent work from my lab has suggested that fluency and informativeness measures, like correct information units, may be most reliable in aphasia especially when collapsing data across different monologic discourse tasks, but that these may vary by task, length of sample, and aphasia severity [144]. A recent study in chronic mild-to-moderate aphasia found that a variety of measures (including propositional and macrostructural measures) had good validity (content, convergent, and groups) [139]. The field's renewed interest in evaluating psychometric properties indicates its commitment to improving the evidence base of discourse, which will in turn improve the extent to which we can sensitively and accurately characterize discourse and also use discourse as an outcome measure of intervention.

Development of Discourse-Specific Treatments

A typical means of treating discourse has been to treat underlying linguistic deficits and identify if they translate into linguistic, propositional, macrostructural and/or pragmatic improvements in discourse (see details in a comprehensive review in 2011 [145]). Relatively few treatments have been specifically developed with discourse-level trained items and outcomes, e.g., using discourse as a treatment stimulus, and training propositional, macrostructural/planning, and pragmatic aspects of discourse. Early work by Ulatowska and colleagues emphasized the need for and importance of discourse therapy in aphasia, which highlights communicative competence rather than only linguistic competence [35]. Recently, two innovative studies have advocated for discourse-specific treatment, both creating and validating protocols for conducting discourse treatment in aphasia [126, 146]. In the Novel Approach to Real-life communication: Narrative Intervention in Aphasia (NARNIA) study, a multilevel intervention was created to increase awareness of word retrieval, sentence structure, and macrostructure across a variety of discourse genres [126]. A single-blind randomized controlled trial in 14 people with mild-to-moderate aphasia demonstrated that certain aspects of macrostructure were significantly improved in the NARNIA group compared to a usual care group, although the changes were relatively restricted to narrative discourse [126]. Recent research has also evaluated NARNIA's efficacy in primary progressive aphasia (in a man with semantic variant and a woman with logopenic variant), finding significant gains across several discourse metrics (e.g., noun and verb usage, overall output, macrostructural elements) [147]. The Language Underpins Narrative in Aphasia (LUNA) protocol targets personal stories of importance to the individual with aphasia whilst simultaneously targeting language production at word, sentence, and discourse (coherence, story grammar) levels [146]. The LUNA project is still ongoing as of this chapter's creation, but early evidence suggests that LUNA is both feasible and effective, with a single case experimental study demonstrating improvements across all language levels (word, sentence, discourse), such as improvements in verb production, predicate argument structure, local coherence, and story grammar/structure [146]. Importantly, the LUNA protocol was co-designed with individuals with aphasia and speech-language pathologists, reflecting yet another up-and-coming future direction for discourse research, which is that of participatory research design [148]. Both the NARNIA and LUNA studies represent promising future directions for using discourse as the primary stimuli and/or learning tool throughout therapy.

Interaction of Culture and Bilingualism in Discourse Production

Discourse elicitation methods have great potential to measure language and communication in more natural settings, yet many have fallen short due to a variety of issues, one of which is a lack of cultural and linguistic sensitivity and appropriateness. Picture descriptions are the most common form of discourse elicitation method conducted in clinical and research settings to acquire a discourse sample from the populations described above [2, 3]. However, the most typically used ones (like the Cookie Theft picture description from the Boston Diagnostic Aphasia Examination and the National Institutes of Health Stroke Scale) have intrinsic issues. In the original version, there are several outdated stereotypes that are perpetuated, e.g., a woman whose role is in the kitchen and who is meant to be "minding" the children whilst the father (a heteronormative assumption) is outside mowing the lawn. A significant update to this picture was recently created and validated [149]. Work by Olness and colleagues also demonstrates that ethnicity may influence discourse in aphasia (beyond age and education), where features of African American dialect were observed in picture descriptions as well as narratives, though the thematic content was similar when compared to a group of 29 Caucasians with aphasia [150]. Speech-language pathologists and researchers in this field recognize that cultural and linguistic irrelevance is a critical flaw in currently available discourse tools. Qualitative feedback from our recent survey cited a critical barrier to discourse assessment and analysis in aphasia as being a lack of culturally and linguistically appropriate stimuli [3]. Typical procedures used to elicit discourse, like picture description instructions ("tell me a story with a beginning, middle, and end"), are grounded in an

Anglo-European understanding of discourse and storytelling. For example, for the Navajo, these instructions would be less appropriate, since Navajo storytelling emphasizes a return to the beginning, or to a new beginning, rather than an ending [151]. Further, one of the most common narrative elicitations in our field, the retelling of the Cinderella story, poses an issue for individuals not raised in the USA or those raised in the USA whose cultural upbringing did not include this fairy tale. As a field, we are slowly moving toward addressing these cultural and linguistic issues because of the clear importance of creating sensitive and appropriate tools with which to elicit discourse.

Another imperative step in discourse analysis in aphasia is the need to understand how discourse breaks down in multilingual speakers, which comprise 40% (with some estimated >50%) of the world's population [152]. In the USA, the number is slightly lower (~20%) though still considerable (based on the 2019 US Census American Community Survey [153]). The great majority of discourse analysis has been conducted on primarily monolingual speakers, as evidenced by the demographic makeup of large databases like AphasiaBank, where the majority are monolingual (as well as non-Hispanic White). Multilingualism may be particularly important to evaluate in discourse because of known linguistic and cognitive characteristics at play, such as code switching. Recent research evaluated main concepts produced for picture stimuli in 83 young English and Spanish bilinguals (without aphasia), demonstrating that more main concepts were produced in the dominant language, but in individuals whose English and Spanish were relatively equal in proficiency, they tended to produce more main concepts in English [154]. This research, though not evaluating discourse in aphasia, clearly demonstrates the importance of acquiring a measure of language proficiency in bilingual speakers. Indeed, research in aphasia has suggested that contextual variation in lexical retrieval is related to premorbid language skill in bilingual aphasia [155]. A recent article points out that cross-language generalization has been reported in about half of all published cases of bilingual aphasia treatment, yet the large majority of these studies evaluate single-word naming, rather than discourse [156]. This study underlines the need to evaluate cross-language generalization during discourse, which, because of its unique involvement of language and cognitive processes, may be sensitive to subtle changes that vary by not only context but also language spoken in those who are multilingual.

A continued focus of our field should be on ensuring that discourse elicitation methods are sensitive and appropriate to culture and language and that discourse analysis is conducted with emphasis on important sociocultural and linguistic variables, such as multilingualism.

Conclusion

Discourse assessment and analysis are a powerful technique and highly informative to clinical application. The treatment of discourse is a particularly important future direction, with interventions specialized to improve language at the discourse level in these neurogenic populations.

Major Takeaways

1. Discourse is the way by which we communicate, and thus discourse analysis offers a way to measure the complex language processes associated with neurogenic communication disorders.
2. Discourse has been studied in neurogenic populations for many years, with a sharp increase in studies in the last 10-20 years evidencing enhanced interest in measuring and remediating discourse.
3. Discourse analysis, and treatment of discourse-related outcomes (e.g., improving word finding during discourse), is of interest to researchers and clinicians, and improving communication at the discourse level has been cited by individuals with aphasia to be of high importance during their recovery process.
4. Recent advances in technology (e.g., speech recognition), perceptual rating scales (e.g., on-

the-ground means of measuring discourse), access to databases and larger populations, interdisciplinary collaboration, a focus on best practices for discourse analysis, and an increase in evidence evaluating the impact of language and culture on discourse in aphasia will hugely benefit the ability to measure and remediate discourse in neurogenic populations.

Acknowledgments Dr. Stark's research has been supported by the American Speech-Language-Hearing Foundation (New Investigator Award), the National Institutes of Health (National Institute on Deafness and Other Communication Disorders), the National Institute on Disability, Independent Living, and Rehabilitation Research, Indiana University Bloomington, and the National Aphasia Association (Barbara Martin Research Grant).

References

1. Worrall L, Sherratt S, Rogers P, et al. What people with aphasia want: their goals according to the ICF. Aphasiology. 2011;25(3):309–22. https://doi.org/10.1080/02687038.2010.508530.
2. Bryant L, Ferguson A, Spencer E. Linguistic analysis of discourse in aphasia: a review of the literature. Clin Linguist Phon. 2016;30(7):489–518. https://doi.org/10.3109/02699206.2016.1145740.
3. Stark BC, Dutta M, Murray LL, et al. Spoken discourse assessment and analysis in aphasia: an international survey of current practices. J Speech Lang Hear Res. 2021;64:4366. https://doi.org/10.1044/2021_JSLHR-20-00708.
4. Ulatowska HK, Olness GS. Discourse. In: The MIT encyclopedia of communication disorders. MIT Press; 2004. p. 300–2.
5. Ska B, Duong A, Joanette Y. Discourse impairments. In: The MIT encyclopedia of communication disorders. MIT Press; 2004. p. 302–4.
6. Armstrong E. Aphasic discourse analysis: the story so far. Aphasiology. 2000;14(9):875–92. https://doi.org/10.1080/02687030050127685.
7. Halliday MAK. An introduction to functional grammar. 3rd ed. Arnold; 2004.
8. Fromm D, Forbes M, Holland A, Dalton G. Discourse characteristics in aphasia beyond the Western aphasia battery cutoff. Am J Speech-Lang Pathol. 2017;26:1–7. https://doi.org/10.1044/2016_AJSLP-16-0071.
9. Richardson JD, Dalton SG, Greenslade KJ, Jacks A, Haley KL, Adams J. Main concept, sequencing, and story grammar analyses of Cinderella narratives in a large sample of persons with aphasia. Brain Sci. 2021;11(1):110. https://doi.org/10.3390/brainsci11010110.
10. Stark BC, Cofoid C. Task-specific iconic gesturing during spoken discourse in aphasia. Am J Speech Lang Pathol. 2022;31(1):30–47.
11. Pritchard M, Dipper L, Morgan G, Cocks N. Language and iconic gesture use in procedural discourse by speakers with aphasia. Aphasiology. 2015;29(7):826–44. https://doi.org/10.1080/02687038.2014.993912.
12. Kong APH, Law SP, Wat WKC, Lai C. Co-verbal gestures among speakers with aphasia: influence of aphasia severity, linguistic and semantic skills, and hemiplegia on gesture employment in oral discourse. J Commun Disord. 2015;56:88–102. https://doi.org/10.1016/j.jcomdis.2015.06.007.
13. Kong APH, Law SP, Chak GWC. A comparison of Coverbal gesture use in Oral discourse among speakers with fluent and nonfluent aphasia. J Speech Lang Hear Res. 2017;60(7):2031–46. https://doi.org/10.1044/2017_JSLHR-L-16-0093.
14. van Nispen K, van de Sandt-Koenderman M, Sekine K, Krahmer E, Rose ML. Part of the message comes in gesture: how people with aphasia convey information in different gesture types as compared with information in their speech. Aphasiology. 2017;31(9):1078–103. https://doi.org/10.1080/02687038.2017.1301368.
15. Cocks N, Byrne S, Pritchard M, Morgan G, Dipper L. Integration of speech and gesture in aphasia. Int J Lang Commun Disord. 2018;53(3):584–91. https://doi.org/10.1111/1460-6984.12372.
16. Cocks N, Dipper L, Middleton R, Morgan G. What can iconic gestures tell us about the language system? A case of conduction aphasia. Int J Lang Commun Disord. 2011;46(4):423–36. https://doi.org/10.3109/13682822.2010.520813.
17. Dipper L, Cocks N, Rowe M, Morgan G. What can co-speech gestures in aphasia tell us about the relationship between language and gesture? Gesture. 2011;11(2):123–47. https://doi.org/10.1075/gest.11.2.02dip.
18. Kistner J, Dipper LT, Marshall J. The use and function of gestures in word-finding difficulties in aphasia. Aphasiology. 2019;33(11):1372–92. https://doi.org/10.1080/02687038.2018.1541343.
19. Mueller KD, Hermann B, Mecollari J, Turkstra LS. Connected speech and language in mild cognitive impairment and Alzheimer's disease: a review of picture description tasks. J Clin Exp Neuropsychol. 2018;40(9):917–39. https://doi.org/10.1080/13803395.2018.1446513.
20. Dipper L, Marshall J, Boyle M, Hersh D, Botting N, Cruice M. Creating a theoretical framework to underpin discourse assessment and intervention in aphasia. Brain Sci. 2021;11(2):183. https://doi.org/10.3390/brainsci11020183.
21. Frederiksen CH, Bracewell RJ, Breuleux A, Renaud A. The cognitive representation and processing of discourse: function and dysfunction. In: Discourse ability and brain damage. New York,

NY: Springer-Verlag; 1990. p. 69–110. https://doi.org/10.1007/978-1-4612-3262-9_4.
22. Sherratt S. Multi-level discourse analysis: a feasible approach. Aphasiology. 2007;21(3–4):375–93. https://doi.org/10.1080/02687030600911435.
23. Van Dijk TA, Kintsch W. Strategies of discourse comprehension. New York: Academic Press; 1983.
24. Cherney L, Coelho CA, Shadden BB. Analyzing discourse in communicatively impaired adults. In: Cherney LR, Coelho CA, Shadden BB, editors. Google books. Gaithersburg, MD: Aspen Publishers; 1998. Accessed December 2, 2020. https://books.google.com/books/about/Analyzing_Discourse_in_Communicatively_I.html?id=DeMLAQAAMAAJ.
25. Nicholas LE, Brookshire RH. A system for quantifying the informativeness and efficiency of the connected speech of adults with aphasia. J Speech Hear Res. 1993;36(2):338–50.
26. Dalton SG, Richardson J. A large-scale comparison of main concept production between persons with aphasia and persons without brain injury. Am J Speech Lang Pathol Published online. 2018;28:1–28.
27. Nicholas L, Brookshire R. Presence, completeness, and accuracy of main concepts in the connected speech of non-brain-damaged adults and adults with aphasia. J Speech Lang Hear Res. 1995;38:145–56.
28. Stein NL, Glenn CG. An analysis of story comprehension in elementary school children: a test of a schema. 1975. Accessed October 28, 2022. https://eric.ed.gov/?id=ED121474
29. Ulatowska HK, North AJ, Macaluso-Haynes S. Production of narrative and procedural discourse in aphasia. Brain Lang. 1981;13(2):345–71. https://doi.org/10.1016/0093-934X(81)90100-0.
30. Ulatowska HK, Allard L, Chapman SB. Narrative and procedural discourse in aphasia. In: Joanette Y, Brownell HH, editors. Discourse ability and brain damage: theoretical and empirical perspectives. Springer series in neuropsychology. Springer; 1990. p. 180–98. https://doi.org/10.1007/978-1-4612-3262-9_8.
31. Fergadiotis G, Wright HH, Capilouto GJ. Productive vocabulary across discourse types. Aphasiology. 2011;25(10):1261–78. https://doi.org/10.1080/02687038.2011.606974.
32. Stark BC, Fukuyama J. Leveraging big data to understand the interaction of task and language during monologic spoken discourse in speakers with and without aphasia. Lang Cogn Neurosci. 2021;36(5):562–85. https://doi.org/10.1080/23273798.2020.1862258.
33. Doyle PJ, Goda AJ, Spencer KA. The communicative Informativeness and efficiency of connected discourse by adults with aphasia under structured and conversational sampling conditions. Am J Speech Lang Pathol. 1995;4(4):130–4. https://doi.org/10.1044/1058-0360.0404.130.
34. Damico JS, Oelschlaeger M, Simmons-Mackie N. Qualitative methods in aphasia research: conversation analysis. Aphasiology. 1999;13:667–79. https://doi.org/10.1080/026870399401777.
35. Ulatowska H, Bond CS. Discourse considerations for aphasia management. Semin Speech Lang. 1989;10(04):298–314. https://doi.org/10.1055/s-2008-1064270.
36. Berthier ML. Poststroke aphasia: epidemiology, pathophysiology and treatment. Drugs Aging. 2005;22(2):163–82. https://doi.org/10.2165/00002512-200522020-00006.
37. Kertesz A. Western aphasia battery—revised. The Psychological Corporation; 2007.
38. Linnik A, Bastiaanse R, Höhle B. Discourse production in aphasia: a current review of theoretical and methodological challenges. Aphasiology. 2016;30(7):765–800. https://doi.org/10.1080/02687038.2015.1113489.
39. Stark BC, Basilakos A, Hickok G, Rorden C, Bonilha L, Fridriksson J. Neural organization of speech production: a lesion-based study of error patterns in connected speech. Cortex. 2019;117:228–46. https://doi.org/10.1016/j.cortex.2019.02.029.
40. Wagenaar E, Snow C, Prins R. Spontaneous speech of aphasic patients: a psycholinguistic analysis. Brain Lang. 1975;2:281–303.
41. Bastiaanse R, Jonkers R. Verb retrieval in action naming and spontaneous speech in agrammatic and anomic aphasia verb retrieval in action naming and spontaneous speech in agrammatic and anomic aphasia. Aphasiology. 1998;12(11):951–69. https://doi.org/10.1080/02687039808249463.
42. Beeke S, Cooper F, Best W, Edwards S, Maxim J. Measuring conversation change in people with agrammatic aphasia. Aphasiology. 2008;22(i):2008.
43. Lavoie M, Black SE, Tang-Wai DF, et al. Longitudinal changes in connected speech over a one-year span in the nonfluent/agrammatic variant of primary progressive aphasia. Aphasiology. 2022:1–12. https://doi.org/10.1080/02687038.2022.2084707.
44. Matchin W, Basilakos A, Stark BC, den Ouden DB, Fridriksson J, Hickok G. Agrammatism and paragrammatism: a cortical double dissociation revealed by lesion-symptom mapping. Neurobiol Lang. 2020;1(2):1–18. https://doi.org/10.1162/nol_a_00010.
45. Butterworth B, Howard D. Paragrammatisms. Cognition. 1987;26:1–37.
46. Kim H, Kintz S, Zelnosky K, Wright HH. Measuring word retrieval in narrative discourse: core lexicon in aphasia. Int J Lang Commun Disord. 2019;54(1):62–78. https://doi.org/10.1111/1460-6984.12432.
47. Leaman MC, Edmonds LA. Revisiting the correct information unit: measuring Informativeness in unstructured conversations in people with aphasia. Am J Speech Lang Pathol. 2019;28(3):1099–114. https://doi.org/10.1044/2019_AJSLP-18-0268.
48. Friedmann N. Speech production in Broca's agrammatic aphasia: syntactic tree pruning. Brocas Reg. 2006:63–82. https://doi.org/10.1093/acprof:oso/9780195177640.003.0005.

49. Armstrong EM. The potential of cohesion analysis in the analysis and treatment of aphasic discourse. Clin Linguist Phon. 1991;5(1):39–51. https://doi.org/10.3109/02699209108985501.
50. Olness GS, Ulatowska HK. Personal narratives in aphasia: coherence in the context of use. Aphasiology. 2011;25(11):1393–413. https://doi.org/10.1080/02687038.2011.599365.
51. Andreeta S, Cantagallo A, Marini A. Narrative discourse in anomic aphasia. Neuropsychologia. 2012;50:1787–93.
52. Armstrong E, Ciccone N, Godecke E, Kok B. Monologues and dialogues in aphasia: some initial comparisons. Aphasiology. 2011;25(11):1347–71. https://doi.org/10.1080/02687038.2011.577204.
53. Bastiaanse R, Bamyaci E, Hsu CJ, Lee J, Duman TY, Thompson CK. Time reference in agrammatic aphasia: a cross-linguistic study. J Neurolinguistics. 2011;24(6):652–73. https://doi.org/10.1016/j.jneuroling.2011.07.001.
54. Bastiaanse R. Why reference to the past is difficult for agrammatic speakers. Clin Linguist Phon. 2013;27(4):244–63. https://doi.org/10.3109/02699206.2012.751626.
55. Faroqi-Shah Y, Friedman L. Production of verb tense in Agrammatic aphasia: a meta-analysis and further data. Behav Neurol. 2015;2015:e983870. https://doi.org/10.1155/2015/983870.
56. Dalton SG, Richardson JD. Core-lexicon and main-concept production during picture-sequence description in adults without brain damage and adults with aphasia. Am J Speech Lang Pathol. 2015;24(4):S923. https://doi.org/10.1044/2015_AJSLP-14-0161.
57. Richardson JD, Dalton SG. Main concepts for three different discourse tasks in a large non-clinical sample. Aphasiology. 2016;30(1):45–73. https://doi.org/10.1080/02687038.2015.1057891.
58. Wright H, Capilouto G. Considering a multi-level approach to understanding maintenance of global coherence in adults with aphasia. Aphasiology. 2012;26:656–72.
59. Galetto V, Kintz S, West T, Mrini A, Wright H. Measuring global coherence in aphasia. Procedia-Soc Behav Sci. 2013;94:198–9.
60. Hazamy AA, Obermeyer J. Evaluating informative content and global coherence in fluent and non-fluent aphasia. Int J Lang Commun Disord. 2020;55(1):110–20. https://doi.org/10.1111/1460-6984.12507.
61. Kong APH, Linnik A, Law SP, Shum WWM. Measuring discourse coherence in anomic aphasia using rhetorical structure theory. Int J Speech Lang Pathol. 2018;20(4):406–21. https://doi.org/10.1080/17549507.2017.1293158.
62. Linnik A, Bastiaanse R, Stede M, Khudyakova M. Linguistic mechanisms of coherence in aphasic and non-aphasic discourse. Aphasiology. 2022;36(2):123–46. https://doi.org/10.1080/02687038.2020.1852527.
63. Richardson JD, Hudspeth SG. Story grammar analysis in persons with mild aphasia. Published 2014. Accessed October 28, 2022. http://aphasiology.pitt.edu/2593/
64. Coelho C, Flewellyn L. Longitudinal assessment of coherence in an adult with fluent aphasia: a follow-up study. Aphasiology. 2003;17(2):173–82. https://doi.org/10.1080/729255216.
65. Olness GS, Matteson SE, Stewart CT. "Let me tell you the point": how speakers with aphasia assign prominence to information in narratives. Aphasiology. 2010;24(6–8):697–708. https://doi.org/10.1080/02687030903438524.
66. Ulatowska HK, Olness GS. Pragmatics in discourse performance: insights from Aphasiology. Semin Speech Lang. 2007;28(2):148–58. https://doi.org/10.1055/s-2007-970572.
67. Doedens W, Bose A, Lambert L, Meteyard L. Face-to-face communication in aphasia: the influence of conversation partner familiarity on a collaborative communication task. Front Commun. 2021;6 https://doi.org/10.3389/fcomm.2021.574051. Accessed October 31, 2022
68. Holland AL. Observing functional communication of aphasic adults. J Speech Hear Disord. 1982;47(1):50–6. https://doi.org/10.1044/jshd.4701.50.
69. Holland A, Forbes M, Fromm D, MacWhinney B. Communicative strengths in severe aphasia: the famous people protocol and its value in planning treatment. Am J Speech Lang Pathol. 2019;28(3):1010–8. https://doi.org/10.1044/2019_AJSLP-18-0283.
70. Chapman SB, Ulatowska HK. Consideration of consciousness: discourse in dementia. In: Stamenov MI, editor. Language structure, discourse and the access to consciousness. Amsterdam: John Benjamins Publishing Company; 1997. p. 155. https://doi.org/10.1075/aicr.12.08cha.
71. Leaman MC, Archer B. "If you just stay with me and wait…You'll get an idea of what I'm saying": the communicative benefits of time for conversational self-repair for people with aphasia. Am J Speech Lang Pathol. 2022;31(3):1264–83. https://doi.org/10.1044/2022_AJSLP-21-00199.
72. Simmons-Mackie N, Raymer A, Armstrong E, Holland A, Cherney LR. Communication partner training in aphasia: a systematic review. Arch Phys Med Rehabil. 2010;91(12):1814–37. https://doi.org/10.1016/j.apmr.2010.08.026.
73. Mesulam MM. Primary progressive aphasia. Ann Neurol. 2001;49(4):425–32. https://doi.org/10.1002/ana.91.
74. Gorno-Tempini ML, Hillis AE, Weintraub S, et al. Classification of primary progressive aphasia and its variants. Neurology. 2011;76(11):1006–14. https://doi.org/10.1212/WNL.0b013e31821103e6.
75. Mesulam M. Slowly progressive aphasia without generalized dementia. Ann Neurol. 1982;11(6):592–8.
76. Wilson SM, Henry ML, Besbris M, et al. Connected speech production in three variants of primary progressive aphasia. Brain. 2010;133:2069–88. https://doi.org/10.1093/brain/awq129.

77. Fraser KC, Hirst G, Graham NL, Meltzer JA, Black SE, Rochon E. Comparison of different feature sets for identification of variants in progressive aphasia. In: Proceedings of the workshop on computational linguistics and clinical psychology: from linguistic signal to clinical reality; 2014. p. 17–26. https://doi.org/10.3115/v1/W14-3203.
78. Sajjadi SA, Patterson K, Tomek M, Nestor PJ. Abnormalities of connected speech in the non-semantic variants of primary progressive aphasia. Aphasiology. 2012;26(10):1219–37. https://doi.org/10.1080/02687038.2012.710318.
79. Marcotte K, Graham NL, Fraser KC, et al. White matter disruption and connected speech in non-fluent and semantic variants of primary progressive aphasia. Dement Geriatr Cogn Disord Extra. 2017;7(1):52–73. https://doi.org/10.1159/000456710.
80. Lavoie M, Black SE, Tang-Wai DF, et al. Description of connected speech across different elicitation tasks in the logopenic variant of primary progressive aphasia. Int J Lang Commun Disord. 2021;56(5):1074–85. https://doi.org/10.1111/1460-6984.12660.
81. Grossman M. Linguistic aspects of primary progressive aphasia. Annu Rev Linguist. 2018;4:377–403. https://doi.org/10.1146/annurev-linguistics-011516-034253.
82. Rogers MA, Alarcon NB. Dissolution of spoken language in primary progressive aphasia. Aphasiology. 1998;12(7–8):635–50. https://doi.org/10.1080/02687039808249563.
83. Ash S, Nevler N, Phillips J, et al. A longitudinal study of speech production in primary progressive aphasia and behavioral variant frontotemporal dementia. Brain Lang. 2019;194:46–57. https://doi.org/10.1016/j.bandl.2019.04.006.
84. Wong SB, Anand R, Chapman SB, Rackley A, Zientz J. When nouns and verbs degrade: facilitating communication in semantic dementia. Aphasiology. 2009;23(2):286–301. https://doi.org/10.1080/02687030801943112.
85. Hameister I, Foxe D, Hodges J, Piguet O, Nickels L. Information selection and information sequencing deficits in two variants of primary progressive aphasia – a connected speech analysis. Front Hum Neurosci. 2017;11:11. https://doi.org/10.3389/conf.fnhum.2017.223.00036.
86. Bruna SL, Naida G, Carol L, et al. The effect of semantic memory deficits on global coherence: an analysis of the discourse of patients with the semantic variant of primary progressive aphasia. Front Psychol. 2016;7:7. https://doi.org/10.3389/conf.fpsyg.2016.68.00073.
87. Cummings L. Narrating the Cinderella story in adults with primary progressive aphasia. In: Capone A, Carapezza M, Lo Piparo F, editors. Further advances in pragmatics and philosophy: part 2 theories and applications. Perspectives in pragmatics. Philosophy & Psychology. Springer International Publishing; 2019. p. 301–29. https://doi.org/10.1007/978-3-030-00973-1_18.
88. Orange JB, Kertesz A, Peacock J. Pragmatics in frontal lobe dementia and primary progressive aphasia. J Neurolinguistics. 1998;11(1):153–77. https://doi.org/10.1016/S0911-6044(98)00011-6.
89. Taylor C, Croot K, Power E, Savage SA, Hodges JR, Togher L. Trouble and repair during conversations of people with primary progressive aphasia. Aphasiology. 2014;28(8–9):1069–91. https://doi.org/10.1080/02687038.2014.930411.
90. Bartels-Tobin LR, Hinckley JJ. Cognition and discourse production in right hemisphere disorder. J Neurolinguistics. 2005;18(6):461–77. https://doi.org/10.1016/j.jneuroling.2005.04.001.
91. Minga J. Discourse production and right hemisphere disorder. Perspect ASHA Spec Interest Groups. 2016;1(2):96–105. https://doi.org/10.1044/persp1.SIG2.96.
92. Rivers DL, Love RJ. Language performance on visual processing tasks in right hemisphere lesion cases. Brain Lang. 1980;10(2):348–66. https://doi.org/10.1016/0093-934X(80)90061-9.
93. Joanette Y, Goulet P, Ska B, Nespoulous JL. Informative content of narrative discourse in right-brain-damaged right-handers. Brain Lang. 1986;29(1) 81–105. https://doi.org/10.1016/0093-934X(86)90035-0.
94. Marini A, Carlomagno S, Caltagirone C, Nocentini U. The role played by the right hemisphere in the organization of complex textual structures. Brain Lang. 2005;93(1):46–54. https://doi.org/10.1016/j.bandl.2004.08.002.
95. Sherratt SM, Penn C. Discourse in a right-hemisphere brain-damaged subject. Aphasiology. 1990;4(6):539–60. https://doi.org/10.1080/02687039008248506.
96. Albyn Davis G, O'Neil-Pirozzi TM, Coon M. Referential cohesion and logical coherence of narration after right hemisphere stroke. Brain Lang. 1997;56(2):183–210. https://doi.org/10.1006/brln.1997.1741.
97. Roman M, Brownell HH, Potter HH, Seibold MS, Gardner H. Script knowledge in right hemisphere-damaged and in normal elderly adults. Brain Lang. 1987;31(1) 151–70. https://doi.org/10.1016/0093-934x(87)90066-6.
98. Brownell H, Martino G. Deficits in inference and social cognition: the effects of right hemisphere brain damage on discourse. In: Right hemisphere language comprehension: perspectives from cognitive neuroscience. Lawrence Erlbaum Associates Publishers; 1998. p. 309–28.
99. Beeman M, Chiarello C, editors. Right hemisphere language comprehension: perspectives from cognitive neuroscience, vol. xii. Lawrence Erlbaum Associates Publishers; 1998. p. 408.
100. Chantraine Y, Joanette Y, Ska B. Conversational abilities in patients with right hemisphere damage. J Neurolinguistics. 1998;11(1):21–32. https://doi.org/10.1016/S0911-6044(98)00003-7.
101. Kennedy MRT. Topic scenes in conversations with adults with right-hemisphere brain damage. Am J

Speech Lang Pathol. 2000;9(1):72–86. https://doi.org/10.1044/1058-0360.0901.72.
102. Minga J, Fromm D, Jacks A, Stockbridge MD, Nelthropp J, MacWhinney B. The effects of right hemisphere brain damage on question-asking in conversation. J Speech Lang Hear Res. 2022;65(2):727–37. https://doi.org/10.1044/2021_JSLHR-21-00309.
103. Coelho CA. Discourse production deficits following traumatic brain injury: a critical review of the recent literature. Aphasiology. 1995;9(5):409–29. https://doi.org/10.1080/02687039508248707.
104. Marini A, Zettin M, Bencich E, Bosco FM, Galetto V. Severity effects on discourse production after TBI. J Neurolinguistics. 2017;44:91–106. https://doi.org/10.1016/j.jneuroling.2017.03.005.
105. Coelho CA, Grela B, Corso M, Gamble A, Feinn R. Microlinguistic deficits in the narrative discourse of adults with traumatic brain injury. Brain Inj. 2005;19(13):1139–45. https://doi.org/10.1080/02699050500110678.
106. Marini A, Galetto V, Zampieri E, Vorano L, Zettin M, Carlomagno S. Narrative language in traumatic brain injury. Neuropsychologia. 2011;49(10):2904–10. https://doi.org/10.1016/j.neuropsychologia.2011.06.017.
107. Liles BZ, Coelho CA, Duffy RJ, Zalagens MR. Effects of elicitation procedures on the narratives of normal and closed head-injured adults. J Speech Hear Disord. 1989;54(3):356–66. https://doi.org/10.1044/jshd.5403.356.
108. Glosser G, Deser T. Patterns of discourse production among neurological patients with fluent language disorders. Brain Lang. 1990;40:67–88.
109. McDonald S. Pragmatic language skills after closed head injury: ability to meet the informational needs of the listener. Brain Lang. 1993;44(1):28–46. https://doi.org/10.1006/brln.1993.1003.
110. Peach RK, Hanna LE. Sentence-level processing predicts narrative coherence following traumatic brain injury: evidence in support of a resource model of discourse processing. Lang Cogn Neurosci. 2021;36:694–710. https://doi.org/10.1080/23273798.2021.1894346.
111. Peach RK. The cognitive basis for sentence planning difficulties in discourse after traumatic brain injury supplement: select papers from the 42nd clinical aphasiology conference. Am J Speech-Lang Pathol N. 2013;22:285–97. https://doi.org/10.1044/1058-0360(2013/12-0081).
112. Galetto V, Andreetta S, Zettin M, Marini A. Patterns of impairment of narrative language in mild traumatic brain injury. J Neurolinguistics. 2013;26(6):649–61. https://doi.org/10.1016/j.jneuroling.2013.05.004.
113. Angeleri R, Bosco FM, Zettin M, Sacco K, Colle L, Bara BG. Communicative impairment in traumatic brain injury: a complete pragmatic assessment. Brain Lang. 2008;107(3):229–45. https://doi.org/10.1016/j.bandl.2008.01.002.
114. Byom L, Turkstra LS. Cognitive task demands and discourse performance after traumatic brain injury. Int J Lang Commun Disord. 2017;52(4):501–13. https://doi.org/10.1111/1460-6984.12289.
115. Snow P, Douglas J, Ponsford J. Procedural discourse following traumatic brain injury. Aphasiology. 1997;11(10):947–67. https://doi.org/10.1080/02687039708249421.
116. Coelho CA, Youse KM, Le KN. Conversational discourse in closed-head-injured and non-brain-injured adults. Aphasiology. 2002;16(4–6):659–72. https://doi.org/10.1080/02687030244000275.
117. Body R, Perkins MR. Validation of linguistic analyses in narrative discourse after traumatic brain injury. Brain Inj. 2004;18(7):707–24. https://doi.org/10.1080/02699050310001596914.
118. Coelho C. Management of Discourse Deficits following traumatic brain injury: Progress, caveats, and needs. Semin Speech Lang. 2007;28(2):122–35. https://doi.org/10.1055/s-2007-970570.
119. MacWhinney B. Understanding spoken language through TalkBank. Behav Res Methods. 2019;51(4):1919–27. https://doi.org/10.3758/s13428-018-1174-9.
120. MacWhinney B. The Talkbank project. In: Beal JC, Corrigan KP, Moisl HL, editors. Creating and digitizing language corpora: volume 1: synchronic databases. Palgrave Macmillan UK; 2007. p. 163–80. https://doi.org/10.1057/9780230223936_7.
121. MacWhinney B. The CHILDES project: tools for analysing talk. 3rd ed. Mahwah NI: Lawrence Erlbaum Associates Inc.; 2000.
122. MacWhinney B, Forbes M, Holland A. AphasiaBank: methods for studying discourse. Aphasiology. 2011;25(11):1286–307. https://doi.org/10.1080/02687038.2011.589893.AphasiaBank.
123. Bogart E, Togher L, Power E, Kenny B. Reporting on TBIBank: a revolutionary clinical tool. In: Speech Pathology Australia National Conference, Hobart; 2012.
124. Minga J, Johnson M, Blake ML, Fromm D, MacWhinney B. Making sense of right hemisphere discourse using RHDBank. Top Lang Disord. 2021;41(1):99–122. https://doi.org/10.1097/TLD.0000000000000244.
125. Marini A, Andreetta S, del Tin S, Carlomagno S. A multi-level approach to the analysis of narrative language in aphasia. Aphasiology. 2011;25(11):1372–92. https://doi.org/10.1080/02687038.2011.584690.
126. Whitworth A, Leitao S, Cartwright J, et al. NARNIA: a new twist to an old tale. A pilot RCT to evaluate a multilevel approach to improving discourse in aphasia. Aphasiology. 2015;29(11):1345–82. https://doi.org/10.1080/02687038.2015.1081143.
127. Bryant L, Spencer E, Ferguson A. Clinical use of linguistic discourse analysis for the assessment of language in aphasia. Aphasiology. 2017;31(10):1105–26. https://doi.org/10.1080/02687038.2016.1239013.
128. Cruice M, Botting N, Marshall J, et al. UK speech and language therapists' views and reported practices of discourse analysis in aphasia rehabilitation.

Int J Lang Commun Disord. 2020;55(3):417–42. https://doi.org/10.1111/1460-6984.12528.
129. Dalton SG, Kim H, Richardson Heather JD, Wright H. A compendium of Core lexicon checklists. Semin Speech Lang. 2020;41(1):45–60.
130. Kim H, Wright HH. Concurrent validity and reliability of the Core lexicon measure as a measure of word retrieval ability in aphasia narratives. Am J Speech Lang Pathol. 2020;29(1):101–10. https://doi.org/10.1044/2019_AJSLP-19-0063.
131. Dalton SG, Stark BC, Fromm D, et al. Comparing automated and manual scoring modalities for core lexicon analysis. Am J Speech Lang Pathol. 2022; https://doi.org/10.31234/osf.io/ex7q5.
132. Casilio M, Rising K, Beeson PM, Bunton K, Wilson SM. Auditory-perceptual rating of connected speech in aphasia. Am J Speech Lang Pathol. 2019;28(2):550–68. https://doi.org/10.1044/2018_AJSLP-18-0192.
133. Le D, Provost EM. Improving automatic recognition of aphasic speech with AphasiaBank. In: Proc Annu Conf Int Speech Commun Assoc INTERSPEECH; 2016. p. 2681–5. https://doi.org/10.21437/Interspeech.2016-213.
134. Dahl DA, Linebarger MC, Berndt RS. Improving automatic speech recognition of aphasic speech through the use of a processing prosthesis. Technol Disabil. 2008;20(4):283–94. https://doi.org/10.3233/tad-2008-20403.
135. Torre IG, Romero M, Álvarez A. Improving aphasic speech recognition by using novel semi-supervised learning methods on AphasiaBank for English and Spanish. Appl Sci. 2021;11(19):8872. https://doi.org/10.3390/app11198872.
136. Dietz A, Boyle M. Discourse measurement in aphasia research: have we reached the tipping point? Aphasiology. 2018;32(4):459–64. https://doi.org/10.1080/02687038.2017.1398803.
137. Dietz A, Boyle M. Discourse measurement in aphasia: consensus and caveats. Aphasiology. 2018;32(4):487–92. https://doi.org/10.1080/02687038.2017.1398814.
138. Stark BC, Bryant L, Themistocleous C, den Ouden DB, Roberts AC. Best practice guidelines for reporting spoken discourse in aphasia and neurogenic communication disorders. Aphasiology. 2022:1–24. https://doi.org/10.1080/02687038.2022.2039372.
139. Pritchard M, Hilari K, Cocks N, Dipper L. Psychometric properties of discourse measures in aphasia: acceptability, reliability, and validity. Int J Lang Commun Disord. 2018;53(6):1078–93. https://doi.org/10.1111/1460-6984.12420.
140. Brookshire RH, Nicholas LE. Speech sample size and test-retest stability of connected speech measures for adults with aphasia. J Speech Hear Res. 1994;37(2):399–407. https://doi.org/10.1044/jshr.3702.399.
141. Boyle M. Test-retest stability of word retrieval in aphasic discourse. J Speech Lang Hear Res. 2014;57(June):966–78. https://doi.org/10.1044/2014.
142. Boyle M. Stability of word-retrieval errors with the AphasiaBank stimuli. Am J Speech Lang Pathol. 2015;24(4):S953. https://doi.org/10.1044/2015_AJSLP-14-0152.
143. Beales A, Whitworth A, Cartwright J, Panegyres PK, Kane RT. Determining stability in connected speech in primary progressive aphasia and Alzheimer's disease. Int J Speech Lang Pathol. 2018;20(3):361–70. https://doi.org/10.1080/17549507.2018.1442498.
144. Stark BC, Alexander JM, Hittson A, Doub A, Igleheart M, Streander T, Jewell E. Test–retest reliability of microlinguistic information derived from spoken discourse in persons with chronic aphasia. J Speech Lang Hearing Res. 2023;66(7):2316–45. https://doi.org/10.1044/2023_JSLHR-22-00266.
145. Boyle M. Discourse treatment for word retrieval impairment in aphasia: the story so far. Aphasiology. 2011;25(11):1308–26. https://doi.org/10.1080/02687038.2011.596185.
146. Dipper L, Cruice M. Personal storytelling in aphasia: a single case study of LUNA therapy. Aphasiology. 2018;32(Suppl. 1):60–1. https://doi.org/10.1080/02687038.2018.1487919.
147. Whitworth A, Cartwright J, Beales A, Leitão S, Panegyres PK, Kane R. Taking words to a new level: a preliminary investigation of discourse intervention in primary progressive aphasia. Aphasiology. 2018;32(11):1284–309. https //doi.org/10.1080/02687038.2017.1390543.
148. Cruice M, Aujla S, Bannister J, et al. Creating a novel approach to discourse treatment through coproduction with people with aphasia and speech and language therapists. Aphasiology. 2021;36(10):1159–81. https://doi.org/10.1080/02687038.2021.1942775.
149. Berube S, Nonnemacher J, Demsky C, et al. Stealing cookies in the twenty-first century: measures of spoken narrative in healthy versus speakers with aphasia. Am J Speech Lang Pathol. 2019;28(1S):321–9. https://doi.org/10.1044/2018_AJSLP-17-0131.
150. Olness GS, Ulatowska HK, Wertz RT, Thompson JL, Auther LL. Discourse elicitation with pictorial stimuli in African Americans and Caucasians with and without aphasia. Aphasiology. 2002;16(4–6):623–33. https://doi.org/10.1080/02687030244000095.
151. Eder DJ. Bringing Navajo storytelling practices into schools: the importance of maintaining cultural integrity. Anthropol Educ Q. 2007;38(3):278–96.
152. Ansaldo AI, Marcotte K, Scherer L, Raboyeau G. Language therapy and bilingual aphasia: clinical implications of psycholinguistic and neuroimaging research. J Neurolinguistics. 2008;21(6):539–57. https://doi.org/10.1016/j.jneuroling.2008.02.001.

153. Dietrich S, Hernandez E. Language Use in the United States. American Community Survey Reports; 2019. p. 37.
154. Rivera A, Hirst J, Edmonds LA. Evaluation of language predictors of Main concept production in Spanish/English bilingual discourse using Nicholas and Brookshire stimuli. Am J Speech Lang Pathol. 2018;27(1):52–70. https://doi.org/10.1044/2017_AJSLP-15-0186.
155. Muñoz ML, Marquardt TP. The influence of language context on lexical retrieval in the discourse of bilingual speakers with aphasia. J Multiling Commun Disord. 2004;2(1):1–17. https://doi.org/10.1080/14769670310001625345.
156. Lerman A, Edmonds LA, Goral M. Cross-language generalisation in bilingual aphasia: what are we missing when we do not analyse discourse? Aphasiology. 2019;33(9):1154–62. https://doi.org/10.1080/02687038.2018.1538493.

Brielle C. Stark, Ph.D., is an Assistant Professor of Speech, Language, and Hearing Sciences at Indiana University Bloomington. She was a Gates Cambridge Trust Scholar during her Ph.D. in Clinical Neurosciences at Cambridge University (UK), where she studied the efficacy and feasibility of tablet-based therapy for individuals with chronic aphasia and the behavioral and neural correlates of inner speech in this population. She completed her postdoctoral work at the University of South Carolina, specializing in understanding the neural bases of impaired language in aphasia. She is interested in language production in poststroke aphasia, and her research evaluates behavioral characteristics (especially spoken discourse) and neural mechanisms. Additionally, she is interested in multimodal attributes of language production in aphasia, especially gesture, and in better understanding the phenomenon of inner speech in this population. Dr. Stark is a co-founder of FOQUSAphasia, a working group revolving around discourse studies in aphasia.

2 Discourse Characteristics in Aphasia

Stephen Kintz

Preview of What Is Currently Known
People with aphasia (PWA) present with impairments to the language systems, but the other cognitive systems, such as attention and memory, are often spared. Due to this, PWA often have intact, complete thoughts but are unable to express these thoughts to others. This reduction in communication ability causes large detrimental effects on activities of daily living, as well as social, vocational, and emotional well-being. This communication impairment extends to discourse abilities, preventing many PWA from producing informative, coherent discourse. Therefore, analyzing the discourse characteristics of PWA will improve the clinicians' or researchers' knowledge about their functional language abilities, as well as provide a better understanding of how to treat them.

Objectives
(a) To identify the different discourse genres and tasks, as well as the different analysis measures used when evaluating discourse in aphasiology
(b) To describe the different levels of discourse (microlinguistic and macrolinguistic) and distinguish between the different linguistic and cognitive systems used for both levels
(c) To summarize the microlinguistic features of discourse for PWA, including productivity, information content, and grammatical complexity
(d) To summarize the macrolinguistic features of discourse for PWA, including cohesion, local coherence, and global coherence
(e) To compare and contrast the discourse characteristics between fluent and non-fluent PWA
(f) To understand the importance of discourse genre and task in the performance of PWA and neurotypical controls

Introduction

Aphasia is defined as a central nervous system impairment acquired from stroke or other brain injury that presents in one or more components of language (i.e., phonology, morphology, semantic, syntax, and pragmatics) during comprehension (i.e., listening or reading) and/or production (i.e., speaking, signing, or writing). The pattern of language impairment divides aphasia into subtypes. This chapter uses the classification system from the American Speech-Language-Hearing Association (ASHA; [1]), where aphasia is divided into fluent and non-fluent. Fluent aphasia is described as having fluent speech that lacks

S. Kintz (✉)
Department of Speech Language Pathology, University of Arkansas at Little Rock, Little Rock, AR, USA
e-mail: sgkintz@ualr.edu

A. P.-H. Kong (ed.), *Spoken Discourse Impairments in the Neurogenic Populations*,
https://doi.org/10.1007/978-3-031-45190-4_2

meaning and includes the following subtypes: (a) anomic, (b) conduction, (c) transcortical sensory, and (d) Wernicke's aphasias. Non-fluent aphasia is described as having halting/effortful and telegraphic speech and includes the following subtypes: (a) Broca's, (b) transcortical motor, and (c) global aphasias [2].

For people with aphasia (PWA), this language impairment extends to discourse [3]. Discourse can be defined in multiple ways. A formalist/structuralist perspective would consider any unit of language above a single utterance to be discourse [4]. A functionalist perspective may consider any language used within a specific context to convey a message to be discourse, regardless of length [5]. This chapter considers discourse as any unit of language beyond a single utterance that conveys information [6]. When analyzing discourse, it reflects more etiological real and functional language tasks compared to confrontational naming tasks or sentence repetitions tasks, and it is already an important, but underutilized, component in the assessment of aphasia [3], since the Boston Diagnostic Aphasia Exam-3rd (BDAE-3; [7]) and the Western Aphasia Battery (WAB; [8]) include a discourse-based subtest to distinguish between fluent and non-fluent aphasia subtypes [9].

Theories of Discourse

There are many models/frameworks for understanding discourse, such as the construction-integration model [10] or the multi-level discourse processing model [11]. These different models/frameworks cause investigators to examine discourse in slightly different ways. However, a common theme across all models/frameworks is that coherent discourse requires multiple levels of representations/processing, with most models specifying, at least, microlinguistic and macrolinguistic processes. Microlinguistic processes include the traditional language components, such as phonology, semantics, and syntax, related to the bottom-up processes required for accessing words and using these words to construct phrases and utterances. Macrolinguistic processes include cohesion, coherence, and pragmatics related to top-down processes arranging these linguistic elements into a meaningful whole. The power of discourse lies in the analysis of both the micro- and macrolinguistic levels.

Of course, discourse can be divided into different genres, including conversation, expository, narrative, and procedural discourse, and these genres can be subdivided into different types (e.g., expository may be descriptive/informative or persuasive). See Table 2.1 for more information on the genres and types of discourse [6]. The different genres and types of discourse require a different menagerie of linguistic and cognitive processes/resources to produce a coherent language sample. For example, a procedural discourse task, such as "How to make a peanut butter and jelly sandwich," would require a simpler syntax and tax memory/organizational skills less than producing a narrative with multiple characters and scenes that jump around both spatially and temporally. This gets to a crucial aspect of discourse analysis. People will perform differently on different discourse tasks. An individual could perform at normative levels on one task but do poorly on another. Therefore, to properly assess discourse in aphasia, clinicians/researchers need to understand not only the different discourse characteristics of fluent and non-fluent aphasia, but also the different discourse tasks used.

In aphasiology, discourse is often investigated by eliciting monologues using pictures or scripts due to the ease of administration and interpretation. Few studies examine conversations or dialogues [22]. Bryant and colleagues conducted a systematic review and found that single-picture expository descriptions, such as the description of the "Cookie Theft" [7] and "Picnic" [8] pictures, were the most common discourse tasks used in research. This was followed by the wordless picture book *Cinderella* [15]. Personal recounts and procedural discourse (e.g., how to plant a flower) are also common. The authors also found that a majority of studies (n = 113) used multiple discourse genres/tasks to elicit language samples. Of these, 77 studies collapsed the different genres/tasks into one large sample

Table 2.1 Summary of the most common discourse genres, types, and tasks in aphasiology

Genres	Types	Tasks
Narrative: Monologues with spatial and temporal information (e.g., a beginning, middle, and end)	Stimuli based	**Single pictures:** *Cookie Theft* from BDAE [7] *Picnic* from WAB [8] **Sequential**: Argument and Flowerpot [12–14] **Wordless picture books**: Cinderella [15] Good Dog Carl [16] Picnic [17]
	Non-stimuli based	**Personal recounts:** Tell me about your stroke [18] Tell me about your holiday [19] Tell me about your weekend [19]
Expository: Monologues used to describe events, facts, or opinions	Informative	**Picture based:** *Cookie Theft* from BDAE [7, 20] *Picnic* from WAB [8]
	Persuasive	Are you for or against home schooling, and please explain why?
Procedural: Monologues used to provide instructions on how to complete a task		How to mail a letter? How to make a peanut butter and jelly sandwich?
Conversation: Dialogues with two or more speakers	Structured	Interviews Role-playing scenarios
	Unstructured	Familiar/unfamiliar conversation partners [21]

before analysis. The most utilized multitask protocols were developed by Nicholas and Brookshire [23], Doyle et al. [24], and AphasiaBank [18]. These protocols and results from Bryant and colleagues indicate that multiple discourse samples should be utilized when assessing discourse for PWA.

Microlinguistic Processing in Aphasia

PWA demonstrate more problems with the microlinguistic aspects of discourse compared to the macrolinguistic aspects of discourse production. Microlinguistic processing is reliant on traditional linguistic processes, with word access difficulty, anomia, being the most prevalent symptom [25]. Nevertheless, while many PWA may present with problems to word access, they may also have problems utilizing morphology or syntactic construction. The next sections will cover the most common microlinguistic aspects of discourse analyzed in PWA: (a) productivity, (b) information content, and (c) grammatical complexity.

Productivity

Productivity is defined as the amount and ease of language produced within a specific sample [26]. This includes count measures, such as the total number of words or utterances, but also includes measures of fluency and lexical diversity. Fluency is defined as the rate and ease at which an individual produces language, such as words per minute [27]. Lexical diversity (LD) is defined as the variety of words produced for a specific language sample, such as type-token ratio [28]. People with non-fluent aphasia (PWNA) consistently produce language samples that are shorter or less productive than neurotypical controls [29], which is driven by their inability to access/produce words or grammatical structures.

Therefore, discourse samples from PWNA are described as halting, effortful, and telegraphic. Excerpt (1) below shows the PWNA producing a narrative from the wordless picture book, *Picnic* [17]:

Excerpt (1):
PAR: all mouse … um … [Gestures: gathering] food and basket … for picnic.
PAR: um … mice … get in truck … trip.

People with fluent aphasia (PWFA) have more variability in productivity. PWFA often produce a similar amount of language compared to neurotypical controls [14], especially for milder forms of aphasia, such as anomic [13]. Some studies have found that PWFA, especially Wernicke's aphasia, produced a higher number of utterances compared to neurotypical controls [30]. This is described as logorrhea, which is defined as excessive but incoherent talkativeness or wordiness. Therefore, discourse samples from PWFA are described as fluent, maybe even excessive, and lacking insight about the topic. Excerpt (2) is from PWFA from the wordless picture book, *Picnic* [17]:

Excerpt (2):
PAR: the mouses … the father, and mother, and … one, two, three, four … all the children … they're preparing the basset [: basket] of watermelon, sandwiches, sweet dea [: tea] and getting on the truck.

While fluent and non-fluent aphasias differ on measures of raw productivity in terms of number of words or utterances, they have similar output when examining fluency and lexical diversity. Fluency measures were first applied to discourse in the 1970s and 1980s to help distinguish between fluent and non-fluent aphasia [9]; see Clough and Gordon [27, 31] for a more in-depth discussion on fluency in aphasia. Overall, PWA produce less fluent narratives with a slower speech rate as determined by words per minute compared to neurotypical controls [27]. This reduction in fluency is even true when PWFA produce a similar/greater number of words/utterances [14] and is even true for mild forms of aphasia, such as anomic aphasia [13].

People with *latent aphasia*, also known as not aphasic as determined by the WAB, also demonstrated a reduction in measures of fluency. Fromm et al. [32] examined narrative from *Cinderella* in latent aphasia, anomic aphasia, and neurotypical controls and found that latent aphasia had discourse samples with fewer utterances, fewer words per minute, and fewer concepts compared to neurotypical controls [32]. This reduction in speech rate was mainly driven by longer pauses compared to neurotypical controls. The rate of articulation (i.e., word fluency) was similar between PWA and neurotypical controls [33]; yet latent aphasia still has better fluency scores than the mildest form of aphasia, anomic aphasia [32]. Therefore, fluency not only distinguishes between fluent and non-fluent aphasias [9] but may be more sensitive to language change compared to standardized assessment methods, such as the WAB.

To explain this reduction in fluency, Clough and Gordon [31] examined how fluency scores were explained by scores on measures of word retrieval, grammatical complexity, and speech production. The researchers found that specific fluency measures are affected differently by these underlying causes. For example, words per minute was best explained by scores for grammatical processing abilities, while fluency scores on the WAB were equally explained by scores for lexical access, grammatical complexity, and speech production [31]. The researchers also found that the different subtypes of aphasia had different causes for their reduction in fluency. For example, when classifying the type of problems that may disrupt fluency, people with latent aphasia produce more pauses, fillers (e.g., "um," "uh," "you know,"), revisions, and repetitions with an increase in the number of phonemic errors compared to neurotypical controls. However, people with latent aphasia still performed better than people with anomic aphasia, who produced more phonemic, semantic, and pronoun errors with less attempts at revisions [32].

Lexical diversity (LD) is another common measure of productivity utilized in aphasiology. LD is defined as the diversity of words produced for a specific language sample, and it requires a store of words (i.e., vocabulary) and the retrieval processes to access said words. There are numerous ways to calculate lexical diversity. This includes older measures, such as the number of different words and type-token ratio, but it also includes newer measures, such as VocD (D), measure of textual lexical diversity (MTLD), and moving-average type-token ratio (MATTR), that address some of the shortfalls of the older methods. See Fergadiotis et al. [34] and Gordon [35] for an in-depth discussion on calculating LD.

PWA produce discourse samples with a lower lexical diversity compared to neurotypical controls [28, 32, 36–38]. Fergadiotis and Wright [36] examined lexical diversity in PWA and neurotypical controls for several discourse tasks: (a) single-picture narratives, (b) sequential picture narratives, and (c) narrative retell tasks from a wordless picture book. The researchers found that LD scores from neurotypical controls generally increased with the complexity of the tasks. The increase in LD was probably the result of the increased complexity required to tell the story. See Example (1) below:

Example (1):
Lexical Diversity in Controls:

(Higher LD--------------------------Lower LD)

Wordless Picture Books > Sequential Pictures > Single Picture.

A similar pattern was seen in PWA. They had lower lexical diversity scores for single pictures compared to sequential pictures, but PWA had similar lexical diversity scores between sequential pictures and wordless picture books. See Example (2) below:

Example (2):
Lexical Diversity in Aphasia:

(Higher-------------------------------------Lower)

Wordless Picture Books = Sequential Pictures > Single Picture.

Therefore, PWA have reduced productivity in terms of sample length [9], fluency [27], and lexical diversity [34, 36]. This is indicative of their language samples being less productive and efficient. This makes productivity a useful group of measures that appear capable of detecting the presence of aphasia [9] and severity of aphasia [35] and distinguishing between fluent/non-fluent subtype [27].

Information Content

Information content is a measure of the informativeness and content of a language sample. This may include measures similar to productivity, such as correct information units (CIUs), propositional density, and number of main ideas, which calculate how informative a sample is, but it also includes measures of lexical and semantic analysis that investigate the types of words produced. Unlike productivity that differed between fluent and non-fluent aphasia, PWA consistently demonstrate discourse that is less informative compared to neurotypical controls [29].

Correct information units (CIUs) are defined as single words, which are considered accurate, informative, and relevant to the language sample being produced [23], and it is the most utilized measure in aphasiology for measuring the informativeness of discourse samples [22, 26]. CIUs are significantly correlated with aphasia severity for both fluent and non-fluent aphasia, and higher CIUs per minute are correlated with better subjective rating of communicative competence from naïve listeners [39] and can classify PWA into different severities [40]. Nicholas and Brookshire [41] found that PWA do produce fewer CIUs compared to neurotypical controls, as well as fewer CIUs per minute. Furthermore, these measures distinguished between PWA and neurotypical controls better than simple counts, such as number of words/utterances [41]. These results have been replicated by other researchers utilizing content units [42], percent information units [43], number of propositions, and main idea/thematic units [12, 13].

So, PWA produce discourse that has less informativeness in terms of overall output, but what about the lexical/semantic content of their samples? An examination of the content of their samples also demonstrates some stark difference compared with neurotypical controls as well as with the different subtypes of aphasia. Content is defined as the concepts and words that make up a discourse sample. When examining the content of a language sample, structuralists often examine the category of words produced, such as nouns, verbs, adjectives, or adverbs.

PWNA often produce language samples with many missing closed-class words and bound affixes, such as plurals or tense endings. Kim and Thompson [44] also found that PWNA had more difficulty accessing verbs than nouns. Verbs are the building blocks of utterances, specifying the number and type of nouns that fill a verb's arguments. A verb's argument is defined as an expression/concept that helps complete a verb meaning. For example, the verb "run" has a required "subject/agent" that is "running" and an optional "location-based" argument. Hence, the utterances, *I run* and *I run to the store*, are both grammatical. The verb "slap" has two required arguments, "subject/agent" that is "slapping" and an "object/receiver" that is "slapped." Therefore, while *the girl slapped the boy* is grammatical, **the girl slapped* is not. Kim and Thompson [44] found that verbs with two or more arguments were harder to access in confrontational naming tasks and used less often in narrative samples compared to verbs with one argument. In Excerpt (1) from above, the PWNA did not produce many closed-class words or verbs in their utterance. For example, the individual used 7 nouns to 1 verb. The individual also gestured "gathering" or "packing" instead of using a lexical item.

Fluent aphasia is more difficult to classify. Some studies have shown that fluent aphasia has a similar pattern to non-fluent aphasia, where closed-class words are more difficult to access [12]. However, fluent aphasia is more likely to produce an error, while non-fluent aphasia is more likely to make an error of omission. Wernicke's aphasia is particularly known for phonological paraphasias. Paraphasias are lexical substitutions where a target word (i.e., intended word) is replaced with a phonological or semantically related word. See Example (3) below:

Example (3):
Semantic paraphasia: Mouse (target) → rat (replacement)
Phonological paraphasia: t<u>r</u>uck (target) → tuck (replacement)

In Excerpt (2) above, the PWFA produce two phonemic errors: "basset" for "basket" and "dea" for "tea." These paraphasias may improve productivity due to the ease that the lexical items were produced, but they prevent the discourse from being informative without further inferencing from the listener. Taken together, PWA produce less informative discourse samples for most discourse tasks. PWFA produce more fluent speech, but it is filled with paraphasias and other errors. PWNA produce less fluent speech that is often missing information, such as verbs and closed-class words.

Grammatical Complexity

Grammatical complexity provides an overall assessment of the type of morphological and syntactic structures/processes utilized when producing utterances [45]. The most common measures include mean length of utterances in terms of morphemes or words, the types of syntactic units produced, the number of complete/grammatical utterances, and the number/type of errors produced. There is a general consensus that PWA have reduced grammatical complexity, with a linear decline in grammatical complexity as severity increases [37].

Ulatowska et al. [46] were some of the first researchers to investigate grammatical complexity in PWA for a procedural discourse task. The authors found that PWA had a significant reduction in the number of utterances, percentage of grammatical utterances, clauses per utterances, and percentage of both dependent and nonfinite clauses. Overall, the authors concluded that PWA produce simple, shorter utterances compared to neurotypical controls. However, PWA did produce a similar number of words per utterance.

These results differ from other researchers who found a significant difference in the mean length of utterances when comparing single- and sequential picture tasks [14], which may be related to the nature of the discourse task. However, Ulatowska and colleagues did find that PWNA produced a lower number of utterances, as well as percentage of correct utterances compared to PWFA. Yet, there was no difference in measures of complexity, such as clause length or embedding, though the authors argue that this may be because of the simple nature of procedural discourse tasks.

The grammar of fluent and non-fluent aphasia is often described as paragrammatic or agrammatic, respectively [47]. Agrammatism is defined as the omission of grammatical morphology and/or function words. Again, consider Excerpt (1), where the PWNA produced few closed-class items helping structure the phrase. Paragrammatism is defined as a substitution of morphology and/or function words. Consider Excerpt (2) where the PWFA produce "mouses" for "mice" or "on the truck" instead of "in the truck." For English speakers, this is a rather straightforward distinction between fluent and non-fluent aphasia. However, in other languages with more morphological inflections, such as German or Italian, both fluent and non-fluent aphasia are more likely to produce morphological substitutions compared to morphological omissions [47].

Syntactic complexity is also measured through the number of morphological and syntactic errors produced. Andreetta and Marini [14] found that PWA do produce fewer complete/grammatical utterances compared to neurotypical controls. Their incomplete/ungrammatical utterances were not driven by morphological issues but by omissions of arguments (i.e., concepts/words) as well as incorrect function words. The authors concluded that the grammatical difficulties faced by PWA have more to do with lexical access problems more so than actual syntactic constructions. Taken together, it is clear that PWA use less complex syntax. Again, PWFA make more errors of substitution, while PWNA are more likely to produce errors of omissions. For example, Broca's aphasia often misses the past tense inflection ending for verbs [48]. Further, most researchers agree that the word access problems due to phonological, semantic, or grammatical processing issues are the main driver of PWA's simple, short utterances. However, working memory has also been implicated [49].

Microlinguistic Summary

PWA present with strong deficits to many microlinguistic processes, including productivity, informativeness, and grammatical complexity. In general, fluent aphasia has more productivity in terms of the number of words or words per minute produced. Non-fluent aphasia is less productive/fluent with fewer grammatical utterances overall. While cognitive deficits related to working memory and attention are possible candidates for driving these findings, most researchers and clinicians agree that anomia (i.e., word access) due to phonological, semantic, or grammatical processing issues is one of the main drivers of these microlinguistic issues. See Table 2.2 for a summary of the microlinguistic processes affected in aphasia.

Table 2.2 Microlinguistic discourse characteristics for aphasia

Discourse measures		Fluent	Non-fluent
Productivity	Raw production	Variable	Reduced
	Fluency	Reduced	Reduced
	Lexical diversity	Reduced	Reduced
Informative content	Informativeness	Reduced	Reduced
	Lexical errors	Substitution errors	Omission errors
Grammatical complexity	Complexity	Simple, shorter syntax	Simple, shorter
	Grammatical errors	Substitution errors	Omission errors

Macrolinguistic Processes for PWA

PWA have less problems with the macrolinguistic processes of discourse compared to the microlinguistic processes, and many researchers believe that microlinguistic impairments contribute to the disruptions at the macrolinguistic level, though attention and executive function are also implicated. Cohesion and coherence are the most studied aspects of the macrolinguistic level, though some researchers consider cohesion a microlinguistic process. Coherence can be further subdivided into local and global coherence. For PWA, cohesion and global coherence are more impaired than local coherence.

Cohesion

Cohesion refers to how semantic information or concepts are connected between different phrases and utterances [50]. Cohesion is maintained through word choice. Specifically, referential language (e.g., pronouns, conjunctions) and grammatical morphemes (e.g., number, gender agreement) coordinate concepts across phrasal/utterance boundaries. Excerpt (3) below illustrates how the pronouns "they" and "her" link/reference the concepts "mice" and "baby mouse" from the previous utterance. It also demonstrates how the conjunction "but" coordinates between the two utterances.

Excerpt (3):
PAR: the **mice** start to look for the baby mouse.
PAR: *but* **they** can't find her.

Cohesion is often viewed as both a microlinguistic and macrolinguistic process [45]. It patterns with other microlinguistic processes due to requiring access to referential language [12], but the coordination of meaning across utterance boundaries is more similar to macrolinguistic processes.

PWA often present with an impairment to cohesion [51]. PWA produce fewer cohesive ties than neurotypical controls [20, 52], though some researchers have found a similar number of cohesive ties [51]. Overall, PWA relied on conjunctions (e.g., *for*, *and*, *nor*, *but*, *or*, *yet*, and *so*) for a large percentage of their cohesive ties, and these conjunctions were mainly additive in nature (e.g., and), not adversative, causal, or temporal [9, 52]. Another research has also shown that non-fluent aphasia may be particularly bad at making temporal reference (48). Excerpt (2) above illustrates the overuse of the conjunction "and." The PWFA simply adds to the information already presented by saying "the mouses" and then naming each mouse included in "the mouses" by saying "and the father … and mother … and … children."

PWA also produce many cohesive errors [12–14]. Andreetta and Marini [14] found that PWA produce more cohesive errors compared to neurotypical controls. The errors included missing/ambiguous pronouns, missing/inappropriate closed-class words, number/gender disagreement, and incomplete utterances. Excerpt (4) below illustrates an ambiguous pronoun. "He" may refer to the "baby mouse" or "older mouse," making it ambiguous.

Excerpt (4):
PAR: The **baby mouse** fell out of the truck.
PAR: *and* the **older mouse** kept driving.
PAR: **He**'s in trouble.

Scores on cohesive errors correlated with measures of missing information (e.g., complete/incomplete utterances), suggesting that anomia/omission explain many of the cohesive errors [12, 14]. A longitudinal case study further illustrates the point. For the individual, cohesion varied across the 12-month period poststroke, but overall, cohesion scores improved as other microlinguistic abilities improved. This improvement was probably again driven by lexical access improvements [53]. Even mild forms of aphasia, such as anomic aphasia, produce more cohesive errors compared to neurotypical controls, and these errors are again driven by problems with word access [13].

There are also differences between fluent and non-fluent aphasia. According to Zhang et al. [52], non-fluent aphasia had trouble with grammatical processes due to the misuse of articles and pronouns. Non-fluent aphasia produced a similar number of lexical cohesive ties compared to neurotypical controls, but this was mainly driven by repetition [29, 52]. Fluent aphasia had more grammatical ties compared to lexical. In fact, PWFA produced almost half the number of lexical ties compared to neurotypical controls. This may be due to semantic/word access issues. Therefore, the main difference between fluent and non-fluent aphasia is that fluent aphasia has problems with lexical ties, while non-fluent aphasia has problems with grammatical ties.

Taken together, these results suggest that cohesion is strongly tied to microlinguistic abilities. Some research have also shown a link between cohesion and coherence, where poor cohesion leads to poor coherence [20]. Other studies have shown a division between the morphological and lexical aspects required for cohesion and the more semantic processes associated with coherence [12–14, 51].

Coherence

Coherence is defined as the integration of different elements in a logical, consistent manner [54]. In aphasiology, coherence refers to the ability to organize different story elements (e.g., utterances) so that the topic/theme (i.e., semantic relationships) is maintained throughout the discourse [51], and it is an important aspect of effective communication. Coherent discourse facilitates a listener's ability to comprehend and extract important information from a sample of language. Coherence is often divided into local and global coherence. Local coherence is concerned with the logical consistency between neighboring, or almost neighboring, utterances. Local coherence measures are often concerned about how/what information is linked, repeated, or elaborated. Global coherence is concerned with the consistency of utterances to the overall theme/purpose of the discourse.

Coherence may be measured in numerous ways [55]. Some researchers measure the percentage of main concepts and details produced, making these measures similar to measures of informativeness. Some researchers measure whether the story grammar is maintained. For example, a narrative typically needs a beginning, middle, and end. However, the most common methods in aphasiology are subjective rating scale [51, 56, 57] and error analyses [12–14] for both local and global coherence.

Local Coherence

PWA consistently perform better on measures of local coherence compared to measures of global coherence [58]. Glosser and Deser [51] examined local and global coherence by utilizing a 5-point rating scale. The authors found no difference between local coherence scores for PWA and neurotypical controls. A case study examining a 55-year-old with mild-to-moderate anomic aphasia also found that the individual had more problems with maintaining global coherence compared to local coherence [53]. So, while PWA have relatively preserved local coherence abilities, Andreetta et al. [13] found that PWA produce more local coherence-disrupting elements compared to neurotypical controls. The authors found that these local coherence errors were driven mainly by missing referents (i.e., missing words/concepts) and not topic shifts. Topic shifts are when an utterance is aborted prematurely, and the next utterance starts a new topic. Therefore, again, local coherence is mainly disrupted through lexical access problems. Due to few topic shifts and adequate scores of informativeness, the authors suggested that PWA are capable of understanding and organizing the gist of the narratives, but lexical access issues cause small disruptions to local coherence [13].

While microlinguistic deficits for PWA cause problems for coherence [57], it is not the only driver of coherence problems. Researchers have found that declines in working memory, as measured by word and reading span tasks, are correlated with declines in local coherence [59]. However, local coherence is less disrupted than global coherence, and local coherence does not appear to correlate with executive function [60]. Hoffman et al. [61] argued that local coherence relies on automatic (i.e., priming) activation of concepts between utterances, and it appears relatively preserved in PWA. Executive function or semantic control processes, which are damaged in aphasia, are more related to global coherence. Due to these reasons, primed/local semantic connections are maintained, but the damage executive systems cause drifts over multiple utterances, impacting global coherence.

Global Coherence

Global coherence has been investigated more thoroughly than local coherence. Again, one of the earliest studies from Glosser and Deser [51] pioneered the rating scale used and adapted by most other researchers investigating global coherence in aphasia. While this study did not find a difference between PWA and neurotypical controls, leading to the conclusion that macrolinguistic skills are more preserved compared to microlinguistic skills [51], most other investigations have found that PWA have reduced global coherence scores [13, 56, 62, 63], including an increase in the number of coherence errors [12, 62, 63].

Andreetta et al. [13] investigated global coherence errors in PWA for single-picture and sequential picture tasks. The authors found that PWA produce more coherence errors, but these errors were not related to tangential or incorrect information. Instead, PWA mainly produced repetitive information and filler utterance (i.e., utterances with a subjective statement or circumlocution). See examples in Excerpts (5) and (6):

Excerpt (5): An Example of Repetition of Utterance:
PAR: the mouse was terrified they lost the baby.
PAR: **the mouse was terrified**.

Excerpt (6): An Example of Filler Utterances:
PAR: the mouse was terrified they lost the baby.
PAR: the mouse was terrified.
PAR: **So scared on such a beautiful, sunny day**.

These errors suggest that PWA are able to maintain the theme/gist of the text. Leaman and Edmonds [63] found that almost 60% of utterances with low coherence scores for their PWA were associated with ambiguous/nonspecific language. Only 26% of low-coherence utterances were considered off-topic, and only 10% were considered as incorrect information. Between mild and severe aphasia, the researchers found that severe aphasia is more likely to use nonspecific language compared to milder aphasia, and mild aphasia uses more off-topic utterances compared to severe aphasia. These results suggest that less severe aphasias have a greater ability to access more specific language that could communicate more pertinent information but also more off-topic information. People with severe aphasia sometimes cannot produce enough information for listeners to understand that the utterance is off-topic.

There are also differences between fluent and non-fluent aphasia. Fluent aphasia may have higher global coherence scores compared to nonfluent aphasia [64]. Unfortunately, most of the research into global coherence has been conducted on fluent aphasia [54]. Christensen [62] investigated global coherence errors for several subtypes of fluent aphasia: (a) Wernicke's, (b) conduction, and (c) anomic. People with Wernicke's aphasia produced discourse samples that alternated between narrating a story and describing items in the picture. The author concluded that Wernicke's presentation may be the result of attentional issues. This is bolstered by the fact that Wernicke's aphasia also produced the most off-topic and incorrect information. Conduction aphasia produced the most repetition errors, by constantly repeating information already provided. Anomic aphasia had more gaps of information (i.e., missing information). Non-fluent aphasia is more likely, again, to produce errors of omissions: single-word utterances or aborted utterances [64].

Most researchers agree that disruptions to the microlinguistic processes cause problems for the macrolinguistic processes. In fact, lexical retrieval scores correlate with reduced informativeness and increased global coherence errors. These errors are not tangential or conceptually incongruent errors, but often repetitive information or filler utterances (i.e., utterances with subjective statements or circumlocutions). Again, this suggests that microlinguistic processes contribute to the problems associated with global coherence [13]. However, declines in other cognitive systems do contribute. Declines in working memory and executive function negatively impact global coherence [59, 64], and preserving these cognitive systems correlates more strongly with preserved communication ability, especially global coherence [65].

Summary of Macrolinguistic Processes

PWA do have problems associated with macrolinguistic processes of discourse production. Cohesion is typically impaired because it relies on linguistic features to link information between utterances. Global coherence is also impaired in most studies, and it correlated with declines in both microlinguistic processes and executive function processes. Local coherence, related to semantic priming, is relatively preserved. See Table 2.3 for a summary of macrolinguistic processes for PWA.

Table 2.3 Macrolinguistic discourse characteristics for aphasia

Discourse measures		Fluent	Non-fluent
Cohesion	Cohesive ties	More grammatical	More lexical
	Cohesive errors	More lexical errors	More grammatical errors
Local coherence	Local rating	Relatively preserved	Relatively preserved
	Local errors	Ambiguous referents	Missing referents
Global coherence	Global rating	Reduced (PWFA better than PWNA)	Reduced (PWFA better than PWNA)
	Global errors	Repetition, filler, and substitution errors	Omission errors

Note: *PWFA* People with fluent aphasia, *PWNA* People with non-fluent aphasia

Discourse Task

The presentation of discourse characteristics for PWA is often based on the specific discourse task since different tasks require differing levels of linguistic and cognitive processing. Therefore, it is important to consider tasks when analyzing discourse. For example, Stark et al. [66] compared three different discourse tasks: procedural, narrative, and expositional discourse. The narrative discourse task had the highest number of ideas per utterance but had the weakest fluency as determined by the number of words per minute. The procedural discourse task had the lowest grammatical complexity and ideas per utterance, but it had similar fluency to the expository tasks and more fluency than the narrative task. See Example (4) below:

Example (4):
Idea Density:
(Higher------------------------Lower)
Narrative > Expository > Procedural
Fluency:
(Faster-------------------------Slower)
Expository = Procedural > Narrative

Cohesion and coherence also vary by discourse task. Unfortunately, most of the research have been conducted on monologues using either single or sequential pictures [26]. This is problematic since a longer narrative, such as wordless picture books, may be more sensitive to changes in cohesion and coherence over time. For cohesion, there is a difference between monologues and conversations. Armstrong et al. [67] examined cohesive ties in monologues and conversations for two individuals with aphasia. Both speakers were able to use cohesive ties and maintain cohesion for both discourse tasks, but the monologue task caused more cohesive problems overall. This suggests that the cues and support provided by a conversational partner are beneficial to the discourse macrostructure for PWA.

For coherence, Wright and Capilouto [56] have even found that the same discourse tasks, narratives from wordless picture books, differ based on content and structure of the task. They found that productivity best explained the global coherence scores for *Picnic* [17], but informativeness best explained the global coherence scores for *Good Dog Carl* [16]. The authors concluded that the structure and content of the story influenced these results. These above results illustrate that it is important to consider the specific discourse task when analyzing discourse samples from neurotypical controls or PWA. Moreover, it is important to have multiple language samples from multiple genres/types of discourse to properly assess the language abilities of PWA.

Conclusion

PWA present with deficits in discourse processing. PWA are generally less productive and less fluent, with a restricted vocabulary that reduces the language sample's informativeness, cohesion, and coherence, especially since cohesion and coherence are mostly related to missing or ambiguous information. Macrolinguistic processes are more preserved due to them relying more on spared cognitive systems, such as attention and executive function, instead of the damaged language system. Throughout the chapter, discourse analysis has been shown to be an excellent way to assess PWA and determine severity and subtype. It is also more functionally real, compared to standardized methods like the WAB. While discourse analysis should become an important component for clinicians and researchers, the variety of aphasia subtypes, discourse tasks, and analysis methods prevents it from being easily digestible and useable for many researchers and clinicians.

Major Takeaways

1. People with aphasia (PWA) have declines in discourse processing associated with both microlinguistic and macrolinguistic processes.
2. Microlinguistic processes include reduced fluency and a restricted vocabulary that may drive PWA's language to be less informative and grammatical.
3. Macrolinguistic processes include poor cohesion and global coherence with relatively spared local coherence.
4. Macrolinguistic processes of cohesion are largely driven by lexical impairments, while global coherence is driven by both word access problems and cognitive declines in working memory and executive function.
5. Fluent aphasia makes more errors of substitution at both the micro- and macrolinguistic levels.
6. Non-fluent aphasia makes more errors of omission at both the micro- and macrolinguistic levels.
7. Discourse task is an important consideration when assessing aphasic discourse due to different genres/types requiring differing levels of linguistic and cognitive processing.

References

1. ASHA. Aphasia: overview. American Speech-Language-Hearing Association; 2019. [cited 2019 Apr 4]. Available from: https://www.asha.org/PRPSpecificTopic.aspx?folderid=8589934663&section=Overview
2. Davis GA. Aphasiology: disorders and clinical practice. 2nd ed. Boston, Mass. Munich: Pearson; 2006. 400 p
3. Armstrong E. Aphasic discourse analysis: the story so far. Aphasiology. 2000;14(9):875–92.
4. Grimes JE. The thread of discourse. Paris: The Hague Mouton; 1975. https://doi.org/10.1515/9783110886474/html.
5. Halliday MAK, Matthiessen CMIM. An introduction to functional grammar. 3rd ed. London/New York: Arnold; Distributed in the United States of America by Oxford University Press; 2004. 689 p
6. Coelho CA, Cherney LR, Shadden BB. Discourse analysis in adults with and without communication disorders: a resource for clinicians and researchers. San Diego, CA: Plural Publishing Inc; 2023. [cited 2022 Nov 8]. Available from: https://www.pluralpublishing.com/publications/discourse-analysis-in-adults-with-and-without-communication-disorders-a-resource-for-clinicians-and-researchers
7. Goodglass H, Kaplan E, Barresi B. The Boston diagnostic aphasia examination. Baltimore, MD: Lippincott, Williams, & Wilkins; 2001.
8. Kertesz A. The Western aphasia battery. New York, NY: Grune & Stratton; 1982.

9. Gleason JB, Goodglass H, Obler L, Green E, Hyde MR, Weintraub S. Narrative strategies of aphasic and normal-speaking subjects. J Speech Hear Res. 1980;23(2):370–82.
10. Kintsch W, Welsch DM. The construction-integration model: a framework for studying memory for text. In: Relating theory and data: essays on human memory in honor of Bennet B. Murdock. Hillsdale, NJ: Lawrence Erlbaum Associates, Inc; 1991. p. 367–85.
11. Sherratt S. Multi-level discourse analysis: a feasible approach. Aphasiology. 2007;21(3–4):375–93.
12. Marini A, Andreetta S, del Tin S, Carlomagno S. A multi-level approach to the analysis of narrative language in aphasia. Aphasiology. 2011;25(11):1372–92.
13. Andreetta S, Cantagallo A, Marini A. Narrative discourse in anomic aphasia. Neuropsychologia. 2012;50(8):1787–93.
14. Andreetta S, Marini A. The effect of lexical deficits on narrative disturbances in fluent aphasia. Aphasiology. 2015;29(6):705–23.
15. Grimes N. Cinderella. New York, NY: Random House Books; 1993.
16. Day A. Good dog Carl. New York, NY: Simon & Schuster; 1986.
17. McCully EA. Picnic. New York, NY: HarperCollins; 1984.
18. MacWhinney B, Fromm D, Forbes M, Holland A. AphasiaBank: methods for studying discourse. Aphasiology. 2011;25(11):1286–307.
19. Wright HH, Capilouto GJ. Discourse processing in healthy aging in the United States. National Archive of computerized data on aging. Ann Arbor, MI: Inter-university Consortium for Political and Social Research [distributor]; 2017. https://doi.org/10.3886/ICPSR36634.v1.
20. Lock S, Armstrong L. Cohesion analysis of the expository discourse of normal, fluent aphasic and demented adults: a role in differential diagnosis? Clin Linguist Phon. 1997;11(4):299–317.
21. Herbert R, Hickin J, Howard D, Osborne F, Best W. Do picture-naming tests provide a valid assessment of lexical retrieval in conversation in aphasia? Aphasiology. 2008;22(2):184–203.
22. Pritchard M, Hilari K, Cocks N, Dipper L. Reviewing the quality of discourse information measures in aphasia. Int J Lang Commun Disord. 2017;52:689.
23. Nicholas LE, Brookshire RH. A system for quantifying the Informativeness and efficiency of the connected speech of adults with aphasia. J Speech Hear Res. 1993;36(2):338–50.
24. Doyle PJ, McNeil MR, Spencer KA, Goda AJ, Cottrell K, Lustig AP. The effects of concurrent picture presentations on retelling of orally presented stories by adults with aphasia. Aphasiology. 1998;12(7):561–74.
25. Goodglass H, Wingfield A, editors. Anomia: neuroanatomical and cognitive correlates. San Diego, CA: Academic Press; 1997.
26. Bryant L, Ferguson A, Spencer E. Linguistic analysis of discourse in aphasia: a review of the literature. Clin Linguist Phon. 2016;30(7):489–518.
27. Gordon JK, Clough S. How fluent? Part B. Underlying contributors to continuous measures of fluency in aphasia. Aphasiology. 2020;34(5):643–63.
28. Harris Wright H, Silverman S, Newhoff M. Measures of lexical diversity in aphasia. Aphasiology. 2003;17(5):443–52.
29. Linnik A, Bastiaanse R, Höhle B. Discourse production in aphasia: a current review of theoretical and methodological challenges. Aphasiology. 2016;30(7):765–800.
30. Pallickal M, N. H. Discourse in Wernicke's aphasia. Aphasiology. 2020;34(9):1138–63.
31. Clough S, Gordon JK. Fluent or nonfluent? Part A. Underlying contributors to categorical classifications of fluency in aphasia. Aphasiology. 2020;34(5):515–39.
32. Fromm D, Forbes M, Holland A, Dalton SG, Richardson J, MacWhinney B. Discourse characteristics in aphasia beyond the Western aphasia battery cutoff. Am J Speech Lang Pathol. 2017;26(3):762–8.
33. DeDe G, Salis C. Temporal and episodic analyses of the story of Cinderella in latent aphasia. Am J Speech Lang Pathol. 2020;29(1S):449–62.
34. Fergadiotis G, Wright HH, West TM. Measuring lexical diversity in narrative discourse of people with aphasia. Am J Speech Lang Pathol. 2013;22(2):S397.
35. Gordon JK. Measuring the lexical semantics of picture description in aphasia. Aphasiology. 2008;22(7–8):839–52.
36. Fergadiotis G, Wright HH. Lexical diversity for adults with and without aphasia across discourse elicitation tasks. Aphasiology. 2011;25(11):1414–30.
37. Bryant L, Spencer E, Ferguson A, Craig H, Colyvas K, Worrall L. Propositional idea density in aphasic discourse. Aphasiology. 2013;27(8):992–1009.
38. Wachal RS, Spreen O. Some measures of lexical diversity in aphasic and normal language performance. Lang Speech. 1973;16:169–81.
39. Jacobs BJ. Social validity of changes in Informativeness and efficiency of aphasic discourse following linguistic specific treatment (LST). Brain Lang. 2001;78(1):115–27.
40. Im EJ, Kwon M, Sim HS, Im EJ, Kwon M, Sim HS. The informativeness and efficiency of the connected speech samples in Korean fluent aphasics. Commun Sci Disord. 2001;6(2):374–91.
41. Nicholas LE, Brookshire RH. Consistency of the effects of rate of speech on brain-damaged adults' comprehension of narrative discourse. J Speech Lang Hear Res. 1986;29(4):462–70.
42. Yorkston KM, Beukelman DR. An analysis of connected speech samples of aphasic and normal speakers. J Speech Hear Disord. 1980;45(1):27–36.
43. McNeil MR, Doyle PJ, Fossett TRD, Park GH, Goda AJ. Reliability and concurrent validity of the information unit scoring metric for the story retelling procedure. Aphasiology. 2001;15(10–11):991–1006.
44. Kim M, Thompson CK. Verb deficits in Alzheimer's disease and agrammatism: implications for lexical organization. Brain Lang. 2004 Jan;88(1):1–20.

45. Bryant L. Analyzing linguistic features of discourse in people with aphasia. In: Coelho CA, Cherney LR, Shadden BB, editors. Discourse analysis in adults with and without communication disorders: a resource for clinicians and researchers. San Diego, CA: Plural Publishing Inc; 2023.
46. Ulatowska HK, Doyel AW, Stern RF, Haynes SM, North AJ. Production of procedural discourse in aphasia. Brain Lang. 1983;18(2):315–41.
47. Bates E, Friederici A, Wulfeck B. Grammatical morphology in aphasia: evidence from three languages. Cortex. 1987;23(4):545–74.
48. Bastiaanse R. Why reference to the past is difficult for agrammatic speakers. Clin Linguist Phon. 2013;27(4):244–63.
49. Wright HH, Fergadiotis G. Conceptualising and measuring working memory and its relationship to aphasia. Aphasiology. 2012;26(3–4):258–78.
50. Halliday MAK, Hasan R. Cohesion in English. London, UK: Longman Group Limited; 1976.
51. Glosser G, Deser T. Patterns of discourse production among neurological patients with fluent language disorders. Brain Lang. 1991 Jan;40(1):67–88.
52. Zhang M, Geng L, Yang Y, Ding H. Cohesion in the discourse of people with post-stroke aphasia. Clin Linguist Phon. 2021;35(1):2–18.
53. Coelho C, Youse K, Le K, Feinn R. Narrative and conversational discourse of adults with closed head injuries and non-brain-injured adults: a discriminant analysis. Aphasiology. 2003 Jan;17(5):499–510.
54. Ellis C, Henderson A, Wright HH, Rogalski Y. Global coherence during discourse production in adults: a review of the literature. Int J Lang Commun Disord. 2016;51(4):359–67.
55. Kintz S, Fergadiotis G, Wright HH. Aging effects on discourse production. In: Wright HH, editor. Cognition, language and aging. Amsterdam: John Benjamins Publishing Company; 2016. p. 81–106. [cited 2018 Jun 12]. Available from: https://benjamins.com/catalog/z.200.04kin.
56. Harris Wright H, Capilouto GJ. Considering a multi-level approach to understanding maintenance of global coherence in adults with aphasia. Aphasiology. 2012;26(5):656–72.
57. Wright HH, Capilouto GJ, Koutsoftas A. Evaluating measures of global coherence ability in stories in adults: global coherence in stories. Int J Lang Commun Disord. 2013;48(3):249–56.
58. Huber W. Text comprehension and production in aphasia: analysis in terms of micro- and macrostructure. In: Joanette Y, Brownell HH, editors. Discourse ability and brain damage: theoretical and empirical perspectives. New York, NY: Springer-Verlag; 1990. p. 154–79.
59. Cahana-Amitay D, Jenkins T. Working memory and discourse production in people with aphasia. J Neurolinguistics. 2018;48:90–103.
60. Rogalski Y, Altmann LJP, Plummer-D'Amato P, Behrman AL, Marsiske M. Discourse coherence and cognition after stroke: a dual task study. J Commun Disord. 2010;43(3):212–24.
61. Hoffman P, Cogdell-Brooke L, Thompson HE. Going off the rails: impaired coherence in the speech of patients with semantic control deficits. Neuropsychologia. 2020;146:107516.
62. Christiansen JA. Coherence violations and propositional usage in narratives of fluent aphasics. Brain Lang. 1995;51:291–317.
63. Leaman MC, Edmonds LA. Measuring global coherence in people with aphasia during unstructured conversation. Am J Speech Lang Pathol. 2020;1–17:359.
64. Hazamy AA, Obermeyer J. Evaluating informative content and global coherence in fluent and nonfluent aphasia. Int J Lang Commun Disord. 2020 Jan;55(1):110–20.
65. Ramsberger G. Achieving conversational success in aphasia by focusing on non-linguistic cognitive skills: a potentially promising new approach. Aphasiology. 2005;19(10–11):1066–73.
66. Stark BC. A comparison of three discourse elicitation methods in aphasia and age-matched adults: implications for language assessment and outcome. Am J Speech Lang Pathol. 2019;28(3):1067–83.
67. Armstrong E, Ciccone N, Godecke E, Kok B. Monologues and dialogues in aphasia: some initial comparisons. Aphasiology. 2011;25(11):1347–71.

Stephen Kintz, Ph.D., is an Assistant Professor at the University of Arkansas at Little Rock in the Department of Speech-Language Pathology, where he serves as Undergraduate Program Coordinator. Dr. Kintz is interested in neurogenic communication disorders, specifically aphasia, traumatic brain injury, and dementia. His research goals are (1) to better understand the relationship between linguistic processes and other cognitive processes (e.g., attention and memory) and (2) to use this information to improve cognitive and language assessments for neurogenic communication disorders.

Discourse and Conversation Impairments in Patients with Dementia

3

Charalambos Themistocleous

Preview of What Is Currently Known
Neurodegeneration characterizes individuals with different dementia subtypes, leading to progressive decline in cognitive, linguistic, and social functioning. Language and communication deficits manifest early in the development of dementia (e.g., Alzheimer's disease, primary progressive aphasia, and Parkinson's disease) affecting the production and understanding of discourse microstructure (e.g., in grammar, semantics, and pragmatics) and macrostructure (e.g., discourse planning, organizing, and structuring). This work discusses findings on discourse impairments and suggests that clinical discourse analysis can provide a comprehensive assessment of language and communication skills in individuals with dementia that complements existing neurocognitive assessments for (differential) diagnosis, prognosis, and treatment efficacy evaluation.

Objectives
(a) To describe the effects of dementia on discourse.
(b) To identify the language and communication biomarkers for dementia assessment, diagnosis, prognosis, and treatment efficacy valuation elicited through clinical discourse analysis.
(c) To determine the impact of dementia on the cognitive representation of *grammar, communicative competence, emotions, empathy,* and *theory of mind.*
(d) To determine whether individuals employ a socially appropriate language communication and follow the turn-taking dynamics and conventions in conversations.

Introduction

Every year, more than ten million individuals develop dementia, with almost fifty-five million people worldwide now living with dementia [1]. Dementia is the progressive deterioration of cognitive, linguistic, and social functioning that affects the quality of life, including the physical, social, and economic conditions of individuals, their families, and society [2–5]. Although there is no treatment for dementia, early-stage identification and assessment of individuals with dementia are of utmost importance to enable interventions that can delay the progression of dementia and support family planning. The neurocognitive assessment aims to evaluate individuals' condition and provide early diagnosis, prognosis, and quantify intervention efficacy.

Speech, language, and communication impairments are early symptoms in individuals with dementia [6–8]. For example, earlier studies have shown that discourse narratives in the autobiog-

C. Themistocleous (✉)
Department of Special Needs Education, University of Oslo, Oslo, Norway
e-mail: charalampos.themistokleous@isp.uio.no

A. P.-H. Kong (ed.), *Spoken Discourse Impairments in the Neurogenic Populations*,
https://doi.org/10.1007/978-3-031-45190-4_3

raphies of Catholic sisters of the School Sisters of Notre Dame congregation can be an exceedingly early predictor of dementia [9]. In addition, studies of the speeches of the US President Ronald Reagan [10, 11] and the comparative analysis of the British novelists Iris Murdoch and Agatha Christie works showed that narratives could provide an early prognosis of dementia development [12].

Clinical discourse analysis (CDA) examines speech, language, and communication impairments in individuals with dementia and elicits language and communication measures. These measures can provide an early, stressless, and comprehensive assessment of individuals' language and neurocognitive functioning (e.g., memory, attention, social interaction) and inform treatment approaches [13, 14]. CDA involves the characterization of texts produced by individuals through language, cooperation, and social interaction in communicative settings such as conversations, semi-structured interviews [15–17], role-plays, and monologues [18]. [1]

In this review, we provide evidence from recent neurolinguistic and computational developments and demonstrate that discourse provides early linguistic biomarkers for (differential) diagnosis and prognosis of individuals with dementia. We discuss the following groups of individuals:

1. Individuals with primary progressive aphasia (PPA), a progressive neurological condition, which primarily affects speech and language. Individuals with PPA are grouped into three variants based on their distinct underlying neuropathology and area of brain damage [20]. According to current classification criteria, their characteristic neuropathology and damage patterns give rise to different discourse deficits across three variants [21, 22], namely in individuals with the non-fluent PPA variant (nfvPPA), individuals with the semantic PPA variant (svPPA), and individuals with the logopenic PPA variant (lvPPA).
2. Individuals with Alzheimer's disease (AD) constitute the larger group of individuals with dementia. They are characterized by a progressive deterioration of memory, language, conversation, and ability to perform everyday activities, unlike individuals with mild cognitive impairment, whose cognitive impairments are incipient and retain their day-to-day functioning.
3. Individuals with Parkinson's disease (PD) are characterized by a progressive deterioration of movement functioning, which impairs balance, speaking, language, chewing, and swallowing.

We identify the effects of brain damage due to neurodegeneration on discourse microstructure (e.g., phonology, morphology, and syntax) and macrostructure (e.g., *cohesion* of linguistic forms to determine whether individuals produce a text that follows the grammar and *coherence* of meanings and whether text productions make sense) [23, 24]. Macrostructure and microstructure are intertwined, and often the attempt to disentangle them is difficult as the same constituents can perform both microstructure and macrostructure functions, yet the distinction is necessary for the description of discourse structure. However, most language impairments associate with left hemisphere damage [21, 25], as discourse involves speech (and writing [26, 27]), language, emotions, social cognition, and cognitive domains, such as memory and attention; discourse impairments can result in neurodegenerative effects on the left and right hemispheres [28–31].

Here, we will discuss findings concerning the following three areas: (i) *language function, cognitive representation,* and *impairment*,[2] and examine how dementia impacts the cognitive representations of grammar (rules and principles)

[1]A more broad scope of CDA, yet uncommon in clinical settings, is the study of meaningful symbolic behavior of individuals in any mode, including social structures expressed through discourse, e.g., the discourse of race and power [19].

[2]Researchers often use the word "errors" to refer to incorrect productions with respect to correct productions (targets) in typical speakers; however, individuals produce language that follows their own grammatical system or interlanguage as it has developed after the brain damage. Moreover, the term error conceals the systematicity of these productions.

that enable speakers to produce grammatically correct sentences [32]; (ii) *communicative competence, emotions, empathy,* and *theory of mind* [33], and evaluate whether individuals employ a socially appropriate language communication; and (iii) *talk in interaction* to identify how individuals with dementia follow the turn-taking dynamics and conventions in conversations [34–36].

Language Function, Cognitive Representation, and Impairment

Discourse Microstructure and Dementia

Individuals with dementia produce speech with deficits that affect speech and articulation (e.g., prosodic patterns and rhythmical patterns), phonology (e.g., phonological errors, such as insertions, deletions, syllable structure simplifications), prosodic phonology (stress, rhythmical errors, intonation), morphology (e.g., morphological errors in verb and noun inflections, tense and number agreement, grammatical and content word production, and parts of speech) [37], lexicon [38], syntax (e.g., phrase structure and embedded phrases) [16, 39, 40], and semantics (e.g., lexical semantics, naming) [6, 41–48]. These deficits can characterize individuals with other speech and language disorders as well, such as stroke aphasia [49–52]. Discourse analysis employs both manual analysis and computational methods, such as acoustic analysis, natural language processing, and machine learning to automate the analysis [20, 53–60].

Traditionally, these discourse microstructure impairments are assessed during conventional neurophysiological examination with standardized language assessment tasks and neurolinguistic batteries, such as the Boston Naming Test (BNT; [61]), Western Aphasia Battery-Revised (WAB-R; Kertesz [62]), Boston Diagnostic Aphasia Examination (BDAE; [63]), Psycholinguistic Assessment of Language Processing in Aphasia (PALPA; [64]); and the Verb and Sentence Test (VAST; [65]). Nevertheless, single-domain standardized tests (cf., articulation and conformation naming) are not meant to assess broad language communication skills (e.g., articulation, morphosyntax, semantics, pragmatics, turn-taking), which alternatively require the application of multiple separate time-consuming and stressful language assessment tests. Thus, CDA aims to provide a comprehensive analysis and assessment of speech and grammar in context without requiring lengthy evaluation tests to target specific language domains. Here, we will review the primary microstructural deficits in individuals with PPA, AD, and PD, using combined information from studies employing discourse and standardized test evaluations.

In *individuals with PPA*, the primary language deficits correspond to the effects of neurodegeneration on the left hemisphere [43, 66–70]. Specifically, neuroimaging data shows that the peak atrophy site in individuals with nfvPPA is the posterior inferior frontal gyrus (pIFG), also known as Broca's area. In individuals with svPPA, the peak atrophy is the left anterior temporal lobe, and in individuals with lvPPA, the peak atrophy is located in the left posterior temporal and inferior parietal regions [21, 44, 71, 72].

More specifically, the individuals with nfvPPA, svPPA, and lvPPA differ in their discourse microstructure deficits. First, the individuals with nfvPPA are characterized by agrammatism resulting in telegraphic speech productions, namely they omit grammatical words, such as conjunctions, particles, and prepositions. Often, their speech is accompanied by Apraxia of Speech (AOS), which is associated with slow effortful speech with speech errors and pauses [73–77]. Individuals with nfvPPA with agrammatism are characterized by substantial deficits in function word production [17, 78, 79]. Consequently, in the context of producing discourse, individuals with nfvPPA produce more filled pauses than individuals with the semantic variant as they strive to construct grammatical structures and words [56]. Studies of the connected speech productions showed impaired production of sentence structure components, such as verb and noun phrases [7, 40]. In addition, individuals with the nfvPPA are characterized by syntactic comprehension impairments, especially during the perception of syntactically complex sentences [80]. Supporting evidence from naming tests showed that single-word comprehension and object naming are retained [21].

Although AOS and agrammatism are the two key diagnostic features in individuals with nfvPPA, agrammatism often occurs without AOS [78] and AOS without agrammatism [81]. Consequently, many studies distinguish individuals with the agrammatic variant of PPA [78] and individuals with PPA and AOS (PPAOS) [82–84]. Often, the classification is unclear as symptoms progress, leading to different degrees of language deterioration [85].

Moreover, individuals with nfvPPA produce selectively fewer verbs than healthy individuals [17, 78, 79], but verb perception can be preserved [86]. Verb production may be preserved in individuals with other PPA variants, although individuals with lvPPA show deficits during discourse in noun production [17, 78, 79]. In a computational study of morphology in individuals with PPA, Themistocleous et al. [37] have shown differential usage of parts of speech in individuals with different PPA variants [20].

Second, individuals with svPPA are characterized by impaired confrontation naming and single-word comprehension, impaired object knowledge, dysgraphia, and dyslexia [37, 43, 87]. However, unlike individuals with nfvPPA, speech production is spared in individuals with svPPA. Individuals with svPPA are also characterized by deficits in inflectional morphology. For example, Wilson et al. [88] showed that individuals with svPPA are impaired in inflecting low-frequency irregular words [89]. Nonetheless, inflectional morphology can be impaired in individuals with the other two PPA variants as individuals with nfvPPA show difficulties in inflecting pseudowords and individuals with lvPPA display morphophonological deficits [88].

Third, individuals with lvPPA are characterized by impaired single-word retrieval in spontaneous speech and naming and impaired sentence and phrase repetition, often with phonological errors. Further analysis of discourse has the potential to reveal interactions between lexical and morphosyntactic categories as suggested by task-based assessments [90].

Individuals with AD and MCI are impaired in discourse microstructure; however, these are incipient deficits in individuals with MCI and become progressively more severe in individuals with AD, which may end into mutism, and this mutism is more common in individuals with frontotemporal dementia [91, 92]. Studies using signal processing have shown that individuals with AD and MCI produce connected speech productions with significantly different patterns in segmental acoustic structure (i.e., vowels and consonants), prosody, voice quality, speech fluency, and speech rate; it was also demonstrated that speech acoustics not only can be employed for both diagnosis and differential diagnosis of individuals with AD and MCI from healthy controls, but also provide classification models for diagnosis or subtyping [54, 93–96]. For example, a recent study by Themistocleous et al. [57] found significantly slower speech productions in Swedish individuals with MCI than healthy controls, manifested as slower speech rate and long syllables. Moreover, they found that the speech of individuals with MCI is characterized by a greater degree of breathy voice, dysphonia, center of gravity, and shimmer than in healthy controls. They argue that the acoustic differences of individuals with MCI from healthy individuals indicate a physiological impairment in the fine control of vocal fold vibration, pulmonary pressure, respiration, and coordination of phonation and articulation [15, 50–53]. However, other studies show mixed results. More specifically, studies on emotional prosody showed impaired prosody in expressive speech productions, such as less pitch modulation and slower speech rate in individuals with dementia than in healthy controls, but their ability to control pitch and speech rate was normal [97].

Although phonology is relatively intact in individuals with MCI and AD, several studies showed phonetic and phonological errors, such as incorrect phoneme production, false starts, phonological paraphasias, and articulatory difficulties [98, 99]. Compared to healthy controls, individuals with AD can exhibit deterioration or simplification of grammar and semantics [100].

For example, an early study of narratives and constrained tasks showed significant errors in open and closed lexical classes, pronouns, and morphosyntax (e.g., inflection and agreement) between individuals with AD and healthy elderly individuals [101]. Similarly, a study with Greek individuals showed that individuals with probable AD were more impaired in verb aspect than in tense and agreement compared to healthy controls, in both production and grammaticality judgement; in contrast, verb agreement was in general retained [102]. Furthermore, individuals with AD can produce discourse with word finding and lexical retrieval difficulties [103], redundant words, and a higher proportion of closed-class words [98, 104].

Individuals with PD are characterized by speech acoustic differences in speech production and intonation identified from both discourse and non-discourse data [105, 106] and in other linguistic domains, such as syntax and sentence production [107]. Moreover, individuals with the behavioral variant of frontotemporal dementia (bvFTD) manifest progressive changes in personality, behavior, and social cognitive functions [108, 109] but can also manifest language impairments in their lexicon, semantics, prosody, reading, and writing [110]. At the same time, they may preserve motor speech production and morphosyntax [110].

Discourse Macrostructure and Dementia

In conversations, individuals with dementia, especially those with PPA, display impairments in discourse planning and macrostructure. Glosser and Deser [111] suggested that individuals with dementia are selectively more impaired in discourse macrostructure (e.g., thematic coherence and cohesion) than microstructure (e.g., phonology, morphology, lexicon, and syntax). Moreover, as dementia develops, text cohesion and coherence [112] become progressively more impaired [113].

Cohesion impairments manifest as irregularities in how individuals establish cohesive relationships in the text [114]. For example, individuals with dementia produce text with impaired lexical cohesion (i.e., lexical repetition and lexical chains, collocation) and discourse markers, which connect post-sentential constituents, having additive (e.g., and, furthermore, in addition), adversative (e.g., but, however, nevertheless), causal (e.g., so, consequently), and temporal meaning (e.g., then, after that, finally). Moreover, they display compromised application of cohesive devices, such as anaphora and cataphora [115], namely referencing usually with pronouns to an earlier (anaphora) or subsequent (cataphora) name or entity in discourse, substitution, conjunction, and replacement [116].

Furthermore, individuals with dementia display deficits in making cohesive associations with adjacency pairs, such as question-answer pairs, enumerations, greeting-greeting pairs, invitation-acceptance or rejection, and request-acceptance or rejection. When speakers employ adjacency pairs, the first part of the adjacency pair creates expectations that an ensuing part should satisfy; for example, in a question-answering pair, listeners expect an answer to a question and in an enumeration, an utterance, such as "I am going to state three things," should be followed by a list of three things; missing these associations is common in patients with dementia. For example, Ramanathan [117] notes that the expectations developed by Tina, an individual with AD, are not fulfilled by her, and the communication collapses:

> *Tina's talk here does not allow stanza parsing. Her talk starts off as a narrative (...) where she talks about how her India trip came about ("I had always wanted to go to India ..."), but she does not sustain her effort. In fact, in some instances she does not respond at all. (...) she does not pick up my prompts as cues for her to keep talking and (...) she is non-responsive to my question (...) but, once again, she does not develop her utterances into narratives* [103].

Coherence is the structuring and continuity of meanings and the semantic relationship of oral (or written) productions to their context including the situational conditions related to space, time, participants, and sociocultural meanings [118]. Coherence deficits reveal impairments in memory and semantic-linguistic interface, including impairments in recalling and organizing semantic meanings, such as past experiences and knowledge about the world [119]. Individuals with AD and MCI produce discourse with impaired semantic meaning and structure [119].

In addition, individuals with svPPA manifest semantic impairments in discourse affecting the production of lexical items and particularly content words [120]. A recent study by Seixas Lima et al. [121] on individuals with svPPA showed that although they produced episodic information related to the discourse topic, the semantic information was unrelated to discourse topic. The authors argue that, for individuals with svPPA, impairment depends on the selection of relevant semantic information and the inhibition of irrelevant ones. These findings are consistent with the evidence from confrontational naming tasks, such as the Boston Naming Test (BNT) [61] and the Hopkins Assessment on Naming Actions (HANA) [122].

Furthermore, individuals with dementia produce speech with impaired information packaging, concerning the new and old information, contrast, and pragmatic implicatures [123]. Specifically, information packaging is achieved using linguistic means such as syntax and prosody [124, 125]. Information packaging using syntax is manifested with cleft structures, where constituents are moved to a different position in the sentence to express contrast, emphasis, etc., as in the following examples in (1):

(1)

(i) It is George[F] [3] who went to the movies last week.
(ii) It was to the movies[F] that George went last week.
(iii) It was yesterday[F] that Jerry went to the movies.
(iv) What I need is a nice milk chocolate.

The cleft structures in the examples above can imply a contrasted constituent as:

(2)

(i) It was GEORGE who went to the movies last week [not Maria].

Moreover, prosody (e.g., intonation and phrasing cues) expresses information structure in English and other languages. For example, new-information focus and contrast are manifested using nuclear pitch accents that highlight the prominent or contrasting constituent [126–129], whereas preceding words, if any, are marked with a different type of accent, a.k.a. prenuclear pitch accents.

In English, syntax expresses information structure (cf. examples above (1) and (2)) combined with a nuclear pitch accent at the end manifesting broad focus (3):

(3)

(i) George went to the movies last week.

These cases demonstrate an interplay between prosody and syntax. Dementia can impair prosody and syntax in individuals with non-fluent PPA with agrammatism [124] and individuals with MCI and AD [54, 95, 110, 130].

Using rhetorical structure theory, Abdalla et al. [131] showed the effects of AD on discourse rhetorical mechanisms [132]. RST evaluates various relationships and how they are constructed in discourse, e.g., elaboration, circumstance, solutionhood, cause, restatement, presentational relations, motivation, background, justify, and concession [132, 133]. Studies of discourse in the nun study, a longitudinal study of cognitive decline, also showed that nuns with AD produced discourse with impaired idea density; in fact, research on the nun study showed that discourse deterioration is a very early predictor of dementia [134].

Overall, discourse macrostructure impairments can correlate with the deterioration of language and cognition, such as working memory, planning, generation, problem-solving, and abstraction [111].

Dementia and Communicative Competence, Emotions, Empathy, and Theory of Mind

Communication assessment aims to determine how individuals employ language in the appropriate social context, follow social norms, and

[3] [F] indicates the focused or highlighted constituent.

make connections with participants and settings. Therefore, Hymes [135] suggests that utterances should be evaluated concerning their discourse context. In other words, the communicative competence of individuals is assessed based on whether they produce utterances that consider the following discourse settings, namely:

1. The other participants.
2. The roles they assume.
3. The conversational topic.
4. The communicative channel (e.g., writing and speaking).
5. The language code (e.g., language variety, dialect, language style).
6. The message form (e.g., lecture, a conversation, a fairy tale, narrative).
7. The situation (e.g., a ceremony, a friendly conversation).
8. The purpose of the speech.
9. The key (e.g., tone and manner).

Therefore, there is a fundamental distinction between CDA and standardized language assessment in that CDA assesses language communication, which involves several distinct components at once, such as the following: (i) the *intentionality of discourse* and whether individuals perceive utterances as intentional and actively make a cooperative effort to produce and understand the discourse content [114, 136]; (ii) *the situationality of discourse* and whether individuals produce utterances that are related to the immediate discourse context; and (iii) the *intertextuality* of discourse and whether individuals' utterances connect discourse productions to the broader intertextual context correctly [114].

Kong et al. [137] employed story grammars, which consider information such as the conversational background, participants, and time and place of conversation to analyze discourse produced by individuals with fluent aphasia, non-fluent aphasia, and AD and healthy controls. Their study showed significant differences in the production of situational discourse information in individuals with AD and healthy controls. Interestingly, their study showed similarities in the use of situational information between individuals with AD and individuals with fluent aphasia.

Individuals with dementia can exhibit discourse impairments in communicative competence [138]. However, individuals with the behavioral variant of frontotemporal dementia (bvFTD) show communicative competence impairments more predominantly than other individuals with dementia. These individuals display impairments in early behavioral disinhibition, which is the distinguishing symptom of individuals with bvFTD clinical syndrome from individuals with AD, dementia with Lewy bodies, and vascular dementia [108]. Inappropriate language accompanies an overall loss of manners of decorum, such as cursing, speaking loudly, expressing offensively and sexually, obscene remarks, jokes, and opinions [108]. In addition, apathy, failure to initiate or sustain a conversation, loss of empathy, insight, and executive dysfunction are associated with frontal and temporal atrophy [108]. The speech of individuals with bvFTD is also characterized by selective impairments linked to an overall degraded communicative competence, as reflected by poor organization discourse, simplification of grammatical production, selective impairments in word use, and changes in acoustic properties [110, 138–142].

Notably, the assessment of communicative competence brings language to the fore as the connecting link between the social context, paralinguistic expression and emotion, empathy/sympathy, and theory of mind (ToM). ToM is the ability of individuals to attribute mental states to other individuals and employ the states to understand and predict actions and discourse contributions. Using standardized tests for memory, comprehension, and general inferencing question, Youmans and Bourgeois [143] found that individuals with mild-to-moderate AD exhibit mild but specific ToM impairment. Again, ToM impairments are more severe in individuals with bvFTD. However, standardized neurocognitive testing of ToM can only modestly distinguish between individuals with FTD and AD [144], as these tests create an artificial environment that does not provide the necessary social context to adequately evaluate ToM. In contrast, discourse can provide a natural environment and comprehensive assessment of ToM.

These findings from discourse provide quantitative measures of communicative competence and assess social and behavioral symptoms using more naturalistic and conversational interactions than standardized language tests (e.g., identifying pictures in cards or picture books and repeating words and sentences).

Dementia and Talk in Interaction (Turn-Taking)

As discourse is used in conversations between individuals and other individuals (e.g., clinicians and other individuals), conversation analysis can be employed as a method to identify how dementia influences both language and social interaction. Conversation analysis studies the social conventions that facilitate the interaction of interlocutors and the passing of conversational turns from one participant to another. The conversational turns are the basic units of any conversation [36]. The aim of conversation analysis in the clinic is twofold: first, it aims to determine whether the basic properties that characterize social interaction break down in individuals with dementia and quantify the communicative characteristics of their speech, and second, it aims to identify how individuals with dementia construct the conversational turn, vis-à-vis other groups of speakers (e.g., healthy controls, individuals with different conditions or with respect to an earlier stage of the same individual). Examining how individuals with dementia engage in conversations in the clinic provides information about the language and social interaction impairments.

First formulated by Sacks et al. [36], conversation analysis aims to determine whether speakers follow the social conventions that regulate the exchange of turns in conversations. In particular, the authors formulated a set of simple principles that determine conversation [36]: speaker change recurs; one party speaks at a time; occurrences, when speakers talk simultaneously, are common but brief; turn transitions with a slight or no gap make the majority of turn transitions; the turn order and size are not fixed; and the length and content of transitions vary. Moreover, the selection of speakers in the conversation follows conventionalized turn-allocation techniques, which are a core component of any conversation. The conversation exchange consists of turns structured from turn-constructional units (cf. sentences consisting of phrases and words). A conversational unit contains turn-transition points where the current speaker can select the next speaker or decide to continue, known as self-selection, using gestures such as prosody or intonation, hand and head gestures, body posture, glance, and eyebrow movement. Lexicogrammar can also indicate transitions, such as specific lexical units or the right end of a sentence. For example, conversation exchange involves the identification of the appropriate places to exchange the conversational turn, such as passing it to the next speaker and resolving conflicts that may occur.

Individuals with PPA display interactional difficulties during communication. For example, a study of individuals with svPPA showed that although these individuals participated actively in the conversation, they had problems maintaining the flow of interaction, such as requesting for confirmation, and displayed an inability to keep with the conversation, such as to initiate or continue the conversational topic [145]. In addition, individuals with AD differ in the construction of turns from healthy controls. For example, a study of conversations in individuals with AD showed that individuals with AD produced fewer word per turn and fewer speech acts—especially, requestives, and assertives—than healthy individuals [146].

The types of conversations, e.g., casual conversations [147], telephone conversations [148], map task navigation, computer-mediated decision-making interactions, and spontaneous dialogue data [149], determines the role of exchange between speakers. However, a common complaint is that individuals with dementia often have difficulty following conventional patterns, such as ring-greeting-message-greeting, that characterize phone conversations [150].

Moreover, reduced conversational skills characterize individuals with dementia, including PPA, MCI, AD, and PD [151–154]. For example, studies showed that individuals with PPA could "maintain turn-taking but had reduced amount of talk and were able to request confirmation and actively repair their own and their partners' trouble in talk" [155]. Nevertheless, studies using conversational analysis usually rely on a few participants. Thus, it is far from straightforward to generalize on the population.

Whitworth et al. [156] employed conversational analysis and showed that individuals with PD display impairments in turn initiation, turn-taking, and repair, such as failing or delaying responding to conversational cues when turns are allocated to them by the current speaker. As a result, in individuals with PD, conversational difficulties arise regarding speaker coordination during turn-taking and turn resolution [157, 158]. These failures may occur due to a failure to perceive a turn-taking cue during the interaction. Several studies in talk in interaction benefit from analyzing multimodal cues from speech language and video. However, these studies generally rely on very few participants [159]; thus, it is essential to employ conversation multimodal analytic research on larger individual groups to safeguard the generalizability of the findings.

Conclusions

This chapter has discussed discourse and conversation in the context of assessment and diagnosis and demonstrated that CDA provides information about speech communication impairments across discourse domains. The multimodal information highlights the value of CDA as an approach that provides measures that can complement those from current standardized language evaluation batteries [160–164] for assessment, diagnosis, prognosis, and therapy efficacy estimation [159, 163–165].

Major Takeaways

1. Dementia affects speech, language, and communication in most individuals with dementia, but these are especially evident in individuals with primary progressive aphasia.
2. Deficits characterize the microstructure (e.g., phonology, morphology, syntax) and discourse macrostructure (e.g., cohesion, coherence), theory of mind, and conversation.
3. Discourse analysis in individuals with dementia provides comprehensive linguistic biomarkers for speech, language, communication, and cognition assessment (differential), diagnosis, prognosis, and treatment efficacy valuation.

References

1. World Health Organization. Global action plan on the public health response to dementia 2017–2025. Geneva: World Health. Organization; 2017.
2. Geda YE, Schneider LS, Gitlin LN, Miller DS, Smith GS, Bell J, Evans J, Lee M, Porsteinsson A, Lanctôt KL, Rosenberg PB, Sultzer DL, Francis PT, Brodaty H, Padala PP, Onyike CU, Ortiz LA, Ancoli-Israel S, Bliwise DL, Martin JL, Vitiello MV, Yaffe K, Zee PC, Herrmann N, Sweet RA, Ballard C, Khin NA, Alfaro C, Murray PS, Schultz S, Lyketsos CG. Neuropsychiatric symptoms in Alzheimer's disease: past progress and anticipation of the future. Alzheimers Dement. 2013;9(5):602–8.
3. Lyketsos CG, DelCampo L, Steinberg M, Miles Q, Steele CD, Munro C, Baker AS, Sheppard JME, Frangakis C, Brandt J. Treating depression in Alzheimer disease: efficacy and safety of sertraline therapy, and the benefits of depression reduction: the DIADS. Arch Gen Psychiatry. 2003;60(7):737.
4. Lyketsos CG, Lopez O, Jones B, Fitzpatrick AL, Breitner J, DeKosky S. Prevalence of neuropsychiatric symptoms in dementia and mild cognitive impairment results from the cardiovascular health study. JAMA. 2002;288(12):1475–83.
5. Lyketsos CG, Steinberg M, Tschanz JT, Norton MC, Steffens DC, Breitner JCS. Mental and behavioral disturbances in dementia: findings from the Cache County study on memory in aging. Am J Psychiatr. 2000;157(5):708–14.
6. Thompson CK, Lukic S, King MC, Mesulam MM, Weintraub S. Verb and noun deficits in stroke-induced and primary progressive aphasia: the northwestern naming battery. Aphasiology. 2012;26(5):632–55.

7. Thompson CK, Mack JE. Grammatical impairments in PPA. Aphasiology. 2014;28(8–9):1018–37.
8. Mesulam MM. Primary progressive aphasia and the language network: the 2013 H. Houston Merritt Lecture. Neurology. 2013;81(5):456–62.
9. Danner DD, Snowdon DA, Friesen WV. Positive emotions in early life and longevity: findings from the nun study. J Pers Soc Psychol. 2001;80(5):804–13.
10. Berisha V, Wang S, LaCross A, Liss J. Tracking discourse complexity preceding Alzheimer's disease diagnosis: a case study comparing the press conferences of presidents Ronald Reagan and George Herbert Walker bush. J Alzheimers Dis. 2015;45(3):959–63.
11. Berisha V, Sandoval S, Utianski R, Liss J, Spanias A. Characterizing the distribution of the quadrilateral vowel space area. J Acoust Soc Am. 2014;135(1):421–7.
12. Le X, Lancashire I, Hirst G, Jokel R. Longitudinal detection of dementia through lexical and syntactic changes in writing: a case study of three British novelists. Literary Linguist Comput. 2011;26(4):435–61.
13. Brown G, Yule G. Discourse analysis. Cambridge: Cambridge University Press; 1983.
14. Armstrong E. Aphasic discourse analysis: the story so far. Aphasiology. 2000;14(9):875–92.
15. Graham NL, Patterson K, Hodges JR. When more yields less: speaking and writing deficits in nonfluent progressive aphasia. Neurocase. 2004;10(2):141–55.
16. Knibb JA, Woollams AM, Hodges JR, Patterson K. Making sense of progressive non-fluent aphasia: an analysis of conversational speech. Brain. 2009;132(10):2734–46.
17. Thompson CK, Ballard KJ, Tait ME, Weintraub S, Mesulam MM. Patterns of language decline in nonfluent primary progressive aphasia. Aphasiology. 1997;11:297.
18. Whitworth A, Cartwright J, Beales A, Leitao S, Panegyres PK, Kane R. Taking words to a new level: a preliminary investigation of discourse intervention in primary progressive aphasia. Aphasiology. 2018;32(11):1284–309.
19. Blommaert J. Discourse. Cambridge: Cambridge University Press; 2005.
20. Themistocleous C, Ficek B, Webster K, den Ouden D-B, Hillis AE, Tsapkini K. Automatic subtyping of individuals with primary progressive aphasia. J Alzheimers Dis. 2021;79:1185–94.
21. Gorno-Tempini ML, Hillis AE, Weintraub S, Kertesz A, Mendez M, Cappa SF, Ogar JM, Rohrer JD, Black S, Boeve BF, Manes F, Dronkers NF, Vandenberghe R, Rascovsky K, Patterson K, Miller BL, Knopman DS, Hodges JR, Mesulam MM, Grossman M. Classification of primary progressive aphasia and its variants. Neurology. 2011;76(11):1006–14.
22. Ash S, Evans E, O'Shea J, Powers J, Boller A, Weinberg D, Haley J, McMillan C, Irwin DJ, Rascovsky K, Grossman M. Differentiating primary progressive aphasias in a brief sample of connected speech. Neurology. 2013;81:329–36.
23. Hall K, Lind C, Young JA, Okell E, van Steenbrugge W. Familiar communication partners' facilitation of topic management in conversations with individuals with dementia. Int J Lang Commun Disord. 2018;53(3):564–75.
24. Botinis A, Bakakou-Orphanou A, Themistocleous C. Multifactor analysis of discourse turn in Greek. In: Proceedings of the 16th International Congress of Phonetic Sciences (ICPhS XVI). Universität des Saarlandes: Saarbrücken, Germany; 2007. p. 1341–4.
25. Peristeri E, Tsimpli IM, Tsapkini K. The local-global dimension in cognitive control after left lateral prefrontal cortex damage: evidence from the verbal and the non-verbal domain. In: Academy of Aphasia—52nd annual meeting. Miami-Florida: Frontiers in Psychology; 2014. p. 1–2.
26. Neophytou K, Themistocleous C, Wiley R, Tsapkini K, Rapp B. Understanding and classifying the different variants of primary progressive aphasia based on spelling performance. Front Hum Neurosci. 2018;12
27. Themistocleous C, Neophytou K, Rapp B, Tsapkini K. A tool for automatic scoring of spelling performance. J Speech Lang Hear Res. 2020;63:4179–92.
28. Hickok G, Wilson M, Clark K, Klima ES, Kritchevsky M, Bellugi U. Discourse deficits following right hemisphere damage in deaf signers. Brain Lang. 1999;66(2):233–48.
29. Afthinos A, Themistocleous C, Herrmann O, Fan H, Lu H, Tsapkini K. The contribution of working memory areas to verbal learning and recall in primary progressive aphasia. Front Neurol. 2022;13:1–11.
30. Winner E, Brownell H, Happé F, Blum A, Pincus D. Distinguishing lies from jokes: theory of mind deficits and discourse interpretation in right hemisphere brain-damaged patients. Brain Lang. 1998;62(1):89–106.
31. Chapman SB, Highley AP, Thompson JL. Discourse in fluent aphasia and Alzheimer's disease: linguistic and pragmatic considerations. J Neurolinguistics. 1998;11(1–2):55–78.
32. Chomsky N. Aspects of the theory of syntax. Cambridge, MA: M.I.T. Press; 1965.
33. Murray L, Timberlake A, Eberle R. Treatment of underlying forms in a discourse context. Aphasiology. 2007;21(2):139–63.
34. Schegloff EA. Reflections on studying prosody in talk-in-interaction. Lang Speech. 1998;41(3–4):235–63.
35. Schegloff EA, Jefferson G, Sacks H. The preference for self-correction in the organization of repair in conversation. Language. 1977;53(2):361–82.
36. Sacks H, Schegloff EA, Jefferson G. A simplest systematics for the organization of turn-taking for conversation. Language. 1974;50:696–735.
37. Themistocleous C, Webster K, Afthinos A, Tsapkini K. Part of speech production in patients with primary progressive aphasia: an analysis based on natural language processing. Am J Speech Lang Pathol. 2020;30:1–15.

38. Fergadiotis G, Wright Heather H, West TM. Measuring lexical diversity in narrative discourse of people with aphasia. Am J Speech Lang Pathol. 2013;22(2):S397–408.
39. Wilson SM, DeMarco AT, Henry ML, Gesierich B, Babiak M, Miller BL, Gorno-Tempini ML. Variable disruption of a syntactic processing network in primary progressive aphasia. Brain. 2016;139(11):2994–3006.
40. Wilson SM, Galantucci S, Tartaglia MC, Gorno-Tempini ML. The neural basis of syntactic deficits in primary progressive aphasia. Brain Lang. 2012;122(3):190–8.
41. Fergadiotis G, Wright HH. Modelling confrontation naming and discourse performance in aphasia. Aphasiology. 2016;30(4):364–80.
42. Fenner AS, Webster KT, Ficek BN, Frangakis CE, Tsapkini K. Written verb naming improves after tDCS over the left IFG in primary progressive aphasia. Front Psychol. 2019;10:1396.
43. Sebastian R, Thompson CB, Wang NY, Wright A, Meyer A, Friedman RB, Hillis AE, Tippett DC. Patterns of decline in naming and semantic knowledge in primary progressive aphasia. Aphasiology. 2018;32(9):1010–30.
44. Tsapkini K, Webster KT, Ficek BN, Desmond JE, Onyike CU, Rapp B, Frangakis CE, Hillis AE. Electrical brain stimulation in different variants of primary progressive aphasia: a randomized clinical trial. Alzheimers Dement (N Y). 2018;4:461–72.
45. Faria A, Meyer A, Tippett D, Sebastian R, Mori S, Friedman R. Decline in naming in patients with Primary Progressive Aphasia is associated with the strength of functional correlation between homologous Pre-Frontal cortices in the initial MRI (P5. 018). Neurology. 2015;84(Suppl. 14) P5. 018
46. Budd MA, Kortte K, Cloutman L, Newhart M, Gottesman RF, Davis C, Heidler-Gary J, Seay MW, Hillis AE. The nature of naming errors in primary progressive aphasia versus acute post-stroke aphasia. Neuropsychology. 2010;24(5):581–9.
47. Newhart M, Davis C, Kannan V, Heidler-Gary J, Cloutman L, Hillis AE. Therapy for naming deficits in two variants of primary progressive aphasia. Aphasiology. 2009;23:823–34.
48. Hillis AE, Oh S, Ken L. Deterioration of naming nouns versus verbs in primary progressive aphasia. Ann Neurol. 2004;55(2):268–75.
49. Salis C, DeDe G. Sentence production in a discourse context in latent aphasia: a real-time study. Am J Speech Lang Pathol. 2022;31(3):1284–96.
50. Salis C, Martin N, Meehan SV, McCaffery K. Short-term memory span in aphasia: insights from speech-timing measures. J Neurolinguistics. 2018;48:176–89.
51. Yoo H, McNeil MR, Dickey MW, Terhorst L. Linguistic and nonlinguistic processing speed across age-matched normal healthy controls and individuals with left-hemisphere damage, with and without aphasia. Aphasiology. 2022;36(2):147–69.
52. Fyndanis V, Themistocleous C. Are there prototypical associations between time frames and aspectual values? Evidence from Greek aphasia and healthy ageing. Clin Linguist Phon. 2019;33(1–2):191–217.
53. Themistocleous C, Fyndanis V, Tsapkini K. Sonorant spectra and coarticulation distinguish speakers with different dialects. Speech Comm. 2022;1–14:1.
54. König A, Satt A, Sorin A, others. Automatic speech analysis for the assessment of patients with predementia and Alzheimer's disease. Alzheimers Dement 2018;1(1):112–124.
55. Satt A, Hoory R, König A, Aalten P, Robert PH. Speech-based automatic and robust detection of very early dementia. In: Proceedings of the Annual Conference of the International Speech Communication Association, INTERSPEECH. Curran Associates, Inc.: Brno, Czech Republic; 2014.
56. Wilson SM, Henry ML, Besbris M, Ogar JM, Dronkers NF, Jarrold W, Miller BL, Gorno-Tempini ML. Connected speech production in three variants of primary progressive aphasia. Brain. 2010;133(Pt 7):2069–88.
57. Themistocleous C, Eckerström M, Kokkinakis D. Voice quality and speech fluency distinguish individuals with mild cognitive impairment from healthy controls. PLoS One. 2020;15(7):e0236009.
58. Themistocleous C. Dialect classification from a single sonorant sound using deep neural networks. Front Commun. 2019;4:1–12.
59. Themistocleous C, Kokkinakis D, Marie E, Kathleen F, Kristina Lundholm F. Effects of cognitive impairment on vowel duration. In: Proceedings of the 9th Tutorial; Research Workshop on Experimental Linguistics (ExLing 2018) 28–30. International Society of Experimental Linguistics: Paris, France; 2018. p. 113–6.
60. Themistocleous C. Dialect classification using vowel acoustic parameters. Speech Comm. 2017;92:13–22.
61. Kaplan E, Goodglass H, Weintraub S. Boston naming test. Austin, TX: Pro-ed; 2001.
62. Kertesz A. Western aphasia battery-revised (WAB-R). New York: Pearson; 2006.
63. Goodglass H, Kaplan E. Boston diagnostic aphasia examination (BDAE). Philadelphia: Lea & Febiger; 1983.
64. Kay J, Lesser R, Coltheart RM. Psycholinguistic assessments of language processing in aphasia (PALPA). New York: Psychology Press; 1992.
65. Bastiaanse R, Edwards S, Rispens J. The verb and sentence test (VAST). Harlow (UK): Thames Valley Test Company; 2002.
66. de Aguiar V, Zhao Y, Ficek BN, Webster K, Rofes A, Wendt H, Frangakis C, Caffo B, Hillis AE, Rapp B, Tsapkini K. Cognitive and language performance predicts effects of spelling intervention

and tDCS in primary progressive aphasia. Cortex. 2020;124:66–84.
67. Hudspeth Dalton SG, Shultz C, Henry ML, Hillis AE, Richardson JD. Describing phonological Paraphasias in three variants of primary progressive aphasia. Am J Speech Lang Pathol. 2018;27:336–49.
68. Tippett DC, Hillis AE, Tsapkini K. Treatment of primary progressive aphasia. Curr Treat Options Neurol. 2015;17(8):362.
69. Tsapkini K, Frangakis C, Davis C, Gomez Y, Chakravarty T, Hillis A. Spelling rehabilitation using transcranial direct current (tDCS) in primary progressive aphasia (PPA). Front Psychol. 2014;5:1.
70. Hillis AE. Deterioration or recovery of selective cognitive function can reveal the role of focal areas within networks of the brain. Behav Neurol. 2013;26(1–2):3–5.
71. de Aguiar V, Zhao Y, Faria A, Ficek B, Webster KT, Wendt H, Wang Z, Hillis AE, Onyike CU, Frangakis C, Caffo B, Tsapkini K. Brain volumes as predictors of tDCS effects in primary progressive aphasia. Brain Lang. 2020;200:104707.
72. Hillis AE, Tsapkini K. Neuroanatomical aspects of reading. In: The handbook of adult language disorders. Philadelphia, PA: Psychology Press; 2015. p. 40–53.
73. Gorno-Tempini ML, Pressman P. Introduction to primary progressive aphasia. In: Small SL, Hickok G, editors. Neurobiology of language. Amsterdam: Academic Press; 2016. p. 935–52.
74. Themistocleous C, Ficek B, Webster K, Tsapkini K. tDCS reduces phonological errors in patients with primary progressive aphasia. In: In: 60th annual academy of aphasia meeting, Philadelphia. Academy of Aphasia. Philadelphia; 2022.
75. Themistocleous C, Webster K, Tsapkini K. Effects of tDCS on sound duration in patients with apraxia of speech in primary progressive aphasia. Brain Sci. 2021;11(3):335.
76. Gorno-Tempini ML, Dronkers NF, Rankin KP, Ogar JM, Phengrasamy L, Rosen HJ, Johnson JK, Weiner MW, Miller BL. Cognition and anatomy in three variants of primary progressive aphasia. Ann Neurol. 2004;55(3):335–46.
77. Ash S, Adamowicz D, McMillan C, Grossman M. Sounds of silence: pauses in the speech of progressive non-fluent aphasics. Neurology. 2010;74(9):A504–A5.
78. Thompson CK, Cho S, Hsu CJ, Wieneke C, Rademaker A, Weitner BB, Mesulam MM, Weintraub S. Dissociations between fluency and Agrammatism in primary progressive aphasia. Aphasiology. 2012;26(1):20–43.
79. Thompson CK, Meltzer-Asscher A, Cho S, Lee J, Wieneke C, Weintraub S, Mesulam MM. Neurocognitive mechanisms of verb argument structure processing. Behav Neurol. 2013;26:141–68.
80. Marcotte K, Graham NL, Fraser KC, Meltzer JA, Tang-Wai DF, Chow TW, Freedman M, Leonard C, Black SE, Rochon E. White matter disruption and connected speech in non-fluent and semantic variants of primary progressive aphasia. Dement Geriatr Cogn Disord Extra. 2017;7(1):52–73.
81. Duffy JR. Apraxia of speech in degenerative neurologic disease. Aphasiology. 2006;20(6):511–27.
82. Duffy JR, Strand EA, Clark H, Machulda M, Whitwell JL, Josephs KA. Primary progressive apraxia of speech: clinical features and acoustic and neurologic correlates. Am J Speech Lang Pathol. 2015;24(2):88–100.
83. Josephs KA, Duffy JR, Strand EA, Whitwell JL, Layton KF, Parisi JE, Hauser MF, Witte RJ, Boeve BF, Knopman DS, Dickson DW, Jack CR Jr, Petersen RC. Clinicopathological and imaging correlates of progressive aphasia and apraxia of speech. Brain. 2006;129(Pt 6):1385–98.
84. Josephs KA, Whitwell JL, Duffy JR, Vanvoorst WA, Strand EA, Hu WT, Boeve BF, Graff-Radford NR, Parisi JE, Knopman DS, others. Progressive aphasia secondary to Alzheimer disease vs FTLD pathology. Neurology 2008;70(1):25–34.
85. Gorno-Tempini ML, Ogar JM, Brambati SM, Wang P, Jeong JH, Rankin KP, Dronkers NF, Miller BL. Anatomical correlates of early mutism in progressive nonfluent aphasia. Neurology. 2006;67(10):1849–51.
86. Wang H, Walenski M, Litcofsky K, Mack JE, Mesulam MM, Thompson CK. Verb production and comprehension in primary progressive aphasia. J Neurolinguistics. 2022;64:101099.
87. Neophytou K, Wiley RW, Rapp B, Tsapkini K. The use of spelling for variant classification in primary progressive aphasia: theoretical and practical implications. Neuropsychologia. 2019;133:107157.
88. Wilson SM, Brandt TH, Henry ML, Babiak M, Ogar JM, Salli C, Wilson L, Peralta K, Miller BL, Gorno-Tempini ML. Inflectional morphology in primary progressive aphasia: an elicited production study. Brain Lang. 2014;136:58–68.
89. Mack JE, Mesulam MM, Rogalski EJ, Thompson CK. Verb-argument integration in primary progressive aphasia: real-time argument access and selection. Neuropsychologia. 2019;134:107192.
90. Stockbridge MD, Matchin W, Walker A, Breining B, Fridriksson J, Hickok G, Hillis AE. One cat, two cats, red cat, blue cats: eliciting morphemes from individuals with primary progressive aphasia. Aphasiology. 2021;35(12):1–12.
91. Barber R, Snowden JS, Craufurd D. Frontotemporal dementia and Alzheimer's disease: retrospective differentiation using information from informants. J Neurol Neurosurg Psychiatry. 1995;59(1):61.
92. van Engelen M-PE, Gossink FT, de Vijlder LS, Meursing JRA, Scheltens P, Dols A, Pijnenburg YAL, Knopman D. End stage clinical features and cause of death of behavioral variant frontotemporal dementia and Young-onset Alzheimer's disease. J Alzheimers Dis. 2020;77(3):1169–80.

93. Meilan JJG, Martinez-Sanchez F, Carro J, Carcavilla N, Ivanova O. Voice markers of lexical access in mild cognitive impairment and Alzheimer's disease. Curr Alzheimer Res. 2018;15(2):111–9.
94. Themistocleous C, Kokkinakis D. Speech and mild cognitive impairment detection. In: Botinis A, editor. Proceedings of the 9th tutorial research workshop on experimental linguistics (ExLing2019). International Society of Experimental Linguistics: Lisbon, Portugal. 2019. p. 201.
95. Themistocleous C, Eckerström M, Kokkinakis D. Identification of mild cognitive impairment from speech in Swedish using deep sequential neural networks. Front Neurol. 2018;9:975.
96. Tóth L, Hoffmann I, Gosztolya G, Vincze V, Szatloczki G, Banreti Z, Pakaski M, Kalman J. A speech recognition-based solution for the automatic detection of mild cognitive impairment from spontaneous speech. Curr Alzheimer Res. 2018;15(2):130–8.
97. Horley K, Reid A, Burnham D. Emotional prosody perception and production in dementia of the Alzheimer's type. J Speech Lang Hear Res. 2010;53(5):1132–46.
98. Sajjadi SA, Patterson K, Tomek M, Nestor PJ. Abnormalities of connected speech in semantic dementia vs Alzheimer's disease. Aphasiology. 2012;26(6):847–66.
99. Croot K, Hodges JR, Xuereb J, Patterson K. Phonological and articulatory impairment in Alzheimer's disease: a case series. Brain Lang. 2000;75(2):277–309.
100. Sanz C, Carrillo F, Slachevsky A, Forno G, Gorno Tempini ML, Villagra R, Ibáñez A, Tagliazucchi E, García AM. Automated text-level semantic markers of Alzheimer's disease. Alzheimers Dement. 2022;14(1):1–10.
101. Altmann LJP, Kempler D, Andersen ES. Speech errors in Alzheimer's disease: reevaluating morphosyntactic preservation. J Speech, Lang Hearing Res. 2001;44(5):1069–82.
102. Fyndanis V, Manouilidou C, Koufou E, Karampekios S, Tsapakis EM. Agrammatic patterns in Alzheimer's disease: evidence from tense, agreement, and aspect. Aphasiology. 2013;27(2):178–200.
103. Pekkala S, Wiener D, Himali J, Beiser A, Obler L, Liu Y, McKee A, Auerbach S, Seshadri S, Wolf P, Au R. Lexical retrieval in discourse: an early indicator of Alzheimer's dementia. Clin Linguist Phon. 2013;27:27.
104. Faroqi-Shah Y, Treanor A, Ratner NB, Ficek B, Webster K, Tsapkini K. Using narratives in differential diagnosis of neurodegenerative syndromes. J Commun Disord. 2020;85:1–13.
105. Tsanas A, Arora S. Data-driven subtyping of Parkinson's using acoustic analysis of sustained vowels and cluster analysis: findings in the Parkinson's voice initiative study. SN Comput Sci. 2022;3(3):232.
106. Troche J, Troche M, Berkowitz R, Grossman M, Reilly J. Tone discrimination as a window into acoustic perceptual deficits in Parkinson's disease. Procedia Soc Behav Sci. 2010;6:130.
107. Troche MS, Altmann LJP. Sentence production in Parkinson disease: effects of conceptual and task complexity. Appl Psycholinguist. 2012;33(2):225–51.
108. Rascovsky K, Hodges JR, Knopman D, Mendez MF, Kramer JH, Neuhaus J, van Swieten JC, Seelaar H, Dopper EGP, Onyike CU, Hillis AE, Josephs KA, Boeve BF, Kertesz A, Seeley WW, Rankin KP, Johnson JK, Gorno-Tempini M-L, Rosen H, Prioleau-Latham CE, Lee A, Kipps CM, Lillo P, Piguet O, Rohrer JD, Rossor MN, Warren JD, Fox NC, Galasko D, Salmon DP, Black SE, Mesulam M, Weintraub S, Dickerson BC, Diehl-Schmid J, Pasquier F, Deramecourt V, Lebert F, Pijnenburg Y, Chow TW, Manes F, Grafman J, Cappa SF, Freedman M, Grossman M, Miller BL. Sensitivity of revised diagnostic criteria for the behavioural variant of frontotemporal dementia. Brain. 2011;134(9):2456–77.
109. Neary D, Snowden JS, Gustafson L, Passant U, Stuss D, Black S, Freedman M, Kertesz A, Robert PH, Albert M, Boone K, Miller BL, Cummings J, Benson DF. Frontotemporal lobar degeneration. Neurology. 1998;51(6):1546.
110. Geraudie A, Battista P, García AM, Allen IE, Miller ZA, Gorno-Tempini ML, Montembeault M. Speech and language impairments in behavioral variant frontotemporal dementia: a systematic review. Neurosci Biobehav Rev. 2021;131:1076–95.
111. Glosser G, Deser T. Patterns of discourse production among neurological patients with fluent language disorders. Brain Lang. 1991;40(1):67–88.
112. St-Pierre M-C, Ska B, Béland R. Lack of coherence in the narrative discourse of patients with dementia of the Alzheimer's type. J Multiling Commun Disord. 2009;3(3):211–5.
113. Obler LK. Chapter 12: language and brain dysfunction in dementia. In: Segalowitz SJ, editor. Language functions and brain organization. Boston: Academic Press; 1983. p. 267–82.
114. Beaugrande RD, Dressler WU. Introduction to text linguistics. London: Longman; 1981.
115. Almor A, Kempler D, MacDonald MC, Andersen ES, Tyler LK. Why do Alzheimer patients have difficulty with pronouns? Working memory, semantics, and reference in comprehension and production in Alzheimer's disease. Brain Lang. 1999;67(3):202–27.
116. Halliday MAK, Hasan R. Cohesion in English. London: Longman; 1976. xv, 374 p
117. Ramanathan V. Narrative well-formedness in Alzheimer's discourse: an interactional examination across settings. J Pragmat. 1995;23(4):395–419.
118. Perkins L, Whitworth A, Lesser R. Conversing in dementia: a conversation analytic approach. J Neurolinguistics. 1998;11(1–2):33–53.

119. Chapman SB, Zientz J, Weiner M, Rosenberg R, Frawley W, Burns MH. Discourse changes in early Alzheimer disease, mild cognitive impairment, and normal aging. Alzheimer Dis Assoc Disord. 2002;16(3):177–86.
120. Garrard P, Rentoumi V, Gesierich B, Miller B, Gorno-Tempini ML. Machine learning approaches to diagnosis and laterality effects in semantic dementia discourse. Cortex. 2014;55(1):122–9.
121. Seixas Lima B, Levine B, Graham NL, Leonard C, Tang-Wai D, Black S, Rochon E. Impaired coherence for semantic but not episodic autobiographical memory in semantic variant primary progressive aphasia. Cortex. 2020;123:72–85.
122. Breining BL, Tippett DC, Davis C, Posner J, Sebastian R, Oishie K, Hillis AE. Assessing dissociations of object and action naming in acute stroke. In: Clinical aphasiology conference. Clinical Aphasiology. Monterey, CA; 2015.
123. Roberts A, Savundranayagam M, Orange JB. Non-Alzheimer dementias. In: Cummings L, editor. Research in clinical pragmatics. Cham: Springer International Publishing; 2017. p. 347–77.
124. Walenski M, Mack JE, Mesulam MM, Thompson CK. Thematic integration impairments in primary progressive aphasia: evidence from eye-tracking. Front Hum Neurosci. 2020;14:587594.
125. Ribu ISB. Language and cognition in healthy aging and dementia. Olslo: University of Oslo; 2019.
126. Themistocleous C, Seeking an Anchorage. Stability and variability in tonal alignment of rising Prenuclear pitch accents in Cypriot Greek. Lang Speech. 2016;59(4):433–61.
127. Themistocleous C. Prosody and information structure in Greek (Prosodia Kai plirophoriaki domi stin Ellinici). Athens: National and Kapodistrian University of Cyprus; 2011.
128. Beckman M, Pierrehumbert J. Intonational structure in Japanese and English. Phonol Yearb. 1986;3:255–309.
129. Pierrehumbert J. Phonology and phonetics of English intonation. Boston: Massachusetts Institute of Technology; 1980.
130. Misiewicz S, Brickman AM, Tosto G. Prosodic impairment in dementia: review of the literature. Curr Alzheimer Res. 2018;15(2):157–63.
131. Abdalla M, Rudzicz F, Hirst G. Rhetorical structure and Alzheimer's disease. Aphasiology. 2018;32(1):41–60.
132. Taboada M, Mann WC. Rhetorical structure theory: looking back and moving ahead. Discourse Stud. 2006;8(3):423–59.
133. Kong AP-H, Linnik A, Law S-P, Shum WW-M. Measuring discourse coherence in anomic aphasia using rhetorical structure theory. Int J Speech-Lang Pathol. 2018;20(4):406–21.
134. Farias ST, Chand V, Bonnici L, Baynes K, Harvey D, Mungas D, Simon C, Reed B. Idea density measured in late life predicts subsequent cognitive trajectories: implications for the measurement of cognitive reserve. J Gerontol B Psychol Sci Soc Sci. 2012;67(6):677–86.
135. Hymes DH. Ethnography, linguistics, narrative inequality toward an understanding of voice critical perspectives on literacy and education. New York: Routledge; 1996.
136. Grice HP. Logic and conversation. In: Cole P, Morgan JL, editors. Syntax and semantics speech acts, vol. 3. Amsterdam: Academic Press; 1975. p. 41–58.
137. Kong AP, Whiteside J, Bargmann P. The Main concept analysis: validation and sensitivity in differentiating discourse produced by unimpaired English speakers from individuals with aphasia and dementia of Alzheimer type. Logoped Phoniatr Vocol. 2016;41(3):129–41.
138. Rosen HJ, Allison SC, Ogar JM, Amici S, Rose K, Dronkers N, Miller BL, Gorno-Tempini ML. Behavioral features in semantic dementia vs other forms of progressive aphasias. Neurology. 2006;67(10):1752–6.
139. Carr AR, Ashla MM, Jimenez EE, Mendez MF. Screening for emotional expression in frontotemporal dementia: a pilot study. Behav Neurol. 2018;2018:1–6.
140. Ducharme S, Pearl-Dowler L, Gossink F, McCarthy J, Lai J, Dickerson BC, Chertkow H, Rapin L, Vijverberg E, Krudop W, Dols A, Pijnenburg Y. The frontotemporal dementia versus primary psychiatric disorder (FTD versus PPD) checklist: a bedside clinical tool to identify behavioral variant FTD in patients with late-onset behavioral changes. J Alzheimers Dis. 2019;67(1):113–24.
141. Nevler N, Ash S, Jester C, Irwin DJ, Liberman M, Grossman M. Automatic measurement of prosody in behavioral variant FTD. Neurology. 2017;89(7):650–6.
142. Ash S, Moore P, Antani S, McCawley G, Work M, Grossman M. Trying to tell a tale. Discourse impairments in progressive aphasia and frontotemporal dementia. Neurology. 2006;66(9):1405–13.
143. Youmans G, Bourgeois M. Theory of mind in individuals with Alzheimer-type dementia. Aphasiology. 2010;24(4):515–34.
144. Bora E, Walterfang M, Velakoulis D. Theory of mind in behavioural-variant frontotemporal dementia and Alzheimer's disease: a meta-analysis. J Neurol Neurosurg Psychiatry. 2015;86(7):714–9.
145. Taylor-Rubin C, Croot K, Power E, Savage SA, Hodges JR, Togher L. Communication behaviors associated with successful conversation in semantic variant primary progressive aphasia. Int Psychogeriatr. 2017;29(10):1619–32.
146. Ripich DN, Vertes D, Whitehouse P, Fulton S, Ekelman B. Turn-taking and speech act patterns in the discourse of senile dementia of the Alzheimer's type patients. Brain Lang. 1991;40(3):330–43.
147. Voutilainen L, Henttonen P, Kahri M, Kivioja M, Ravaja N, Sams M, Peräkylä A. Affective stance, ambivalence, and psychophysiological responses

during conversational storytelling. J Pragmat. 2014;68:1–24.
148. Shimoda A, Li Y, Hayashi H, Kondo N. Dementia risks identified by vocal features via telephone conversations: a novel machine learning prediction model. PLoS One. 2021;16(7):e0253988.
149. de la Fuente GS, Ritchie CW, Luz S. Protocol for a conversation-based analysis study: PREVENT-ED investigates dialogue features that may help predict dementia onset in later life. BMJ Open. 2019;9(3):e026254.
150. Orange JB, Lubinski RB, Higginbotham J. Conversational repair by individuals with dementia of the Alzheimer's type. J Speech Hear Res. 1996;39(4):881–95.
151. Bohling HR. Communication with Alzheimer's patients: an analysis of caregiver listening patterns. Int J Aging Hum Dev. 1991;33(4):249–67.
152. Kindell J, Sage K, Keady J, Wilkinson R. Adapting to conversation with semantic dementia: using enactment as a compensatory strategy in everyday social interaction. Int J Lang Commun Disord. 2013;48(5):497–507.
153. Watson CM. An analysis of trouble and repair in the natural conversations of people with dementia of the Alzheimer's type. Aphasiology. 1999;13(3):195–218.
154. Myrberg K, Hydén L-C, Samuelsson C. Instances of trouble in aphasia and dementia: an analysis of trouble domain and interactional consequences. Aphasiology. 2022;36(11):1333–50.
155. Taylor C, Croot K, Power E, Savage SA, Hodges JR, Togher L. Trouble and repair during conversations of people with primary progressive aphasia. Aphasiology. 2014;28(8–9):1069–91.
156. Whitworth A, Lesser R, McKeith I. Profiling conversation in Parkinson's disease with cognitive impairment. Aphasiology. 1999;13(4–5):407–25.
157. Saldert C, Bauer M. Multifaceted communication problems in everyday conversations involving people with Parkinson's disease. Brain Sci. 2017;7(10)
158. Saldert C, Ferm U, Bloch S. Semantic trouble sources and their repair in conversations affected by Parkinson's disease. Int J Lang Commun Disord. 2014;49(6):710–21.
159. Thilakaratne R, Loftus AM, Cocks N. Assessing and treating conversations with partners in Parkinson's disease: a scoping review of the evidence. Int J Speech Lang Pathol. 2022;24(4):427–36.
160. Aliakbari M, Faraji E, Pourshakibaee P. Investigation of the proxemic behavior of Iranian professors and university students: effects of gender and status. J Pragmat. 2011;43(5):1392–402.
161. Stark BC, Bryant L, Themistocleous C, den Ouden D-B, Roberts AC. Best practice guidelines for reporting spoken discourse in aphasia and neurogenic communication disorders. Aphasiology. 2022;1-24:761.
162. Stark Brielle C, Dutta M, Murray Laura L, Bryant L, Fromm D, MacWhinney B, Ramage Amy E, Roberts A, den Ouden DB, Brock K, McKinney-Bock K, Paek Eun J, Harmon Tyson G, Yoon Si O, Themistocleous C, Yoo H, Aveni K, Gutierrez S, Sharma S. Standardizing assessment of spoken discourse in aphasia: a working group with deliverables. Am J Speech Lang Pathol. 2020:1–12.
163. Marangolo P, Fiori V, Calpagnano MA, Campana S, Razzano C, Caltagirone C, Marini A. tDCS over the left inferior frontal cortex improves speech production in aphasia. Front Hum Neurosci. 2013;7:539.
164. Marangolo P, Fiori V, Caltagirone C, Marini A. How conversational therapy influences language recovery in chronic non-fluent aphasia. Neuropsychol Rehabil. 2013;23(5):715–31.
165. Gartner-Schmidt J, Gherson S, Hapner ER, Muckala J, Roth D, Schneider S, Gillespie AI. The development of conversation training therapy: a concept paper. J Voice. 2016;30(5):563–73.

Charalambos Themistocleous, Ph.D., is an Associate Professor of speech, language, and communication at the Department of Special Needs Education at the University of Oslo. He served as a postdoctoral researcher in computational neurolinguistics at the Department of Neurology at Johns Hopkins University. He is a computational linguist with research interests in speech, language, and communication. He is also interested in the relationship between the brain and language and in providing opportunities to patients with aphasia by developing automated, personalized, high-quality speech and language assessments, diagnoses, and prognoses. He has developed Open Brain AI an automatic platform for analyzing discourse and communication and machine learning models for treatment, monitoring, and diagnosis of individuals with primary progressive aphasia, Alzheimer's disease, and mild cognitive impairment.

Using Discourse as a Measure of Early Cognitive Decline Associated with Alzheimer's Disease Biomarkers

4

Kimberly D. Mueller

Preview of What Is Currently Known
Both retrospective and prospective studies of individuals at risk for dementia have shown linear declines in discourse measures across stages of cognitive decline and dementia [1–3]. While many studies on discourse changes in people with mild cognitive impairment (MCI) and dementia have been based on clinical signs and symptoms, a smaller subset of evidence has linked discourse changes with the etiology of cognitive decline from participants with either autopsy- or in vivo biomarker-confirmed AD [1, 4, 5]. By studying discourse changes in individuals with biomarker-confirmed AD, particularly before the onset of clinical symptoms, we may be able to intervene earlier, measure disease progression, and monitor response to treatment in clinical trials.

Objectives
(a) To present the current knowledge about AD biomarker detection and progression.
(b) To discuss what is known about cognitive decline and AD biomarker progression.
(c) To describe the discourse measures that are likely to be sensitive to pathological amyloid, tau, and neurodegeneration.
(d) To propose potential future applications of discourse analysis across the AD biomarker continuum.

K. D. Mueller (✉)
Department of Communication Sciences and Disorders, University of Wisconsin, Madison, WI, USA

Division of Geriatrics in School of Medicine and Public Health, University of Wisconsin, Madison, WI, USA
e-mail: kdmueller@wisc.edu

Discourse Analysis Within the Alzheimer's Disease Research Framework

Alzheimer's disease (AD) is defined neuropathologically by the presence of amyloid-beta (Aβ) plaques and tau neurofibrillary tangles. The staging of AD according to neuropathology was established by Braak and Braak in 1991 [6] and is determined at autopsy. Clinical criteria for "probable" and "possible" AD were first introduced in 1984 and include a gradual onset of memory and other cognitive decline, leading to a loss of independent function and dementia [7]. Criteria for mild cognitive impairment (MCI), often a precursor to AD dementia, include a decline in cognition with concern, but without loss of independence in activities of daily living [8]. Definitions and key terms for defining AD and MCI are presented in Table 4.1.

Most studies examining discourse in AD thus far have been based on clinical definitions of AD, i.e., "probable AD dementia" or "MCI due to probable AD," where participants are diagnosed

A. P.-H. Kong (ed.), *Spoken Discourse Impairments in the Neurogenic Populations*,
https://doi.org/10.1007/978-3-031-45190-4_4

Table 4.1 Key terms and neuropathological versus clinical definitions of Alzheimer's disease

Term or concept	Definition
Alzheimer's disease (AD)—neuropathological definition	The presence of extracellular accumulations of amyloid-beta (Aβ) peptides in the form of plaques, and intracellular tangles, consisting of hyperphosphorylated tau proteins [6]
"Probable" or "possible" Alzheimer's disease—clinical definition	Cognitive impairment in at least two domains (memory, executive function, language, visuospatial skills, problem-solving, personality/behavior) severe enough to interfere with independent activities of daily living; must have an insidious onset and must not be due to any other causes [7, 8]
Mild cognitive impairment (MCI)	A syndrome defined by clinical, cognitive, and functional criteria, including (1) concern regarding a change in cognition; (2) impairment in one or more cognitive domains; and (3) preservation of independence in functional activities [8]
Amyloid-beta (Aβ)	Misfolded peptide proteins that clump together to form plaques, which collect between neurons and may disrupt brain cell function [6]
Neurofibrillary tau tangles	Insoluble, twisted fibers containing tau protein that collect inside neurons [6]
Neurodegeneration	Neuronal injury leading to cell death; may be due to a variety of etiologies including AD processes and/or cerebrovascular injury [15]

based on the signs and symptoms and progression of cognitive impairment [9–14]. These studies have led to a detailed understanding of the stages of speech, language, and communication declines across the symptomatic dementia continuum and have undoubtedly contributed to the development of successful cognitive-communication interventions. For example, discourse studies have informed communication caregiver training interventions that empower caregivers with education about communication changes along the disease continuum and provide strategies for success. Although it is possible that the participants in these studies may have had a dementia etiology different from or in addition to AD, such as vascular or Lewy body disease, the understanding of how MCI and dementia impact discourse and communication have led to major advances in dementia diagnosis and care.

Other studies have examined discourse changes retrospectively in individuals with autopsy-confirmed AD. In these instances, the discourse changes can be viewed as specific to the neuropathology of AD using the "gold standard" diagnostic criteria. For example, Ahmed et al. [1] collected longitudinal discourse samples in life from 15 participants with autopsy-confirmed AD and showed linear declines in semantic, lexical, and syntactic content across the progression from MCI to moderate AD dementia. Similarly, Garrard et al. [2] retrospectively analyzed the writing of renowned British novelist, Iris Murdoch, who also had autopsy-confirmed AD, and showed a similar deterioration of lexical and syntactic content years prior to diagnosis. The latter example may be considered as one of the first studies to show changes in discourse—in this case, written prose—in the asymptomatic phase of AD, or "preclinical AD."

The potential benefits of evaluating discourse changes in the preclinical phase of AD are numerous. First, because discourse depends upon a complex interplay of multiple cognitive processes, including semantic and episodic memory, working memory, and executive function, discourse may in fact be a more sensitive measure of cognitive decline due to AD than other neuropsychological tests that work to isolate various cognitive functions. The ability to identify individuals who are most at risk for developing cognitive decline and dementia, early on the AD continuum, may help to identify individuals who will reap the most benefit from clinical trials. Second, despite the dozens of metrics and functions that discourse analysis can yield for research, the task presents relatively low time and cognitive burden on the research participant. The tasks lend themselves to mobile technology and can be done in an unsupervised, home-based setting; as a result, discourse sampling can lead to increased diversity of research participants due to the removal of logistic and other barriers. Third, because discourse is an ecologically valid tool for measuring speech, language, and communication, it may serve as an ideal functional outcome measure of response to treatment in clinical trials.

An Alzheimer's Disease Research Framework: Rationale

In 2018, the National Institute on Aging and the Alzheimer's Association (NIA-AA) developed a research framework for defining and studying AD [15]. Importantly, because of the changing landscape of biomarker development, i.e., the development of new assays and the need to further refine and validate existing ones, this framework was not designed to be implemented in clinical practice; rather, it was meant to be utilized solely for research, particularly longitudinal cohort studies and randomized placebo-controlled trials. Rationale for this approach is rooted in the fact that the historical approach to diagnosing "probable AD" based on clinical signs and symptoms is not always specific to AD. Between 10% and 30% of individuals diagnosed with probable AD based on this approach do not display AD neuropathology at autopsy [16]. Furthermore, since it is well established that AD pathology often begins at least 10 years prior to the onset of clinical symptoms [17–19], the ability to define preclinical AD with biomarkers, before an individual has experienced significant neurodegeneration and resulting cognitive impairment, provides a crucial window for studying the temporal relationships between disease progression, cognitive change, and pharmacological interventions.

What Are AD Biomarkers?

Various imaging, cerebrospinal fluid (CSF), and blood plasma AD biomarkers are widely used in research studies, and new discoveries are rapidly emerging. The NIA-AA framework organizes these biomarkers with the descriptive classification scheme labeled AT(N): Aβ plaques (A), fibrillar tau (T), and neurodegeneration, which is notated as (N) due to the lack of specificity of neurodegeneration biomarkers to AD [15]. Below is a list of currently validated AD biomarkers; also see Table 4.2.

Amyloid-beta biomarkers. Multiple validation studies comparing amyloid positron-emission tomography (PET) to autopsy results show that amyloid PET is a valid in vivo proxy for Aβ deposits in the parenchymal and vessel walls of the brain [20–22]. PET imaging of amyloid deposits utilizes radioligands that cross the blood-brain barrier and bind to amyloid in the brain; two commonly used ligands include ^{11}C-Pittsburgh compound B (PiB) [23] and ^{18}F-florbetapir [24]. Another type of amyloid biomarker includes assays that measure $A\beta_{42}$ in CSF acquired by lumbar puncture, which have shown good concordance with amyloid PET [25]. At the time the NIA-AA research framework was released in 2018, PET and CSF biomarkers were the only biomarkers for "A" listed; however, at the time of this writing, there have been major advances in assays for measuring amyloid in blood plasma [26]. Plasma collection offers a more available and tolerable means of measurement for patients and clinicians than PET imaging or lumbar puncture. Although assays continue to be validated, the present research suggests that plasma measures of phosphorylated tau at Thr181 (p-tau$_{181}$), Thr217 (p-tau$_{217}$), and Thr231 (p-tau$_{231}$) have high diagnostic accuracy in differentiating AD from other forms of dementia, are concordant with amyloid PET [26], and have been validated against autopsy-confirmed AD [27].

Fibrillar tau biomarkers. One widely used biomarker of tau pathology includes elevated levels of p-tau in the CSF [28]. P-tau$_{231}$ has been shown to correlate with postmortem neurofibrillary tangles and neuritic plaques [29], and CSF p-tau$_{181}$ has been correlated with both amyloid PET and incipient cognitive decline [30]. Tau PET is a newer tau marker: radioligand tracers have been developed to bind to pathologic tau in the brain, including ^{18}F-flortaucipir, ^{18}F-THK5351, and ^{18}F-MK6240 [31–33]. Plasma assays of tau (p-tau181, p-tau217, and p-tau231)

Table 4.2 Examples of currently validated and/or potential Alzheimer's disease biomarkers by modality

Alzheimer's disease component	Modality	Biomarker measure
Amyloid-beta (Aβ)	Positron-emission tomography (PET)	Continuous or dichotomous value denoting the degree of binding to a distribution volume ratio average across AD-specific regions of interest; tracers include *^{11}[C] Pittsburgh compound B; 18F-florbetaben*
	Cerebrospinal fluid (CSF)	$A\beta_{42}$ or $A\beta_{42/40}$ ratio (lower values indicate increased levels of Aβ in the brain)
	Blood plasma	$A\beta_{1-42}$ and $A\beta_{1-40}$ using mass spectrometry or immunoassays
Tau	PET	Continuous or dichotomous value denoting the degree of binding to a distribution volume ratio average across AD-specific regions of interest; tracers include *^{18}[F] R0948; ^{18}F-flortaucipir; MK6240*
	CSF	Phosphorylated tau: p-tau$_{181}$; p-tau$_{217}$; total tau (t-tau)
	Blood plasma	p-tau$_{181}$; p-tau$_{217}$; p-tau$_{231}$; may be more strongly correlated with early Aβ-PET pathology
Neurodegeneration	Magnetic resonance imaging (MRI)	T1- and T2-weighted imaging; gray matter volume, cortical thickness
	PET	^{18}[F] fluorodeoxyglucose (FDG) regional glucose metabolism
	CSF	Neurofilament light (NfL); neurogranin
	Blood plasma	NfL
Genetics[a]		*Apolipoprotein ε-4 (APOE-ε-4)*

Note. Adapted from Hansson, O. (2021). Biomarkers for neurodegenerative diseases. *Nature medicine, 27*(6), 954–963

[a]Genetic biomarkers only for Late Onset Alzheimer's Disease (LOAD); *PSEN-1, PSEN-2 and APP mutations are deterministic for Dominantly Inherited Alzheimer's Disease*

are a proxy of cortical tau and do not represent the same components of tau accumulation processes as those measured with tau-PET; furthermore, plasma tau markers appear to represent early pathological presentation and have been recommended as a screening tool for identifying Aβ-positive individuals [26, 34].

Neurodegeneration or neuronal injury biomarkers. Extensively used measures of neurodegeneration include measuring volumetric changes on magnetic resonance imaging (MRI), particularly in the medial temporal lobes and posterior cingulate and temporoparietal cortices [35, 36]. Fluorodeoxyglucose-PET (FDG-PET) measures metabolic dysfunction via glucose uptake and has been a valid predictor of neurodegeneration in AD [37, 38]. In the CSF, total tau (t-tau) has been correlated with neuronal injury across multiple degenerative conditions, including AD [39]. In plasma, longitudinal p-tau$_{181}$ and neurofilament light (NFL) have been associated with progressive neurodegeneration in AD [40].

Genetic AD biomarkers. Genetic factors play an important role in late-onset AD as evidenced by twin data indicating heritability in the range of 58–79% [41]. The epsilon 4 allele of the *APOE* gene (*APOE-ε4*) confers up to a 50% increased risk of developing AD dementia and is associated with higher rates of Aβ and tau positivity in cognitively unimpaired adults [42]. Considerably rarer (<1% of all cases) is the early-onset, autosomal dominant form of AD resulting from fully penetrant mutations in the Aβ precursor protein (*APP*) and presenilin genes (*PSEN1, PSEN2)* [43, 44].

The NIA-AA Framework for Biomarker Profiles and Cognitive Staging

The 2018 NIA-AA research framework defines AD as the presence of abnormal levels of *both* Aβ and pathologic tau defined by in vivo biomarkers (A+, T+). Individuals who are biomarker amyloid positive and tau negative are classified as showing "Alzheimer's pathologic change," and those who are amyloid negative but tau positive are defined as having "non-Alzheimer's pathologic change" [15]. Neurodegenerative/neuronal injury biomarkers and cognitive symptoms are not exclusive to Alzheimer's disease and are utilized solely to gauge the degree of severity rather than to confirm the existence of the Alzheimer's continuum.

Cognitive syndrome categories in this model for the purpose of research are defined as cognitively unimpaired (CU), MCI, or dementia, the definitions of which are similar to the NIA-AA 2011 guidelines [8] but are independent of biomarker status. The framework also provides cognitive staging to those whose biomarker profiles place them on the Alzheimer's continuum. Of note, while Stage 1 describes individuals who are cognitively unimpaired with no measurable decline, Stage 2 is described as "transitional cognitive decline," whereby the individual's performance is normal based on test norms, but there are subtle declines in cognition evidenced by longitudinal testing or self- or care partner reports. This stage has also been referred to as "cognitively unimpaired-declining" in longitudinal cohort studies [45] and embodies the concept of "preclinical" cognitive decline associated with biomarker-defined AD.

Known Associations Between Biomarker Positivity and Cognitive Decline

Verbal learning and memory and language. Accruing evidence shows associations with various biomarkers and cognitive decline, even in individuals who are cognitively unimpaired according to test norms and self-report. For example, in multiple longitudinal cohort studies, higher [^{11}C]PiB retention has been linked to lower scores or steeper declines in verbal learning and memory [46–49] and in tests of semantic verbal fluency [50]. Such rates of decline were shown to accelerate in individuals with elevations in both amyloid and tau PET imaging [42, 51]. Furthermore, a sample of 282 individuals with both CSF and PET amyloid and tau found that tau PET alone was the strongest predictor of decline on a memory composite than any of the other biomarker modalities [52].

Executive function. A study including 316 CU individuals with multimodal AD biomarkers suggested that elevated Aβ, regardless of modality (CSF or PET), was independently associated with worse performance on an executive measure (trail making test) but not with memory performance, while tau pathology was independently associated with worse memory. These findings were confirmed in a separate cohort of 361 CU individuals [53].

Visuospatial skills. Evidence for associations between amyloid and tau biomarkers in CU individuals and performance on tests of visuospatial function is limited, but more recently developed measures, such as the digital clock drawing test, have shown promising results linking spatial reasoning with early amyloid PET accumulation [54].

Discourse Analysis and AD Biomarkers

Early pathologic tau accumulation in AD tends to occur in the hippocampal complex but not in the hippocampus itself. Evidence for lexical-semantic deficits early in the AD continuum, as well as in the semantic variant of primary progressive aphasia, shows direct correlations between severity of neuronal injury in perirhinal cortices and severity of lexical-semantic retrieval [55]. Thus, it stands to reason that discourse analysis may be an excellent candidate for measuring cognitive and communication declines in preclinical, biomarker-defined AD.

Discourse studies linking linguistic measures with in vivo AD biomarkers are beginning to emerge at the time of this writing. Following is a list of discourse features that have been associated with AD biomarkers in people who are CU or diagnosed with MCI. Figure 4.1 depicts these early discourse findings on a hypothetical AD biomarker continuum.

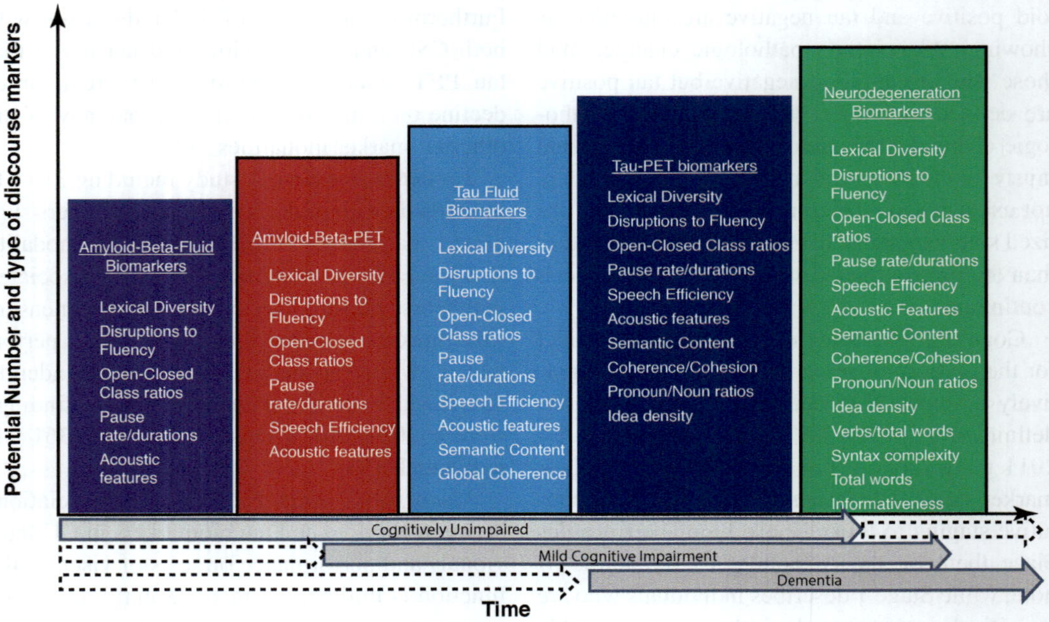

Fig. 4.1 Potential discourse markers across a hypothetical Alzheimer's disease biomarker and cognitive continuum
Note. The filled gray arrows indicate a hypothetical cognitive status across the biomarker continuum; the arrows with dashed lines indicate that each cognitive status could potentially exist anywhere along the hypothetical biomarker continuum. Potential discourse measures are hypothesized from the extant literature on discourse in Alzheimer's disease and dementia
Figure adapted from Jack Jr., C. R., Knopman, D. S., Jagust, W. J., Petersen, R. C., Weiner, M. W., Aisen, P. S., ... & Trojanowski, J. Q. (2013). Update on hypothetical model of Alzheimer's disease biomarkers. *Lancet Neurology*, *12*(2), 207

Lexical-semantic measures from discourse. Hajjar et al. (2022) collected discourse samples, neuropsychological testing, and CSF markers of $A\beta_{42}$, total tau, and p-tau_{181} from 92 CU individuals and 114 individuals with MCI (mean age = 64 years). Using machine learning approaches, results showed that lexical-semantic features distinguished MCI participants from CU (area under the curve = 0.80) and those with higher CSF-$A\beta_{42}$; these same features were significant predictors of change in functional cognition at a 2-year follow-up visit [56].

Similarly, both Verfaillie et al. (2019) and Mueller et al. (2021) showed that in CU individuals with either CSF-$A\beta_{42}$ or amyloid PET, lexical-semantic indices from picture description were significantly associated with amyloid positivity [4, 5]. Another study showed associations with fewer prepositions, nouns, and word frequency indices and levels of CSF-p-tau [57].

Macrolinguistic measures. "Global coherence," or the ability to organize discourse around a central theme or topic [58], is an example of a macrolinguistic skill that has been linked to individuals with evidence of AD biomarkers. Mazzon et al. (2019) studied narrative discourse production in individuals with MCI, 15 of whom had CSF biomarker-confirmed AD. The authors found that global coherence and lexical informativeness identified individuals with AD CSF biomarker positivity versus those without [59]. Similarly, Pistono et al. (2019) showed that individuals with MCI and CSF biomarker-confirmed AD produced less informative utterances with less global coherence than controls without AD.

Fluency measures from discourse. Fluency measures including pause rate, pause duration, filled pauses, and words per minute likely reflect lexical-semantic retrieval, executive function, or both. Therefore, the theoretical neural bases for declines in semantic processing in preclinical AD may be reflected in disruptions to fluency in discourse, but frontotemporal regions involved in planning and working memory may also be indicated. For example, a study showed that elevated levels of CSF-p-tau were correlated with lower speech segment durations and higher pause rates in CU individuals [57]; early pathologic tau tends to accumulate in entorhinal cortices and association cortices [60], which may explain these disruptions. Another study showed that the location of pauses—specifically, between-utterance pauses—was higher for individuals with MCI and positive AD biomarkers than control participants [61]. This study also showed that pause use was negatively correlated with the frontopolar gray matter density, suggesting a compromised executive function component to discourse planning.

Syntax, pragmatics and other measures from discourse. At the time of this writing, there is limited exploration of relationships between in vivo AD biomarkers in cognitively unimpaired individuals and other measures of discourse, such as syntax complexity, pragmatic language measures, and discourse comprehension. It is possible that these functions remain stable during the preclinical AD phase; however, as discourse sampling becomes more widely implemented in longitudinal cohort studies, these facets may in fact show subtle declines and are worth exploring.

Caveats, Summary, and Future Directions for Discourse Analysis in Preclinical Alzheimer's Disease

The sections above describe the most studied AD biomarkers in 2023 and place them in a 2018 framework proposed by the National Institute on Aging-Alzheimer's Association working group [15]. Even within the past two years, validation studies of blood plasma assays of amyloid, tau, and neurodegeneration have multiplied in number [62]. Thus, the field of identifying and understanding Alzheimer's disease is changing at a rapid pace, and researchers who are interested in exploring discourse changes within an AD biomarker framework are encouraged to stay abreast of the new developments that are sure to come.

A biomarker framework for research in Alzheimer's disease is not without criticism; although intended only for research and not for clinical practice, some fear that the adoption of this nomenclature and way of thinking about AD may seep into clinical practice before enough validation has occurred. One of the inherent dangers of labeling someone who is amyloid and tau positive but cognitively unimpaired with "Alzheimer's disease" is that there are numerous autopsy studies showing individuals with AD pathology who never went on to experience symptoms. Thus, an individual labeled as "cognitively unimpaired, with AD," while there is no cure or known prevention for AD, could be psychologically or emotionally damaging to the individual, with harmful downstream physical effects [63].

Another potential problem with viewing biomarker-defined AD as a gold standard for research is that of access to collection and analysis of these biomarkers. Groups with important research questions for individuals with clinical evidence of disease, but who do not have the resources or access to lumbar puncture, MRI, PET, or advanced blood plasma assays, should not be discouraged from studying individuals with subtle or overt cognitive decline or genetic risk based on family history, particularly with respect to discourse analysis. The complexity of discourse coupled with the increased number of open-access tools for analysis can yield new discoveries globally. Furthermore, there is an urgent need for understanding declines in discourse in MCI and dementia in diverse populations; discourse is a culture-fair means of measuring within-person change, regardless of etiology.

Focusing on biomarker-defined Alzheimer's disease, if utilized in a clinical setting without further validation, could also harmfully shift clinicians' focus from the individual's signs, symptoms, subjective concerns, and objective test results to a biomarker profile that may or may not be validated or accurate. This can lead to a lack of personalized care and could potentially lead to missed opportunities for early intervention for cognitive decline.

While keeping these caveats in mind, researchers who have the opportunity to study aspects of discourse alongside AD biomarkers, particularly in the preclinical phase, may be able to make great contributions to the field. First, as noted above, since discourse samples can be collected frequently and remotely with little burden placed on participants and staff, validated discourse metrics with early AD pathology can improve reach to participants who are most likely to benefit from pharmacological and nonpharmacological clinical trials. Importantly, several new protocols have been proposed to add discourse procedures to longitudinal cohort studies involving CU individuals and biomarker collection [64, 65]. Specifically, the Alzheimer's Disease Neuroimaging Initiative-4 (ADNI-4) will implement a "digital biomarker" component to remote testing, in which the Novoic Ltd. "Storyteller task" will be self-administered by ADNI participants at home. The task, similar to other story recall tasks, is embedded in a mobile application and utilizes automatic speech recognition and machine learning approaches for analyzing transcripts [64, 66]. Some of the speech-language data collected from ADNI-4, along with all other data such as AD biomarkers and neuropsychological testing data, will be available to researchers worldwide to utilize for analyses (https://adni.loni.usc.edu/data-samples/access-data/). Similarly, the Speech on the Phone Assessment (SPeAk) study is a prospective observational study recruiting patients who are aged 50 and older from a cohort of individuals who previously provided MRI, PET, and CSF biomarkers. Participants will complete cognitive and speech tasks over the phone which will be digitally recorded; speech tasks include responding to conversational prompts, such as "What animal makes the best pet?" and engaging in a game of "20 Questions." Cognitive testing will also be recorded and used for acoustic and linguistic analyses; the study plans to utilize automatic speech recognition and other automated procedures for acoustic analyses [65].

Another potential benefit of studying discourse alongside AD biomarkers is the potential development of outcome measures: the FDA emphasizes the need for performance-based, functional outcome measures for drug trials, versus global cognition measures such as the MMSE [67], in order to really know if a drug is improving daily life [68]. Developing discourse analysis to serve as a functional outcome measure for clinical trials that may be targeting amyloid and tau accumulation could substantially move the fields of AD and discourse analysis forward. Finally, discourse analysis early in the AD continuum has the potential to uncover aspects of communication change that could serve as early targets for speech-language pathology assessments and interventions.

Major Takeaways

1. This chapter provided a brief introduction to Alzheimer's disease biomarkers and a research framework for studying discourse in the context of biologically defined AD.
2. Evidence for what is known about the validity of each type of biomarker was presented.
3. Emerging studies showing subtle changes to discourse in cognitively unimpaired participants with evidence of AD neuropathology were discussed. Only a handful of studies have shown early declines in discourse in cognitively unimpaired participants, but the findings thus far are promising.
4. The cautions and caveats for using biological versus clinical AD frameworks were described. Advantages of the biological framework include being able to link the specific etiology of cognitive decline, MCI, and dementia to discourse changes, as well as the ability to identify at-risk individuals who may not be showing frank cognitive decline. Advantages of the clinical framework include taking advantage of widely accessible technologies to develop new ways of analyzing discourse in people with MCI and dementia, to further elucidate targets for assessment and intervention, as well as ensuring a more person-centered approach in clinical settings. Future studies using discourse analysis along the AD continuum are needed under both frameworks.

Acknowledgements Special appreciation to research participants in Alzheimer's disease studies, as their dedication to ending Alzheimer's disease is unmatched. Gratitude to Dr. Mark Sager and Dr. Bruce Hermann, for their early vision to study individuals at risk for AD. Thanks to Olivia Goulette for her assistance with the contents of this chapter.

References

1. Ahmed S, Haigh AM, de Jager CA, Garrard P. Connected speech as a marker of disease progression in autopsy-proven Alzheimer's disease. Brain. 2013;136(Pt 12):3727–37.
2. Garrard P, Maloney LM, Hodges JR, Patterson K. The effects of very early Alzheimer's disease on the characteristics of writing by a renowned author. Brain. 2005;128(2):250–60.
3. Mueller KD, Koscik RL, Hermann BP, Johnson SC, Turkstra LS. Declines in connected language are associated with very early mild cognitive impairment: results from the Wisconsin Registry for Alzheimer's Prevention. Front Aging Neurosci. 2018;9:437.
4. Verfaillie SC, Witteman J, Slot RE, Pruis IJ, Vermaat LE, Prins ND, et al. High amyloid burden is associated with fewer specific words during spontaneous speech in individuals with subjective cognitive decline. Neuropsychologia. 2019;131:184–92.
5. Mueller KD, Van Hulle CA, Koscik RL, Jonaitis E, Peters CC, Betthauser TJ, et al. Amyloid beta associations with connected speech in cognitively unimpaired adults. Alzheimers Dement (Amst). 2021;13(1):e12203.
6. Braak H, Braak E. Neuropathological staging of Alzheimer-related changes. Acta Neuropathol. 1991;82(4):239–59.
7. McKhann G, Drachman D, Folstein M, Katzman R, Price D, Stadlan EM. Clinical diagnosis of Alzheimer's disease: report of the NINCDS-ADRDA Work Group* under the auspices of Department of Health and Human Services Task Force on Alzheimer's Disease. Neurology. 1984;34(7):939–44.
8. Albert MS, DeKosky ST, Dickson D, Dubois B, Feldman HH, Fox NC, et al. The diagnosis of mild cognitive impairment due to Alzheimer's disease: recommendations from the National Institute on Aging-Alzheimer's Association workgroups on diagnostic guidelines for Alzheimer's disease. Alzheimers Dement. 2011;7(3):270–9.
9. Duong A, Tardif A, Ska B. Discourse about discourse: what is it and how does it progress in Alzheimer's disease? Brain Cogn. 2003;53(2):177–80.
10. Tomoeda CK, Bayles KA. Longitudinal effects of Alzheimer disease on discourse production. Alzheimer Dis Assoc Disord. 1993;7(4):223–36.
11. Chapman SB, Zientz J, Weiner M, Rosenberg R, Frawley W, Burns MH. Discourse changes in early Alzheimer disease, mild cognitive impairment, and normal aging. Alzheimer Dis Assoc Disord. 2002;16(3):177–86.
12. Forbes-McKay K, Shanks MF, Venneri A. Profiling spontaneous speech decline in Alzheimer's disease: a longitudinal study. Acta Neuropsychiatr. 2013;25(6):320–7.
13. Fraser KC, Meltzer JA, Rudzicz F. Linguistic features identify Alzheimer's disease in narrative speech. J Alzheimers Dis. 2016;49(2):407–22.
14. Ripich DN. Functional communication with AD patients: a caregiver training program. Alzheimer Dis Assoc Disord. 1994;8:95–109.
15. Jack CR Jr, Bennett DA, Blennow K, Carrillo MC, Dunn B, Haeberlein SB, et al. NIA-AA research framework: toward a biological definition of Alzheimer's disease. Alzheimers Dement. 2018;14(4):535–62.
16. Nelson PT, Head E, Schmitt FA, Davis PR, Neltner JH, Jicha GA, et al. Alzheimer's disease is not "brain aging": neuropathological, genetic, and epidemiological human studies. Acta Neuropathol. 2011;121:571–87.
17. Sperling RA, Jack CR Jr, Aisen PS. Testing the right target and right drug at the right stage. Sci Transl Med. 2011;3(111):111cm33.
18. Sperling R, Mormino E, Johnson K. The evolution of preclinical Alzheimer's disease: implications for prevention trials. Neuron. 2014;84(3):608–22.
19. Jack CR Jr, Lowe VJ, Weigand SD, Wiste HJ, Senjem ML, Knopman DS, et al. Serial PIB and MRI in normal, mild cognitive impairment and Alzheimer's disease: implications for sequence of pathological events in Alzheimer's disease. Brain. 2009;132(Pt 5):1355–65.
20. Ikonomovic MD, Klunk WE, Abrahamson EE, Mathis CA, Price JC, Tsopelas ND, et al. Post-mortem correlates of in vivo PiB-PET amyloid imaging in a typical case of Alzheimer's disease. Brain. 2008;131(6):1630–45.
21. Fleisher AS, Chen K, Liu X, Roontiva A, Thiyyagura P, Ayutyanont N, et al. Using positron emission tomography and florbetapir F 18 to image cortical amyloid in patients with mild cognitive impairment or dementia due to Alzheimer disease. Arch Neurol. 2011;68(11):1404–11.
22. Seo SW, Ayakta N, Grinberg LT, Villeneuve S, Lehmann M, Reed B, et al. Regional correlations between [11C] PIB PET and post-mortem burden of amyloid-beta pathology in a diverse neuropathological cohort. NeuroImage: Clin. 2017;13:130–7.
23. Klunk WE, Lopresti BJ, Ikonomovic MD, Lefterov IM, Koldamova RP, Abrahamson EE, et al. Binding of the positron emission tomography tracer Pittsburgh compound-B reflects the amount of amyloid-β in Alzheimer's disease brain but not in transgenic mouse brain. J Neurosci. 2005;25(46):10598–606.
24. Clark CM, Schneider JA, Bedell BJ, Beach TG, Bilker WB, Mintun MA, et al. Use of florbetapir-PET for imaging β-amyloid pathology. JAMA. 2011;305(3):275–83.

25. Blennow K, Mattsson N, Schöll M, Hansson O, Zetterberg H. Amyloid biomarkers in Alzheimer's disease. Trends Pharmacol Sci. 2015;36(5):297–309.
26. Milà-Alomà M, Ashton NJ, Shekari M, Salvadó G, Ortiz-Romero P, Montoliu-Gaya L, et al. Plasma p-tau231 and p-tau217 as state markers of amyloid-β pathology in preclinical Alzheimer's disease. Nat Med. 2022;28(9):1797–801.
27. Palmqvist S, Janelidze S, Quiroz YT, Zetterberg H, Lopera F, Stomrud E, et al. Discriminative accuracy of plasma phospho-tau217 for Alzheimer disease vs other neurodegenerative disorders. JAMA. 2020;324(8):772–81.
28. Mattsson N, Zetterberg H, Hansson O, Andreasen N, Parnetti L, Jonsson M, et al. CSF biomarkers and incipient Alzheimer disease in patients with mild cognitive impairment. JAMA. 2009;302(4):385–93.
29. Buerger K, Ewers M, Pirttilä T, Zinkowski R, Alafuzoff I, Teipel SJ, et al. CSF phosphorylated tau protein correlates with neocortical neurofibrillary pathology in Alzheimer's disease. Brain. 2006;129(11):3035–41.
30. Brier MR, Gordon B, Friedrichsen K, McCarthy J, Stern A, Christensen J, et al. Tau and Aβ imaging, CSF measures, and cognition in Alzheimer's disease. Sci Transl Med. 2016;8(338):338ra66.
31. Gobbi LC, Knust H, Körner M, Honer M, Czech C, Belli S, et al. Identification of three novel radiotracers for imaging aggregated tau in Alzheimer's disease with positron emission tomography. J Med Chem. 2017;60(17):7350–70.
32. Johnson KA, Schultz A, Betensky RA, Becker JA, Sepulcre J, Rentz D, et al. Tau positron emission tomographic imaging in aging and early Alzheimer disease. Ann Neurol. 2016;79(1):110–9.
33. Wang L, Benzinger TL, Su Y, Christensen J, Friedrichsen K, Aldea P, et al. Evaluation of tau imaging in staging Alzheimer disease and revealing interactions between β-amyloid and tauopathy. JAMA Neurol. 2016;73(9):1070–7.
34. Petersen RC. Are plasma markers for Alzheimer's disease ready for clinical use? Nature Aging. 2022;2(2):94–6.
35. Seab J, Jagust W, Wong S, Roos M, Reed B, Budinger T. Quantitative NMR measurements of hippocampal atrophy in Alzheimer's disease. Magn Reson Med. 1988;8(2):200–8.
36. Fox NC, Crum WR, Scahill RI, Stevens JM, Janssen JC, Rossor MN. Imaging of onset and progression of Alzheimer's disease with voxel-compression mapping of serial magnetic resonance images. Lancet. 2001;358(9277):201–5.
37. Minoshima S, Giordani B, Berent S, Frey KA, Foster NL, Kuhl DE. Metabolic reduction in the posterior cingulate cortex in very early Alzheimer's disease. Ann Neurol. 1997;42(1):85–94.
38. Knopman DS, Jack CR, Wiste HJ, Weigand SD, Vemuri P, Lowe VJ, et al. Selective worsening of brain injury biomarker abnormalities in cognitively normal elderly persons with β-amyloidosis. JAMA Neurol. 2013;70(8):1030–8.
39. Blennow K, Hampel H, Weiner M, Zetterberg H. Cerebrospinal fluid and plasma biomarkers in Alzheimer disease. Nat Rev Neurol. 2010;6(3):131–44.
40. Moscoso A, Grothe MJ, Ashton NJ, Karikari TK, Rodríguez JL, Snellman A, et al. Longitudinal associations of blood phosphorylated Tau181 and neurofilament light chain with neurodegeneration in Alzheimer disease. JAMA Neurol. 2021;78(4):396–406.
41. Saykin AJ, Shen L, Foroud TM, Potkin SG, Swaminathan S, Kim S, et al. Alzheimer's Disease neuroimaging initiative biomarkers as quantitative phenotypes: Genetics core aims, progress, and plans. Alzheimers Dement. 2010;6(3):265–73.
42. Betthauser TJ, Koscik RL, Jonaitis EM, Allison SL, Cody KA, Erickson CM, et al. Amyloid and tau imaging biomarkers explain cognitive decline from late middle-age. Brain. 2020;143(1):320–35.
43. Levy-Lahad E, Wasco W, Poorkaj P, Romano DM, Oshima J, Pettingell WH, et al. Candidate gene for the chromosome 1 familial Alzheimer's disease locus. Science. 1995;269(5226):973–7.
44. Goate A, Chartier-Harlin MC, Mullan M, Brown J, Crawford F, Fidani L, et al. Segregation of a missense mutation in the amyloid precursor protein gene with familial Alzheimer's disease. Nature. 1991;349(6311):704–6.
45. Langhough Koscik R, Hermann BP, Allison S, Clark LR, Jonaitis EM, Mueller KD, et al. Validity evidence for the research category, "cognitively unimpaired–declining," as a risk marker for mild cognitive impairment and Alzheimer's disease. Front Aging Neurosci. 2021;13:688478. https://doi.org/10.3389/fnagi.2021.688478.
46. Resnick S, Sojkova J, Zhou Y, An Y, Ye W, Holt D, et al. Longitudinal cognitive decline is associated with fibrillar amyloid-beta measured by [11C] PiB. Neurology. 2010;74(10):807–15.
47. Donohue MC, Sperling RA, Petersen R, Sun C-K, Weiner MW, Aisen PS, et al. Association between elevated brain amyloid and subsequent cognitive decline among cognitively normal persons. JAMA. 2017;317(22):2305–16.
48. Sperling RA, Donohue MC, Raman R, Sun C-K, Yaari R, Holdridge K, et al. Association of factors with elevated amyloid burden in clinically normal older individuals. JAMA Neurol. 2020;77(6):735–45.
49. Mueller KD, Koscik RL, Du L, Bruno D, Jonaitis EM, Koscik AZ, et al. Proper names from story recall are associated with beta-amyloid in cognitively unimpaired adults at risk for Alzheimer's disease. Cortex. 2020;131:137–50.
50. Papp KV, Mormino EC, Amariglio RE, Munro C, Dagley A, Schultz AP, et al. Biomarker validation of a decline in semantic processing in preclinical Alzheimer's disease. Neuropsychology. 2016;30(5):624–30.
51. Ossenkoppele R, Pichet Binette A, Groot C, Smith R, Strandberg O, Palmqvist S, et al. Amyloid and tau PET-positive cognitively unimpaired individuals are

at high risk for future cognitive decline. Nat Med. 2022;28(11):2381–7.
52. Bucci M, Chiotis K, Nordberg A, AsDN I. Alzheimer's disease profiled by fluid and imaging markers: tau PET best predicts cognitive decline. Mol Psychiatry. 2021;26(10):5888–98.
53. Tideman P, Stomrud E, Leuzy A, Mattsson-Carlgren N, Palmqvist S, Hansson O, et al. Association of β-Amyloid accumulation with executive function in adults with unimpaired cognition. Neurology. 2022;98(15):e1525–e33.
54. Rentz DM, Papp KV, Mayblyum DV, Sanchez JS, Klein H, Souillard-Mandar W, et al. Association of digital clock drawing with PET amyloid and tau pathology in normal older adults. Neurology. 2021;96(14):e1844–e54.
55. Venneri A, McGeown WJ, Hietanen HM, Guerrini C, Ellis AW, Shanks MF. The anatomical bases of semantic retrieval deficits in early Alzheimer's disease. Neuropsychologia. 2008;46(2):497–510.
56. Hajjar I, Okafor M, Choi JD, Moore E, Abrol A, Calhoun VD, et al. Development of digital voice biomarkers and associations with cognition, cerebrospinal biomarkers, and neural representation in early Alzheimer's disease. Alzheimers Dement (Amst). 2023;15(1):e12393.
57. Cho S, Cousins KAQ, Shellikeri S, Ash S, Irwin DJ, Liberman MY, et al. Lexical and acoustic speech features relating to Alzheimer disease pathology. Neurology. 2022;99(4):e313–e22.
58. Ellis C, Henderson A, Wright HH, Rogalski Y. Global coherence during discourse production in adults: A review of the literature. Int J Lang Commun Disord. 2016;51(4):359–67.
59. Mazzon G, Ajčević M, Cattaruzza T, Menichelli A, Guerriero M, Capitanio S, et al. Connected speech deficit as an early hallmark of CSF-defined Alzheimer's disease and correlation with cerebral hypoperfusion pattern. Curr Alzheimer Res. 2019;16(6):483–94.
60. Furman JL, Vaquer-Alicea J, White CL, Cairns NJ, Nelson PT, Diamond MI. Widespread tau seeding activity at early Braak stages. Acta Neuropathol. 2017;133:91–100.
61. Pistono A, Jucla M, Barbeau EJ, Saint-Aubert L, Lemesle B, Calvet B, et al. Pauses during autobiographical discourse reflect episodic memory processes in early Alzheimer's disease. J Alzheimers Dis. 2016;50(3):687–98.
62. Leuzy A, Mattsson-Carlgren N, Palmqvist S, Janelidze S, Dage JL, Hansson O. Blood-based biomarkers for Alzheimer's disease. EMBO Mol Med. 2022;14(1):e14408.
63. Dubois B, Villain N, Frisoni GB, Rabinovici GD, Sabbagh M, Cappa S, et al. Clinical diagnosis of Alzheimer's disease: recommendations of the International Working Group. Lancet Neurol. 2021;20(6):484–96.
64. Weiner MW, Veitch DP, Miller MJ, Aisen PS, Albala B, Beckett LA, et al. Increasing participant diversity in AD research: plans for digital screening, blood testing, and a community-engaged approach in the Alzheimer's Disease Neuroimaging Initiative 4. Alzheimers Dement. 2023;19(1):307–17.
65. Gregory S, Linz N, König A, Langel K, Pullen H, Luz S, et al. Remote data collection speech analysis and prediction of the identification of Alzheimer's disease biomarkers in people at risk for Alzheimer's disease dementia: the Speech on the Phone Assessment (SPeAk) prospective observational study protocol. BMJ Open. 2022;12(3):e052250.
66. Fristed E, Skirrow C, Meszaros M, Lenain R, Meepegama U, Cappa S, et al. A remote speech-based AI system to screen for early Alzheimer's disease via smartphones. Alzheimers Dement (Amst). 2022;14(1):e12366.
67. Folstein MF, Folstein SE, McHugh PR. "Mini-mental state": a practical method for grading the cognitive state of patients for the clinician. J Psychiatr Res. 1975;12(3):189–98.
68. Gold M, Amatniek J, Carrillo MC, Cedarbaum JM, Hendrix JA, Miller BB, et al. Digital technologies as biomarkers, clinical outcomes assessment, and recruitment tools in Alzheimer's disease clinical trials. Alzheimers Dement (N Y). 2018;4:234–42.

Kimberly D. Mueller, M.S., Ph.D., is an Assistant Professor in the Department of Communication Sciences and Disorders at the University of Wisconsin–Madison and affiliate faculty in the Division of Geriatrics at the University of Wisconsin School of Medicine and Public Health. Dr. Mueller is a speech-language pathologist and received her M.S. at Teacher's College, Columbia University, and her Ph.D. from the University of Wisconsin–Madison. Her research includes studying discourse changes across the AD continuum, including in participants with AD biomarkers. Dr. Mueller's research is funded by the National Institute on Aging (R01-AG070940; R33-AG069827; R21-DC020257; R01-AG04732721).

Discourse Characteristics in Traumatic Brain Injury

5

Karen Lê and Carl Coelho

Preview of What Is Currently Known
Traumatic brain injury (TBI) causes disruption to communication at the level of discourse. Discourse impairments following TBI are now well characterized in the literature across multiple genres, such as conversational, narrative, procedural, expository, and written discourse. These impairments are distinct from those observed in aphasia. Deficiencies in discourse ability impact functioning across multiple life domains, including socialization, work/school, psychosocial functioning, and quality of life. Discourse impairments often do not resolve over time and have been shown to persist for decades after TBI. Over the past 20 years, the development of discourse treatments (further explored in Chap. 24) has emerged as a new frontier.

Objectives
(a) To describe major discourse characteristics in TBI.
(b) To explain the functional impact of discourse impairments on life domains.
(c) To examine discourse impairments in TBI across common discourse genres.
(d) To review the cognitive bases of discourse impairments.
(e) To present the structure building framework (SBF) as a cognitive discourse model with potential utility in TBI.
(f) To discuss relationships among discourse and mental health (MH) factors and considerations for veterans with TBI and comorbid MH conditions.

Introduction

The incidence of traumatic brain injury (TBI) in the United States increased more than 50% from almost two million per year to almost three million per year from 2006 to 2014 [1]. The overall lifetime economic burden of TBI is estimated at $76.5 billion [2]. Civilians living with a long-term TBI-related disability account for 1–2% of the US population [3]. However, TBI disproportionately affects veterans at higher rates and, consequently, has been deemed the "signature wound" of the Iraq and Afghanistan wars [4]. An estimated 20% of military service members have sustained a TBI [5, 6]. Cognitive-communication disorders following TBI occur in an estimated 80–100% of cases and disrupt communication at the level of discourse and related social interaction [7].

K. Lê (✉)
Audiology and Speech Pathology Service, VA Connecticut Healthcare System,
West Haven, CT, USA
e-mail: karen.le2@va.gov

C. Coelho
Department of Speech, Language, and Hearing Sciences, University of Connecticut, Storrs, CT, USA
e-mail: carl.coelho@uconn.edu

A. P.-H. Kong (ed.), *Spoken Discourse Impairments in the Neurogenic Populations*,
https://doi.org/10.1007/978-3-031-45190-4_5

Discourse refers to "a series of connected sentences or related linguistic units that convey a message" [8]. As such, discourse impairments are breakdowns in meaningful, connected language, such as narratives and conversation, beyond the level of words and sentences and are a hallmark of cognitive-communication disorders in TBI. Discourse impairment is common across all levels of TBI severity, including mild TBI (mTBI), which comprises the largest TBI severity group in both veterans and civilians. A national study of Iraq and Afghanistan veterans with TBI found that more than 85% had mTBI [9]. Prior prevailing wisdom was that individuals with mTBI return to baseline functioning shortly after injury. However, emerging literature has challenged this notion and shown that while individuals with mTBI may perform comparably to neurotypical peers on isolated cognitive or linguistic tasks, they consistently demonstrate breakdowns at the level of discourse [10, 11]. Cognitive-communication disorders, such as discourse impairments, are undertreated in mTBI [12].

Discourse impairments often do not resolve over time. Various studies have shown that impaired discourse persists several years post-injury. Discourse impairments present at 2 years post-injury have been found to persist at 10-year follow-up [13]. In a study of Vietnam War veterans with TBI, almost 50% of the group had impaired discourse more than three decades after injury [14]. MacDonald's model of cognitive-communicative competence (Fig. 5.1) provides a framework for understanding the functional impact of discourse impairments on individuals with TBI and offers guidance for evidence-based cognitive-communication interventions after TBI [15]. The model identifies seven interconnected domains of functioning that influence communication success: the individual, context/environment, cognition, communication, physical/

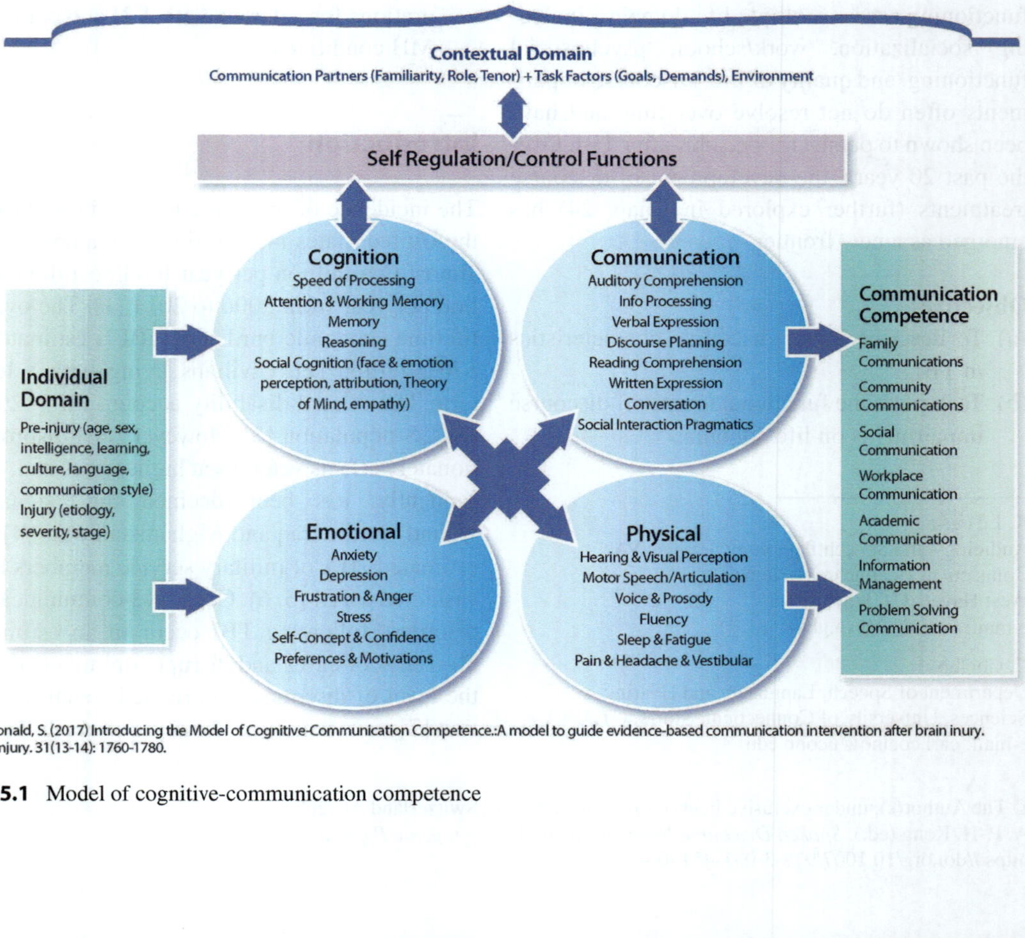

Fig. 5.1 Model of cognitive-communication competence

sensory functioning, and emotional/psychosocial functioning, all of which contribute to the last domain of communication competence. "Functional communication" can be operationalized based on MacDonald's definition of communication competence as "the strategic and effective employment of communication perception and production skill … to meet the individual's participation goals within family, community, social, work, academic, and problem-solving contexts." In contrast to people with aphasia following a stroke who are often described as communicating better than they speak because they can often convey their message despite significant deficits in language fundamentals (e.g., syntax or lexical skills), people with discourse impairments following TBI have been described as speaking better than they communicate because they often do not get their message across to communication partners despite seemingly preserved language fundamentals. Discourse skills require the integration of multiple skills, including linguistic, cognitive, and social abilities, deployed in the individual's natural environments, to achieve functional communication. Consistent with MacDonald's model, the disruption to discourse ability following TBI has predictably and systematically resulted in failures of functional communication in the literature as described in the following section.

Discourse impairments impact functioning across a number of life domains, presenting significant challenges to occupational functioning, social reintegration, and quality of life (QoL) following TBI. Discourse impairments have been shown to predict hospital length of stay and overall disability outcome in people with TBI [16]. A systematic review study found that less than half of individuals with TBI secure stable work after their injury [17]. Discourse functioning has been tied to return to work and job stability [18, 19]. For example, in one study, discourse ability in combination with auditory processing ability classified employment status of individuals with TBI with 85% accuracy [18].

In parallel with the loss of work and difficulty maintaining employment associated with discourse impairments, many struggle with finding another role that provides a sense of purpose and meaning [20]. Individuals with discourse impairments after TBI also routinely report struggles with maintaining social relationships, loss of social contact, and social isolation [21, 22] (see Table 5.1). Empirical research now also shows that effective discourse skills play an important role in social reintegration [21, 22]. In one study, not only did discourse variables predict social reintegration and QoL after TBI, but also only discourse variables, rather than psychosocial variables, predicted social reintegration following TBI [22]. Social communication measures reflecting discourse ability have uniquely accounted for employment and social reintegration outcomes over and above the contribution of cognitive measures [28]. A recent randomized controlled trial (RCT) involving both veterans and civilians with TBI provided training of discourse skills as a key part of social competence treatment; the collective TBI group demonstrated gains in social and functional communication, reduction in psychological distress, and improved QoL following treatment [29].

Examination of discourse ability in TBI can identify communicative impairments, which are sometimes subtle, that often elude traditional standardized language tests. Frank aphasias are rare in TBI, and decontextualized language batteries that focus on word- and sentence-level performance often overestimate communication ability in TBI. Non-standardized, functional assessments (e.g., discourse analyses, pragmatic rating scales, and communication checklists), further explored in Chap. 14, have offered a more fruitful evaluation approach to the detection and characterization of discourse impairments and determination of treatment goals.

Discourse impairments have been observed across multiple genres and modalities. The two most common and studied genres are conversation and narrative, but people with TBI also have challenges with procedural, expository, and descriptive discourse. While the majority of studies have focused on spoken discourse, there is now emerging evidence that TBI disrupts written

Table 5.1 Common characteristics and functional impact of discourse impairments in TBI

Common discourse impairments	Life domains	Functional impact on people with TBI
Word- and sentence-level (microlinguistic) problems: • Fewer propositions • Frequent mazes • Reduced productivity and communicative efficiency • Inadequate cohesion *Global (macrolinguistic and superstructural) problems:* • Omission of critical information • Reduced coherence • Poor topic management • Choppy, disconnected utterances • Disorganized information *Pragmatic problems:* • Inappropriate comments • Reduced ability to understand and address communication partners' needs • Paucity or verbosity of speech • Problems understanding social cues *Reading and writing problems:* • Difficulty with paragraph comprehension • Slower reading speed • Sparser writing • Challenges with complex writing (e.g., expository discourse)	• Family • Community • Social relationships	• Strained relationships with family members due to communication problems [23] • Fear and anxiety related to communication and communicative situations [23, 24] • Social exclusion [23, 24] • Difficulties developing friendships and romantic relationships • Problems navigating the legal system
	• Work • Employment • Academic	• Difficulties using language for context-dependent communicative intents (e.g., negotiating, collaborating) [25] • Conflicts with peers and colleagues due to communication problems [26] • Problems with using complex language in presentations and discussions • Challenges with writing essays and reports • Difficulty securing and keeping work
	• Quality of life	• Reduced participation in life activities • Poorer psychosocial outcomes [27] • Mental health factors may influence and exacerbate communicative functioning • Reduced quality of life

discourse as well. Although discourse production impairments are now well characterized, less is known about discourse comprehension ability in TBI.

Discourse Comprehension

Discourse comprehension studies in TBI, while limited, have identified problems in understanding auditory-verbal, written, and pragmatic information. TBI impacts the ability to understand spoken stories, especially for implicit information [30, 31]. A review of reading ability in TBI found significant deficits in comprehension and speed of reading [32]. Furthermore, individuals with TBI have difficulty with understanding paraphrases of written expository text and are less productive during free recall of read passages [33]. In complicated mTBI, lower Glasgow Coma Scale (GCS) scores have predicted poorer reading comprehension with right frontal lobe damage associated with worse auditory and reading comprehension [34]. Preliminary electroencephalogram (EEG) findings suggest that TBI alters neural activity associated with sentence processing as evidenced by lack of a reliable P600 response, a language-relevant event-related potential [35]. Moreover, reading comprehension deficits can affect academic and vocational functioning in TBI. A related concern is the impact of discourse comprehension impairments on navigating the legal system given that people with TBI have demonstrated reduced accuracy and speed in grasping legal language and social-legal interactions [36, 37]. Individuals with TBI are also less discerning of written social cues [38]. Pragmatic deficits in TBI are well documented, revealing problems with processing the context and paralinguistics of discourse interactions, including theory of mind (ToM), tone of voice (e.g., sincerity, sarcasm), figurative language, and communicative intent [39–41]. In summary, analogous to findings on expressive discourse ability, the evidence suggests that receptive discourse skills are also disrupted following TBI.

Narrative Discourse

Narrative involves the telling of a story in which characters and actions are presented following a logical sequence constructed through temporal and causal links [42]. Narrative discourse impairments are common in TBI and can manifest at the word- and sentence-level (microlinguistic), global text-level (macrolinguistic), and global organizational-level (superstructural) overarching. Studies examining discourse at the microlinguistic level often involve lexical, semantic, and grammatical analyses or productivity and efficiency measures, and findings from these studies have been inconsistent. Some studies found no significant differences in syntactic ability as reflected on measures of sentential complexity and grammatical accuracy [43–45], while others challenged this notion [46, 47].

In contrast, propositional analyses have yielded greater consensus that individuals with TBI struggle on informational measures. Propositions refer to the set of semantic relations (i.e., meaning) specified by an utterance's predicate and associated arguments. At the microlinguistic level, essential content is often measured by essential propositions or content information units (CIUs). Several studies have demonstrated that individuals with TBI consistently omit critical microlinguistic elements of information in narrative discourse [48, 49]. Furthermore, studies have also revealed that stories from individuals with TBI contain fewer propositions overall [46, 50, 51]. These results are somewhat tempered by findings of another study in which people with TBI and a neurotypical comparison group produced comparable numbers of explicit propositions [52]. However, the TBI group performed more poorly in producing implicit propositions, suggesting particular difficulty with information that must be inferred, which is a common observation in TBI.

Findings on productivity and communicative efficiency in narrative discourse TBI have been somewhat variable. A review of discourse production in TBI identified consistent reductions in verbal output and decreased communicative efficiency in monologic discourse, which includes narratives [53]. A variety of productivity and communicative efficiency measures (e.g., tallies of total words, T-unit or C-unit counts, lexical errors, tangential utterances) have distinguished discourse functioning between individuals with TBI and neurotypical individuals [45, 54, 55]. However, some studies have found no differences in similar measures [56]. Elicitation task may also influence productivity and communicative efficiency as demonstrated by a study in which participants with TBI produced more utterances and fewer words per utterance on monologic narratives but were on par with neurotypical participants on cooperative narratives produced with a familiar communication partner [48].

Cohesion refers to the extent to which utterances are meaningfully linked in a text and reflects inter-sentential organization that lies at the intersection of discourse microstructure and macrostructure. Cohesive markers or ties bridge meaning between utterances and can only be understood by searching another utterance for the meaning (e.g., The *curry* is too spicy. I'll make *it* milder next time.). Cohesion measures can include counts of cohesive ties and adequacy ratings [57]. Examinations of narrative cohesion in TBI have been inconclusive. Preserved cohesion has been found in some studies [43, 58, 59] and impaired cohesion in others [48, 60].

Macrolinguistic discourse deficits are a consistent finding in TBI. Global coherence, gist summarization (i.e., extrapolation of key information and meaning), and story completeness are macrolinguistic components that are often evaluated when assessing narrative discourse for story content. Global coherence, which identifies meaningful relationships between an utterance and the discourse as a whole, has been studied extensively in TBI. With few exceptions [58], the literature substantiates disruption in global coherence in discourse following TBI [45, 61]. Individuals with TBI struggle with establishing logical connections between their utterances and the topic of discussion, resulting in poorer global coherence.

Deficiencies in story completeness and accuracy of story information are a frequent occurrence after TBI, reflecting impaired discourse. Individuals with TBI have difficulty judging the importance of story information [62, 63]. During storytelling, they frequently omit critical information and key details and provide irrelevant or inaccurate information [14, 30, 64]. On a picture story sequencing task, individuals with impaired discourse following TBI performed more poorly than neurotypical peers on arranging the pictures in logical order [65]. Even when the pictures were presented in correct order, the people with discourse impairments following TBI still produced inaccurate accounts that reflected a failure to identify the important components of the picture story.

Beyond story content, TBI also disrupts story organization ability, which is considered a global aspect of discourse referred to as the superstructural level. Global analyses of story organization focus primarily on the overarching framework that organizes discourse content (i.e., story schema). Story grammar, the causal and temporal rules that specify and guide the connections between characters and events, provides the logical ordering of story information that aids comprehension and production and gives rise to the narrative framework [42]. The episode, a sequence of events, is central to many measures of story grammar. A complete episode consists of three main elements:

1. An *initiating event* that provides the impetus for a character's action (e.g., "The farmer's prize tomato plant was not growing due to the surrounding bushes blocking the sunlight.")
2. An *attempt* by the character to achieve the goal (e.g., "So, he chopped down the bushes to allow the plant more light.")
3. A *direct consequence* of the attempt (e.g., "The plant flourished, much to the relief of the farmer.")

Breakdowns in story organization, as evidenced by poor performance on story grammar measures, are frequently observed following TBI. Narratives produced by individuals with TBI often contain fewer story grammar elements and a lower proportion of utterances organized into episodes [46, 59]. Story organization may vary depending on elicitation condition with some evidence showing that in people with TBI, the extent of disorganization for the generation of spontaneous stories is greater than that in story retelling [59].

Impairments in story content and story organization in TBI diminish the overall goodness of narratives. Story goodness has been operationalized as the combination of story content and story organization [66]. The analysis of narrative discourse integrating measures of story content and story organization has demonstrated utility. Such an approach has provided a way to quantify diminished goodness of story following TBI and enabled identification of categories of disordered discourse [14]. While some individuals have greater deficiencies in story content, others have greater deficiencies in story organization, and some have comparably poor performance in both content and organization. The quantification and categorization of story goodness in TBI have potential clinical implications as they can help focus treatment and monitor discourse changes over time. Ecological validity of diminished story goodness has been supported by listener perceptions of narratives produced by individuals with TBI as deficiencies in story content and story organization have been associated with poorer ratings in overall story quality [62].

One long-standing view of discourse impairments is the construct of a dissociation between microlinguistic and global discourse (macrolinguistic and superstructural) ability in TBI with impairments primarily affecting the former and sparing the latter. More recently, a compelling alternative view has emerged, offering a more unifying construct [67, 68]. Through a series of studies, Peach and colleagues demonstrated support for a resource allocation model of discourse production in TBI. They identified an association between sentence planning deficits in narratives and problems in working memory (WM) and executive functions (EF) [69]. They then found a significant relationship between inter-sentential (i.e., cohesion) and intra-sentential (e.g., pauses, mazes, errors) measures, as characterized by synchrony of typical cohesion and well-formed utterances, with disruption to intra-sentential processing. In a recent study, they found that cohesive adequacy and sentence planning ability highly predicted story grammar outcomes, strongly implicating that the various layers of discourse processing are dependent on one another [68]. The collective findings from the studies support a resource allocation model of discourse performance and highlight the potential cost to aspects of discourse processing (e.g., microlinguistic) to achieve meaningful and organized discourse in TBI.

Conversational Discourse

Conversation is discourse in which two or more people exchange thoughts and feelings, or discuss ideas. Conversation enables individuals to negotiate their needs and wants. Proficiency in conversation is critical not only in education and vocational performance but also for establishing and maintaining social relationships [22, 70]. It is well established that individuals with TBI generally present with cognitive-communication disorders characterized by discourse deficits [71–73]. In casual interactions, individuals with TBI are often perceived as being off-target, disorganized, and tangential, and, in some cases, they offer little specific information. These deficits are particularly apparent in conversational discourse.

The success of any conversational interaction is dependent on the mutual contributions of all participants. The conversation of individuals with TBI is characterized by decreased initiation, problems maintaining the topic of discussion, and content errors [74, 75] as well as a greater number of turns and shorter, less complex utterances [76]. Due to these difficulties, interactions involving individuals with TBI may evolve into interviews, that is, a question/answer format, as opposed to natural conversation. The effectiveness of such interactions is frequently more a function of the skill of the neurotypical communication partner at sustaining the flow of the conversation than that of the person with TBI. Consistent with this notion, recent work in TBI rehabilitation has focused on the training of neurotypical conversational partners to improve such interactions [77].

There are a number of issues to consider when a clinician is preparing to sample and analyze conversational discourse. These include conversational partners, topic, where the interaction takes place, duration of the conversation, how it is recorded, and length of the interaction. For example, a conversation between an individual with a brain injury and a clinician during a diagnostic evaluation will be very different from one involving family members or close friends discussing a favorite activity at home. In addition, the use of audio-video recording devices may impact the comfort and naturalness of a conversation. If conversation samples are to be used to monitor communicative change longitudinally, it is critical that the format of each conversation remains the same (i.e., participants, topic, locale).

Once a sample of conversation is obtained, there are a myriad of analyses that can be applied. The particular measure selected will be determined by the purpose of the language assessment. Analyses of conversation can be relatively informal such as pragmatic rating scales [78, 79] or formal, more complex multicomponent procedures such as conversational analysis or systemic functional linguistics [80, 81]. Regardless of the approach taken, key aspects of conversation should always be considered such as turn taking, response appropriateness and adequacy, topic management, and conversation repair [82].

Turn taking in conversation involves frequent speaker changes, ideally with one individual speaking at a time. If two individuals speak simultaneously, it should be of short duration. As speakers shift from one to another, there should be minimal delay. The overall length of a conversation is variable, as is the order of speakers and duration of turns. Typically, allocation of turns and content are not established prior to the conversation. Turns may follow in succession (continuous talk) or there may be pauses during which no one talks (discontinuous talk). Measures of turn taking include number and length of speaking turns for each participant and appropriateness of the alternation of turns. Ineffectual turn taking can disrupt communication. Therefore, instances of faulty turn taking should be noted in transcripts of conversational samples to help identify potential sources of breakdowns.

Response adequacy refers to the appropriateness of an utterance within the context of an ongoing conversation. The concept of response appropriateness (and adequacy) has been studied within the psychiatric literature on neurotic and psychotic patients [83] and more recently in research on rehabilitation of cognitive-communication disorders following brain injury [76, 84]. Once again, transcripts should be coded to identify the adequacy of speaker responses over the course of the conversation.

Topics pertain to what is talked about in a conversation and how the topic may shift during the interaction. Topic management pertains to how a topic is initiated and how it is maintained. A topic may be introduced by a single speaker or in conjunction with the conversational partner. Topics may be changed by one of the following means, and the examination of conversation should include tallies of such topic management behaviors [82]:

1. Novel introduction, either at the beginning of a conversation or at the ending of a discussion of one topic and initiating another.
2. A smooth shift, in which the topic of discussion is subtly changed to another.
3. A disruptive shift in which the transition is abrupt or irrational.

Finally, conversational repair pertains to how effectively a speaker can modify or clarify an utterance when their dyadic partner does not fully understand the message. Four types of repair mechanisms have been described [85]:

1. Other-initiated other-repair: the listener indicates a problem and repairs it.
2. Other-initiated self-repair: a clarification is requested by the listener and the speaker provides it.
3. Self-initiated other-repair: the speaker recognizes a problem and the listener repairs it.
4. Self-initiated self-repair: the speaker recognizes a breakdown and explains the message.

The ability to manage communication breakdowns is critical for independent functioning in a variety of everyday environments. Highlighting such skills in conversational transcripts is particularly helpful for monitoring change and treatment planning.

Descriptive, Procedural, and Expository Discourse

While the majority of discourse studies in TBI have focused on narrative and conversation, findings from examinations of other discourse genres (e.g., descriptive, procedural, and expository) have provided further insights into cognitive-communicative functioning following TBI. Descriptive discourse involves the enumeration of features and concepts about an item (e.g., picture, object) or experience (e.g., hobby). Procedural discourse entails explanations of a series of actions to perform a task and instructs the communication partner about how to carry out an activity. Expository discourse is meant to inform the listener about a topic through facts or interpretation and encompasses comparison and contrast, cause and effect, and generalization [8] that are critical to academic success.

Findings from investigations of descriptive, procedural, and expository discourse are analogous to those of narrative discourse with more variable findings at the microlinguistic level and more consistent evidence of disruption at the macrolinguistic level. In descriptive discourse, minimal differences have been discerned on grammatical complexity or cohesive adequacy between TBI and neurotypical comparison groups, but deficits in global coherence were identified, underscoring a pattern of greater impairment in macrolinguistic processing [45, 86]. Propositional analyses in procedural discourse have yielded conflicting results, with some studies finding typical performance [87] and others finding impaired performance, such as too few or too many propositions [62]. Reductions in communicative efficiency have been observed in the face of typical productivity (i.e., words, utterances) and consistent challenges with delineation of essential steps of a procedure [88].

Studies of expository discourse in TBI have revealed both sentence- (e.g., poorer sentence planning, sparser discourse) and global-level (e.g., poorer overall quality of text) impairments [89, 90]. These collective findings would support a resource allocation model of discourse production as proposed by Peach and colleagues [68]. Drawing upon more complex reasoning ability, expository discourse often places greater cognitive demands on the individual in comparison to procedural or descriptive discourse, thus resulting in disruption to multiple levels of discourse processing.

Written Discourse

Despite the importance of written communication across life domains, written discourse ability following TBI is still an emerging area of research. Early work in this area found written discourse in TBI to be sparser in words and impaired in local coherence (thematic unity between sentences) but on par with neurotypical participants for other indices, such as cohesion and global coherence [91]. These findings are consistent with reports from individuals with TBI themselves, who endorse substantial challenges with writing that interfere with daily functioning [92, 93]. Analogous to spoken discourse, the application of multi-level assessment of written discourse has revealed various profiles of impairment, highlighting the importance of examining different aspects of writing [94]. College students with mild TBI have improved aspects of their writing in preliminary evidence from early-stage interventions [93, 95]. However, those with moderate and severe TBI and limited awareness of deficits are unlikely to be successful in learning and implementing writing strategies while insight into their functioning is impaired [96].

Cognitive Factors Underlying Discourse

Discourse can be considered as the intersection of cognition and communication, and multiple cognitive processes are deployed at various stages (microlinguistic, macrolinguistic, superstructural) in the synthesis and comprehension of discourse. It is widely accepted that discourse impairments have cognitive underpinnings. Like discourse impairments, cognitive impairments are also a hallmark of TBI and encompass but are not limited to disruption in major cognitive domains, including attention, memory, and executive functions (EFs). The research literature has strongly substantiated a relationship between discourse ability and each of these cognitive domains.

A recent systematic review identified several research studies that linked discourse with attention [97]. Given the multifaceted nature of attention, multiple types of attention were connected with discourse, including attention control, executive attention, working memory (WM), and information processing. Problems with sustained attention, in particular, were associated with tangentiality as well as deficits in verbal reasoning, topic maintenance, and social inference. Further support for attention as a key factor in discourse performance emerged from a recent narrative discourse treatment study that resulted in greater generalization when combined with attention process training [98].

Similar to attention, various aspects of memory are associated with discourse functioning in TBI with WM being the most well studied. WM involves storage and transformation of information and has been implicated in both discourse production and comprehension in TBI. WM has correlated with measures of cohesion, content, and organization in narrative discourse produced by people with TBI [46, 99, 100]. There is evidence to support WM as a constraining factor in grammatical and figurative language processing [101, 102], and individuals with TBI who have higher WM scores are better discourse comprehenders than those with lower WM scores [103]. Although less well studied in relation to discourse, declarative memory is also thought to underlie discourse performance in TBI. In particular, episodic memory, related to event knowledge, has predicted narrative completeness of critical information and narrative organization (i.e., story grammar) [55, 104]. In a meta-analysis, declarative memory surpassed other major cognitive domains in accounting for pragmatic comprehension [41].

Executive functions (EF) are higher order cognitive processes that underpin goal-directed behavior and include components, such as planning, monitoring, inhibition, and flexible problem-solving. In several constructs of EF, EF subsumes WM. EF measures are numerous and diverse, tapping components of EF differently, and exemplar tasks comprise card-sorting, verbal learning and fluency, and trail-making. As discourse synthesis is a goal-directed process, EF impairments should cause disruption to discourse functioning. Indeed, relationships between various EF measures and multiple aspects of discourse production have been identified at both the microlinguistic and global levels and across genres [69, 105, 106]. For example, card-sorting, which involves monitoring and flexible problem-solving, has correlated with narrative organization [107], and trail-making has correlated with conversational abilities [106].

In summary, the research evidence across major cognitive domains of attention, memory, and EF highly substantiates the cognitive bases of discourse ability. The relationships between cognition and discourse have been observed at multiple levels of discourse processing and across multiple discourse genres. Given the co-occurrence of and relationship between cognitive deficits and discourse processing impairments, a discourse model that accounts for the cognitive-communicative impairments in TBI and harmonizes with the construct of resource allocation would be of immense theoretical and clinical utility.

The Structure Building Framework (SBF)

One discourse model with the potential to explain discourse impairments in TBI is the Structure Building Framework (SBF) [108]. The SBF is a cognitive discourse processing model that posits that discourse comprehension involves creation of mental representations (i.e., structures) through the following processes: (1) laying a foundation, (2) mapping relevant information onto that foundation, and (3) shifting, as needed, to initiate a new substructure when incoming information is unrelated to the currently activated substructure. Enhancement of relevant information and suppression of irrelevant information are purported to be the general mechanisms at work in creating mental structures. Applied to discourse, mental structures could represent microlinguistic aspects of discourse, such as formation of single sentences, or global aspects, such as story grammar.

The SBF is a normative discourse comprehension model that was developed to account for how neurotypical individuals understand discourse, but it has been argued that the same mechanisms function in discourse production [109]. SBF is the only cognitive model that has been applied to explain both discourse comprehension and production in neurologic and psychiatric populations and has gained increasing attention in accounting for discourse impairments in TBI [33, 104]. Such a cognitive model would also be compatible with the construct of resource allocation as cognitive resources are finite. If cognitive demands are exceeded and resources for enhancement and suppression are inadequate, this could potentially result in incomplete or poorly formed mental structures.

Discourse Ability, Mental Health, and Considerations for Veterans with TBI

Although TBI is a known disruptor of discourse ability, other factors can potentially influence discourse production and exacerbate discourse impairments, including premorbid factors, such as education and premorbid language ability, and comorbidities, such as mental health (MH) concerns [59, 110–112]. MH disorders, such as PTSD, anxiety, and depression, often co-occur with TBI in veterans and may further exacerbate, or even be a primary cause of, discourse impairments in this population. Research on the relationships among discourse, TBI, and MH is in a nascent stage, but the few studies on this topic suggest that it may be a promising area for further exploration. Veterans with comorbid TBI and PTSD produce narratives with fewer words than their peers with TBI only or neurotypical peers and perform more poorly on neuropsychological measures than those with only a singular diagnosis of TBI or PTSD [113, 114]. Veterans with PTSD take longer to read paragraphs and answer questions about them compared to those without this condition, despite comparable test accuracy between groups [115]. These findings implicate PTSD as a potential factor in changes in language comprehension, production, and cognitive performance following TBI.

There is evidence that telling well-formed stories may have therapeutic effects and facilitating particular aspects of language production in trauma narratives may improve outcomes in trauma recovery [116, 117]. For example, in a nonclinical sample where participants were asked to write about the most traumatic event of their lives repeatedly over intervals, coherence increased over time [117]. Increased organization and decreased fragmentation have been associated with reduction in PTSD symptoms [118]. Findings from such studies may be of particular importance to veterans with TBI and concomitant PTSD, as their MH challenges may concurrently impact their discourse functioning and their discourse impairments may impact their ability to benefit from MH treatment.

The manner in which discourse tasks are implemented in intervention may also influence MH outcomes. In a study examining expressive writing in veterans with self-reported reintegration difficulties following return from deployment, veterans in the expressive writing group were asked to describe their transition to civilian life through expression of feelings and insights into challenges [119]. Those in the factual writing group were instructed to describe information needs of veterans in transition. Veterans who wrote expressively experienced greater reductions in physical, psychiatric, and emotional symptoms than those who wrote factually or not at all, underscoring the potential influence of discourse expression on functioning. In summary, the implications from these studies for TBI are twofold. One implication is that PTSD and other MH factors may influence and exacerbate discourse functioning in TBI, and the other implication is that the use of discourse tasks may be therapeutic for improving not only communication but also MH outcomes.

Conclusions, Future Directions, Implications for Treatment

Discourse impairments are characteristic of the disruption to cognitive-communicative functioning prevalent following TBI. Competence in discourse has a clear and significant impact on functioning, social reintegration, QoL, and life satisfaction in people with TBI. Breakdowns in discourse ability in TBI occur at multiple levels of processing, across genres, and in both comprehension and production. Discourse performance is dependent on the integrity of various cognitive networks. The SBF is a cognitive discourse model that may have potential utility in explaining discourse deficits in TBI and guiding treatment. Consideration of factors that may influence discourse ability, such as PTSD and other MH challenges, is an area for further exploration.

Given the functional impact of discourse impairments, development of discourse intervention in TBI is a needed and growing area of research. Further discussion of discourse treatment is explored in Chap. 24. A recent systematic review of discourse and social communication interventions in TBI identified five "essential" treatment components that were found in interventions with durable treatment effects [120]. These treatment "building blocks" comprised feedback, simulated or actual social contexts, functional practice, training in metalinguistic/metacognitive strategies, and hierarchical training. Inclusion of these components is likely to increase efficacy and extent of therapeutic effects.

In addition to discourse treatment development, current gaps in the literature present opportunities for further investigation in understanding discourse ability following TBI. Potentially promising areas for continued exploration in TBI include spoken discourse and reading comprehension, writing impairments and writing interventions, relationships between discourse and other less well-studied cognitive factors (e.g., declarative memory), and potential influences of TBI comorbidities.

Major Takeaways

1. Discourse impairments are a hallmark of TBI, disrupting communication at multiple levels, across genres, and across modalities.
2. Reduced discourse competence negatively impacts the ability to participate in a number of major life activities.
3. Discourse impairments are thought to have cognitive underpinnings, which may be explained through the lens of resource allocation and the structure building framework.
4. There is emerging evidence that mental health conditions may affect discourse functioning in TBI. The manner in which discourse tasks are implemented may have potential effects on mental health in addition to cognitive-communicative functioning.

Acknowledgements Research reported in this publication was supported by the U.S. Department of Veterans Affairs, Veterans Health Administration, Office of Research and Development, Rehabilitation Research and Development Service (award #: 1 IK2 RX003494-01A2) awarded to Karen Lê. The content is solely the responsibility of the authors and does not necessarily represent the official views, position, or policy of the Department of Veterans Affairs or the U.S. Government.

References

1. CDC. TBI-Related Emergency Department Visits, Hospitalizations, and Deaths (EDHDs) 2019 [updated 03/29/2019]. Available from: https://www.cdc.gov/traumaticbraininjury/data/tbi-edhd.html.
2. CDC. Severe TBI 2019 [updated 04/02/19]. Available from: https://www.cdc.gov/traumaticbraininjury/severe.html.
3. Zaloshnja E, Miller T, Langlois JA, Selassie AW. Prevalence of long-term disability from traumatic brain injury in the civilian population of the United States, 2005. J Head Trauma Rehabil. 2008;23(6):394–400.
4. Snell FI, Halter MJ. A signature wound of war: mild traumatic brain injury. J Psychosoc Nurs Ment Health Serv. 2010;48(2):22–8.
5. DVBIC. DoD Worldwide Numbers for TBI 2018. Available from: https://dvbic.dcoe.mil/dod-worldwide-numbers-tbi.
6. Swanson TM, Isaacson BM, Cyborski CM, French LM, Tsao JW, Pasquina PF. Traumatic brain injury incidence, clinical overview, and policies in the US Military Health System Since 2000. Public Health Rep. 2017;132(2):251–9.
7. MacDonald S, Wiseman-Hakes C. Knowledge translation in ABI rehabilitation: a model for consolidating and applying the evidence for cognitive-communication interventions. Brain Inj. 2010;24(3):486–508.
8. Cherney LR, Coelho CA, Shadden BB. Analyzing discourse in communicatively impaired adults. Gaithersburg, MD: Aspen Publishers; 1998.
9. Lindquist LK, Love HC, Elbogen EB. Traumatic brain injury in Iraq and Afghanistan veterans: new results from a national random sample study. J Neuropsychiatry Clin Neurosci. 2017;29(3):254–9.
10. Stockbridge MD, Newman R. Enduring cognitive and linguistic deficits in individuals with a history of concussion. Am J Speech Lang Pathol. 2019;28(4):1554–70.
11. Gallagher K, Azuma T. Analysis of story recall in military veterans with and without mild traumatic brain injury: preliminary results. Am J Speech Lang Pathol. 2018;27(1s):485–94.
12. Duff MC, Proctor A, Haley K. Mild traumatic brain injury (MTBI): assessment and treatment procedures used by speech-language pathologists (SLPs). Brain Inj. 2002;16(9):773–87.
13. Ponsford JL, Downing MG, Olver J, Ponsford M, Acher R, Carty M, et al. Longitudinal follow-up of patients with traumatic brain injury: outcome at two, five, and ten years post-injury. J Neurotrauma. 2014;31(1):64–77.
14. Lê K, Coelho C, Mozeiko J, Krueger F, Grafman J. Measuring goodness of story narratives: implications for traumatic brain injury. Aphasiology. 2011;25(6–7):748–60.
15. MacDonald S. Introducing the model of cognitive-communication competence: a model to guide evidence-based communication interventions after brain injury. Brain Inj. 2017;31(13/14):1760–80.
16. Gauthier S, LeBlanc J, Seresova A, Laberge-Poirier A, Correa JA, Alturki AY, et al. Acute prediction of outcome and cognitive-communication impairments following traumatic brain injury: the influence of age, education and site of lesion. J Commun Disord. 2018;73:77–90.
17. van Velzen JM, van Bennekom CA, Edelaar MJ, Sluiter JK, Frings-Dresen MH. How many people return to work after acquired brain injury?: a systematic review. Brain Inj. 2009;23(6):473–88.
18. Isaki E, Turkstra L. Communication abilities and work re-entry following traumatic brain injury. Brain Inj. 2000;14(5):441–53.

19. Rietdijk R, Simpson G, Togher L, Power E, Gillett L. An exploratory prospective study of the association between communication skills and employment outcomes after severe traumatic brain injury. Brain Inj. 2013;27(7–8):812–8.
20. Douglas JM. Placing brain injury rehabilitation in the context of the self and meaningful engagement. Semin Speech Lang. 2010;31(3):197–204.
21. Dahlberg C, Hawley L, Morey C, Newman J, Cusick CP, Harrison-Felix C. Social communication skills in persons with post-acute traumatic brain injury: three perspectives. Brain Inj. 2006;20(4):425–35.
22. Galski T, Tompkins C, Johnston MV. Competence in discourse as a measure of social integration and quality of life in persons with traumatic brain injury. Brain Inj. 1998;12(9):769–82.
23. Douglas J. Elizabeth Usher memorial lecture: placing therapy in the context of the self and social connection. Int J Speech Lang Pathol. 2015;17(3):199–210.
24. Douglas JM. So that's the way it is for me—Always being left out' acquired pragmatic language impairment and social functioning following traumatic brain injury. Brain Impairment. 2017;18(3):321–31.
25. Meulenbroek P, Cherney LR. The voicemail elicitation task: functional workplace language assessment for persons with traumatic brain injury. J Speech Lang Hear Res. 2019;62(9):3367–80.
26. Wyse JJ, Pogoda TK, Mastarone GL, Gilbert T, Carlson KF. Employment and vocational rehabilitation experiences among veterans with polytrauma/traumatic brain injury history. Psychol Serv. 2020;17(1):65–74.
27. Elbourn E, Kenny B, Power E, Togher L. Psychosocial outcomes of severe traumatic brain injury in relation to discourse recovery: a longitudinal study up to 1 year post-injury. Am J Speech Lang Pathol. 2019;28(4):1463–78.
28. Struchen MA, Clark AN, Sander AM, Mills MR, Evans G, Kurtz D. Relation of executive functioning and social communication measures to functional outcomes following traumatic brain injury. NeuroRehabilitation. 2008;23(2):185–98.
29. Harrison-Felix C, Newman JK, Hawley L, Morey C, Ketchum JM, Walker WC, et al. Social competence treatment after traumatic brain injury: a multicenter, randomized controlled trial of interactive group treatment versus noninteractive treatment. Arch Phys Med Rehab. 2018;99(11):2131–42.
30. Ferstl EC, Walther K, Guthke T, von Cramon DY. Assessment of story comprehension deficits after brain damage. J Clin Exp Neuropsychol. 2005;27(3):367–84.
31. Nicholas LE, Brookshire RH. Comprehension of spoken narrative discourse by adults with aphasia, right-hemisphere brain damage, or traumatic brain injury. Am J Speech Lang Pathol. 1995;4(3):69–81.
32. Pei Y, O'Brien KH. Reading abilities post traumatic brain injury in adolescents and adults: a systematic review and meta-analysis. Am J Speech Lang Pathol. 2021;30(2):789–816.
33. Sohlberg MM, Griffiths GG, Fickas S. An evaluation of reading comprehension of expository text in adults with traumatic brain injury. Am J Speech Lang Pathol. 2014;23(2):160–75.
34. LeBlanc J, Seresova A, Laberge-Poirier A, Tabet S, Alturki AY, Feyz M, et al. Cognitive-communication performance following mild traumatic brain injury: Influence of sex, age, education, site of lesion and bilingualism. Int J Lang Commun Disord. 2021;56(1):130–44.
35. Key-DeLyria SE. Sentence processing in traumatic brain injury: evidence from the P600. J Speech Lang Hear Res. 2016;59(4):759–71.
36. Wszalek JA, Turkstra LS. Comprehension of legal language by adults with and without traumatic brain injury. J Head Trauma Rehabil. 2019;34(3):E55–e63.
37. Wszalek JA, Turkstra LS. Comprehension of social-legal exchanges in adults with and without traumatic brain injury. Neuropsychology. 2019;33(7):934–46.
38. Meulenbroek P, Turkstra LS. Response to text-based social cues in the formation of causal attributions in adults with traumatic brain injury. Brain Inj. 2018;32(13–14):1720–4.
39. McDonald S. Impairments in social cognition following severe traumatic brain injury. J Int Neuropsychol Soc. 2013;19(3):231–46.
40. McDonald S, Gowland A, Randall R, Fisher A, Osborne-Crowley K, Honan C. Cognitive factors underpinning poor expressive communication skills after traumatic brain injury: theory of mind or executive function? Neuropsychology. 2014;28(5):801–11.
41. Rowley DA, Rogish M, Alexander T, Riggs KJ. Cognitive correlates of pragmatic language comprehension in adult traumatic brain injury: a systematic review and meta-analyses. Brain Inj. 2017;31(12):1564–74.
42. Stein NL, Glenn CG. An analysis of story comprehension in elementary school children: a test of a schema. New Direct Discourse Process. 1979;2:53–120.
43. Coelho C, Le K, Mozeiko J, Hamilton M, Tyler E, Krueger F, et al. Characterizing discourse deficits following penetrating head injury: a preliminary model. Am J Speech Lang Pathol. 2013;22(2):S438–48.
44. Chapman SB, Levin HS, Wanek A, Weyrauch J, Kufera J. Discourse after closed head injury in young children. Brain Lang. 1998;61(3):420–49.
45. Glosser G, Deser T. Patterns of discourse production among neurological patients with fluent language disorders. Brain Lang. 1991;40(1):67–88.
46. Hay E, Moran C. Discourse formulation in children with closed head injury. Am J Speech Lang Pathol. 2005;14(4):324–36.
47. Peach RK, Schaude BA, Peach RK, Schaude BA. Reformulating the notion of 'preserved' syntax following closed head injury [Paper presentation]. Detroit, MI, USA: American Speech-Language-Hearing Association. https://www.academia.edu/43534021/reformulating_the_notion_

of_preserved_syntax_following_closed_head_injury; 1986.
48. Jorgensen M, Togher L. Narrative after traumatic brain injury: a comparison of monologic and jointly-produced discourse. Brain Inj. 2009;23(9):727–40.
49. Stout CE, Yorkston KM, Pimentel JI. Discourse production following mild, moderate, and severe traumatic brain injury: a comparison of two tasks. J Med Speech-Lang Pathol. 2000;8(1):15–25.
50. Chapman SB, Culhane KA, Levin HS, Harward H, Mendelsohn D, Ewing-Cobbs L, et al. Narrative discourse after closed head injury in children and adolescents. Brain Lang. 1992;43(1):42–65.
51. Coelho CA, Grela B, Corso M, Gamble A, Feinn R. Microlinguistic deficits in the narrative discourse of adults with traumatic brain injury. Brain Inj. 2005;19(13):1139–45.
52. Biddle KR, McCabe A, Bliss LS. Narrative skills following traumatic brain injury in children and adults. J Commun Disord. 1996;29(6):447–68.
53. Coelho C, Ylvisaker M, Turkstra LS. Nonstandardized assessment approaches for individuals with traumatic brain injuries. Semin Speech Lang. 2005;26(4):223–41.
54. Aguilar JM, Elleman CB, Cassedy AE, Mercuri Minich N, Zhang N, Owen Yeates K, et al. Long term effects of early childhood traumatic brain injury on narrative discourse gist and psychosocial functioning. Disabil Rehabil. 2020;42(17):2383–92.
55. Lindsey A, Mozeiko J, Krueger F, Grafman J, Coelho C. Changes in discourse structure over time following traumatic brain injury. Neuropsychologia. 2018;119:308–19.
56. Power E, Weir S, Richardson J, Fromm D, Forbes M, MacWhinney B, et al. Patterns of narrative discourse in early recovery following severe traumatic brain injury. Brain Inj. 2020;34(1):98–109.
57. Liles BZ, Coelho C. Cohesion analyses. In: Cherney LR, Shadden BB, Coelho CA, editors. Analyzing discourse in communicatively impaired adults. Gaithersburg, MD: Aspen; 1998. p. 65–83.
58. Van Leer E, Turkstra L. The effect of elicitation task on discourse coherence and cohesion in adolescents with brain injury. J Commun Disord. 1999;32(5):327–49.
59. Coelho CA. Story narratives of adults with closed head injury and non-brain-injured adults: Influence of socioeconomic status, elicitation task, and executive functioning. J Speech Lang Hear Res. 2002;45(6):1232–48.
60. Carlomagno S, Giannotti S, Vorano L, Marini A. Discourse information content in non-aphasic adults with brain injury: a pilot study. Brain Inj. 2011;25(10):1010–8.
61. Ellis C, Henderson A, Wright HH, Rogalski Y. Global coherence during discourse production in adults: a review of the literature. Int J Lang Commun Disord. 2016;51(4):359–67.
62. McDonald S. Pragmatic language skills after closed head injury: ability to meet the informational needs of the listener. Brain Lang. 1993;44(1):28–46.
63. Chapman SB, Gamino JF, Cook LG, Hanten G, Li X, Levin HS. Impaired discourse gist and working memory in children after brain injury. Brain Lang. 2006;97(2):178–88.
64. Kintz S, Hibbs V, Henderson A, Andrews M, Wright HH. Discourse-based treatment in mild traumatic brain injury. J Commun Disord. 2018;76:47–59.
65. Tucker FM, Hanlon RE. Effects of mild traumatic brain injury on narrative discourse production. Brain Inj. 1998;12(9):783–92.
66. Lê K, Coelho C, Mozeiko J, Grafman J. Measuring goodness of story narratives. J Speech Lang Hear Res. 2011;54(1):118–26.
67. Peach RK, Coelho CA. Linking inter- and intrasentential processes for narrative production following traumatic brain injury: Implications for a model of discourse processing. Neuropsychologia. 2016;80:157–64.
68. Peach RK, Hanna LE. Sentence-level processing predicts narrative coherence following traumatic brain injury: evidence in support of a resource model of discourse processing. Lang Cogn Neurosci. 2021;36(6):694–710.
69. Peach RK. The cognitive basis for sentence planning difficulties in discourse after traumatic brain injury. Am J Speech Lang Pathol. 2013;22(2):S285–S97.
70. Coelho CA, Liles BZ, Duffy RJ, Clarkson JV. Conversational patterns of aphasic, closed-head-injured, and normal speakers. Clin Aphasiol. 1992;21:183–92.
71. Coelho CA. Discourse production deficits following traumatic brain injury: a critical review of the recent literature. Aphasiology. 1995;9(5):409–29.
72. Snow PC, Douglas JM. Conceptual and methodological challenges in discourse assessment with TBI speakers: towards an understanding. Brain Inj. 2000;14(5):397–415.
73. Togher L. Discourse sampling in the 21st century. J Commun Disord. 2001;34(1–2):131–50.
74. Coelho CA, Liles BZ, Duffy RJ. Analysis of conversational discourse in head-injured adults. J Head Trauma Rehabil. 1991;6(2):92–8.
75. Mentis M, Prutting CA. Analysis of topic as illustrated in a head-injured and a normal adult. J Speech Hear Res. 1991;34(3):583–95.
76. Coelho CA, Youse KM, Le KN. Conversational discourse in closed-head-injured and non-brain-injured adults. Aphasiology. 2002;16(4–6):659–72.
77. Togher L, McDonald S, Tate R, Power E, Rietdijk R. Training communication partners of people with severe traumatic brain injury improves everyday conversations: a multicenter single blind clinical trial. J Rehabil Med. 2013;45(7):637–45.
78. Halper AS, Cherney LR, Burns MS. Clinical management of right hemisphere dysfunction. Aspen Publishers; 1996.

79. Ehrlich J, Barry P. Rating communication behaviours in the head-injured adult. Brain Inj. 1989;3(2):193–8.
80. Azios JH, Simmons-Mackie N. Clinical application of conversation analysis in aphasia. In: Coelho CA, Cherney LR, Shadden BB, editors. Discourse analysis in adults with and without communication disorders: a resource for clinicians and researchers. San Diego: Plural; 2023. p. 109–30.
81. Halliday MAK. An introduction to functional grammar. London: Edward Arnold; 1985.
82. Brinton B, Fujiki M. Conversational management with language-impaired children: pragmatic assessment and intervention. Aspen Publishers; 1989.
83. Blank M, Franklin E. Dialogue with preschoolers: a cognitively-based System of assessment. Appl Psycholinguist. 1980;1(2):127–50.
84. Keegan LC, Behn N, Power E, Howell S, Rietdijk R. Assessing conversation after traumatic brain injury. In: Coelho CA, Cherney LR, Shadden BB, editors. Discourse analysis in adults with and without communication disorders: a resource for clinicians and researchers. San Diego: Plural; 2023.
85. Schegloff EA, Jefferson G, Sacks H. The preference for self-correction in the organization of repair in conversation. Language. 1977;53(2):361–82.
86. Hough MS, Barrow I. Descriptive discourse abilities of traumatic brain-injured adults. Aphasiology. 2003;17(2):183–91.
87. Cruse N, Piotto V, Coelho C, Behn N. Telehealth administration of narrative and procedural discourse: A UK and US comparison of traumatic brain injury and matched controls. Int J Lang Commun Disord. 2022; https://doi.org/10.1111/1460-6984.12813. Epub ahead of print
88. Stubbs E, Togher L, Kenny B, Fromm D, Forbes M, MacWhinney B, et al. Procedural discourse performance in adults with severe traumatic brain injury at 3 and 6 months post injury. Brain Inj. 2018;32(2):167–81.
89. Lundine JP, Harnish SM, McCauley RJ, Zezinka AB, Blackett DS, Fox RA. Exploring summarization differences for two types of expository discourse in adolescents with traumatic brain injury. Am J Speech Lang Pathol. 2018;27(1):247–57.
90. Lundine JP, Barron HD. Microstructural and fluency characteristics of narrative and expository discourse in adolescents with traumatic brain injury. Am J Speech Lang Pathol. 2019;28(4):1638–48.
91. Wilson BM, Proctor A. Written discourse of adolescents with closed head injury. Brain Inj. 2002;16(11):1011–24.
92. Dinnes C, Hux K, Holmen M, Martens A, Smith M. Writing changes and perceptions after traumatic brain injury: "Oh, by the way, I can't write". Am J Speech Lang Pathol. 2018;27(4):1523–38.
93. Ledbetter AK, Sohlberg MM, Fickas SF, Horney MA, McIntosh K. Evaluation of a computer-based prompting intervention to improve essay writing in undergraduates with cognitive impairment after acquired brain injury. Neuropsychol Rehabil. 2019;29(8):1226–55.
94. Dinnes CR, Hux K. Informal written language analysis methods: case examples of adults with traumatic brain injury. Am J Speech Lang Pathol. 2022;31(1):203–20.
95. Dinnes C, Hux K. A multicomponent writing intervention for a college student with mild brain injury. Commun Disord Q. 2018;39(4):490–500.
96. Dinnes CR, Hux K. Perceptions about writing by adults with moderate or severe traumatic brain injury. Am J Speech Lang Pathol. 2022;31(2):838–53.
97. VanSolkema M, McCann C, Barker-Collo S, Foster A. Attention and communication following TBI: making the connection through a meta-narrative systematic review. Neuropsychol Rev. 2020;30(3):345–61.
98. Henderson A, Roeschlein MA, Wright HH. Improving discourse following traumatic brain injury: a tale of two treatments. Semin Speech Lang. 2020;41(5):365–82.
99. Hartley LL, Jensen PJ. Narrative and procedural discourse after closed head injury. Brain Inj. 1991;5(3):267–85.
100. Youse KM, Coelho CA. Working memory and discourse production abilities following closed-head injury. Brain Inj. 2005;19(12):1001–9.
101. Moran CA, Nippold MA, Gillon GT. Working memory and proverb comprehension in adolescents with traumatic brain injury: a preliminary investigation. Brain Inj. 2006;20(4):417–23.
102. Turkstra LS, Holland AL. Assessment of syntax after adolescent brain injury: effects of memory on test performance. J Speech Lang Hear Res. 1998;41(1):137–49.
103. Barbey AK, Colom R, Grafman J. Neural mechanisms of discourse comprehension: a human lesion study. Brain J Neurol. 2014;137(1):277–87.
104. Le K, Coelho C, Mozeiko J, Krueger F, Grafman J. Predicting story goodness performance from cognitive measures following traumatic brain injury. Am J Speech Lang Pathol. 2012;21(2):S115–25.
105. Coelho CA, Liles BZ, Duffy RJ. Impairments of discourse abilities and executive functions in traumatically brain-injured adults. Brain Inj. 1995;9(5):471–7.
106. Snow P, Douglas J, Ponsford J. Conversational discourse abilities following severe traumatic brain injury: a follow-up study. Brain Inj. 1998;12(11):911–35.
107. Mozeiko J, Le K, Coelho C, Krueger F, Grafman J. The relationship of story grammar and executive function following TBI. Aphasiology. 2011;25(6–7):826–35.
108. Gernsbacher MA. Language comprehension as structure building. Psychology Press; 1990.
109. Gernsbacher MA, Tallent KA, Bolliger CM. Disordered discourse in schizophrenia described by the structure building framework. Discourse Stud. 1999;1(3):355–72.

110. Ramírez-Esparza N, Pennebaker JW. Do good stories produce good health? Exploring words, language, and culture. Narrat Inq. 2006;16(1):211–9.
111. Bryant L, Ferguson A, Spencer E. Linguistic analysis of discourse in aphasia: a review of the literature. Clin Linguist Phon. 2016;30(7):489–518.
112. Koebli JR, Balasubramanian V, Zipp GP. An exploration of higher-level language comprehension deficits and factors influencing them following blast TBI in US veterans. Brain Inj. 2020;34(5):630–41.
113. Combs HL, Berry DT, Pape T, Babcock-Parziale J, Smith B, Schleenbaker R, et al. The effects of mild traumatic brain injury, post-traumatic stress disorder, and combined mild traumatic brain injury/post-traumatic stress disorder on returning veterans. J Neurotrauma. 2015;32(13):956–66.
114. Myers JR, Solomon NP, Lange RT, French LM, Lippa SM, Brickell TA, et al. Analysis of discourse production to assess cognitive communication deficits following mild traumatic brain injury with and without posttraumatic stress. Am J Speech Lang Pathol. 2022;31(1):84–98.
115. Sullivan MP, Griffiths GG, Moore SM. Effect of posttraumatic stress on study time in a task measuring four component processes underlying text-level reading. J Speech Lang Hear Res. 2014;57(5):1731–9.
116. Sloan DM, Thompson-Hollands J, Hayes AM, Lee DJ, Alpert E, Marx BP. Sudden gains in two trauma-focused treatments for posttraumatic stress disorder. Behav Ther. 2022;53(2):255–66.
117. Vrana SR, Bono RS, Konig A, Scalzo GC. Assessing the coherence of narratives of traumatic events with latent semantic analysis. Psychol Trauma. 2019;11(5):521–4.
118. Foa EB, Molnar C, Cashman L. Change in rape narratives during exposure therapy for posttraumatic stress disorder. J Trauma Stress. 1995;8(4):675–90.
119. Sayer NA, Noorbaloochi S, Frazier PA, Pennebaker JW, Orazem RJ, Schnurr PP, et al. Randomized controlled trial of online expressive writing to address readjustment difficulties among U.S. Afghanistan and Iraq War Veterans. J Trauma Stress. 2015;28(5):381–90.
120. Lê K, Coelho C, Fiszdon J. Systematic review of discourse and social communication interventions in traumatic brain injury. Am J Speech Lang Pathol. 2022;31(2):991–1022.

Karen Lê, Ph.D., CCC-SLP, is a research and clinical speech-language pathologist in the VA Connecticut Healthcare System and serves on the Polytrauma Support Clinic Team. She completed her Ph.D. at the University of Connecticut. Her research interests encompass discourse ability following traumatic brain injury (TBI), clinically feasible discourse assessment tools, discourse intervention, and relationships between TBI comorbidities and cognitive-communicative functioning. Her research has been funded by the National Institutes of Health, National Institute on Deafness and Other Communication Disorders, and the U.S. Department of Veterans Affairs, Veterans Health Administration, Office of Research and Development, Rehabilitation Research and Development Service.

Carl Coelho Ph.D., BC-ANCDS, is Professor Emeritus and former Department Head of the Speech, Language, and Hearing Sciences Department at the University of Connecticut. Prior to beginning his academic career, he worked as a clinician and department director of speech-language pathology and audiology in rehabilitation hospitals. His research on cognitive-communication disorders has been published in numerous journal articles and chapters. Dr. Coelho is a Fellow of the American Speech-Language-Hearing Association.

Spoken Discourse Production Following Right Hemisphere Damage

6

Ronelle Hewetson and Petrea Cornwell

Preview of What Is Currently Known
Spoken discourse can be disrupted at multiple levels leading to changes that impact the lives of people with right hemisphere damage (RHD). "He seems to go well with old friends but add their partners to the mix with unfamiliar topics and he is lost. He then tends to just change the topic and can say embarrassing things." Some of the impairments that occur following RHD related to discourse meaning, appropriateness, cohesion, and efficiency are evident in this quote from the partner of a person with RHD. This chapter summarizes the current and emerging evidence related to spoken discourse impairments in people with RHD. It also emphasizes the need for future research to adopt standardized approaches to assessing discourse in this population to support work that aims to establish profiles of impairment, or subtypes, and establishing intervention efficacy.

Objectives
(a) To define the scope of spoken discourse within right hemisphere damage (RHD).
(b) To describe the presenting spoken discourse features following RHD.
(c) To discuss considerations related to assessment of spoken discourse post-RHD.
(d) To highlight the impact of spoken discourse deficits.

R. Hewetson (✉) · P. Cornwell
School of Health Sciences and Social Work, Griffith University, Gold Coast, QLD, Australia
e-mail: r.hewetson@griffith.edu.au; p.cornwell@griffith.edu.au

Introduction

Our understanding of the role the right hemisphere of the brain plays in the comprehension and production of language is in its relative infancy. First reports suggesting that right hemisphere damage (RHD) results in unique communication impairments compared to those caused by left hemisphere damage (LHD) emerged in the 1960s [1, 2]. Descriptions of communicative interactions with people with RHD paint a picture of someone disinterested, concrete, or literal in their use of language, verbose, and tangential, and unable to respond to or use emotion in conversations [3]. These post-injury communication changes occur in more complex linguistic constructs such as discourse and pragmatics despite deceptively normal foundation linguistic skills (e.g., phonology, morphology, and syntax) [2, 4].

Communication is more than the words and sentences we produce to express our thoughts and ideas; it is an interactive, complex task reliant on discourse and pragmatic abilities [5]. Pragmatics refers to the context-determined use of linguistic, paralinguistic, and extralinguistic skills during communicative interactions, while

A. P.-H. Kong (ed.), *Spoken Discourse Impairments in the Neurogenic Populations*,
https://doi.org/10.1007/978-3-031-45190-4_6

discourse draws on a person's ability to sequentially and logically convey or comprehend linguistic content beyond the level of the sentence [5, 6]. There is a close relationship between these concepts, with intact pragmatics being fundamental to meaningful and appropriate spoken discourse [7]. A multitude of meanings from various fields of study exist for the term discourse, but the ensuing discussion will draw on a multidisciplinary framework incorporating the fields of linguistic, cognitive, and social sciences. Discourse is a multilevel representation of our thoughts situated within a given context (genre). A meaningful, appropriate, cohesive, and efficient spoken discourse utilizes cognitive strategies to organize linguistic and interactional structures [8]. Discourse is multimodal with comprehension and production occurring in both spoken and written modalities. This chapter explores how spoken discourse in people with RHD is impaired considering context (genre), linguistic skills, and structural influences. An overview of assessment options to determine if spoken discourse is meaningful, appropriate, cohesive, and efficient in individuals with RHD is provided.

Heterogeneity of RHD Communication Presentation

The communication presentations of the RHD population are known to be heterogeneous and evident across communication domains of discourse, prosody, semantics, and pragmatics [5, 9]. The centrality of spoken discourse deficits, as a characteristic of communication disorder after RHD, is evident in four clinical communication profiles [9, 10]. Changes in narrative and/or conversational discourse production were evident, to different degrees, in three of the four profiles [10]. Differing discourse impairments across the four clinical profiles highlight the importance of considering discourse production abilities across discourse genres with several reports that the elicitation task, stimulus, and manner of analysis can impact the deficits that are identified [11–14]. On analysis across discourse genres, further heterogeneity is evident. Blake and colleagues [3] noted varying patterns of efficiency and appropriateness of spoken discourse in their hyperresponsive (e.g., verbosity, talkative, tangential, impulsive, disinhibited) and hyporesponsive (e.g., paucity of speech, slow responses, poor initiation, unelaborated speech) profiles. The prevalence rate of each profile was relatively equal at 41.5% and 39%, respectively, and replicated earlier findings of variation across different genres. Earlier work on discourse profiles on a descriptive task that analyzed the efficiency and appropriateness of content identified five patterns of discourse production: (1) irrelevant, (2) paucity, (3) digressive, (4) verbose, and (5) normal [15]. Additionally, in a study of narrative discourse, Joanette and colleagues [16] described two distinct profiles of production based on an analysis of informativeness.

Context in Spoken Discourse

Discourse grouping into different types or genres is based on "recurrent actions" [17 , p. 181] associated with a specific communication goal. These typified forms of discourse constitute the contextual level of spoken discourse. Discourse genres are goal-oriented social processes that have sets of conventions or expectations that inform not only the required elements but also the sequence of such elements [18]. There are four key discourse genres to consider when describing spoken discourse after RHD: procedural, descriptive, narrative, and conversational. The conventions for each genre are relatively stable and based on social life or nature of interpersonal interactions in a particular culture or historical time. For example, narratives may be identified based on the presence of typical parts such as an orientation, a complicating action, an evaluation, and a resolution [19]. Each of the discourse genres provides different contextual support for the speaker ranging from the relatively constrained tasks of procedural and descriptive discourse through narrative tasks to conversational discourse, which involves the interaction with at least one communication partner. Investigation of discourse production after RHD has led to an understanding that not only genre [20] but also method of elicitation including stimulus and instruction influence performance [13]. To explore further the types of genre and stimuli that have been used to elicit them, please refer to Appendix 1.

The following will summarize key points from our current understanding of how spoken discourse abilities differ across context (genres) after RHD with reference to the meaning, appropriateness, cohesion, and efficiency of output.

Exploring Meaningful, Appropriate, Cohesive, and Efficient Discourse Production

Meaningful

People with RHD have been described as producing concrete and literal discourse, which Myers [21] succinctly summarizes as they *talk better than they communicate*. This points towards people with RHD unsuccessfully imparting their intended meaning despite apparently intact linguistic skills. It is, however, acknowledged that the linguistic domain of semantics is often impaired in this population [10, 11]. In fact, multiple theories of semantic processing such as coarse coding, suppression deficit, and graded salience hypotheses have been proposed to explain difficulties in comprehension of meaning (see Blake [5] for an overview), yet the extension of these models to production of meaning occurs less frequently.

Conceptualizing the impact of semantic deficits on discourse production requires us to consider two sub-areas: lexical semantics and structural semantics. Lexical semantics focuses on the meaning of words considering the semantic features, fields, and ambiguity [22]. Structural semantics is how we create meaning at the level of the sentence including word order and grammatical markers. Early work seeking to explore the linguistic basis of communication breakdown after RHD explored the role of lexical-semantics in verbal output through picture naming [12, 23–25] and sentence completion tasks [2]. Significantly lower scores on picture naming were recorded for those with RHD compared to non-brain-damaged (NBD) people [12, 23, 24]. Despite beliefs that co-occurring visual neglect and visuoperceptual deficits were the cause of errors, error analysis identified a visuosemantic or semantic basis [24]. Furthermore, the complexity of the linguistic task influenced performance with generation of abstract concepts causing the most difficulty [2]. Divergent naming tasks have also shown that people with RHD perform significantly worse than controls [12, 26] with additional evidence of a task complexity effect [12]. These divergent naming studies highlighted that people with RHD used fewer strategies when completing the tasks which may reflect a disruption in cognitive processes rather than lexical deficit.

The relevance of findings at the single-word level to the structural semantics (i.e., meaning conveyed at sentence level) or spoken discourse production has rarely been investigated. The structural units within sentences (e.g., phrase, clause, or sentence) carry key content or information, thus playing a crucial role in expressing meaning. Examining links between lexical-semantics and structural semantics at the discourse level, Diggs and Basili [12] identified the number of message units conveyed by individuals with RHD across convergent and divergent discourse tasks. As with convergent and divergent naming tasks, units carrying informative content at the discourse level was significantly less than controls. They also found a task complexity effect mirroring early findings that discourse produced using an abstract stimulus was less informative (fewer message units) than for concrete stimuli [2].

Descriptions of the ability to convey meaning in spoken discourse have centered around the accuracy of these information units, with limited investigation of the lexical-semantic content (e.g., concrete versus abstract words). To date, information on the use of vocabulary to convey meaning in discourse is limited; however, people with RHD are less likely to include emotional content [27]. Limited research has also been conducted to describe discourse production based on communication profiles. The absence of literature documenting discourse production based on profiles perhaps not surprisingly has resulted in mixed findings. Some studies have reported that people with RHD are able to include the essential steps for a procedural discourse as one way of considering task accuracy [20, 28], but others have found the opposite [29, 30]. These latter findings align with accuracy ratings for procedural discourse when using correct information units (CIUs) [20, 28], main concept analysis (MCA) [31], and inclusion of unnecessary or irrelevant detail as the measures [32, 33] with people with RHD less accurate in conveying meaning. This same inaccuracy in meaningfulness has been noted in narrative discourse using story generation stimuli [11, 13, 20, 31].

Appropriate

Appropriate discourse production is linked to how meaningful content is organized to achieve a communication goal. Different constructs such as the genre structure (e.g., story grammar), relevance of content to the topic (global coherence), and use of interactional structures (e.g., providing or taking turns) contribute to the perception of appropriate discourse. The inclusion of off-topic comments, responding in ways that did not align with questions posed, and failing to follow turn-taking conventions during conversations are examples of difficulties with appropriate discourse reported following RHD [7, 34].

Global Coherence

Discourse described as tangential, unrelated, or egocentric likely contributes to problems with topic maintenance reflecting breakdown at the level of global coherence. Considering conversational discourse, topic maintenance and turn-taking quantity were impaired in 40% and 50% of a group of ten people with RHD, respectively [35]. Other studies have reinforced this finding of heterogeneity where global coherence was not an issue for all individuals with RHD at a conversational discourse level. In Kennedy's study, approximately a quarter of individuals with RHD included off-topic or misplaced content [36, 37], while Brady and colleagues observed the use of meta-statements (comment on the topic, about the task, or task performance) and topic shading (relevant antidote or personal opinion) as issues of global coherence [37].

Procedural, descriptive, and picture sequence-based narrative discourse tasks provide greater constraints around structure and topics to be discussed. Task constraints have been proposed as an explanation to the absence of issues with topic coherence and management across these genres [28]. As with much of the literature on communication after RHD, there is however variation in reports of how global coherence is impacted at the group versus individual level. Despite topic maintenance being essentially intact during procedural and descriptive discourse, Brady and colleagues noted differences when examining how topic maintenance occurred. In comparison to NBD individuals, people with RHD used either an increased number of modalizing fillers (i.e., personal comments, or comments about the task) or fewer utterances per topic due to failure to introduce subtopics to continue the broad topic of discussion. Kim and colleagues [38] in a structured conversation task similarly noted that people with RHD were less likely to add related content to the conversation, rather than changing to a new topic. The result of using modalizing fillers would be discourse that could be perceived as overly personalized or inappropriate for the context. Failing to extend conversation on a topic might make the speaker appear disengaged or bored with the topic which is a characteristic reported in the RHD population. Using the Global Coherence Rating Scale (GCRS) [39], Minga and colleagues [31] found that people with RHD presented with global coherence deficits that were significantly below those of NBD individuals on a procedural task and approaching significance on story generation, although the error profiles were quite different across tasks. Approximately one-third of people with RHD produced a procedural discourse marked by content unrelated to the stimuli, tangential or egocentric information, while for the narrative task, the same issues were only evident in around 17%.

Adhering to Expected Genre Structure

Conventions that underpin the structures used to produce discourse across discourse genres vary, are dependent on the speaker's knowledge of societal expectations of the task, and are reliant on different cognitive and linguistic skills [40]. Narrative and conversational discourses both have consistent structures and expectations; however, procedural and descriptive structures are less clear and dependent on individual task instructions [13, 40].

Narrative discourse generally consists of three elements such as the setting, complicating event, and resolution. Difficulty in aspects of the narrative structure may result in a loss of meaning and coherence. The accuracy or completeness of narrative elements has been explored in people with RHD on a story generation task with varying results. Impairments were found in the complicating event only [16], the resolution component only, or both elements leading to discourse being evaluated as inaccurate or confused [41]. Conversational discourse also tends to contain three broad elements: the initiation phase, topic maintenance, and termination phase [36]. Similar to the narrative discourse findings, it has been suggested that structural components of conversational discourse are retained after RHD, but where the emphasis is placed in the conversation may differ. Observations have shown inequal production of content in the topic maintenance and termination phases when compared to NBD individuals [36]. Little to no literature has focused on adherence to the structural frameworks for procedural and descriptive discourse, most likely due to lack of clarity around expectations.

Interactional Level

The appropriateness of discourse may also be determined at an interactional level by analyzing interactional structures that allow for or signal opportunities for recipient contributions. Impairments at an interactional level would be most evident in conversational discourse; however, it might also be seen during other genres. During story production, we would expect to see evidence that the listener understands that a particular cue will signal the end of the story and to wait for the speaker to complete the story before taking their own turn. Beyond these contextualizing cues that signal turn change, we can also consider self- and other-repair strategies when analyzing interactional level difficulties.

There is an order to interactional sequences that includes turn construction and expansions of turns [42]. A turn constructional unit (TCU) [43] consists of grammar, prosody, and action that allows speakers to anticipate completion of a turn to achieve smooth transitions in discourse. Speakers and listeners use and interpret linguistic (e.g., the use of a personal name), paralinguistic (e.g., rising intonation to signal a question), and extralinguistic (e.g., gaze directed to a particular individual during small group conversations) to signal that a turn should be taken. Normative expectations associated with well-known actions exist such as greetings in the initiation phase of a conversation [44]. Most spontaneous interactions beyond structured sequences require a greater degree of processing of mutually communicated interactional structures. Inappropriate interactional structures may be evident when a failure of interpretation of and/or adjustment to interpersonal variables (such as conversational partner familiarity) and situational variables (such as the goal of the interaction) occurs.

Speech acts are verbal utterances that convey meaning and perform an action with an underlying intention and likely effect. Speech acts could be an apology, a complaint, a greeting, or a request. In a study of five people with RHD, it was found that three produced less explanatory supportive material and one more information than required compared to NBD individuals [45]. Failure to clarify, or excessive clarification of why a request is made, had a negative impact on the appropriateness and efficiency exchanges. Question-use is another TCU where individuals with RHD perform differently to NBD controls. Frequency of question use has been found to be significantly reduced [46], while Minga and colleagues [47] noted different patterns of question use on an unfamiliar object task, with the RHD group using more content questions (what/where) and fewer polar (yes/no) questions than control participants.

Repair strategies are efforts made to counter problems in signaling or taking a communication turn, which can be initiated within the same turn or after, by the speaker (self-initiated) or listener (other-initiated), and similarly resolved by either self-repair or communication partner repair [48]. Communication breakdown patterns and repair strategies of individuals with RHD have not received much research attention. In one study, a conversational breakdown index was used with 11 individuals with RHD to analyze performance on a structured conversational discourse task [38]. Individuals with RHD had higher rates of conversation overlap (one partner interferes with the other's turn) than NBD individuals. Findings from an examination of 112 individuals with RHD using the Protocole Montréal d'Evaluation de la Communication (Protocole MEC) [49] revealed that conversational discourse, together with aprosodia, is the most frequent impairment highlighting the importance of assessing this genre including the use of interactional structures [9].

Cohesive

Cohesion in spoken discourse is achieved when a speaker not only produces the correct words within a syntactically correct sentence but also ensures reference to previously introduced content to support the listener in making accurate connections between sentences [6]. In examining cohesion within discourse, we look for the use of words such as conjunctions (and, but), demonstrative (this, that), personal (he, together), and lexical (e.g., the cat) referents that create a link across sentences [6]. Evidence suggests that individuals with RHD use similar numbers of complete cohesive ties to their NBD and LHD counterparts; however, the type or patterns of use differ [6, 11, 13, 50]. Cognitive and linguistic skills together have been proposed as integral to achieving cohesion in discourse, with Balaban and colleagues [50] finding a potential relationship between theory of mind and referential cohesion difficulties. Their finding links to previous proposals that social cognitive theory offers one explanation for some of the communication changes after RHD (see Blake [5] for an overview).

Discourse cohesion relates to how words or phrases are used across sentence; therefore, it could be suggested that syntactic level deficits may play a role. Research to date has failed to identify syntactic deficits in people with RHD [13] including those with diagnosed impaired cohesion [51]. People with RHD tend to use shorter sentences during discourse production [6]; however, the number of cohesive markers was comparative to both NBD and LHD groups [6, 11, 13]. Different patterns in use of cohesive markers are noted with a tendency in the RHD group to use lexical markers to create cohesive ties, while those with LHD use conjunctions or personal pronouns [6]. Overuse of lexical markers would be considered an error in cohesive tie contributing to a perception of excessive detail where other cohesive markers would suffice. People with RHD made significantly more cohesive errors than NBD individuals in narrative discourse based on story retell [6, 11] but not story generation using picture stimuli [11]. Again, these findings highlight the importance of choice of discourse elicitation method and analysis in the assessment of the RHD population.

Efficient

Hypo- and hyper-responsive discourse patterns have been identified in people with RHD alluding to impairment at an efficiency level of spoken discourse production. To examine efficiency, we should consider time and quantity of content. Examples of time-based efficiency measures include total length of sample in minutes, syllables per minute, and content units per minute, while quantity-based measures might include total number of words and syllables per content unit.

Limited information is available on time-based efficiency measures with significantly more research focus dedicated to quantity. With regard to *time*, Minga and colleagues [31] analyzed performance of a single individual with RHD and found that overall words per minute were above an NBD control group on a narrative discourse task. Despite findings of the ability to produce many words in a specified time, producing accurate content in a timely manner (correct information units per minute: CIU/min) was significantly reduced following RHD compared to NBD controls on narrative discourse [20, 52].

Efficiency measures looking at *quantity* of content have shown mixed results across discourse genres, with early studies finding RHD speakers to be less efficient than controls based on total syllable/word count, lower numbers of content units (CUs), or more syllables required to produce essential content (SyllCU) [12, 15]. A greater number of syllables per content unit found during a descriptive discourse task (Cookie Theft) was associated with topic digressions and tangential content in one subgroup and replicated in another study on the same picture (Cookie Theft) [15, 51]. Discourse genre or elicitation method may be contributing to variation in reported findings. Only a potentially emotive personal narrative resulted in substantially longer samples in RHD participants than controls, while sample lengths were comparable across groups on procedural and narrative tasks using picture sequences [30]. Berube and colleagues [52] reported a significant group difference on total syllables on the Modern Cookie Theft picture descriptive discourse task for a large sample of individuals with acute RHD compared to NBD controls. Within the RHD group, impaired quantity of information occurred with varying frequency seen in lower total syllables (28%) and lower CUs (45%), while an abnormally high quantity of content or verbosity (syllCU) was seen in 19% of the RHD participants [52]. The presence of potential clinical subgroups is highlighted by such patterns of either verbosity/digressiveness or paucity of verbal output [15, 52].

A different pattern of efficiency was found on narrative discourse where quantity, using total number of words, was similar between people with RHD and NBD controls and between RHD and LHD groups [20, 50]. While individuals with RHD produced a comparable total number of words to NBD controls on a narrative task using an abstract stimulus (where participants were instructed to suppose they are living in the world where only feet are visible through dense fog), RHD participants' productions were considered insufficient in meaning units and due to inclusion of nonessential content [12]. Similarly, although total number of words and T units did not distinguish between an RHD and control group on a sequential image narrative task, a significant difference was found when considering the inclusion of essential content, with the RHD group producing fewer core or essential pieces of information [16].

Assessment of Spoken Discourse in RHD

The heterogeneous presentation of communication post-RHD and the multidimensional nature of discourse require assessment to be comprehensive with inclusion of a range of tools and tasks. A comprehensive assessment will support differential diagnosis and provide specific guidance on treatment targets. As noted by Tompkins [53 , p. 120], cognitive impairments that often co-occur with communication impairments following RHD necessitate an assessment approach that gathers information across genres representing varying levels of complexity—"Multiple narrative discourse samples, elicited with multiple methods, will help provide a complete picture of patients' abilities, especially since deficits in perceptual, attentional, or memorial domains may confound performance on any single elicitation task." An account of these co-occurring and contributing factors is beyond the scope of this chapter—the reader is referred to Blake [54]. This section considers assessment tools and tasks that have been used to diagnose and describe spoken discourse in those with RHD with a particular focus on aspects of discourse discussed in the preceding sections.

In the field of speech-language pathology, the assessment of discourse after an acquired brain injury may involve gathering samples of different discourse genres followed by quantification of linguistic elements, and determining if discourse is efficient and effective in meeting contextual requirements. Some tasks (such as descriptive discourse) may use a standard picture, offering a consistent referent, thus enabling quantification and comparison against normative data. However, such highly constrained tasks may not identify impairments across all genres, notably in those that place higher cognitive demand on the speaker such as conversations. Blake [54] described a myriad of measures (e.g., productivity, coherence, cohesion, content, structure, appropriateness, and pragmatics), using a variety of tasks including storytelling, picture description, procedural discourse, and conversation being used in clinical practice. As highlighted in this chapter, research seeking to describe spoken discourse in the RHD population has failed to find consistent deficits across discourse genres likely due to the existence of subgroups or profiles [9, 37] highlighting the need to consider what discourse assessment should look like in clinical practice. The Protocole MEC assesses two discourse genres: conversational and narrative [49], and through its application to the RHD population, four clinical profiles of communication have emerged with three including impairment in discourse production [9]. A standard assessment battery has until recently not been present that would ensure that all aspects of discourse known to be impaired in this population were systematically evaluated. In the absence of standardized approaches, speech-language pathologists have relied on clinical judgement and opinion of what normal performance might look like in discourse [55]. The establishment of RHDBank (https://rhd.talkbank.org) in 2015 was motivated by the need to systematically evaluate discourse. RHDBank consists of a standard protocol representing different genres with recommended analyses drawing on previously established protocols and methods [31].

An important overarching consideration when evaluating spoken discourse is the premorbid abilities of the person with RHD. Achievement of a shared meaning or communication outcome through discourse should be evaluated beyond structure and content, incorporating information on appropriateness and efficiency from a communication partner's perspective. Consequently, comprehensive discourse assessment warrants inclusion of information drawn from communication partners based on communication occurring in naturalistic settings to supplement clinician observations. Clinical experts in a study supporting the development of a screening assessment for the RHD population rated communication partner rating of conversational discourse as more important than clinician evaluation of procedural and narrative discourse [56]. Based on family report using the Communicative Effectiveness Index [57], supplemented by five items relevant to RHD, a quarter of people with RHD had impaired discourse abilities [58]. Participating in a fast conversation with multiple communication partners was the most frequently identified communication impairment by family members [58]. Replication of discourse production in a fast-paced group conversation in most clinical contexts creates challenges, highlighting the need to support clinical discourse assessment with either naturalistic observation or informant report. Examples of assessment tasks and analyses that have been used to describe spoken discourse post-RHD are provided in Appendix 2.

Throughout this chapter, we highlighted how different analysis methods have been used to describe spoken discourse production of people with RHD as meaningful, appropriate, cohesive, and efficient. Clinically, we may be tempted to make judgements about "normality" of someone's discourse. It is worth noting that while a clinician's judgement of impairment after RHD is relatively accurate in highly deviant samples, accuracy reduced for individuals with milder changes or where other relevant factors such as age of the individual were not considered [55]. To diagnose discourse impairment and inform treatment planning, it is imperative that a systematic approach be undertaken which might incorporate a structural approach by analyzing the constituents of discourse or a functional approach focusing on the information conveyed [59]. The nature of impairments seen in spoken discourse after RHD summarized to date suggests that analysis that focuses on informativeness, global coherence, use of cohesive markers, and efficiency appears particularly relevant. Discourse informative measures examine the meaning of discourse by quantifying the amount of information relayed. Analysis can be undertaken using measures such as correct information units (CIUs) or by recording the presence of main concepts or propositions [60]. Measures of efficiency seek to determine whether the speaker uses too much, too little, or just the right amount of content to be considered. It needs to be noted that the evaluation of efficiency such as quantity of information produced, without inclusion of significant other input on pre-injury communication style, might result in false positives or false negatives [55]. Global coherence analysis examines the speaker's ability to organize discourse and to maintain the theme, which could be analyzed using a tool such as the 4-Point Global Coherence Rating Scale [31, 39]. At a conversational level, an analysis of TCUs holds value. Tools can be grouped across action (normative expectation), design (use of prosody to signal a question), allocation (active selection of next speaker), and embodiment (positioning, gaze towards a recipient) [44]. Beyond determining the presence or absence of a TCU, consideration should also be given to whether use was timely or delayed, appropriate or misaligned with the interactional requirements.

Summary and Future Directions

Undoubtedly, consensus exists that discourse-level impairments develop for some individuals after RHD and, importantly, such impairments are not uniform for those affected and vary across discourse genres. At present, many studies include participants based on the presence of RHD irrespective of lesion site and size, diagnosis of communication change, or profile of communication impairment. Moving forward, it is imperative that a diagnosis of communication impairment is confirmed, and specific communication profiles are considered when investigating the existence, characteristics and impact of discourse deficits. Additionally, use of a systematic approach to discourse assessment and analysis, utilizing normative data, will progress the field to more effectively support people who have communication impairment after RHD. As Mackenzie suggested, it is not possible to appropriately recommend intervention without knowledge of normality [61]. Furthermore, the lack of clarity around the basis of discourse deficits, in particular the role of co-occurring cognitive impairment, in this population has led to a relative dearth of evidence to guide clinicians on intervention.

Preserved discourse ability is important for long-term outcomes following an acquired brain injury, but to date, there have been limited reports about the impacts of communication impairment after RHD. Literature focused on the traumatic brain injury population found moderate disability arising in those with communication disorder, with conversational discourse being predictive of social outcomes inclusive of return-to-work success [62]. While the presence of communication impairment after RHD has been shown to be predictive of poor social participation, most notably in maintaining interpersonal relationships, the exact role of spoken discourse impairments is unknown [63]. Furthermore, there is evidence that many people with communication difficulties after RHD are not identified during hospital stays [3] and not referred for speech-language pathology services in the community [64]. Ongoing work to categorize the discourse profiles of this population and standardized approaches to diagnosing the communication impairment that occurs subsequent to RHD is important to ensure that the *right* rehabilitation is received.

Major Takeaways

1. Spoken discourse impairments exist in people with RHD, and access to speech-language pathology services for assessment and management should be provided.
2. Comprehensive assessment of RHD requires elicitation of spoken discourse across genres.
3. Analysis of spoken discourse needs to incorporate measures targeted to address concerns related to meaning, appropriateness, cohesion, and efficiency.

4. Further exploration of spoken discourse after RHD with detailed assessments is required to progress our understanding of communication and discourse profiles.

Appendix 1. Overview of Discourse Genres

A *procedural discourse* is a form of expository discourse that is generally brief with a specific focus on explaining how something is done in a chronological or logical order [65]. The cognitive-linguistic demands of this discourse genre relate to its purpose to inform or instruct, which consequently influences its structure and cohesion characteristics [66]. Elicitation procedures for procedural discourse usually involve asking the speaker to explain either a simple or a complex everyday task such as how to make a sandwich, although modifications to this are required based on cultural considerations.

Descriptive discourse, a further form of expository discourse, centers around presenting information (e.g., outlining facts, properties, or functions) about a referent such as an object or a picture. A picture description task is commonly used in clinical practice to elicit this genre [67]. The generic structure of verbal output required for this type of task is sensitive to the use of cohesive ties but less clear than for narrative discourse [66]. The most reported picture used to elicit a descriptive discourse for research purposes is the Cookie Theft (CT) [68] with Berube and colleagues [52] updating the image to remove outdated biases and is known as the Modern Cookie Theft (MCT) picture.

Narrative discourse involves conveying an experience or a series of events as a story. The elicitation of narrative discourse can be undertaken across two broad approaches: story retell and story generation. Many different instructions and stimuli are used for story generation, e.g., generating a story about a personal experience, using pre-ordered picture sequences versus unordered pictures, and concrete versus abstract images. Compared to picture-based discourse tasks, personal narratives are considered more representative of spontaneous communication [69]. The cognitive processing demands for the different tasks should be considered in interpreting the discourse produced. As an example, telling a story based on a series of novel images requires interpretation of each image and integration across the images to formulate a coherent narrative, as opposed to generating a story about a single static image.

Conversational discourse. Levelt [70] highlighted aspects that are key to the nature of conversation, that a conversation is an interaction between speakers with a particular purpose. In most conversations, there is an interdependence as one person's contributions are based not only on what has been said previously but also on the verbal and nonverbal contributions made by conversational partner(s). Conversations occur in multiple settings, be that email exchanges, telephone calls, or intake interviews in a hospital setting. Each of these conversational settings will require slightly different skills. As an example, turn sequences are faster paced during face-to-face conversations and highly reliant on in-the-moment interpretation and revision than during asynchronous email conversations [71]. Despite variation in planning, timing, and revision across conversational settings, all conversations are assumed to be organized along principles that allows conversational partners to achieve a common purpose through sequences of actions such as a question-answer sequence [72].

Appendix 2. Example Assessment Tools and Task Used in the Literature to Diagnose Impaired Verbal Discourse Post-RHD

Task/tool	Task overview and citation examples	*Analysis*: method (source/protocol listed if stated)
Procedural discourse		
How to change a lightbulb/make your favorite sandwich [73]?	The person is asked to describe how they would change a lightbulb or make their favorite sandwich [28, 75]	*Appropriate*: Topic introduction and maintenance [74], macro- and micro-level analyses of topic use, e.g., % on-topic, off-topic, and intrusive utterances [75]
How would you change a tire/ replace the glass in a window/ teach someone to ride a bike [6]?	The person, who is not familiar with the task in the absence of visual stimuli, is asked to describe how to, e.g., change a tire [31, 70]	*Appropriate*: Relevance [76], discourse grammar [69], cohesion [77] *Efficient*: Total words, mean T-unit length, clarity disruptors (e.g., empty phrases, repeated words) [69]
How to make a peanut butter and jelly sandwich [47]?	The person is asked to describe how he/she would make a peanut butter and jelly sandwich [31, 48]	*Appropriate*: Global coherence [47], main concept analysis (MCA) [60]
Descriptive discourse		
Concrete: Descriptive Cookie theft picture [68]	After being shown a black-and-white line drawing, the person is asked to tell the examiner everything that he/she sees happening in the picture [6]	*Meaningful*: Content units [78], MCA [79] *Appropriate*: Cohesive ties—Adequacy and count [80] *Efficient*: Word count [79], content units/minute [78]
Concrete: Descriptive Modern cookie theft picture [81]	After being shown a color line drawing, the person is asked to tell the examiner everything that he/she sees happening in the picture [52]	*Meaningful*: Total content units (if included in discourse produced by at least three healthy controls) [81] *Efficient*: Total number of syllables (Syll count), SyllCU [81] *Other*: Left/right CUs (LRCU) to explore the impact of neglect [52, 81]
Abstract: Descriptive/problem solution Just suppose activity from the Torrance test of creative thinking [82]	After being shown a picture of fog covering the world with only feet visible, the person is asked to consider how life might change and what would happen if this picture represented the world [12]	*Meaningful:* Number of information units [12] *Efficient:* Total number of words [12] *Other:* Divergent thinking [12]
Narrative discourse		
Personal narrative Personal experience narratives [69]	The person is asked to tell the examiner about a frightening/ embarrassing/happy/funny experience that he/she has had at any time in their life [30, 70]	*Appropriate*: Clausal structures, relevance [76], number and types of cohesive ties *Efficient*: Length in total words, T-unit length

Task/tool	Task overview and citation examples	*Analysis*: method (source/protocol listed if stated)
Story generation with one composite image Cat Rescue picture [83]	While shown a black-and-white line drawing, the person is instructed to look at everything that is happening and to tell a story with a beginning, a middle, and an end of what they see [31, 47]	RHDBank discourse protocol [47] *Meaningful:* Communicative informativeness (CIU) [84], MCA [6, 79] *Cohesive*: Number or % of parts of speech/cohesive ties *Appropriate:* Story grammar components [85], global coherence [39] *Efficient:* Total words and words/minute [47]
Story generation with sequential visual stimuli Cinderella story [78]	After being encouraged to look at sequential visual stimuli from the Cinderella storybook, the person is asked to tell the Cinderella story in own words [20, 31]	RHDBank discourse protocol [47] *Meaningful:* Communicative informativeness (CIU) [84], MCA [6, 79] *Cohesive*: Number or % of parts of speech/cohesive ties *Appropriate:* Story grammar components [85], global coherence [39] *Efficient:* Total words and words/minute [47]
Story generation with sequential visual stimuli The cowboy story [16]	After being shown a black-and-white 8-frame drawing, the person is asked to tell a story about the 8 pictures [16]	*Meaningful:* Propositional analysis [86], core propositions [16] *Appropriate*: Story grammar [87] *Efficient:* T-units [16]
Story generation with sequential visual stimuli Six picture sequences depicting a father and his son	After being shown a picture sequence, the person is asked to tell a story about the father and son that is seen in the picture sequence [70]	*Appropriate*: Relevance [76], discourse grammar [69], cohesion [77] *Efficient*: Total words, mean T-unit length, clarity disruptors (e.g., empty phrases, repeated words) [69]
Story generation Old McDonald had an apartment house [88]	After being shown a 16-frame story sequence, the person is asked to tell a story [91]	*Appropriate*: Macrostructural, coherence, and superstructural (story grammar) *Cohesive*: Microlinguistic, microstructural, intersentential cohesion
Story generation with 13 sets of pictures, each representing a situation (e.g., a boy picking flowers) and its development (giving them to his mother) [20]	The pictures are placed side by side, one pair at a time, and the person is asked to tell the examiner what is happening in the first picture and then how the story ends based on the second picture [20]	*Meaningful*: Microlinguistic analysis, e.g., % lexical informativeness *Appropriate*: Macrolinguistic analysis, e.g., % global coherence errors *Efficient*: Number of words, MLU
Story retell MEC [89]	Task 1: a story is read out, one paragraph at a time, with the person asked to retell it. Task 2: Then the person retells the story again, this time in its entirety [89]	*Meaningful*: MCA [79] with comparison against norms across age and years of education *Appropriate*: Qualitative observations of appropriateness and story grammar *Efficient*: Qualitative observations of efficiency
Conversational discourse		
Semi-structured Topic structured clinical conversation [90]	10-minute topic-directed interview in which three topics are introduced as open-ended questions [75]	*Appropriate*: Verbal disruption; cohesion [90]; topic coherence [74] *Efficient*: Number of words, total time

Task/tool	Task overview and citation examples	*Analysis*: method (source/protocol listed if stated)
Semi-structured Hallym conversation and pragmatics Protocol [38]	Three topics are sequentially introduced, supported by associated picture stimuli, and followed by open-ended questions [38]	*Appropriate*: Conversational participation index [38] (#turns, #utterances/turn); topic manipulation index [38] (#topics, #turns/topic, % topics initiated, % topics maintained, % topics switched), conversational breakdown index [38] (% overlap, % discontinuance)
Unstructured First encounter conversation with a stranger [46]	After being introduced to an unfamiliar person and instructed that it is not an interview, the person is told to get to know the stranger [31, 46]	*Appropriate:* Interactional level—Conversational turn-taking skills, e.g., frequency of introducing, maintaining, or terminating a topic [42]; turn construction units, e.g., question asking [47]
Unstructured Conversation with assessor (e.g., D-MEC conversation discourse subtest: MEC) [89]	Ten-minute conversation with assessor on everyday topics [95]	*Appropriate*: Scales of conversational parameters that are present/absent, e.g., initiation, turn taking, topic maintenance, intonation, eye contact
Informant report Communication screening questionnaire [89, 91]	14-item questionnaire that can be administered as an interview [97]	*Appropriate*: Rating scales of conversational parameters scored as present or not by significant other
Unstructured with familiar communication partner	Evaluation of a recorded conversation with a familiar communication partner [98, 99]	*Appropriate:* Conversational analysis (CA) to identify impairments at an interactional level [92]

Note: This table is not intended to be a comprehensive summary of prior literature or assessment tools; rather, it offers examples of assessment tasks and analyses/methods across discourse genres

References

1. Critchley M. Speech and speech-loss in relation to duality of the brain. In: Mountcastle VB, editor. Interhemispheric relations and cerebral dominance. Baltimore: John Hopkins Press; 1962. p. 208–13.
2. Eisenson J. Language and intellectual modifications associated with right cerebral damage. Lang Speech. 1962;5(2):49–53.
3. Blake ML, Duffy JR, Myers PS, Tompkins CA. Prevalence and patterns of right hemisphere cognitive/communicative deficits: retrospective data from an inpatient rehabilitation unit. Aphasiology. 2002;16(4–6):537–47.
4. Wapner W, Hamby S, Gardner H. The role of the right hemisphere in the apprehension of complex linguistics materials. Brain Lang. 1981;14(1):15–33.
5. Blake ML. Communication deficits associated with right hemisphere brain damage. In: Damico JS, Muller N, Ball MJ, editors. The handbook of language and speech disorders. 1st ed. Oxford: John Wiley & Sons Ltd.; 2021. p. 571–89.
6. Stockbridge MD, Berube S, Goldberg E, Suarez A, Mace R, Ubellacker D, et al. Differences in linguistic cohesion within the first year following right-and left-hemisphere lesions. Aphasiology. 2021;35(3):357–71.
7. García EL, Ferré P, Joanette Y. Right-hemisphere language disorders. In: Cummings L, editor. Handbook of pragmatic language disorders: complex and underserved populations. Cham, Switzerland: Springer; 2021. p. 313–34.
8. Van Dijk T. Discourse studies: a multidisciplinary introduction. 2nd ed. Thousand Oaks: Sage Publications; 2011.
9. Ferré P, Fonseca RP, Ska B, Joanette Y. Communicative clusters after a right-hemisphere stroke: are there universal clinical profiles? Folia Phoniatr Logop. 2012;64(4):199–207.
10. Ferré P, Joanette Y. Communication abilities following right hemisphere damage: prevalence, evaluation, and profiles. Perspect ASHA Spec Interest Groups. 2016;1(2):106–15.
11. Davis GA, O'Neil-Pirozzi TM, Coon M. Referential cohesion and logical coherence of narration after right hemisphere stroke. Brain Lang. 1997;56(2):183–210.
12. Diggs CC, Basili AG. Verbal expression of right cerebrovascular accident patients: convergent and divergent language. Brain Lang. 1987;30(1):130–46.

13. Marini A, Carlomagno S, Caltagirone C, Nocentini U. The role played by the right hemisphere in the organization of complex textual structures. Brain Lang. 2005;93(1):46–54.
14. Ska B, Joanette Y. Discourse in older adults: influence of text, task, and participant characteristics. J Speech Lang Pathol Audiol. 1996;20:101–8.
15. Hillis Trupe E, Hillis A. Paucity vs. verbosity: another analysis of right hemisphere communication deficits. Clin Aphasiology. 1985;15:83–96.
16. Joanette Y, Goulet P, Ska B, Nespoulous JL. Informative content of narrative discourse in right-brain-damaged right-handers. Brain Lang. 1986;29(1):81–105.
17. Johnstone B. Discourse analysis. 2nd ed. Maldon: Wiley Blackwell; 2008.
18. Rose D, Martin JR. Learning to write, reading to learn: genre, knowledge and pedagogy in the Sydney school. London: Equinox; 2012.
19. Hodges A. Intertextuality in discourse. In: Tannen D, Hamilton HE, Schiffrin D, editors. The handbook of discourse analysis. Oxford: John Wiley & Sons; 2015.
20. Bartels-Tobin LR, Hinckley JJ. Cognition and discourse production in right hemisphere disorder. J Neurolinguistics. 2005;18(6):461–77.
21. Myers PS. Profiles of communication deficits in patients with right cerebral hemisphere damage: implications for diagnosis and treatment. In: Clinical aphasiology: proceedings of the conference; Minneapolis, Minn. 1979. p. 38–46.
22. McAllister J, Miller JE. Introductory linguistics for speech and language therapy practice. Hoboken: John Wiley & Sons; 2013.
23. Adamovich BL, Brooks RL. A diagnostic protocol to assess the communication deficits of patients with right hemisphere damage. In: Clinical aphasiology: proceedings of the conference; 1981. p. 244–53.
24. Gainotti G, Caltagirone C, Miceli G. Selective impairment of semantic-lexical discrimination in right-brain-damaged patients. In: Perecman E, editor. Cognitive processing in the right hemisphere. New York: Academic Press; 1983. p. 149–67.
25. Myers PS, Linebaugh CW. The perception of contextually conveyed relationships by right brain-damaged patients. In: A paper presented to the annual convention of the American Speech-Language-Hearing Association; 1980.
26. Varley R. Lexical-semantic deficits following right hemisphere damage: evidence from verbal fluency tasks. Int J Lang Commun Disord. 1995;30(3):362–71.
27. Bloom RL, Borod JC, Obler LK, Gerstman LJ. Discourse following right and left brain damage. J Speech Hear Res. 1983;36:1227–35.
28. Brady M, Armstrong L, Mackenzie C. Further evidence on topic use following right hemisphere brain damage: procedural and descriptive discourse. Aphasiology. 2005;19(8):731–47.
29. Hill C, Marquardt T. The effects of right cerebral hemisphere damage on communication effectiveness and speech and language performance. In: Clinical aphasiology conference; 2005.
30. Sherratt S, Bryan K. Discourse production after right brain damage: gaining a comprehensive picture using a multi-level processing model. J Neurolinguistics. 2012;25(4):213–39.
31. Minga J, Johnson M, Blake ML, Fromm D, McWhinney B. Making sense of right hemisphere discourse using RDHBank. Top Lang Disorders. 2021;41(1):99–122.
32. Cummings L. On making a sandwich: procedural discourse in adults with right-hemisphere damage. In: Further advances in pragmatics and philosophy: part 2 theories and applications. Springer; 2019. p. 331–55.
33. McDonald S. Exploring the cognitive basis of right-hemisphere pragmatic language disorders. Brain Lang. 2000;75(1):81–107.
34. Chantraine Y, Joanette Y, Ska B. Conversational abilities in patients with right hemisphere damage. J Neurolinguistics. 1998;11(1–2):21–32.
35. Prutting CA, Kittchner DM. A clinical appraisal of the pragmatic aspects of language. J Speech Lang Hear. 1987;52(2):105–19.
36. Kennedy MR. Topic scenes in conversations with adults with right-hemisphere brain damage. Am J Speech Lang Pathol. 2000;9(1):72–86.
37. Brady M, Mackenzie C, Armstrong L. Topic use following right hemisphere brain damage during three semi-structured conversational discourse samples. Aphasiology. 2003;17(9):881–904.
38. Kim YJ, Jeong HY, Choi HC, Sohn JH, Kim C, Lee SH, et al. Effect of right hemispheric damage on structured spoken conversation. PLoS One. 2022;17(8):e0271727.
39. Wright HH, Capilouto GJ, Koutsifras A. Evaluating measures of global coherence ability in stories in adults. Int J Lang Commun Disord. 2013;48(3):249–56.
40. Lundine J, McCauley RJ. A tutorial on expository discourse: structure, development and disorders in children and adolescents. Am J Speech Lang Pathol. 2016;25(3):306–20.
41. Sherratt SM, Penn C. Discourse in right-hemisphere brain-damaged subject. Aphasiology. 1990;4(6):539–60.
42. Ford CE. At the intersection of turn and sequence: negation and what comes next. In: Selting M, Couper-Kuhlen E, editors. Studies in interactional linguistics. J. Benjamins Pub; 2001.
43. Selting M. The construction of units in conversational talk. Lang Soc. 2000;29(4):477–517.
44. Stivers T, Rossano F. Mobilizing response. Res Lang Soc Interact. 2010;43:3–31.
45. Brownell H, Stringfellow A. Making requests: illustrations of how right-hemisphere brain damage can affect discourse production. Brain Lang. 1999;68(3):442–65.
46. Kennedy MRT, Strand EA, Burton W, Peterson C. Analysis of first-encounter conversations of right-hemisphere-damaged adults. Clin Aphasiol. 1994;22:67–80.

47. Minga J, Stockbridge MD, Durfee A, Johnson M. Clinical guidelines for eliciting discourse using the RHDBank protocol. A J Speech Lang Pathol. 2022;31(5):1949–62.
48. Schegloff EA, Jefferson G, Sacks H. The preference for self-correction in the organization of repair in conversation. Language. 1977;53(2):361–82.
49. Joanette Y, Ska B, Coté H. Protocole Montréal d'Evaluation de la communication. Isbergues: Ortho Edition; 2004.
50. Balaban N, Friedmann N, Ariel M. The effect of theory of mind impairment on language: referring after right-hemisphere damage. Aphasiology. 2016;30(12):1424–60.
51. Agis D, Goggins MB, Oishi K, Oishi K, Davis C, Wright A, et al. Picturing the size and site of stroke with an expanded National Institutes of Health stroke scale. Stroke. 2016;47(6):1459–65.
52. Berube SK, Goldberg E, Sheppard SM, Durfee AZ, Ubellacker D, Walker A, Stein CM, Hillis AE. An analysis of right hemisphere stroke discourse in the modern cookie theft picture. A J Speech Lang Pathol. 2022;31(5S):2301–12.
53. Tompkins CA. Right hemisphere communication disorders: theory and management. San Diego: Singular; 1995.
54. Blake ML. The right hemisphere and disorders of cognitive and communication: theory and clinical practice. San Diego: Plural Publishing; 2018.
55. Blake ML. Clinical relevance of discourse characteristics after right hemisphere brain damage. American Speech Language Hearing Association; 2006.
56. Love A, Cornwell P, Hewetson R, Shum D. Test item priorities for a screening tool to identify cognitive-communication disorder after right hemisphere stroke. Aphasiology. 2022;36(6):669–86.
57. Lomas J, Oickard L, Bester S, Elbard H, Finalyson A, Zoghaib C. The communicative effectiveness index: development and psychometric evaluation of a functional communication measure for adult aphasia. J Speech Hear Disord. 1989;54:113–24.
58. Mackenzie C, Brady M, Begg T, Less KR. Communication ability following right brain damage: the family perspective. Advances Speech Lang Pathol. 2001;2(3):81–95.
59. Ellis C, Henderson A, Wright HH, Rogalski Y. Global coherence during discourse production in adults: a review of the literature: global coherence during discourse production in adults: a review. Int J Lang Commun Disord. 2016;51(4):359–67.
60. Dalton SG, Richardson JD. A large-scale comparison of main concept production between persons with aphasia and persons without brain injury. Am J Speech Language Pathol. 2019;28(1S):293–320.
61. Mackenzie C. The relevance of education and age in the assessment of discourse comprehension. Clin Linguist Phon. 2000;14(2):151–61.
62. LeBlanc J, de Guise E, Champoux MC, Couturier C, Lamoureux J, Marcoux J, Maleki M, Feyz M. Acute evaluation of conversational discourse skills in traumatic brain injury. Int J Speech Lang Path. 2014;16(6):582–93.
63. Hewetson R, Cornwell P, Shum D. Social participation following right hemisphere stroke: influence of a cognitive-communication disorder. Aphasiology. 2018;32(2):164–82.
64. Hewetson R, Cornwell P, Shum D. Cognitive-communication disorder following right hemisphere stroke: exploring rehabilitation access and outcomes. Top Stroke Rehabil. 2017;24(5):330–6.
65. Ulatowska HK, Doyel AW, Stern RF, Haynes SM, North AJ. Production of procedural discourse in aphasia. Brain Lang. 1983;18(2):315–41.
66. Ulatowska HK, Allard L, Chapman SB. Narrative and procedural discourse in aphasia. In: Discourse ability and brain damage. New York: Springer; 1990. p. 180–98.
67. Giles E, Patterson K, Hodges JR. Performance on the Boston cookie theft picture description task in patients with early dementia of the Alzheimer's type: missing information. Aphasiology. 1996;10(4):395–408.
68. Goodglass H, Kaplan E, Barresi B. Boston diagnostic aphasia examination. 3rd ed. Philadelphia: Lippincott Williams & Wilkins; 2001.
69. Sherratt SM. Oral discourse: right-brain damage, demographic variables and sampling effects. UK: University College London; 2001.
70. Levelt WJM. Speaking: from intention to articulation. Cambridge, MA: The MIT Press; 1989.
71. Horton WS. Theories and approaches to the study of conversation and interactive discourse. In: Schober MF, Rapp DN, Britt MA, editors. The Routledge handbook of discourse processes. 2nd ed. Taylor and Francis group; 2017.
72. Clark HH. Using language. Cambridge University Press; 1996.
73. Ulatowska HK, North AJ, Macaluso-Haynes S. Production of narrative and procedural discourse in aphasia. Brain Lang. 1981;13(2):345–71.
74. Mentis M, Prutting CA. Analysis of topics as illustrated in a head-injured and normal adult. J Speech Hear Res. 1991;34:583–95.
75. Orange JB, Kertesz A, Peacock J. Pragmatics in frontal lobe dementia and primary progressive aphasia. J Neurolinguistics. 1998;11(1–2):153–77.
76. Sperber D, Wilson D. Précis of relevance: communication and cognition. Behav Brain Sci. 1987;10(4):697–710.
77. Halliday MA, Hasan R. Cohesion in English. Routledge; 2014.
78. Yorkston KM, Beukelman DR. An analysis of connected speech samples of aphasic and normal speakers. J Speech Hear Disord. 1980;45(1):27–36.
79. Nicholas LE, Brookshire RH. Presence, completeness, and accuracy of main concepts in the connected speech of non-brain-damaged adults and adults with aphasia. J Speech Lang Hear Res. 1995;38(1):145–56.
80. Coelho CA. Analysis of story grammar. In: Analyzing discourse in communicatively impaired adults; 1998. p. 115–22.

81. Berube S, Nonnemacher J, Demsky C, Glenn S, Saxena S, Wright A, Tippett DC, Hillis AE. Stealing cookies in the twenty-first century: measures of spoken narrative in healthy versus speakers with aphasia. Am J Speech Lang Pathy. 2019;28(1S):321–9.
82. Torrance EP. Torrance test of creative thinking. Princeton: Personnel Press; 1966.
83. Nicholas LE, Brookshire RH. A system for quantifying the informativeness and efficiency of the connected speech of adults with aphasia. J Speech Lang Hear Res. 1993;36(2):338–50.
84. Fromm D, Forbes M, Holland A, MacWhinney B. Using AphasiaBank for discourse assessment. Semin Speech Lang. 2020;41(1):10–9.
85. Richardson JD, Dalton SG, Greenslade KJ, Jacks A, Haley KL, Adams J. Main concept, sequencing, and story grammar analyses of Cinderella narratives in a large sample of persons with aphasia. Brain Sci. 2021;11(1):110.
86. Kintsch W, Van Dijk TA. Toward a model of text comprehension and production. Psychol Rev. 1978;85(5):363.
87. Van Dijk TA, editor. Discourse as structure and process. Sage; 1997.
88. Barret J. Old Macdonald had an apartment house. Artheneum; 1998.
89. Joanette Y, Ska B, Côté H, Ferré P, LaPointe L, Coppens P, Small SL. Montreal protocol for the evaluation of communication. Sydney, Australia: ASSBI Resources; 2015.
90. Ripich DN, Terrell BY. Patterns of discourse cohesion and coherence in Alzheimer's disease. J Speech Hear Dis. 1988;53:8–15.
91. Ferreres A, Abusamra V, Cuitiño M, Côté H, Ska B, Joanette Y. Protocole Para La Evaluatión de la Communicación de Montreal. Buenos Aires: NeuroPSI; 2007.
92. Barnes S, Armstrong E. Conversation after right hemisphere brain damage: motivations for applying conversation analysis. Clin Ling Phon. 2010;24(1):55–69.
93. Brady M, Armstrong L, Mackenzie C. An examination over time of language and discourse production abilities following right hemisphere brain damage. J Neurolinguistics. 2006;19(4):291–310.
94. Coelho C, Lê K, Mozeiko J, Krueger F, Grafman J. Discourse production following injury to the dorsolateral prefrontal cortex. Neuropsychologia. 2012;50(14):3564–72.
95. Rodriguez E, Belan AF, Radanovic M. Cognitive-communication disorder following right hemisphere damage: narrative production. Cerebral Circ-Cogn Behav. 2022;3:100147.
96. Mackenzie C, Brady M. Communication ability in non-right handers following right hemisphere stroke. J Neurolinguistics. 2004;17(4):301–13.
97. Ferré P, Fonseca RP, Ska B, Joanette Y. Communicative clusters after a right-hemisphere stroke: are there universal clinical profiles? Folia Phoniatr Logo. 2012;64(4):199–207.
98. Barnes S, Toocaram S, Nickels L, Beeke S, Best W, Bloch S. Everyday conversation after right hemisphere damage: a methodological demonstration and some preliminary findings. J Neurolinguistics. 2019;52:100850.

Ronelle Hewetson, Ph.D., is a speech pathology lecturer at Griffith University, Queensland, Australia, with clinical and teaching experience across Australia and South Africa. Her research interests relate to acquired communication disorders with a particular focus on right hemisphere brain damage, student preparation for service provision to older adults, and the use of technology in speech pathology practice. As a founding member of the International Right Hemisphere Collaborative she works to progress the evidence base related to cognitive communication disorders and to support people affected by right hemisphere stroke.

Petrea Cornwell, Ph.D., is the Academic Lead (Speech Pathology) at Griffith University, Queensland, Australia, and leads the Study of Cognition and Communication for Participation and Engagement (SCCoPE) Research Group. Her clinical and research interests focus on improving the participation and engagement outcomes for people with acquired brain injury, particularly those with cognitive-communication disorders.

TalkBank Methods for Studying Spoken Discourse

7

Brian Macwhinney and Davida Fromm

Preview of What Is Currently Known

Language sample analysis (LSA) for clinical populations has relied for decades on careful, but difficult, methods for hand analysis of transcripts with limited access to samples for comparisons. To address these problems, TalkBank provides open access to hundreds of samples of spoken discourse from participants with neurogenic impairments and methods for automatic analysis of the transcripts of these interactions. Disorders being covered include aphasia, dementia, stuttering, traumatic brain injury (TBI), and right hemisphere brain damage (RHD). These methods have resulted in a flowering of research on spoken discourse in these populations, much of which is described in this volume.

Objectives

(a) To explain the structure and goals of TalkBank.
(b) To show how TalkBank methods improve on earlier approaches to language sample analysis (LSA).
(c) To describe the TalkBank principles of open data sharing, a consistent transcription format, software that relies on the format, interoperability, responsivity to research group needs, and adoption of international standards.
(d) To illustrate uses of TalkBank methods for the analysis of spoken discourse.
(e) To describe TalkBank methods for creating individual profiles of participants with language disorders.
(f) To present new methods for Collaborative Commentary and database analysis.

Introduction

Language sample analysis (LSA) provides an ecologically valid way to understand and assess language disorders. However, when done by hand, LSA can be tedious, incomplete, unreplicable, and inaccurate. The TalkBank Project (https://talkbank.org) has provided a series of methods that automate and systematize many of the most tedious steps in this process. These open and free methods can be applied to language samples from any clinical population (e.g., child language disorders, stuttering, aphasia, dementia, traumatic brain injury, psychosis, and right hemisphere brain damage), as well as to control participants without communication impairments.

TalkBank is a shared, multimedia database for the study of spoken language [1]. It includes separate databanks for 15 population types. Of these, the six that focus on adult neurogenic language disorders are AphasiaBank, DementiaBank,

B. Macwhinney (✉) · D. Fromm
Department of Psychology, Carnegie Mellon University, Pittsburgh, PA, USA
e-mail: macw@cmu.edu; fromm@andrew.cmu.edu

A. P.-H. Kong (ed.), *Spoken Discourse Impairments in the Neurogenic Populations*,
https://doi.org/10.1007/978-3-031-45190-4_7

FluencyBank, PsychosisBank, RHDBank, and TBIBank. The data and methods contained in these banks have been used in thousands of publications, many of which focus on spoken discourse in neurogenic populations—the topic of this volume. In this chapter, rather than summarizing all this work, we will focus on reviewing the methods that support the research. In the three major sections of this chapter, we will review (a) the six core principles guiding TalkBank, (b) the current shape of the TalkBank clinical databanks, and (c) the different analytic tools provided by TalkBank.

TalkBank Principles

The TalkBank system is grounded on six basic principles: maximally open data sharing, use of the CHAT transcription format, CHAT-consistent software, interoperability, responsivity to research group needs, and adoption of international standards.

Maximally Open Data Sharing

In the physical and biological sciences, the process of data sharing is taken as a given. However, data sharing has not yet been adopted as the norm in the social sciences and particularly in the study of language disorders. This failure to share research results—much of it supported by public funds—represents a huge loss to science. Researchers often cite privacy concerns as reasons for not sharing data on spoken interactions. However, as explained at http://talkbank.org/share/irb/options.html, TalkBank provides many ways in which data can be made available to other researchers while still preserving participant anonymity (e.g., de-identification, audio bleeping, password protection, controlled viewing). Fortunately, many researchers have managed to conform to these standards, allowing them to contribute large amounts of data to TalkBank.

CHAT Transcription Format

Individual researchers and research groups often develop idiosyncratic methods for language transcription and analysis, thereby complicating cross-corpus analysis. To provide maximum harmonization across these formats, TalkBank has created an inclusive transcription standard, called CHAT, that recognizes the many features of spoken language. These features and codes are documented in the CHAT manual, which can be downloaded from https://talkbank.org/manuals/chat.pdf. Although the overall system is quite extensive, individual projects usually only need to use specific subsections of the full format.

CHAT-Compatible Software

Because all transcripts in TalkBank use the same format, it is possible to create analysis programs and facilities that make maximally systematic use of the format. These include 24 CLAN analysis commands, a system for automatic morphosyntactic tagging, eight programs to produce clinical profiles, methods for automatic speech recognition (ASR) processing, Phon program for phonological analysis, a system for doing conversation analysis (CA) transcription, TalkBank Browser for study of transcripts in the web browser, TalkBankDB database search system, a system for Collaborative Commentary, and Grand Rounds web pages with teaching tools.

Interoperability

TalkBank emphasizes the use of CHAT format. However, there are other important transcript formats that are well adapted to uses in specific communities. To unify the data coming from these other formats, we have created a series of 14 programs for translating to and from these formats to CHAT. These other formats include Anvil, CA, CONLL, DataVyu, ELAN, LAB, LENA, LIPP, Praat, RTF, SALT, SRT, Text, and XMARaLDA.

Responsivity to Research Community Needs

TalkBank seeks to be maximally responsive to the needs of individual researchers and their research communities. Our most basic principle is that we attempt to implement all features that are suggested by users in terms of software features, data coverage, documentation, and user support. We provide this support through construction of web pages for each corpus, index pages for databanks, manuals for CHAT and CLAN, YouTube screencast tutorials, Google Groups mailing lists, article publications, conference presentations, and conference workshops. We receive overall guidance for the project from the TalkBank Governing Board.

International Standards

The sixth basic TalkBank principle is adherence to international standards for database and language technology. In particular, we strive to adhere to the FAIR standards [2] for open access to data. These standards hold that data should be *Findable, Accessible, Interoperable,* and *Reusable*.

TalkBank promotes *findability* by making data discoverable through Google Search, Virtual Linguistic Observatory (VLO), Open Language Archives Community (OLAC), Digital Object Identifiers (DOIs), and permanent identifiers (PIDs) and by providing index pages in each databank with descriptions of datasets and cross-listings to related datasets.

TalkBank promotes *accessibility* by providing fully open access to all TalkBank tools, codes, and programs, by documenting all aspects of the tools in online manuals and YouTube tutorial screencasts and by readily providing passwords for data access. In no cases are any special data use agreements (DUAs) required for data access.

TalkBank promotes *interoperability* through the 14 data conversion programs mentioned earlier. It supports *reusability* through methods for analysis replication. In accord with recent emphases on reproducibility of experimental [3] and computational analyses [4], TalkBankDB is configured to allow researchers to download data for accurate replication from any given time in the past back to 2018.

TalkBank also adheres to the TRUST standards [5] for maintenance of reliable digital databases. These standards require *transparency, responsibility, user focus, sustainability,* and *technology*. To comply with these and other standards, TalkBank conforms to the 16 requirements for peer-reviewed CoreTrustSeal certification (https://www.coretrustseal.org).

The Databanks

To understand the ways in which the TalkBank tools automate LSA, it helps to understand the current contents of the databanks. We will focus here on AphasiaBank, although the features we describe for AphasiaBank apply equally well to the other clinical databanks. AphasiaBank [6] is the only openly available data source for spoken language and communication in aphasia. It has served as a model for the development of several other adult language databases: TBIBank, RHDBank, and DementiaBank. Currently, AphasiaBank has over 1280 members from more than 55 countries. Hundreds of published research articles have utilized AphasiaBank data and methods (e.g., see https://aphasia.talkbank.org/publications/). Additionally, many conference presentations (https://aphasia.talkbank.org/posters/) and graduate theses/dissertations have relied on the use of the AphasiaBank database and methods.

AphasiaBank contains corpora that use a standard discourse protocol and test battery with large numbers of participants, allowing for the development of new discourse assessment tools and norms. Briefly, the discourse protocol includes personal narratives, picture descriptions, storytelling, and a procedural task. Detailed administration instructions and a script for the investigator were developed to ensure consistent implementation across sites. Most of the data collected since AphasiaBank's initial funding in 2007 is in English and includes over 450 videos and transcripts of people with aphasia (PWA) and more than 250 videos and transcripts for controls. The participants come from 26 different sites in the United States and one site in Canada. The standard discourse protocol has been translated into Cantonese, Croatian, French, German, Italian, Japanese, Mandarin, Romanian, and Spanish. These corpora are smaller but also available at the website.

Originally, the standard discourse protocol was administered in person and with materials downloaded from the website. It has recently been adapted for computer-based administration, making it easier and more efficient for clinicians and researchers to collect data using these tasks. A web page (https://aphasia.talkbank.org/protocol/english/) provides various scenarios and hyperlinks for administering the protocol to PWA and controls using web-based or PowerPoint instructions and materials. Recording can be done directly from the program (e.g., Zoom) or the computer, avoiding the need to acquire and manage recording equipment and transfer media files. Currently, this is available for English only.

In addition to the large corpus of data using the standard discourse protocol, AphasiaBank contains over 20 corpora contributed by researchers who collected language data specific to their research goals. Examples include (a) the QAB corpus, which contains video files for 19 PWA doing the Quick Aphasia Battery with transcripts for the 5-min conversation segment (Wilson et al. 2018); (b) the Olness corpus, which contains transcripts and audio files from 50 PWA and 30 controls, half of whom are Caucasian and half African American, doing a wide variety of discourse tasks and an ethnographic semi-structured interview; and (c) the SouthAL corpus, which contains transcripts and media files for 9 PWA and 8 controls reading passages from the Gray Oral Reading Test (Wiederholt and Bryant 2012).

TalkBank Tools

We now turn next to a description of the ways in which TalkBank tools can facilitate LSA for adult neurogenic language disorders. Due to space limitations, we will not discuss the use of TalkBank's Phon program (https://phonbank.talkbank.org) for detailed phonological analysis [7], although researchers interested in analyzing phonology will find that program indispensable.

CLAN Commands

CLAN is the core desktop program for analysis of TalkBank data. It can be freely downloaded from https://dali.talkbank.org. It includes 30 analysis commands and 25 utility commands, each documented in the CLAN manual that is freely downloadable from https://talkbank.org/manuals/clan.pdf. CLAN commands can be divided into five groups:

1. Analysis commands: These provide basic corpus linguistic analysis functions, such as frequency lists, pattern searches, n-gram analysis, keyword and line (KWAL), mean length of utterance (MLU), lexical diversity, and others for a total of 27 commands.
2. Profiling commands: These include EVAL, KIDEVAL, FluCalc, C-NNLA, C-QPA, IPSyn, and DSS. Each of these will be discussed in detail below.
3. Morphosyntactic commands: These include the MOR, PREPOST, POST, POSTMORTEM, and MEGRASP commands, which will be discussed in detail below.
4. Interoperability commands: These include the 14 commands for format conversion that were mentioned earlier.
5. Utility commands: These include 19 commands used to check, adjust, and improve the format of CHAT files.

The CLAN Editor and CHAT

In addition to providing access to these various commands, CLAN can also serve as an editor. As much as possible, the functions of the CLAN editor mirror those that are familiar to users from MS Word. However, unlike MS Word, the files created by the CLAN editor are pure text files

```
/Users/macw/Desktop/adler14a.cha
1  @Begin
2  @Languages: eng
3  @Participants: PAR adler14a Participant, INV Investigator
4  @ID:    eng|Adler|PAR|71;04.|male|Conduction||Participant||83.0|
5  @ID:    eng|Adler|INV|||||Investigator|||
6  @Media: adler14a, video
7  @G: Speech
8  *INV:   I'm gonna be asking you to do some talking . •
9  %mor:   pro:sub|I~aux|be&1S part|go&PRESP~inf|to aux|be part|ask-PRESP pro:per|you inf|to v|do qn|some
10         n:gerund|talk-PRESP .
11 %gra:   1|3|SUBJ 2|3|AUX 3|0|ROOT 4|6|INF 5|6|AUX 6|3|COMP 7|9|SUBJ 8|9|INF 9|6|COMP 10|11|QUANT
12         11|9|OBJ 12|3|PUNCT
13 *PAR:   +< &=head:yes . •
14 *INV:   how do you think your speech is these days ? •
15 %mor:   pro:int|how mod|do pro:per|you v|think det:poss|your n|speech cop|be&3S det:dem|these n|day-PL ?
16 %gra:   1|4|JCT 2|4|AUX 3|4|SUBJ 4|0|ROOT 5|6|DET 6|7|SUBJ 7|4|COMP 8|9|DET 9|7|PRED 10|4|PUNCT
17 *PAR:   my speaks [: speech] [* s:r:der] is (.) &=ges:okay &-um (.) fifty fifty . [+ gram] •
18 %mor:   det:poss|my n|speech cop|be&3S det:num|fifty det:num|fifty .
19 %gra:   1|2|DET 2|3|SUBJ 3|0|ROOT 4|5|QUANT 5|3|PRED 6|3|PUNCT
20 *PAR:   sometime I speak fairly vrɛl@u [: well] [* p:n] . •
21 %mor:   adv:tem|sometime pro:sub|I v|speak adv|fair&dadj-LY adv|well .
22 %gra:   1|3|JCT 2|3|SUBJ 3|0|ROOT 4|3|JCT 5|3|JCT 6|3|PUNCT
23 *PAR:   sometime it's in a rush . •
24 %mor:   adv:tem|sometime pro:per|it~cop|be&3S prep|in det:art|a n|rush .
25 %gra:   1|3|JCT 2|3|SUBJ 3|0|ROOT 4|3|JCT 5|6|DET 6|4|POBJ 7|3|PUNCT
26 *PAR:   gotta slow [/] slow down my spits@u [: speech] [* p:n] &=head:yes . [+ gram] •
27 %mor:   mod|got~inf|to v|slow adv|down det:poss|my n|speech .
28 %gra:   1|3|AUX 2|3|INF 3|0|ROOT 4|3|JCT 5|6|DET 6|3|OBJ 7|3|PUNCT
```

Fig. 7.1 An AphasiaBank transcript opened in the CLAN editor

encoded in UTF-8 that can be read directly by other text editors. Figure 7.1 displays a CLAN editor window with a transcript from AphasiaBank.

The first 6 lines in this example display header tiers that describe the participants and media. Line 7 indicates the beginning of the segment of the AphasiaBank protocol that asks the participant to describe "how your speech is these days." The "@G:" is a gem marker that facilitates later retrieval and analysis of specific segments from one or multiple transcripts. After that, the lines marked as *INV for the investigator and *PAR for the participant give the spoken words. Speaker IDs like *INV and *PAR can be quickly inserted through keystroke shortcuts. Each utterance ends with a little bullet mark that encodes the beginning and end time of the utterance in milliseconds for direct playback from the audio or video. The actual time stamp can be shown if these bullets are expanded, and the bullet on the investigator's first utterance would look like this: •0_2927•. Under each utterance are dependent tiers. In this transcript, they include the %mor and %gra lines, which provide the automatically computed morphological and grammatical relation analysis, respectively, both of which are explained below.

Transcript files in TalkBank have a ".cha" or CHAT extension, which allows them to be opened directly in CLAN by double-clicking. The editor provides four methods to speed transcription through direct linkage to the audio, a system for checking the correct use of CHAT, and a variety of other methods to speed transcription. The default font for CHAT files is Arial Unicode, which allows for representation of the characters of all languages. Entry of characters from languages that write from right to left is possible. However, combining right-to-left script with the left-to-right features of CHAT can be tricky. For that reason, we recommend the use of romanization for languages with right-to-left orthographies.

CHAT has many other codes for special features of spoken language, some of which can be seen in Fig. 7.1. Commonly used codes in AphasiaBank transcripts include &- for fillers, & + for sound fragments, & = for gestures, [/] for repetitions, [//] for revisions, +... for a trailed-off utterance, xxx for unintelligible content, @u placed at the end of phonetic transcriptions, + < to indicate overlapping speech, [*] to indicate an error production, [: target] for the target word following an error production, [+] for optional utterance-level coding, and (.) for a short pause. In addition, there are 32 special Unicode characters with keystroke entry methods (https://ca.talkbank.org/codes.html) for CA coding. There is also a comprehensive system for coding errors using the [* code] format shown in Fig. 7.1.

Compared with other computer-based programs, word/text files, or spreadsheets, transcription in CHAT has several advantages. First, because morphology and syntax can be automatically analyzed through the MOR program discussed below, there is no need for special marking of these features, and transcription can just use standard orthography. Second, because the CLAN editor allows direct linkage to the media, transcription can be faster and more accurate. Third, the use of consistent systems for marking of behaviors such as revisions, repetitions, fillers, and sound fragments allows for tabulations and searches of these features. Most importantly, transcription in CHAT makes it possible to include the results of the work in the shared open science TalkBank database with all its additional methods for analysis and profiling.

ASR and Transcription

For many years, practical use of automatic speech recognition (ASR) seemed like a promise that was always disappearing over the horizon. However, in the last 8 years, there have been steady improvements in the word-level accuracy of ASR, driven by new computational methods implemented on increasingly powerful hardware that uses huge collections of spoken language derived from web platforms. These advances now make it possible to use web-based ASR systems to create the initial version of a transcript for further human-driven checking and formatting. There are various commercial systems for this. We have tested ten of them and found that Rev-AI ASR was able to provide the best accuracy for our purposes. Our methods for going from Rev-AI output to CHAT transcripts can be found at https://talkbank.org/info/batchalign.docx/. However, these methods only work for well-recorded audio from nonclinical adult participants speaking standard American English (SAE). When recording quality goes down, when other versions of English are involved, or when the participants are children or adults with a language disorder, ASR accuracy is no longer acceptable. Once large training sets for these other populations become available [8], we hope that this situation can continue to improve.

MOR/Post/MEGRASP

After creating a transcript, the user can run CLAN's MOR command to automatically insert two lines under each utterance: the %mor tier, which has morphological and part-of-speech parsing, and the %gra tier, which encodes pairwise grammatical relations between words. To illustrate how to read items on the %mor line, consider the first word in line 9 in Fig. 7.1. This code analyzes the word *I'm* as *pro:sub|I ~ aux|be&1 s*. The tilde sign (~) in the middle of this analysis indicates that this is a cliticization of the auxiliary onto the pronoun. The first person pronoun is coded as *pro:sub|I* where *pro:sub* stands for subject pronoun and the form after the bar is the lemma or stem. For the auxiliary, the form after the bar is the lemma *be*, which is marked as being in the first person singular.

In the %gra tier on line 11, the first word is tagged as 1|3|SUBJ. Here, the "1" indicates that this is the first word. The "3" indicates that the word is grammatically related to the third word which is the verb "go." For the syntactic analysis, the cliticized auxiliary is treated as an item. One can double-click the %gra line to fire up a web service that throws a graphic display to the screen

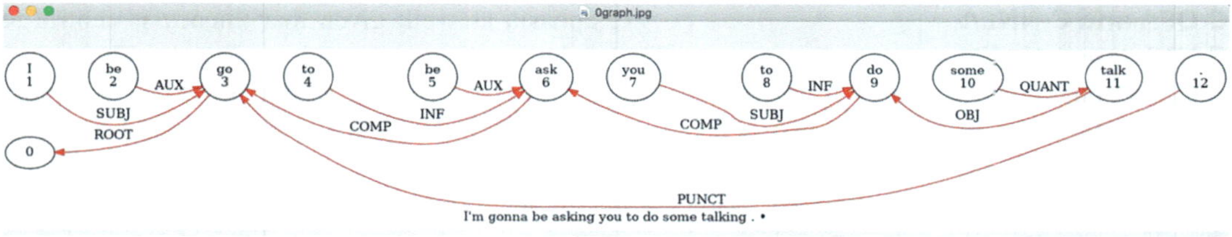

Fig. 7.2 Dependency graph for the first utterance in Fig. 7.1

of the utterance's dependency structure with arcs labeled for the relevant grammatical relations, as in Fig. 7.2.

The creation of the %mor and %gra lines depends on the automatic running of a series of five commands (MOR, PREPOST, POST, POSTMORTEM, and MEGRASP). This whole series of commands can analyze a single file in seconds or a folder with 100 CHAT files in 2 min.

Profiling

Clinical profiling has a long history in the field of speech-language pathology with systems such as DSS [9], IPSyn [10], and LARSP [11, 12] targeting child language and systems like NNLA [13] and QPA [14] targeting language in aphasia. These systems are based on hand analysis of specific lexical and structural items found in an LSA transcript. The results for the target participant are compared with a control reference group matched for age, gender, and other features. However, these reference groups generally included as few as 20–30 subjects. CLAN's profiling commands offer automated versions of these earlier commands, along with comparison to a much larger comparison database. For adult neurogenic populations, the relevant systems include EVAL, C-NNLA, C-QPA, CoreLex, and FluCalc.

EVAL

EVAL produces a language profile for PWA with 34 output measures such as total utterances, total words, mean length of utterance, type-token ratio, words per minute, percent or raw number of various parts of speech, noun-verb ratio, and open-class to closed-class word ratio [15]. An important aspect of this command is the option to compare an individual's performance to the full AphasiaBank database for any of the six tasks in the standard AphasiaBank discourse protocol. For example, one could compare a client's description of the Cat in Tree picture [16] to controls or to other PWA with the same type of aphasia. The comparison group can also be specified by age and sex. Results, in spreadsheet format, show means and standard deviations for the client and the comparison group, with asterisks indicating where the target transcript differs from the group mean by one or two standard deviations. Another feature of this command is the option of comparing a given individual's performance pretreatment and posttreatment to see where changes occurred. Researchers have used this command to generate large datasets and select the variables of interest for their studies. For example, Boucher et al. [17] assessed the relationship between quantitative measures of connected speech and performance in confrontation naming in 20 individuals with early poststroke aphasia and 20 controls. EVAL was used to extract 10 microlinguistic variables such as duration, speech rate, total number of words, mean length of utterance, and lexical diversity from CHAT transcriptions of a picture description task. Stark [18] used the EVAL command to extract six primary linguistic measures including propositional density, verbs per utterance, and type-token ratio in her large study comparing three discourse elicitation methods in 90 PWA and 84 controls.

C-QPA and C-NNLA

C-NNLA and C-QPA commands automatically compute outcome measures from two well-established grammatical analysis systems, the Northwestern Narrative Language Analysis [19] and the Quantitative Production Analysis [14, 20]. These systems have been used in aphasia research for decades, providing highly detailed analyses of aspects of morphological content (number of regular and irregular plurals, possessives), general language measures (mean length of utterance, number of words and utterances), lexical variables (e.g., number of nouns, verbs, pronouns), and structural analysis (e.g., number of utterances, embeddings, verb phrases, subject noun phrases) that have advanced the science, specifically in our understanding of agrammatic speech. When scored by hand, both systems require considerable training, linguistic expertise, and time. The automated commands can be of huge benefit to researchers for efficient and reliable analyses of large numbers of discourse samples. These analyses require CHAT transcription with full error coding and may therefore be less practical for busy clinicians.

CoreLex

CoreLex computes the number of core lexicon words used based on normed core lexicon lists for the five AphasiaBank discourse protocol tasks [21]. This command produces a spreadsheet showing how many and specifically which core lexicon words were used in a language sample or a set of language samples. These results can be used to assess typical language usage [22, 23]. A recent study compared automated and manual CoreLex scoring and found them to be highly correlated, with automated scoring again requiring a small fraction of the time that it takes to train scorers and score manually [24].

FluCalc

FluCalc provides analysis of raw and proportioned counts of disfluencies (e.g., prolongations, silent pauses, filled pauses, phonological fragments) marked in the transcript. This command was originally developed for use in studies of childhood stuttering [25], but can be applied to aphasia as well, given that fluency is central to aphasia diagnosis and treatment. Transcripts need to have specific markings in them to capture the behaviors such as prolongations, blocks, filled pauses, and unfilled pauses. The FluCalc command then provides an analysis of raw and proportioned counts of individual types of dysfluencies, average repetition unit frequency for word and part-word repetitions, and overall counts and proportions of dysfluencies. In addition to providing data on fluency behaviors in aphasia, FluCalc could be used on transcripts from individuals with apraxia of speech, where speech may be slow and halting, with effortful groping, lengthened and repeated sound segments, and disturbed prosody [26]. Automated analyses of larger shared datasets may contribute useful information to the differential diagnosis of these and related disorders.

Advantages of Automated Analyses

The advantages of automated analysis of the types described above cannot be overstated. They allow for faster analysis (in seconds) on one or as many transcripts as desired, less demand for training and expertise of coders and scorers, excellent replicability, and comparisons to existing databases. For researchers, the combination of large datasets and automated analyses has allowed for the application of multivariate and machine learning approaches to aphasia classification [27–29]. In the DementiaBank database, the Pitt corpus [30] has been used in hundreds of projects to create tools that automate the detection of dementia directly from audio files using various computational speech processing and machine learning methods [31, 32].

The combination of large, shared databases and automated analyses has allowed researchers to develop new tools and norms, examine psychometric properties of discourse measures, and answer some basic questions with robust, powerful statistics. For example, Richardson and Dalton [33] created checklists of main concepts (MCs) from the five discourse tasks in the AphasiaBank discourse protocol by using the large set of control data. The checklists show the MCs used by 33%, 50%, and 66% of the respondents. Clinicians can use these checklists to get an objective measure of a PWA's ability to provide "essential content" on these tasks. Fergadiotis et al. [34] were able to use Cinderella storytelling transcripts from 101 PWA in the AphasiaBank database to examine the validity of four measures of lexical diversity and determine which ones yielded the strongest evidence for producing unbiased scores. Their findings led to a strong recommendation for using either the moving-average type-token ratio (MATTR) or the measure of textual lexical diversity (MTLD) as the best measures of lexical diversity in aphasia. Stark [18] explored differences in language produced in three different AphasiaBank standard discourse tasks in 90 PWA and 84 controls. Results demonstrated that each discourse type tapped different aspects of language output in both groups. For example, propositional density was highest and speech rate was reduced in narrative discourse (Cinderella storytelling) compared with the expository (picture description) and procedural discourse tasks. These are just a few examples of the ways researchers have advanced the science of discourse in aphasia by taking advantage of these rich resources.

Finally, an overarching advantage of shared databases is also the greater transparency it afford for clinical and scientific endeavors. The media files, transcripts, and analyses are available for purposes of replication or testing alternative theories and analysis methods.

Conversation Analysis (CA)

When it was introduced in the 1960s [35], conversation analysis (CA) relied on transcription through either pen and paper or typewriter. To mark special features such as overlaps, the typewritten transcript was marked up afterwards by hand. The introduction of Unicode made it possible to create a fully computerized approach to CA by using Unicode symbols for CA features. The web page at https://ca.talkbank.org/codes.html presents 32 Unicode symbols for marking changes in volume, tempo, and pitch, along with markings for whispering, creaky voice, laughter, yawning, and other vocal characteristics. By using these features, CA transcriptions can be analyzed by all TalkBank facilities.

TalkBank Browser

The custom TalkBank Browser (https://sla.talkbank.org/TBB/aphasia) provides direct access to the entire collection of media files (video and audio) and transcripts. After a transcript is selected, the user enters the database password. Then the linked audio or video can be played by pressing the play arrow on the video screen or by pressing the play arrow at the end of any speaker tier in the transcript. As the video plays, a yellow highlighting line shows the transcript line that corresponds to what the speaker is saying. This facility opens the entire TalkBank database to direct analysis for both teaching and research.

Collaborative Commentary (CC)

Collaborative Commentary (CC) allows researchers, instructors, and clinicians to form groups to comment directly on materials in the TalkBank Browser. A step-by-step manual in the browser walks users through the various CC functions; a set of CC screencasts also provides instructions with demonstrations (https://talkbank.org/screencasts/). Group members and managers can create a set of codes for features they need to tag. For example, the code $SUP could be used to mark a contribution by a clinician that provides support for a production by a PWA. The code is inserted by clicking on the line number for the relevant utterance or range of utterances and selecting the relevant code from the set. Once the code is inserted, the user can add a comment explaining how that conversational or linguistic feature functions at that point in the dialog. The codes and comments can then be searched by comment creator or code type for reliability and agreement checks, development of coding systems, detailed CA analysis, and various quantitative analyses. Figure 7.3 shows the insertion of an interesting comment made by a student who

```
40    INV: can you tell about changes you've made in your life since the stroke ? ▶
41 (C) PAR: yeah &=head:shake +... ▶
42    INV: nothing's the same . ▶

$GESX conflict of positive "yeah" with negative head nod, but the
yeah really represents uptake of the question and the head nod
the fact that nothing is the same.
```

Fig. 7.3 A comment in the Collaborative Commentary system

noticed that the PWA was saying "yeah" while shaking her head "no."

This is a new technology with many potential applications. For example, a clinic director may ask her clinical staff to watch the videos of aphasia group therapy sessions and identify (by marking directly in the transcript) behaviors that contribute to effective group management. A professor teaching a course on aphasia may give students a set of videos and transcripts representing different types and severities of aphasia and ask students to identify specific examples of behaviors such as word-finding difficulties, agrammatisms, paragrammatisms, phonemic paraphasias, semantic paraphasias, jargon, neologisms, perseverations, circumlocutions, empty speech, self-corrections, conduite d'approche behaviors, and comprehension difficulties. A research team may use this to establish reliability for identifying and scoring measures of interest such as correct information units, main concepts, local coherence, global coherence, story grammar components, and gestures. All of these and many other applications of this technology will directly and positively impact the field and ultimately the quality of care provided to PWA and their families.

TalkBankDB

To provide support for quantitative analysis of the entire TalkBank database, we have developed a web-based PostgreSQL system called TalkBankDB at https://talkbank.org/DB. This system supports structured queries, as well as downloading of large segments of the database in spreadsheet format in seconds. The manual for this tool can be accessed by clicking on the manual icon in the upper right next to the Login button. For example, a search for all the tokens (words) produced by English-speaking PWA AphasiaBank matches 926,626 words. Clicking on the Save button downloads this matched set in 4 s in spreadsheet form to the desktop, and it then takes another 5 s to open in Excel or 12 s to open in R.

TalkBankDB supports n-gram and CQL (Corpus Query Language) searches across all tiers in CHAT and allows for a variety of visualizations and analyses of data. Users can download datasets directly from Python or R. Features such as utterance length, lexical variables, morphological content, or error production for different demographics or aphasia types can easily be selected, output, plotted, and analyzed through the web interface.

Learning Resources

Beginning users may find themselves overwhelmed by all the methods, data, and resources available in TalkBank. To help guide users toward the methods and data most relevant to their interests and to help them learn how to use the tools, we provide six types of learning resources.

1. **Grand Rounds**: For each of the clinical databases, we provide a set of Grand Rounds pages to familiarize students with various presentations of the disorders. For AphasiaBank, these include case histories of individuals with different types and severities of aphasia, 40 captioned video clips of these individuals' discourse and performance on different tasks,

as well as clinically oriented questions to stimulate thought and discussion. For TBIBank, the Grand Rounds learning modules begin with a pre-learning quiz that allows for measurement of new knowledge and skills.

2. **Examples**: To further supplement the materials in Grand Rounds, AphasiaBank provides a page at https://aphasia.talkbank.org/education/examples/ linked to short video examples of common features from the connected speech of PWA at the word level (e.g., anomia, circumlocution, paraphasias) and at the sentence level (agrammatism, empty speech). Two additional examples at the discourse level highlight how PWA manage to communicate successfully despite having language filled with neologisms and jargon (the one with Wernicke's aphasia) and very limited language output (the one with Broca's aphasia). Further development of these types of examples of common behaviors can be useful for the other clinical language banks as well. Instructors have contributed additional materials and assignments that use the Grand Rounds, examples, and Collaborative Commentary systems.
3. **Screencast tutorials**: To guide learning about the database and tools themselves, we have constructed over 50 screencast tutorials that last between 3 and 8 min (https://talkbank.org/screencasts/). These are available both from our website and through YouTube. Topics covered include transcribing, linking transcripts to media files, running various commands, and more.
4. **Manuals**: We have produced detailed manuals for CHAT, CLAN, and MOR, along with a special manual for speech-language pathologist (SLP) practitioners and translations of the manuals into other languages. These materials are updated regularly as new tools are added to the program.
5. **Discussion lists**: We maintain Google Groups mailing lists for aphasia, child language, bilingualism, and CA. These have proven to be very useful in a variety of ways, such as keeping users up to date on new features and new recording technologies, discussing IRB issues around new ASR technologies, answering questions from users about analysis command options, and receiving bug reports or requests for new features.

Conclusion

Construction of the TalkBank databases has benefited from the commitment of participants and scores of colleagues to open data sharing. Development of the programs and systems described here has also benefited from advances in computer software and hardware, hard work of our programmers, and support from NIH and NSF. These automated analyses provide many advantages that can improve the quality and quantity of information clinicians and researchers obtain from language samples. As a result, important strides are being made in understanding learning, recovery, disfluency, and problems in language disorders. We encourage a wide range of academic and clinical communities to contribute datasets to these shared databases and to make use of these tools to advance science.

Major Takeaways

1. TalkBank provides data and methods to support a wide range of uses in research, education, and clinical practice for spoken discourse in neurogenic impairments.
2. TalkBank resources are open and free.
3. The movement in many fields toward open science is also impacting clinical studies, which must now emphasize open data sharing, along with clear informed consent.
4. TalkBank subscribes to the FAIR and TRUST principles for data validity and accessibility.
5. Reliance on a uniform transcription system (CHAT) has made possible the construction of a wide range of TalkBank tools.
6. The CLAN programs permit automatic construction of analyses that would take hours by hand and which are easily replicated.
7. The systems of Collaborative Commentary and TalkBankDB open up possibilities for new ways of viewing language disorders and therapy.

Acknowledgments This work was supported by NIDCD grant (R01-DC008524) for AphasiaBank and NICHD grant (R01-HD082736) for CHILDES. We are indebted to Audrey Holland for inspiration and direction in the construction of AphasiaBank and to Margie Forbes for her work on constructing the database and tools. We are similarly indebted to Catherine Snow and Nan Bernstein Ratner for their ongoing contributions and support for CHILDES. We also gratefully acknowledge the scores of other researchers, teachers, and clinicians who have contributed data to the shared database and the participants who have consented to sharing their data.

References

1. MacWhinney B. Understanding spoken language through TalkBank. Behav Res Methods. 2019;51(4):1919–27.
2. Wilkinson MD, Dumontier M, Aalbersberg IJ, Appleton G, Axton M, Baak A, et al. The FAIR guiding principles for scientific data management and stewardship. Scientific data. 2016;3(1):1–9.
3. Munafò MR, Nosek BA, Bishop DV, Button KS, Chambers CD, du Sert NP, et al. A manifesto for reproducible science. Nat Hum Behav. 2017;1:0021.
4. Donoho DL. An invitation to reproducible computational research. Biostatistics. 2010;11(3):385–8.
5. Lin D, Crabtree J, Dillo I, Downs RR, Edmunds R, Giaretta D, et al. The TRUST principles for digital repositories. Scientific Data. 2020;7(1):1–5.
6. MacWhinney B, Fromm D, Forbes M, Holland A. AphasiaBank: methods for studying discourse. Aphasiology. 2011;25(11):1286–307.
7. Rose Y, Hedlund GJ. The Phonbank database within Talkbank, and a practical overview of the Phon program. In: Ball MJ, editor. Manual of clinical phonetics. London: Routledge; 2021.
8. Lea C, Mitra V, Joshi A, Kajarekar S, Bigham J. A dataset for stuttering event detection from podcasts with people who stutter. In: ICASSP 2021–2021 IEEE International Conference on Acoustics, Speech and Signal Processing (ICASSP). IEEE; 2021.
9. Lee L. Developmental sentence types: a method for comparing normal and deviant syntactic development. J Speech Hear Disord 1966;31:331–0.
10. Scarborough H. Index of productive syntax. Appl Psycholinguist. 1990;11(1):1–22.
11. Crystal D. Profiling linguistic disability. London: Edward Arnold; 1982.
12. Ball MJ, Crystal D, Fletcher P. Assessing grammar: the languages of LARSP. Clevedon, UK: Multilingual Matters; 2012.
13. Thompson CK, Shapiro LP, Tait ME, Jacobs BJ, Schneider SL, Ballard KJ. A system for the linguistic analysis of agrammatic language production. Brain Lang. 1995;51:124–9.
14. Rochon E, Saffran E, Berndt R, Schwartz M. Quantitative analysis of aphasic sentence production: further development and new data. Brain Lang. 2000;72:193–218.
15. Forbes M, Fromm D, MacWhinney B. AphasiaBank: a resource for clinicians. Semin Speech Lang. 2012;33(3):217–22.
16. Brookshire RH, Nicholas LE. Test-retest stability of measures of connected speech in aphasia. Clin Aphasiol. 1994;22:119–33.
17. Boucher J, Marcotte K, Brisebois A, Courson M, Houzé B, Desautels A, et al. Word-finding in confrontation naming and picture descriptions produced by individuals with early post-stroke aphasia. Clin Neuropsychol. 2020;36:1422–37.
18. Stark B. A comparison of three discourse elicitation methods in aphasia and age-matched adults: implications for language assessment and outcome. Am J Speech Lang Pathol. 2019;28(3):1067–83.
19. Thompson CK, Shapiro LP, Li L, Schendel L. Analysis of verbs and verb-argument structure: a method for quantification of aphasic language production. Clin Aphasiol. 1995;23:121–40.
20. Saffran E, Berndt R, Schwartz M. The quantitative analysis of agrammatic production: procedure and data. Brain Lang. 1989;37(3):440–79.
21. Dalton SG, Kim H, Richardson J, Wright HH. A compendium of core lexicon checklists. Semin Speech Lang. 2020;41(01):045–60.
22. Dalton SG, Richardson J. Core-lexicon and main-concept production during picture sequence description in non-brain-damaged adults and adults with aphasia. Am J Speech Lang Pathol. 2015;24(4):S923–38.
23. Kim H, Kintz S, Wright HH. Development of a measure of function word use in narrative discourse: Core lexicon analysis in aphasia. Int J Lang and Commun Disord. 2019;56:6–19.
24. Dalton SG, Stark B, Fromm D, Apple K, MacWhinney B, Rensch B, et al. Comparing automated and manual scoring modalities for core lexicon analysis. Am J Speech Lang Pathol. 2022;65:2996–3003
25. Bernstein-Ratner N, MacWhinney B. Fluency Bank: a new resource for fluency research and practice. J Fluen Disord. 2018;56:69–80.
26. Peach RK. Acquired apraxia of speech: features, accounts, and treatment. Top Stroke Rehabil. 2004;11(1):49–58.
27. Day M, Dey RK, Baucum M, Paek EJ, Park H, Khojandi A. Predicting severity in people with aphasia: a natural language processing and machine Learning approach. In: 2021 43rd Annual International Conference of the IEEE Engineering in Medicine & Biology Society (EMBC). IEEE; 2021.
28. Fraser KC, Hirst G, Meltzer JA, Mack JE, Thompson CK. Using statistical parsing to detect agrammatic aphasia. In: Proceedings of BioNLP 2014. Baltimore, MD: ACL; 2014. p. 134–42.

29. Fromm D, Greenhouse J, Pudil M, Shi Y, MacWhinney B. Enhancing the classification of aphasia: a statistical analysis using connected speech. Aphasiology. 2021;36:1492.
30. Becker JT, Boller F, Lopez OL, Saxton J, McGonigle KL. The natural history of Alzheimer's disease: description of study cohort and accuracy of diagnosis. Arch Neurol. 1994;51(6):585–94.
31. de la Fuente GS, Ritchie C, Luz S. Artificial intelligence, speech, and language processing approaches to monitoring Alzheimer's disease: a systematic review. J Alzheimers Dis. 2020(Preprint):1–27.
32. Luz S, Haider F, de la Fuente GS, Fromm D, MacWhinney B. Editorial: Alzheimer's dementia recognition through spontaneous speech. Front Aging Neurosci. 2021;3:3.
33. Richardson J, Dalton SG. Main concepts for three different discourse tasks in a large non-clinical sample. Aphasiology. 2016;30(1):45–73.
34. Fergadiotis G, Wright H, West TM. Measuring lexical diversity in narrative discourse of people with aphasia. Am J Speech Lang Pathol. 2013;22(2):397–408.
35. Sacks, H. Lectures on conversation: Volume 1. 1992, Malden, Massachusetts: Blackwell.

Brian MacWhinney, Ph.D., Teresa Heinz Professor of Psychology, Computational Linguistics, and Modern Languages at Carnegie Mellon University, has developed a model of first and second language acquisition, processing, and disorders called the Competition Model. He is also the organizer of the TalkBank system for spoken language data sharing (https://talkbank.org). Recent edited books include *The Handbook of Language Emergence* (Wiley) and *Competing Motivations in Grammar and Usage* (Oxford).

Davida Fromm, Ph.D., is a research faculty member at Carnegie Mellon University. Her research interests in the field of speech-language pathology focus on aphasia, dementia, apraxia of speech, and other neurologically based communication disorders in adults. She has been involved in the development and management of AphasiaBank since its inception in 2007 as a new adult clinical language bank in the TalkBank system. This work has also led to the establishment of three other adult language banks—DementiaBank, TBIBank, and RHDBank—which are dramatically expanding the resources and tools available to researchers, clinicians, and educators worldwide.

The Structural Neural Correlates of Spoken Discourse

8

Reem S. W. Alyahya

Preview of What Is Currently Known

There is a dearth of neuroimaging studies on discourse production, with a particular shortage of studies that have assessed multiple aspects of spoken discourse and/or considered the interconnected processes that underpin the production of discourse. Furthermore, the discourse features that have been used as behavioral measures of interest in structural neuroimaging studies are heterogeneous and tap into different linguistic and cognitive processes, making it challenging to compare the limited number of existing studies. Nevertheless, the available literature indicates that spoken discourse relies on a widely distributed neural network that involves an array of brain regions, which extend beyond the traditional left perisylvian areas, and includes frontal, anterior and posterior temporal, and parietal regions, and their underlying white matter tracts. This suggests that spoken discourse is supported by interconnected mechanisms of language and cognitive domains.

Objectives

(a) To outline the neuroimaging methods used to study language and cognitive processing.
(b) To provide an overview of the mechanisms associated with the production of spoken discourse.
(c) To synthesize and discuss the structural neuroimaging literature on the neural correlates of spoken discourse.
(d) To consider the reasons behind the limited literature on the neural correlates of spoken discourse.
(e) To highlight the challenges that should be addressed when conducting experiments aiming to investigate the neural underpinnings of discourse production and challenges to be considered when interpreting findings from these experiments.

Background

Research into the neural underpinnings of language processing has spanned over a century. Initially, the focus of this field of research was language comprehension, whereas studies on language production were relatively scarce and often limited to single word production rather than spoken discourse (for a review, see [1]). Although understanding the neural underpinnings of spoken discourse has important theoretical and clinical implications, it has received less

R. S. W. Alyahya (✉)
Department of Language and Communication Sciences, School of Health and Psychological Sciences, City, University of London, London, UK

Department of Communication and Swallowing Disorders, King Fahad Medical City, Riyadh, Saudi Arabia

A. P.-H. Kong (ed.), *Spoken Discourse Impairments in the Neurogenic Populations*, https://doi.org/10.1007/978-3-031-45190-4_8

attention in the literature. This is due to methodological challenges related to the complexity of the processes associated with discourse production and the neuroimaging techniques used to investigate language production tasks. In this chapter, the different neuroimaging methods used to study language processing are outlined. Furthermore, an overview of the mechanisms that support the production of spoken discourse are provided. This is followed by a highlight on, and a discussion of, the challenges associated with investigating the neural underpinnings of spoken discourse. Finally, the neuroimaging literature on the structural neural correlates of spoken discourse in relation to the mechanisms that support discourse production are synthesized and discussed.

Neuroimaging Methods

A key source of data to understand the structural neural correlates of language processing has been individuals with language deficits post-brain damage. Early studies that related language deficits to brain lesions were obtained through postmortem dissection [2, 3]. Original models of the structural and functional underpinnings of language processing had attributed production to the anterior parts of the left perisylvian brain regions and comprehension to the posterior parts of these regions [2–5]; these models were precise but oversimplified. It has been realized that the neural correlates of language processing, both production and comprehension, are more complex [6, 7]. More recently, the technological advancements of neuroimaging have allowed researchers to precisely correlate certain anatomical brain areas with specific language processes noninvasively using computerized tomography (CT) and magnetic resonance imaging (MRI). These methods allow identification of the structural neural correlates of language by characterizing the neural regions that have been damaged in brain-injured populations and relating these lesioned regions to language deficits using lesion-symptom mapping techniques, such as voxel-based morphometry (VBM: [8]), voxel-based lesion-symptom mapping (VLSM: [9]), and other multivariate methods (e.g., support-vector regression lesion symptom mapping: [10]). These sophisticated techniques have been developed to identify the structural relationships between brain lesions and impaired cognitive processes. Typically, a structural anatomical scan is acquired from all participants using CT or MRI; these images are then processed, and abnormal, damaged brain regions are identified, before the impact of the lesion is related to performance on a cognitive or language function. In the context of spoken discourse, the presence of damage in a brain region might be correlated with a discourse measure extracted from out-of-scanner discourse samples.

In contrast to structural lesion methods, the functional neural correlates of language are typically assessed using functional neuroimaging methods with healthy and/or brain-injured populations. Specifically, changes in brain activities during cognitive or language processing can be estimated, in vivo, using functional MRI (fMRI), positron-emission tomography (PET), magnetoencephalography (MEG), or electroencephalography (EEG). Functional neuroimaging methods typically identify brain regions that activate during a given task, but do not demonstrate that such regions are necessary for the performance of that cognitive or language process, as they might identify neural regions that are unrelated to that process but which are inadvertently involved with the task due to peculiarities of the in-scanner task (e.g., processes related to decision-making or attention required to perform a demanding in-scanner task, or related to error monitoring if the individual has impaired performance on that task). Conversely, lesion-symptom mapping techniques provide critical evidence on whether certain brain regions are necessary to perform a given cognitive or language function. The focus of this chapter is the structural neural correlates of spoken discourse, whereas the use of functional neuroimaging methods to identify the functional neural correlates of spoken discourse is addressed in Chap. 9.

The Mechanisms of Spoken Discourse

Producing discourse is highly demanding; as several complex processes need to be engaged, including conceptual preparation of the intended message, activation of semantic knowledge, word retrieval, syntactic processing, phonological encoding, and motor articulation [11–14]. This is in addition to engaging other cognitive processes that are involved with organizing and regulating the content of spoken discourse and monitoring spoken output as the discourse unfolds to ensure that it is informative and relevant to the topic under discussion [15, 16].

The mechanisms that support spoken discourse production can be divided into two sets of interconnected processes: (i) microlinguistics, related to phonological, lexical, and syntactic processing, and (ii) macrolinguistics, which are concerned with processes at the message level to organize and maintain appropriate and meaningful concepts that convey a coherent and informative discourse [15–17]. Impairments at the level of microlinguistics and/or macrolinguistics can contribute to deficits in discourse production. For instance, individuals with aphasia and disruptions to language skills at the microlinguistic level could also present with limited discourse production (e.g., [14, 18, 19]). Other patient groups with cognitive impairments could experience discourse deficits at the macrolinguistic level (e.g., reduced discourse coherence) in the absence of deficits to microlinguistic language processes, such as those with right hemisphere stroke (e.g., [20, 21]), traumatic brain injury (e.g., [15, 22]), Alzheimer's disease (e.g [15]), and schizophrenia (e.g., [23]). This suggests that higher cognitive functions might be more relevant to discourse at the macrolinguistic level. Other cognitive processes not typically associated with language production, such as working and declarative memory, might be involved with certain types of discourse such as storytelling or personal narrative (e.g. [24, 25]). It has been shown that patients with bilateral hippocampal damage and severe selective memory impairment can also experience deficits in spoken discourse [24]. Perhaps this is because they have severe memory loss and might not remember the events related to the spoken narrative.

Challenges Using Neuroimaging to Study Spoken Discourse

There is a dearth of neuroimaging studies that have investigated the neural underpinnings of spoken discourse. The limited number of studies might be due to technical and methodological challenges related to investigating connected speech production. The conventional approach utilized in structural and functional neuroimaging studies involves using highly structured tasks that require a single response to a linguistic stimulus (e.g., picture naming, semantic judgement). Other studies have employed sentential stimuli and have identified the neural correlates associated with processing sentences that possess a complex syntactic structure (e.g., [26, 27]), which is more closely related to naturalistic language production than single words. Such well-controlled tasks have expanded our understanding of the relationship between brain regions and language processing. However, they do not reflect the entirety of the complex processes associated with connected speech production, and particularly spoken discourse, which extends beyond the level of single words and sentences. Thus, it is likely that such studies, which have correlated brain regions with language production at the level of single words and sentences, might fail to identify the neural underpinnings of higher level aspects related to spoken discourse.

Studies into the neural correlates of spoken discourse should consider the full array of microlinguistic and macrolinguistic processes involved in spoken discourse. Moreover, researchers studying the neural correlates of spoken discourse must pay special attention to the discourse measures they opt to use to quantify discourse production, and they must consider the linguistic and cognitive processes that tap into each discourse measure. Additionally, one should take these processes into account when interpreting findings from neuroimaging experiments that aim to identify the neural correlates of spoken discourse. Furthermore, cautions must be taken when interpreting findings from some neuroimaging studies that have employed interview tasks to explore the neural correlates of discourse production (e.g., [28]), as these tasks typically involve autobiography, and thus the revealed brain areas might be related to memory processes rather than spoken discourse per se [29]. The vast majority of studies have limited their investigation to exploring only one aspect of discourse production and have typically related structural neuroimaging to microlinguistic features, such as speech fluency (e.g., [30–33]) and syntactic complexity (e.g., [34, 35]), with few studies addressing macrolinguistic features, such as discourse coherence (e.g., [20, 36]). It could be argued that no neuroimaging study has fully captured all aspects of spoken discourse. The current body of research on this topic is discussed in the next section.

The Neural Correlates of Spoken Discourse

Microlinguistic Features

The vast majority of neuroimaging studies that have explored the structural neural correlates of spoken discourse, beyond single words and sentences, have focused on speech fluency. Speech fluency relates to the smoothness, speed, and effortlessness with which words and sentences are produced. This focus on speech fluency is perhaps due to difficulties measuring the other levels of processes involved in spoken discourse, especially in patient populations where language deficits can vary considerably across the patient cohort, and researchers might want to design tasks that can be attempted by both mildly and severely impaired individuals. Earlier lesion studies associated reduced fluency with frontal lesions in the left hemisphere covering the frontal operculum, anterior insula, cortical motor areas, and their underlying white matter tracts [37–39]. Studies using advanced lesion-symptom mapping techniques have supported but enhanced these findings and identified a relationship between reduced fluency in people with post-stroke aphasia and damage to the left frontal lobe including the middle and inferior frontal gyri (pars operculum) and precentral and premotor cortices, as well as the anterior insula, supramarginal gyrus, and anterior and superior temporal regions [30, 40]. The involvement of the left insula and precentral gyrus with speech fluency was identified again in a recent meta-analysis of lesion-symptom mapping studies, which included coordinate-based structural neuroimaging data for 2007 individuals with post-stroke aphasia from 25 studies [41]. Additionally, the same left frontal regions have been implicated with verbal fluency tasks (e.g., [42, 43]). The brain regions that have been identified in association with discourse fluency are illustrated in Fig. 8.1a. Lesions to certain white matter tracts were also identified as predictors of reduced fluency in people with post-stroke aphasia, apraxia of speech, and primary progressive aphasia [31–33]; this includes:

(i) The anterior and long segments of the arcuate fasciculus (white matter tracts connecting the parietal and temporal lobes to the inferior frontal gyrus and precentral gyrus).
(ii) The frontal aslant tract (a white matter tract connecting the superior and inferior regions of the frontal lobe and supplementary motor areas).
(iii) The left uncinate fasciculus (a white matter tract connecting the middle and anterior temporal lobe with the pars triangularis of the inferior frontal lobe).

These studies, however, have used a single fluency measure, such as words per minute (e.g., [32]), or a fluency rating scale from the Western Aphasia Battery [44] (e.g., [31, 33, 45]). To account for this limitation, other lesion-symptom mapping studies have used a combination of microlinguistic measures, including token counts, words per minute, and utterance length (e.g., [30, 34]). These studies found an association between the ability to produce more words and to produce words quickly with left frontal regions. Since neuroimaging techniques are extremely task sensitive, studies using fluency

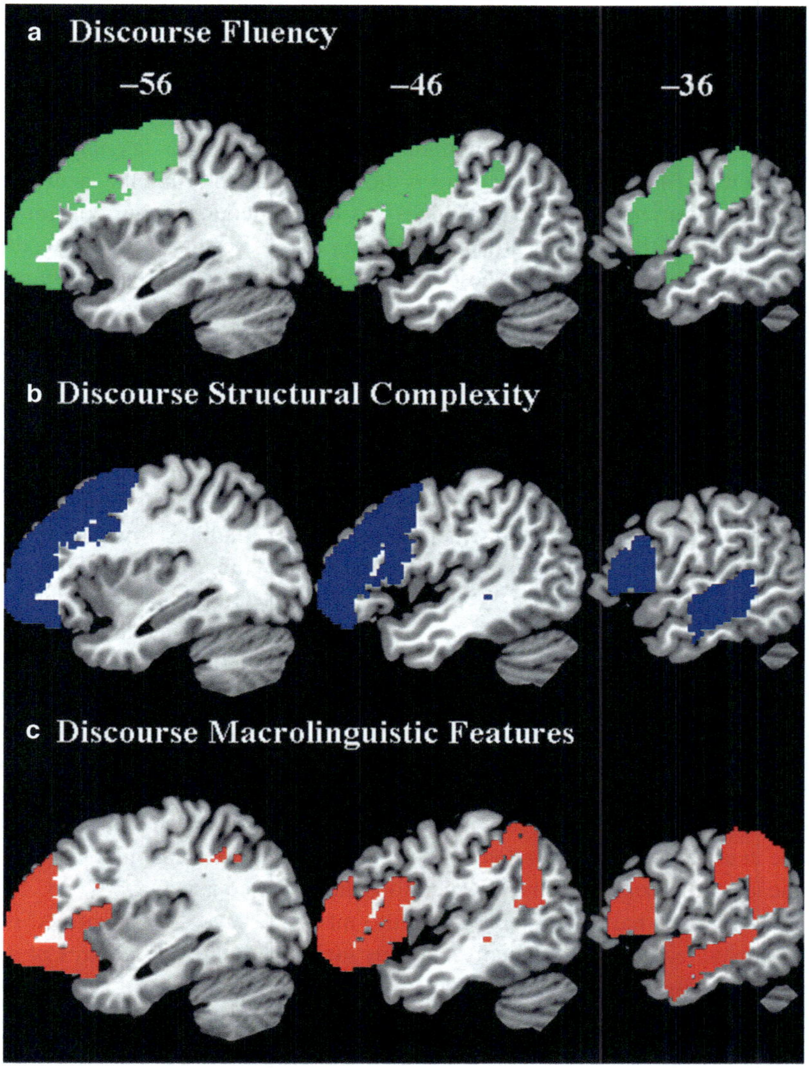

Fig. 8.1 An illustration of the structural brain regions related to discourse production, based on the findings from the studies reviewed in this chapter: (**a**) fluency during spoken discourse; (**b**) structural and syntactic complexity during spoken discourse; (**c**) macrolinguistic features of spoken discourse including informativeness, coherence, semantic diversity, and content word production
Note. The figures were created using masks from the Harvard-Oxford atlas

measures might reflect the speed and amount of connected speech produced, but they are unlikely to capture other microlinguistic and macrolinguistic processes involved with spoken discourse, such as lexical retrieval, semantic diversity, structural complexity, and discourse content. Thus, while they provide certain information, they might be insufficient to capture the neural correlates that underpin the entirety of spoken discourse.

Other microlinguistic processes involved with spoken discourse have been the focus of relatively few lesion-symptom mapping studies. Recent investigations have explored the structural complexity of spoken narratives in stroke patients using a combination of measures related to the mean length of utterance, proportion of grammatical words, and production of complex sentences [30, 34, 35]. Impaired grammatical complexity during discourse production was associated with damage to the left inferior and middle frontal cortices, insular cortex [30, 34, 46], left frontal aslant tract [35], left temporal and parietal regions including the inferior parietal lobule, posterior superior temporal gyrus, and middle temporal gyrus [30, 34]. Similar left frontal regions were also identified in association with syntactic structure and sentence complexity during discourse production in people with primary progressive aphasia [47]. Other studies have identified the superior longitudinal fasciculus (a white matter tract that connects the frontal, temporal, parietal, and occipital lobes), as being associated with syntactic processing during discourse production [48, 49]. These studies suggest that the structural neural correlates associated with syntactic processing during spoken discourse align with the large body of evidence on the involvement of an extensive left frontal, temporal, and parietal network in producing sentences with accurate syntactic structure (for a review, see [1]). The brain regions that have been identified in association with structural complexity during spoken discourse are illustrated in Fig. 8.1b.

Macrolinguistic Features

Studies utilizing measures of structural complexity might capture the syntactic aspects of spoken discourse, but they do not provide information on the neural correlates that relate to the content and meaning of spoken discourse. Therefore, further lesion studies have attempted to capture macrolinguistic features of spoken discourse by including content-related measures, such as:

(i) Informativeness, a measure of information accuracy and appropriateness during discourse production [14].
(ii) Global coherence, a measure of the degree to which each statement of the discourse relates to the current topic under discussion [36, 50, 51].
(iii) Semantic diversity, a measure of the number of words in the discourse that carry different meanings [30, 34].
(iv) Narrative words, a measure of the number of words that directly contribute to the narrative [34].
(v) Content words, a measure of content/relevant word retrieval during spoken discourse [18].

A couple of these studies have accounted for the possible interconnection between different language processes using principal component analysis, in an attempt to tease apart the influence of other language and cognitive process while exploring the neural correlates of spoken discourse using content-related measures [14, 34]. Results from these studies found an association between reduced semantic diversity during spoken discourse and lesions to posterior regions, including the middle and superior temporal gyri, angular and supramarginal gyri, posterior insula, and inferior fronto-occipital fasciculus in people with post-stroke aphasia [30, 52]. Furthermore, damage to the insula had been associated with impaired lexical selection [34, 53]. Moreover, the findings from these studies have related a wide range of cortical regions spanning the left frontal, temporal, and parietal lobes and their white matter connections to the macrolinguistic features of spoken discourse. Specifically, lesions to the left inferior frontal gyrus (pars triangularis and pars opercularis), frontal orbital and operculum cortices, insular cortex, superior temporal gyrus, and frontal aslant tract have been associated with deficits in content word production, informativeness, and global coherence during spoken discourse [14, 18, 36, 51]. The brain regions that have been identified in association with macrolinguistic features of spoken discourse are illustrated in Fig. 8.1c. The role of the left inferior frontal gyrus with spoken discourse has been further explored in an experiment that applied an acute virtual lesion through neuro-stimulation to the left inferior frontal gyrus, which led to reduced coherence and informativeness during discourse production in healthy adults [54].

The involvement of the left prefrontal cortex with macrolinguistic processes of spoken discourse might be related to higher cognitive functions, including attention and executive functions [55, 56]. Executive control processes are essential to ensure that spoken discourse contains the intended information and that it remains focused on the topic being discussed by avoiding the production of irrelevant information [57]. It has been suggested that regulating and organizing the content of spoken discourse depend, at least partially, on representational and executive processes [20, 58] and that the left inferior frontal gyrus is involved in regulating and organizing the content of spoken discourse [36, 50, 51]. Indeed, nonlinguistic cognitive processes, including executive functions and attention, are implicated in the conceptual preparation, organization, and generation of spoken discourse. Studies have highlighted the role of domain-general cognitive and executive systems in the planning and regulation of spoken discourse [59].

Conclusions

There is a dearth of neuroimaging studies not only probing spoken discourse, but also tapping into the numerous aspects of discourse production and considering the interconnected processes that underpin the production of discourse. Furthermore, discourse measures that have been used in structural neuroimaging studies have been heterogeneous and tapped into different linguistic and cognitive processes, making it challenging to compare across the limited number of existing studies. Nevertheless, the available literature indicates that spoken discourse relies on a widely distributed network of neural regions that extends beyond the traditional left perisylvian areas, which are typically associated with the production of single words and sentences. This extensive network includes frontal, anterior and posterior temporal, and parietal regions, as well as their underlying white matter tracts. This suggests that spoken discourse is supported by interconnected mechanisms of language and other cognitive domains. These processes relate to semantic processing, lexical retrieval, syntactic complexity, speech fluency, and organizing and maintaining coherent, informative, and accurate discourse.

The compelling findings from the structural neuroimaging literature tend to indicate that widespread and shared brain regions subserve different features of spoken discourse. For instance, the left inferior frontal gyri, insular cortex, and frontal aslant tract have all been associated with fluency, lexical and semantic diversity, syntactic processing, informativeness, and global coherence of spoken discourse. Moreover, the left superior temporal gyrus has been associated with content word production, informativeness, lexical and semantic diversity, structural complexity, and speech fluency during spoken discourse, while the left supramarginal gyrus is involved with fluency and semantic diversity during discourse production. While the conclusion drawn from existing literature has not identified specific brain regions that uniquely support specific aspects of spoken discourse, it is not possible to conclude that such associations might not exist. This conclusion could not be made unless all processes of spoken discourse are well controlled and investigated in a single study; this could be the aim of future research.

Major Takeaways

1. There is a dearth of neuroimaging studies on spoken discourse.
2. Discourse production relies on a widely distributed neural network that covers an array of brain regions, which extend beyond the traditional left perisylvian areas, and includes frontal, anterior and posterior temporal, and parietal regions, as well as their underlying white matter tracts.
3. Spoken discourse is supported by interconnected mechanisms that involve language and cognitive domains.
4. Several features of spoken discourse that tap into different language and cognitive processes must be considered when interpreting findings from neuroimaging studies.

Acknowledgements The author is grateful to Dr. James Stefaniak and Professor Lucy Dipper for providing peer review of this chapter.

References

1. Price CJ. A review and synthesis of the first 20 years of PET and fMRI studies of heard speech, spoken language and reading. NeuroImage. 2012;62:816–47.
2. Broca P. Loss of speech, chronic softening and partial destruction of the anterior left lobe of the brain. Bulletin de la Sociétè Anthropologique. 1861;2:235–8.
3. Der WC. Aphasische symptomen complex. Breslau: Cohn and Weigert; 1874.
4. Benson DF, Geschwind N. Aphasia and related cortical disturbances. In: Baker AB, Baker LH, editors. Clinical neurology. Philadelphia: Harper & Row; 1971.
5. Geschwind N. Language and the brain. Sci Am. 1972;226:76–83.
6. Hickok G, Poeppel D. Dorsal and ventral streams: a framework for understanding aspects of the functional anatomy of language. Cognition. 2004;92:67–99.
7. Hagoort P, Indefrey P. The neurobiology of language beyond single words. Annu Rev Neurosci. 2004;366:55–8.
8. Ashburner J, Friston KJ. Voxel-based morphometry—the methods. NeuroImage. 2000;11:805–21.
9. Bates E, Wilson SM, Saygin AP, Dick F, Sereno MI, Knight RT, et al. Voxel-based lesion-symptom mapping. Nat Neurosci. 2003;6:448–50.
10. DeMarco AT, Turkeltuab PE. A multivariate lesion symptom mapping toolbox and examination of lesion-volume biases and correction methods in lesion-symptom mapping. Hum Brain Mapp. 2018;39:4169–82.
11. Dell GS. A spreading-activation theory of retrieval in sentence production. Psychol Rev. 1986;93:283–321.
12. Garrett MF. The organization of processing structure of language production: application to aphasic speech. In: Caplan D, Lecours A, Smith AM, editors. Biological perspectives on language. Cambridge, MA: MIT Press; 1984. p. 172–93.
13. Levelt WJM, Roelofs A, Meyer AS. A theory of lexical access in speech production. Behav Brain Sci. 1999;22:1–75.
14. Alyahya RSW, Halai AD, Conroy P, Lambon Ralph MA. A unified model of post-stroke language deficits including discourse production and their neural correlates. Brain. 2020;143:1541–54.
15. Glosser G, Desai R. Patterns of discourse production among neurological patients with fluent language disorders. Brain Lang. 1990;40:67–88.
16. Glosser G, Deser T. A comparison of changes in macrolinguistic and microlinguistic aspects of discourse production in normal aging. J Gerontol. 1992;47:P266–P72.
17. Kintsch W, van Dijk TA. Toward a model of text comprehension and production. Psychol Rev. 1978;85:363–94.
18. Alyahya RSW, Halai AD, Conroy P, Lambon Ralph MA. Content word production during discourse in aphasia: deficits in word quantity, not lexical-semantic complexity. J Cogn Neurosci. 2021;5:2494–511.
19. Stark B. A comparison of three discourse elicitation methods in aphasia and age-matched adults: implications for language assessment and outcome. Am J Speech Lang Pathol. 2019;28:1067–83.
20. Barker MS, Young B, Robinson GA. Cohesive and coherent connected speech deficits in mild stroke. Brain Lang. 2017;168:23–36.
21. Davis G, O'Neil-Pirozzi T, Coon M. Referential cohesion and logical coherence of narration after right hemisphere stroke. Brain Lang. 1997;56:183–210.
22. Marini A, Zettin M, Galetto V. Cognitive correlates of narrative impairment in moderate traumatic brain injury. Neuropsychologia. 2014;64:282–8.
23. Marini A, Spoletini I, Rubino IA, Ciuffa M, Bria P, Martinotti G, et al. The language of schizophrenia: an analysis of micro and macrolinguistic abilities and their neuropsychological correlates. Schizophr Res. 2008;105:144–55.
24. Kurczek J, Duff MC. Cohesion, coherence, and declarative memory: discourse patterns in individuals with hippocampal amnesia. Aphasiology. 2011;1:700–12.
25. Cahana-Amitay D, Jenkins T. Working memory and discourse production in people with aphasia. J Neurolinguistics. 2018;48:90–103.
26. Bavelier D, Corina D, Jezzard P, Padmanabhan S, Clark VP, Karni A. Sentence reading: a functional MRI study at 4 tesla. J Cogn Neurosci. 1997;9:664–86.
27. Just MA, Carpenter PA, Keller TA, Eddy WF, Thulborn KR. Brain activation modulated by sentence comprehension. Science. 1996;274:144–16.
28. Blank SC, Scott JG, Murray K, Warburton. Speech production: Wernicke, Broca and beyond. Brain. 2002;125:1829–38.
29. Awad M, Warren JE, Scott SK, Turkheimer FE, Wise R. A common system for the comprehension and production of narrative speech. J Neurosci. 2007;27(43):11455–64.
30. Borovsky A, Saygin AP, Bates E, Dronkers N. Lesion correlates of conversational speech production deficits. Neuropsychologia. 2007;45:2525–33.
31. Basilakos A, Fillmore P, Rorden C, Rorden C, Guo D, Bonilha L, et al. Regional white matter damage predicts speech fluency in chronic post-stroke aphasia. Front Hum Neurosci. 2014;8:1–9.
32. Catani M, Mesulam MM, Jakobsen E, Malik F, Martersteck A, Wieneke C, et al. A novel frontal pathway underlies verbal fluency in primary progressive aphasia. Brain. 2013;136:2619–28.
33. Fridriksson J, Guo D, Fillmore P, Holland A, Rorden C. Damage to the anterior arcuate fasciculus predicts non-fluent speech production in aphasia. Brain. 2013;136:3451–60.
34. Ding J, Martin RC, Hamilton AC, Schnur TT. Dissociation between frontal and temporal-parietal contributions to connected speech in acute stroke. Brain. 2020;143:862–76.

35. Ding J, Schnur T. Anterior connectivity critical for recovery of connected speech after stroke. Brain. Communications. 2022;4:fcac266.
36. Alyahya RSW, Lambon Ralph M, Halai AD, Hoffman P. The cognitive and neural underpinnings of discourse coherence in post-stroke aphasia. Brain. Communications. 2022;4:fcac147.
37. Dronkers NF. A new brain region for coordinating speech articulation. Nature. 1996;14(384):159–61.
38. Mohr JP, Pessin MS, Finkelstein S, Funkenstein HH, Duncan GW, Davis KR. Broca aphasia: pathologic and clinical. Neurology. 1978;28(4):311–24.
39. Damasio AR. Aphasia. N Engl J Med. 1992;8:531–9.
40. Yourganov G, Fridriksson J, Rorden C, Gleichgerrcht E, Bonilha L. Multivariate connectome-based symptom mapping in post-stroke patients: networks supporting language and speech. Neuroscience. 2016;22(36):6668–79.
41. Na Y, Jung J, Tench CR, Auer DP, Pyun S-B. Language systems from lesion-symptom mapping in aphasia: a meta-analysis of voxel-based lesion mapping studies. Neuroimage Clin. 2022;35:103038.
42. Henseler I, Regenbrecht F, Obrig H. Lesion correlates of patholinguistic profiles in chronic aphasia: comparisons of syndrome-, modality- and symptom-level assessment. Brain. 2014;137:918–30.
43. Baldo JV, Schwartz S, Wilkins D, Dronkers NF. Role of frontal versus temporal cortex in verbal fluency as revealed by voxel-based lesion symptom mapping. J Int Neuropsychol Soc. 2006;12:896–900.
44. Kertesz A. The western aphasia battery: test manual, stimulus cards, and test booklets. New York: Grune & Stratton; 1982.
45. Thompson-Schill SL, D'Esposito M, Aguirre GK, Farah MJ. Role of left inferior prefrontal cortex in retrieval of semantic knowledge: a reevaluation. Proc Natl Acad Sci. 1997;94:14792–7.
46. Mirman D, Kraft AE, Harvey DY, Brecher AR, Schwartz M. Mapping articulatory and grammatical subcomponents of fluency deficits in post-stroke aphasia. Cogn Affect Behav Neurosci. 2019;19:1286–98.
47. Wilson MA, Henry ML, Besbris M, Ogar JM, Dronkers N, Jarrold W, et al. Connected speech production in three variants of primary progressive aphasia. Brain. 2010;133:2069–88.
48. Mills BD, Lai J, Brown TT, Erhart M, Halgren E, Reilly J, et al. White matter microstructure correlates of narrative production in typically developing children and children with high functioning autism. Neuropsychologia. 2013;51(10):1933–41.
49. Friederici AD, Bahlmann J, Heim S, Schubotz RI, Anwander A. The brain differentiates human and non-human grammars: functional localization and structural connectivity. Proc Natl Acad Sci U S A. 2006;103(7):2458–63.
50. Morales M, Patel T, Tamm A, Pickering MJ, Hoffman P. Similar neural networks respond to coherence during comprehension and production of discourse. Cereb Cortex. 2022;32:4317–30.
51. Schneider F, Marcotte K, Brisebois A, Martins Townsend SA, Smidarle AD, Loureiro F, et al. Neuroanatomical correlates of macrolinguistic aspects in narrative discourse in unilateral left and right hemisphere stroke: a voxel-based morphometry study. Int J Lang Commun Disord. 2022;64:1650.
52. Wilmskoetter J, Fridriksson J, Gleichgerrcht E, Stark B, Delgaizo J, Hickok G, et al. Neuroanatomical structures supporting lexical diversity, sophistication, and phonological word features during discourse. Neuroimage: Clinical. 2019;24:101961.
53. Alyahya RSW, Halai AD, Conroy P, Lambon Ralph MA. Mapping psycholinguistic features to the neuropsychological and lesion profiles in aphasia. Cortex. 2020;124:260–73.
54. Marini A, Urgesi C. Please get to the point! A cortical correlate of linguistic informativeness. J Cogn Neurosci. 2012;24:2211–22.
55. Badre D, Wagner A. Frontal lobe mechanisms that resolve proactive interference. Cereb Cortex. 2005;15:2003–12.
56. Gough PM, Nobre AC, Devlin JT. Dissociating linguistic processes in the left inferior frontal cortex with transcranial magnetic stimulation. J Neurosci. 2005;25:8010–6.
57. Marini AA. Age-related effects on language production. In: Wright HH, editor. Cognition, language and aging. Amsterdam: John Benjamins; 2016. p. 55–79.
58. Kintz S, Fergadiotis G, Wright HH. Aging effects on discourse production. In: Wright HH, editor. Cognition, language and aging. Amsterdam/Philadelphia: John Benjamins Publishing Company; 2016. p. 81–106.
59. Alexander MP. Impairments of procedures for implementing complex language are due to disruption of frontal attention processes. J Int Neuropsychol Soc. 2006;12(2):236.

Reem Alyahya, Ph.D., FHEA, M.Sc., B.Sc.-SLP, is a consultant of speech-language pathology, associate professor, cognitive neuroscientist, and clinical researcher. Dr. Alyahya has extensive leadership, research and clinical experience, sub-specializing in neurogenic communication disorders, with main expertise in aphasia. She is an expert in clinical training and research supervision. Dr. Alyahya's research focuses on aphasia deficits and rehabilitation, the neural correlates of language, developing efficient and clinically applicable assessments and outcome measures, language recovery, noninvasive brain stimulation, and tele-rehabilitation. She secured multiple scholarships and research grants, received numerous national and international excellence awards, and has several peer-reviewed publications and invited conference talks. Dr. Alyahya obtained an M.Sc. from University College London and a Ph.D. from the University of Manchester and completed a postdoctoral fellowship at the University of Cambridge.

9 The Functional Neural Correlates of Spoken Discourse

Tatiana T. Schnur, Danielle A. Brown, and Kennedy K. Guess

Preview of What Is Currently Known
Functional neuroimaging studies of the macrolinguistic properties of spoken discourse have primarily focused on the brain regions associated with the ability to maintain the main topic across the discourse, known as global coherence. The brain regions associated with global coherence during spoken discourse include bilateral frontal cortices, which contribute to the selection of semantic representations and the sequencing and organization of discourse, while temporal and parietal regions support semantic representations, retrieval of episodic memories, and potentially self-monitoring. Behavioral evidence converges with functional neuroimaging evidence implicating differential involvement of cognitive and linguistic processes during discourse production. However, smaller sample sizes, differences in age between subject populations, elicitation methods, and derived discourse properties all point to a rich path forward to continue to explore the cognitive and linguistic processes and brain regions involved when producing discourse.

Objectives
(a) To describe discourse elicitation methods used in functional neuroimaging studies.
(b) To outline approaches which quantify higher level discourse properties.
(c) To contrast cognitive and linguistic task demand differences across discourse elicitation methods.
(d) To provide overview of functional neuroimaging methods.
(e) To summarize brain regions and their functional roles during higher level discourse production.
(f) To relate functional neuroimaging with converging behavioral evidence.

Background

When combining multiple utterances to convey a message during language production, which brain regions and their interactions are functionally involved? How is the ability to produce coherent discourse assessed when mapping behavior with brain function? In this chapter, the behavioral and neuroimaging methods and evidence which address the functional brain topography related to discourse production are

T. T. Schnur (✉) · D. A. Brown · K. K. Guess
Department of Physical Medicine and Rehabilitation, University of Texas Health Science Center at Houston McGovern Medical School, Houston, TX, USA
e-mail: Tatiana.Schnur@uth.tmc.edu; Danielle.Brown@uth.tmc.edu; Kennedy.K.Guess@uth.tmc.edu

A. P.-H. Kong (ed.), *Spoken Discourse Impairments in the Neurogenic Populations*,
https://doi.org/10.1007/978-3-031-45190-4_9

discussed. Mapping functional brain correlates provides converging evidence with brain structure and behavioral studies to identify the cognitive and linguistic abilities we use to successfully produce discourse. This information is relevant to theoretical models of language use. Further, it can address the clinically important question of why different clinical populations have varying difficulties with discourse production.

Eliciting and Measuring Discourse in Functional Neuroimaging Studies

Elicitation Methods

In functional neuroimaging studies, discourse is elicited using different methods which differentially influence the produced discourse. Consequently, elicitation methods vary in the degree of cognitive and linguistic demands, which affects the patterns of brain activation we observe during functional neuroimaging of spoken discourse. For example, one approach to elicit discourse involves presenting visual stimuli. Participants describe objects (e.g., [1]) and scenes (e.g., [2]) or produce fictional narratives (e.g., [3]) prompted by a picture or a series of pictures. Eliciting discourse using picture prompts reduces cognitive load as it provides a visual aid to support discourse generation [4]. In another approach, discourse is elicited through non-picture prompts which vary in the type of knowledge required. For example, participants may produce personal narratives recounting an autobiographical experience (e.g., "Tell me about your last holiday" [5]) or provide exposition in the form of opinion (e.g., "Which is your favorite season and why?"), procedural instructions about completing a task (e.g., preparing a cup of coffee [6]), or conversation [7]. Elicitation methods differ in the linguistic demands they place on speakers. For example, when describing a pictured scene in comparison to producing a fictional narrative, unimpaired participants produced fewer and less lexically diverse words [8–10] and participants in the acute phase of stroke produced less syntactically and structurally complex language [11]. Thus, by virtue of their varying cognitive and linguistic demands, elicitation methods can differentially recruit brain regions involved in vision, memory, emotion, language, and motor processing.

Discourse Quantification

Despite varying methods, the different elicited discourse types share features which one can quantitatively assess to measure discourse quality. At the microlinguistic level, we can measure the degree of structural and syntactic complexity (e.g., the number of words and the number of embedded clauses within a sentence; cf. [12, 13]), lexical diversity (e.g., the variety of the type of words used such as words with higher or lower age of acquisition or different grammatical class), and fluency (e.g., the number of words produced per minute). At the macrolinguistic level, we can assess discourse quality by quantifying the degree to which a person effectively conveys a message. For example, discourse informativeness can be assessed by measuring the proportion of words produced that convey relevant information, the proportion of themes produced like the required steps for a procedural discourse, or the number of predetermined main concepts essential to a fictional narrative (cf. analyses of discourse structure through story grammar analysis [14, 15]; for a review, see Stephens et al. [16]).

However, the most common macrolinguistic dependent measure in functional neuroimaging studies is related to global coherence, the ability to maintain the main topic across the discourse [17]. In behavioral studies of impaired discourse, global coherence has been defined by the proportion of utterances that contained tangents, conceptually incongruent information, and fillers or were repetitive [18–20]. However, functional neuroimaging discourse studies quantified global discourse using measures related to a qualitative scale whereby utterances are rated as to how closely related they are to the intended topic on a 1–4 scale ([21]; cf. Van Leer and Turkstra [22] for a 1–5 scale; see section "Studies Correlating Discourse Properties with BOLD fMRI Signal" for further detail). In sum, although there are different approaches to assess discourse quality, functional neuroimaging studies of the macrolinguistic level have primarily focused on the brain patterns associated with discourse global coherence.

Functional Neuroimaging of Discourse Production

In this section, studies that examined the functional neural correlates of macrolinguistic properties of overt, unrehearsed multi-utterance speech are reviewed. We focused on adult nonclinical populations to capture the functional neural correlates of discourse without the influence of reorganization of function as a result of brain injury or disorder (cf. [23, 24]). The review is constrained to studies focused on higher level processes during discourse production (for a list, see Table 9.1) beyond what is involved when retrieving words and combining them to produce phrases and sentences (for a list, see Table 9.2). For systematic reviews of the latter, see Indefrey [25] and Walenski et al. [26] as well as more recent functional neuroimaging studies of sentence production (e.g., [27, 28]).

Functional Neuroimaging Methods

Studies mapping brain regions functionally related to discourse production use methods that estimate neuronal activity via changes in brain blood flow based on the degree of oxygen uptake. The most common method is blood oxygen level-dependent (BOLD) functional magnetic resonance imaging (fMRI). fMRI detects differences in the magnetic properties of oxygenated and deoxygenated blood. BOLD signal is measured during tasks or alternatively at rest. When task related, participants perform a task while BOLD signal is measured. This task-related neural activity is often contrasted with activity recorded during another task to control for baseline processes that are incidental, researchers assume, to the processes of interest during the primary task. In block designs, activity is averaged across blocks of presentations of a single type of trial. In event-related designs, activity is time-locked to events within a specific trial and condition, like the presentation of a stimulus, and then averaged across trials for each subject. Spontaneous activity can also be measured using resting-state (rs) fMRI. Here, participants leave their eyes open or, alternatively, closed while not participating in a task. Analyses using rsfMRI often measure the

Table 9.1 Functional neuroimaging studies of macrolinguistic features of discourse production

Study	Method	Participant no.	Discourse task	Discourse prompt(s)	Contrast baseline(s)
Hoffman (2019) [6]	fMRI	15	Expository discourse	For example: "What would it be like to live in Antarctica?" "What sort of things do you have to do to look after a dog?"	Automatic speech (nursery rhyme)
Morales et al. (2022) [29]	fMRI	25	Expository discourse	For example: "Describe how you would make tea or coffee." "Do you think the internet has improved people's lives?"	Automatic speech (nursery rhyme)
Tagamets et al. (2014) [24]	fMRI	11 (controls)	Expository discourse	"Who or what do you think god is, and why do you think people believe in god?"	One-back word-matching task
Troiani et al. (2008) [3]	fMRI	13	Fictional narrative	Narrative picture sequence	Picture description; pseudoword production
Wu et al. (2022) [30]	fMRI	25	Expository discourse	For example: "Which is your favorite season and why?" "Describe the steps you would need to take if going somewhere by train."	Automatic speech (nursery rhyme)

Table 9.2 Functional neuroimaging studies of discourse production

Study	Method	Participant no.	Discourse task	Discourse prompt(s)	Contrast baseline(s)
AbdulSabur et al. (2014) [31]	PET, fMRI	PET = 17; fMRI = 18	Fictional narrative	Narrative sequences of black and white illustrations	Automatic speech (nursery rhyme)
Awad et al. (2007) [32]	PET	13	Personal narrative	For example: "Tell me what you did last weekend."	Automatic speech (counting)
Blank et al. (2002) [5]	PET	8	Personal narrative	For example: "Tell me about your last holiday."	Automatic speech (counting, nursery rhymes)
Cannizzaro et al. (2019) [7]	fNIRS	10	Procedural discourse; personal narrative; fictional narrative; conversation	For example: Prompts related to planning a trip to new York City, telling a story about an injury, creating a story from a painting, conversing with examiner	Automatic speech (counting)
Geranmayeh et al. (2012) [1]	fMRI	19	Object description	Monosyllabic, concrete nouns, e.g., cake	Nonspeech tongue movements
Grande et al. (2012) [2]	fMRI	18	Scene description	Black-and-white illustrations	Rest
Kuhlen et al. (2017) [33]	fMRI	17	Expository discourse with visual feedback from partner	Instruct partner to move pieces on a gameboard	Expository discourse without visual feedback from partner
Simmonds et al. (2014) [34]	fMRI	16	Object description	Monosyllabic, concrete nouns, e.g., branch	Automatic speech (counting)
Spiegelhalder et al. (2014) [35]	fMRI	22	Personal narrative	For example: "Please speak about: Winning an award"	Narrative speech comprehension
Wilbers et al. (2012) [36]	fMRI	17	Personal narrative	For example: Describe a time you met an important person/partner	Fictional narrative

degree to which spontaneous activity in one brain region varies with the activity in others. Functional connectivity across brain regions can also be measured during task-related fMRI. Other fMRI approaches include fMRI adaptation, correlation, and univariate and multivariate pattern analyses.

A second most common method to measure brain functional activity is positron-emission tomography (PET). This technique also measures changes in blood flow in experimental vs. control tasks but measures the absorption of radioactive isotopes related to neuronal energy consumption like oxygen or glucose. Researchers inject radioactive tracers into participants' blood streams immediately before the beginning of a block of trials of the same type of task (i.e., experimental and baseline). The PET regional cerebral blood flow (rCBF) method has disadvantages in comparison to BOLD fMRI in that it is more invasive, limited by the maximum amount of radioactive tracers safe for humans, and is significantly lower in spatial (centimeter vs. a few millimeters) and temporal resolution (~30 s vs. ~1 s). However, PET may be advantageous to some degree as it can better reveal activation in brain regions for which fMRI has problems measuring BOLD signal, referred to as susceptibility artifacts. For example, BOLD signal drops in brain regions near air-filled cavities like frontal orbital cortex (adjacent to the sinuses) and ventral anterior temporal lobes (near the ears) and can be sensitive to motion artifacts, particularly problematic when producing speech. That said, advanced fMRI analytic techniques continue to be developed to deal with these issues [37, 38].

The assumption across functional neuroimaging methods is that regional changes in brain blood flow are indicative of increased processing in that region required for executing the task at hand. It should be noted that the relationship between task performance and brain blood flow changes is correlational, not causal. Although brain regions may be more active, it remains unknown as to whether these identified regions are epiphenomenal, that is, incidentally involved but not required for the task. Thus, it continues to be important to establish converging evidence from brain structure-behavior studies (e.g., studies using voxel-based lesion symptom mapping, voxel/surface-based morphometry, diffusion tensor imaging), which reveal a more direct relationship between brain and behavior by demonstrating the necessity, not just the involvement, of a region for a specific behavior.

Functional Neural Correlates of Discourse Production

In the first functional neuroimaging study isolating the functional brain correlates of higher macrolinguistic level properties of discourse, Troiani and colleagues [3] compared fictional narrative production with baseline tasks which controlled for lower level lexical-semantic, syntactic, phonological, and articulatory language processes. Among other conditions, 13 participants narrated a story from a sequence of 24 pictures (*Frog, Where Are You?* [39]), described the events within the pictures when randomly presented, and repeatedly produced a pseudoword while instructed to pay attention to the pictures presented in narrative order. Comparing semi-structured story narration with picture description better localized the processes unique to narrative production while reducing the influence of lower level processes. It should, however, be noted that previous work using PET examined the production of discourse via autobiographical prompts [5, 40] but did not isolate higher level discourse properties as the discourse condition was compared with much lower level baseline conditions targeting simple to complex motor movements or overlearned speech acts (e.g., random movements of the articulatory apparatus, nonsense syllable production, and learned nursery rhyme production; cf. [26]).

At the time Troiani and colleagues [3] conducted the experiments, BOLD fMRI approaches to control for susceptibility-related artifacts during longer duration speech acts were less advanced compared to today. Consequently, the researchers adopted the continuous arterial spin labeling (CASL) MRI approach to measure changes in blood perfusion. The CASL MR technique directly measures cerebral blood flow (similar to PET), but noninvasively, by magnetically labeling blood before it reaches brain regions of interest. Labeled and unlabeled blood signal is then compared to provide an estimate of regional blood flow. When comparing semi-structured story narration to picture description, blood flow increased in bilateral inferior frontal and orbitofrontal cortices, Brodmann areas (BAs) 47 and 11, respectively. Other comparisons were less targeted where narrative vs. pseudoword production revealed, unsurprisingly, general language areas including left inferior frontal and precentral gyri (BAs 44, 6), bilateral temporal-parietal regions (BAs 39, 22), and left temporal-parietal (BAs 21, 40) and right temporal-occipital (BAs 22, 19) specific regions (cf. [31, 32]). In sum, a subtraction analysis approach using perfusion fMRI comparing narrating a story from pictures to describing those pictures out of order suggests that bilateral ventral inferior frontal regions are involved when we organize and sequence ideas for narrative production.

Studies Correlating Discourse Properties with BOLD fMRI Signal

Subsequent studies directly related changes in BOLD fMRI with discourse properties estimated via semantic distribution model-related approaches (latent semantic analysis, LSA [41]). Distributional semantic models (DSMs) [42, 43] like LSA analyze how words are distributed across different contexts. These models estimate the likelihood of a word appearing in a natural language corpus (e.g., the British National Corpus) by considering the context of the preceding and following words. DSMs calculate the semantic similarity between words by examining how frequently words co-occur with surrounding words that exhibit similar global distributional patterns [44]. Each word is embedded as a vector in space, where words with similar distributional contexts are closer together in geometric terms. To determine similarity, the angular distance (usually cosine similarity) between word vectors is measured. According to the distributional hypothesis [45, 46], words that appear in similar contexts are likely to have similar meanings, sharing similar semantic properties. In support of this hypothesis, these kinds of word similarity estimates predict behavioral performance and subjective ratings related to lexical-semantic knowledge (e.g., [47–50]). Taking this approach a step further, the linear combination of the vectors of words produced together within a narrative discourse provides an estimate of the overall semantic similarity or meaning space of the narrative. The DSM similarity metric for a narrative is generally understood to reflect macrolinguistic properties that relate to the underlying conceptual organization of the discourse (cf. [6, 24]).

Adopting the DSM-LSA approach as part of a study examining formal thought disorder and executive control in people with schizophrenia, Tagamets and colleagues evaluated discourse in a group of 11 control participants outside the scanner [24]. Semantic similarity vectors of answers to the prompt "Who or what do you think God is, and why do you think people believe in God" were compared with the averaged vectors for the words "myself" and "ourselves." The comparison similarity score was argued to reflect the degree to which the discourse integrated these two themes. To target speech monitoring brain regions potentially disrupted in formal thought disorder, Tagamets et al. measured BOLD fMRI activity as participants completed one-back word-matching tasks (matching the identity, written forms, or sounds of words) in comparison with a baseline fixation condition. Critically, discourse similarity scores from control performance outside the scanner correlated with BOLD fMRI during one of the three word-matching tasks, matching the sounds of words, primarily in regions of the right hemisphere: the right inferior to middle frontal gyri (BAs 45/46), right anterior insula (BA 13), and right anterior cingulate cortex (BA 24). Although consistent with Troiani et al. [3] in terms of general lobule laterality (i.e., right frontal cortex), foci were in different regions, potentially because the fMRI task involved a word reading identification task, as opposed to language production.

In a series of studies in older and younger adults, Hoffman and colleagues related LSA-derived discourse semantic similarity scores with BOLD fMRI activity during an overt discourse production task [6, 29, 30]. Twenty-five younger participants (average age 24 years; reported in both Morales et al. [29] and Wu et al. [30]) and 15 older adults (average age 78 years [6]) read either 12 or 20 discourse-eliciting prompts, respectively (five overlapped with Hoffman [6]). Participants produced 50 seconds of discourse to expository prompts (e.g., "Describe how you would make a cup of tea or coffee"; "What sort of things usually happen at a wedding?"). For the baseline condition, participants repeated a common English nursery rhyme, "Humpty Dumpty" for 15 sec (cf. [31]). By subtracting the memorized nursery rhyme baseline from the discourse task, differences in BOLD fMRI reflected discourse production for both microlinguistic processes including word meaning retrieval, lexical-selection, and phonological processing and macrolinguistic processes including maintaining the main theme across the discourse (global coherence). Of interest here is where these BOLD signal changes were modulated by changes in the global coherence of the participants' responses.

Hoffman and colleagues estimated global coherence properties in multiple steps which are outlined here to allow the reader to compare the coherence measure with other approaches for estimating global coherence [6, 29, 30]. First, each participant's response was compared to a "typical" response. To generate the LSA-derived semantic similarity value of a "typical" response to a prompt, for each participant, word vectors were averaged across words that constituted the participant's response, and then these word vectors were averaged across all participants. To estimate the semantic similarity vector of an individual participant's response, responses were first divided into moving windows of 20 words, advancing one word at a time. The vectors for words within a window were calculated, averaged across the window, compared with the semantic similarity vector of the typical response (the average of the group *not* including the participant), and then assigned to the last word of the window. Hoffman et al. [51] validated this approach with ratings from a group of 20 naïve raters who qualitatively scored responses from a different group of participants on a 1–4 scale following Wright et al. [21]. LSA-derived semantic similarity scores were positively correlated with human ratings of global coherence ($r = 0.68$). However, to create the global coherence-dependent measure to correlate with BOLD signal, the 50-s narratives were divided into 5-s blocks, and the similarity values for words within the 5-s block were averaged, constituting about 10 words per block.

When participants produced discourse in comparison to reciting a nursery rhyme, changes in the global coherence score correlated with changes in BOLD activity bilaterally in frontal regions in older adults, but for younger adults, changes were observed in left hemisphere temporoparietal regions [6, 29, 30]. In older adults, increasing discourse coherence was correlated with increased activation in both right and left hemispheres [6]. Bilaterally, coherence related to parts of the inferior frontal cortex, pars triangularis on the right (BA 45), and pars triangularis/orbitalis on the left (BAs 45/47). Specific to the right hemisphere, regions included frontopolar cortex (BA 10) and more laterally in anterior middle frontal cortex (BA 46). In the left hemisphere, the inferior frontal region extended near to the anterior cingulate (BA 32) and anterior insula (BA 48). Although Morales et al. [29] did not publish the specific neural foci for the same contrast in younger adults, the general reported pattern was different, localized posteriorly in the left hemisphere. Increasing coherence was correlated with increasing activation in left hemisphere temporal-parietal regions (supramarginal gyrus, posterior inferior, and middle temporal gyri) and a frontal focus in the precentral gyrus. Further, in contrast to older participants who demonstrated no negative correlations, decreasing coherence in younger participants correlated with increasing activity in temporal-parietal regions including the angular gyrus, anterior middle, and superior temporal cortex, as well as posterior cingulate and ventromedial prefrontal cortex. In individual difference analyses uncorrected for comparisons across voxels (exploratory analyses), the relationship between coherence (averaged across the discourse for each participant) and BOLD signal yielded again a right hemisphere inferior frontal locus in older adults (pars triangularis and orbitalis, BAs 45/47 [6]) but a left hemisphere inferior frontal locus in younger adults (pars triangularis, BA 45 [29]). In sum, voxel-level whole-brain analyses demonstrated that producing increased global coherence during overt responses to prompts increases activation in bilateral frontal regions in older adults and decreases activation in temporal-parietal regions in younger adults.

To provide a broader view of the contribution of distal but functionally connected brain regions to discourse coherence, Morales et al. [29] and Wu et al. [30] examined the relationship between changes in global discourse and BOLD signal in the principal connectivity gradient, a network of brain regions differentiated from other brain networks by varying degrees of connectivity similarity (gradient connectivity analysis; cf. [51, 52]). The different brain regions within the principal connectivity gradient proceed from primary sensory and motor regions and move to more medial and posterior regions involved in abstract processing, the latter set identified as part of the default mode network (e.g., middle temporal gyrus, anterior angular gyrus, and middle and superior frontal gyri) [53]. Morales et al. [29] found that greater activation near the gradient's primary sensory and motor regions was associated with greater coherence during discourse production, while decreased coherence was associated with greater activation in regions associated with the default mode network. Wu et al. conducted similar but exploratory analyses controlling for the contribution of microlinguistic features of discourse which yielded a generally similar pattern of results.

Summary and Future Directions

Across the functional neuroimaging studies reviewed here, three patterns of associations between functional activity and discourse coherence can be highlighted. First, regions within the general language network were associated with global coherence during discourse production, including left inferior frontal gyrus (LIFG) and left anterior and posterior temporal cortex. The LIFG may be responsible for the selection of semantic content appropriate to maintain the general theme when producing discourse (e.g., [54]). Regions in the left temporal cortex likely support the conceptual world knowledge representations we access to generate the overall message we wish to convey during discourse [55, 56], although the specific roles of anterior vs. posterior cortex in global coherence need to be differentiated.

Second, several regions outside the language network were also associated with global discourse. In both younger [3] and older speakers [6, 24], the right inferior frontal gyrus related to global coherence, although this was not seen in the other group of younger adults [29, 30]. Future research should explore whether the RIFG provides compensatory support when discourse becomes more difficult. The orbitofrontal regions may support the organization and sequencing of discourse (cf. [57]). However, the small sample sizes of several studies (n's ≤ 15) [3, 6, 24] suggest future efforts to replicate effects in right frontal regions with larger samples to understand whether they are typically involved for both younger and older adults and how these regions contribute to global coherence of discourse.

Third, what to make of the default mode network's increased activation when speakers produced less globally coherent discourse? The negative correlation may relate to processes related to self-monitoring, intrusion of unrelated thoughts, or difficulties generating a general schema for discourse [29]. The left angular gyrus in the parietal lobe may be involved in episodic/autobiographical memory retrieval (e.g., [58]) or alternatively semantic events more broadly (e.g., [56, 59]). However, other studies also point to a role of the angular gyrus and posterior temporal regions in semantic control (e.g., [60, 61]; cf. [62, 63]) in addition to the LIFG, so their roles in the global coherence of discourse will need to be more specifically determined, such as in patient lesion studies or by creating virtual lesions using for example transcranial magnetic stimulation in unimpaired speakers (cf. [64]).

Behavioral evidence converges with functional neuroimaging evidence implicating differential involvement of cognitive and linguistic processes during discourse production. Healthy older and younger adults demonstrated significant correlations between discourse coherence, executive function, and semantic skills [50], and for older adults, a relationship between off-topic comments and attention problems [65]. In individuals with mild traumatic brain injury, the informativeness of narratives related to executive functioning [66], and for stroke survivors, attention abilities significantly correlated with global coherence [67, 68] and completeness of narratives [69]. The ability to rapidly process information correlated with global coherence after stroke [68] and was the strongest predictor of global coherence scores in a mixed group of individuals with Parkinson's disease without dementia and healthy older adults [70]. Further, certain discourse genres lead to differences in macrolinguistic processing. For example, producing personal narratives yielded the lowest overall global coherence scores compared to single-picture description and story retell [4], while conversation yielded higher informativeness than either personal or fictional narratives [7]. Macrolinguistic differences may be due to task differences in cognitive demands (e.g., attention and retrieval from episodic and long-term memory) [9] as well as general differences in task demands. For example, personal narratives tend to have less clearly established beginnings and endings, making them more susceptible to tangential utterances, whereas narratives elicited from picture descriptions are more predictable (cf. [4]). Because speaker age and discourse genre affect the cognitive and linguistic processes recruited during discourse, future investigations should experimentally vary in how these differences affect functional involvement of different brain regions.

Conclusions

The functional neuroimaging studies reviewed here point to a network of regions which support both linguistic and cognitive processes involved during the production of coherent discourse. This network involves bilateral frontal cortices, which contribute to the selection of semantic representations and the sequencing and organization of discourse, while temporal and parietal regions support semantic representations, retrieval of episodic memories, and potentially self-monitoring. However, smaller sample sizes and differences across studies in subject population age, elicitation methods, and derived discourse properties all point to a rich path forward to continue to explore the cognitive and linguistic processes and brain regions involved when producing discourse.

Major Takeaways

1. Elicitation methods vary in the degree of cognitive and linguistic demands, which affects the patterns of brain activation observed during functional neuroimaging of spoken discourse.
2. Functional neuroimaging studies which relate discourse changes with BOLD fMRI used semantic distribution model-related approaches to estimate global discourse coherence.
3. The brain regions associated with global coherence during discourse production include bilateral frontal cortices, which contribute to the selection of semantic representations and the sequencing and organization of discourse, while temporal and parietal regions support semantic representations, retrieval of episodic memories, and potentially self-monitoring.
4. Behavioral evidence converges with functional neuroimaging evidence implicating differential involvement of cognitive and linguistic processes during discourse production.
5. Smaller sample sizes and differences across studies in subject population age, elicitation methods, and derived discourse properties suggest multiple research avenues to better understand the cognitive and linguistic processes and brain regions involved when producing discourse.

Acknowledgements This work was supported by R01DC014976 and R01DC019828 awards to the Baylor College of Medicine from the National Institute on Deafness and Other Communication Disorders and the Institute for Rehabilitation and Research Foundation (TIRR) Mission Connect (PI Schnur). We thank Yanchao Bi for reviewing a previous version of this chapter.

References

1. Geranmayeh F, Brownsett SLE, Leech R, Beckmann CF, Woodhead Z, Wise RJS. The contribution of the inferior parietal cortex to spoken language production. Brain Lang. 2012;121(1):47–57.
2. Grande M, Meffert E, Schoenberger E, Jung S, Frauenrath T, Huber W, et al. From a concept to a word in a syntactically complete sentence: an fMRI study on spontaneous language production in an overt picture description task. NeuroImage. 2012;61(3):702–14.
3. Troiani V, Fernández-Seara MA, Wang Z, Detre JA, Ash S, Grossman M. Narrative speech production: an fMRI study using continuous arterial spin labeling. NeuroImage. 2008;40(2):932–9.
4. Wright H, Koutsoftas A, Capiluto G, Fergadiotis G. Global coherence in younger and older adults: influence of cognitive processes and discourse type. Aging Neuropsychol Cognit. 2014;21(2):174–96.
5. Blank SC. Speech production: Wernicke. Broca and beyond Brain. 2002;125(8):1829–38.
6. Hoffman P. Reductions in prefrontal activation predict off-topic utterances during speech production. Nat Commun. 2019;10(1):515.
7. Cannizzaro MS, Stephens SR. Discourse formulation and neurovascular activation across four genres. Clinical Archives of Communication Disorders. 2019;4(1):10–20.

8. Fergadiotis G, Wright HH. Lexical diversity for adults with and without aphasia across discourse elicitation tasks. Aphasiology. 2011;25(11):1414–30.
9. Stark BC. A comparison of three discourse elicitation methods in aphasia and age-matched adults: implications for language assessment and outcome. Am J Speech Lang Pathol. 2019;28(3):1067–83.
10. Wright HH, Capilouto GJ. Manipulating task instructions to change narrative discourse performance. Aphasiology. 2009;23(10):1295–308.
11. Schnur TT, Wang S. Differences in connected speech outcomes across elicitation methods. PsyArXiv gbvqk [Preprint]. 2022. [cited 2023 Jun 23].
12. Rochon E, Saffran EM, Berndt RS, Schwartz MF. Quantitative analysis of aphasic sentence production: further development and new data. Brain Lang. 2000;72(3):193–218.
13. Saffran EM, Berndt RS, Schwartz MF. The quantitative analysis of agrammatic production: procedure and data. Brain Lang. 1989;37(3):440–79.
14. Pritchard M, Hilari K, Cocks N, Dipper L. Psychometric properties of discourse measures in aphasia: acceptability, reliability, and validity. Int J Lang Commun Disord. 2018;53(6):1078–93.
15. Ulatowska HK, North AJ, Macaluso-Haynes S. Production of narrative and procedural discourse in aphasia. Brain Lang. 1981;13(2):345–71.
16. Stephens SR, Coelho C, Cannizzaro MS. Pragmatics: discourse assessment and treatment in traumatic brain injury. In: Guverich N, Grindrod CM, editors. Clinical applications of linguistics to speech language pathology: a guide for clinicians. 1st ed. New York (NY): Routledge; 2022. p. 163–87.
17. Kintsch W, van Dijk TA. Toward a model of text comprehension and production. Psychol Rev. 1978;85(5):363–94.
18. Andreetta S, Cantagallo A, Marini A. Narrative discourse in anomic aphasia. Neuropsychologia. 2012;50(8):1787–93.
19. Marini A, Boewe A, Caltagirone C, Carlomagno S. Age-related differences in the production of textual descriptions. J Psycholinguist Res. 2005;34(5):439–63.
20. Marini A, Andreetta S, Del Tin S, Carlomagno S. A multi-level approach to the analysis of narrative language in aphasia. Aphasiology. 2011;25(11):1372–92.
21. Wright HH, Capilouto GJ, Koutsoftas A. Evaluating measures of global coherence ability in stories in adults. Int J Lang Commun Disord. 2013;48(3):249–56.
22. Van Leer E, Turkstra L. The effect of elicitation task on discourse coherence and cohesion in adolescents with brain injury. J Commun Disord. 1999;32(5):327–49.
23. Kircher TTJ, Liddle PF, Brammer MJ, Williams SCR, Murray RM, McGuire PK. Neural correlates of formal thought disorder in schizophrenia: preliminary findings from a functional magnetic resonance imaging study. Arch Gen Psychiatry. 2001;58(8):769–74.
24. Tagamets MA, Cortes CR, Griego JA, Elvevåg B. Neural correlates of the relationship between discourse coherence and sensory monitoring in schizophrenia. Cortex. 2014;55:77–87.
25. Indefrey P. The relationship between syntactic production and comprehension. In: Rueschemeyer SA, Gaskell MG, editors. The Oxford handbook of psycholinguistics. 2nd ed. Oxford (GB): Oxford University Press; 2018. p. 481–505.
26. Walenski M, Europa E, Caplan D, Thompson CK. Neural networks for sentence comprehension and production: an ALE-based meta-analysis of neuroimaging studies. Hum Brain Mapp. 2019;40(8):2275–304.
27. Giglio L, Ostarek M, Weber K, Hagoort P. Commonalities and asymmetries in the neurobiological infrastructure for language production and comprehension. Cereb Cortex. 2022;32(7):1405–18.
28. Hu J, Small H, Kean H, Takahashi A, Zekelman L, Kleinman D, et al. Precision fMRI reveals that the language-selective network supports both phrase-structure building and lexical access during language production. Cereb Cortex. 2023;33(8):4384–404.
29. Morales M, Patel T, Tamm A, Pickering MJ, Hoffman P. Similar neural networks respond to coherence during comprehension and production of discourse. Cereb Cortex. 2022;32(19):4317–30.
30. Wu W, Morales M, Patel T, Pickering MJ, Hoffman P. Modulation of brain activity by psycholinguistic information during naturalistic speech comprehension and production. Cortex. 2022;155:287–306.
31. AbdulSabur NY, Xu Y, Liu S, Chow HM, Baxter M, Carson J, et al. Neural correlates and network connectivity underlying narrative production and comprehension: a combined fMRI and PET study. Cortex. 2014;57:107–27.
32. Awad M, Warren JE, Scott SK, Turkheimer FE, Wise RJS. A common system for the comprehension and production of narrative speech. J Neurosci. 2007;27(43):11455–64.
33. Kuhlen AK, Bogler C, Brennan SE, Haynes JD. Brains in dialogue: decoding neural preparation of speaking to a conversational partner. Soc Cogn Affect Neurosci. 2017;12(6):871–80.
34. Simmonds AJ, Leech R, Collins C, Redjep O, Wise RJS. Sensory-motor integration during speech production localizes to both left and right plana temporale. J Neurosci. 2014;34(39):12963–72.
35. Spiegelhalder K, Ohlendorf S, Regen W, Feige B, Tebartz van Elst L, Weiller C, et al. Interindividual synchronization of brain activity during live verbal communication. Behav Brain Res. 2014;258:75–9.
36. Wilbers L, Deuker L, Fell J, Axmacher N. Are autobiographical memories inherently social? Evidence from an fMRI study. PLoS One. 2012;7(9):e45089.
37. Kundu P, Voon V, Balchandani P, Lombardo MV, Poser BA, Bandettini PA. Multi-echo fMRI: a review of applications in fMRI denoising and analysis of BOLD signals. NeuroImage. 2017;154:59–80.
38. Willems RM, Van Gerven MAJ. New FMRI methods for the study of language. In: Rueschemeyer SA, Gaskell MG, editors. The Oxford handbook of psy-

cholinguistics [internet]. Oxford University Press; 2018. p. 974–91.
39. Mayer M. Frog, where are you? New York: Dial Books for Young Readers; 1969. p. 31.
40. Landauer TK, Dumais ST. A solution to Plato's problem: the latent semantic analysis theory of acquisition, induction, and representation of knowledge. Psychol Rev. 1997;104(2):211–40.
41. Andrews M, Vigliocco G, Vinson D. Integrating experiential and distributional data to learn semantic representations. Psychol Rev. 2009;116(3):463–98.
42. Lenci A. Distributional semantics in linguistic and cognitive research. Italian Journal of Linguistics. 2008;20(1):1–31.
43. Günther F, Rinaldi L, Marelli M. Vector-space models of semantic representation from a cognitive perspective: a discussion of common misconceptions. Perspect Psychol Sci. 2019;14(6):1006–33.
44. Firth JR. A synopsis of linguistic theory, 1930-1955. In: Studies in linguistic analysis. Basil Blackwell; 1957. p. 1–32.
45. Harris ZS. Distributional structure. Word. 1954;10(2–3):146–62.
46. Pereira F, Gershman S, Ritter S, Botvinick M. A comparative evaluation of off-the-shelf distributed semantic representations for modelling behavioural data. Cogn Neuropsychol. 2016;33(3–4):175–90.
47. Mandera P, Keuleers E, Brysbaert M. Explaining human performance in psycholinguistic tasks with models of semantic similarity based on prediction and counting: a review and empirical validation. J Mem Lang. 2017;92:57–78.
48. Schnur TT, Lei CM. Assessing naming errors using an automated machine learning approach. Neuropsychology. 2022;36(8):709–18.
49. Wang X, Xu Y, Wang Y, Zeng Y, Zhang J, Ling Z, et al. Representational similarity analysis reveals task-dependent semantic influence of the visual word form area. Sci Rep. 2018;8(1):3047.
50. Hoffman P, Loginova E, Russell A. Poor coherence in older people's speech is explained by impaired semantic and executive processes. elife. 2018;7:e38907.
51. Margulies DS, Ghosh SS, Goulas A, Falkiewicz M, Huntenburg JM, Langs G, et al. Situating the default-mode network along a principal gradient of macroscale cortical organization. Proc Natl Acad Sci. 2016;113(44):12574–9.
52. Smallwood J, Karapanagiotidis T, Ruby F, Medea B, de Caso I, Konishi M, et al. Representing representation: integration between the temporal lobe and the posterior cingulate influences the content and form of spontaneous thought. PLoS One. 2016;11(4):e0152272.
53. Raichle ME, MacLeod AM, Snyder AZ, Powers WJ, Gusnard DA, Shulman GL. A default mode of brain function. Proc Natl Acad Sci. 2001;98(2):676–82.
54. Thompson-Schill SL, Schnur TT, Hirshorn E, Schwartz MF, Kimberg D. Regulatory functions of prefrontal cortex during single word production. Brain Lang. 2007;103(1–2):171–2.
55. Bi Y. Dual coding of knowledge in the human brain. Trends Cogn Sci. 2021;25(10):883–95.
56. Binder JR, Desai RH. The neurobiology of semantic memory. Trends Cogn Sci. 2011;15(11):527–36.
57. Badre D, Nee DE. Frontal cortex and the hierarchical control of behavior. Trends Cogn Sci. 2018;22(2):170–88.
58. Wagner AD, Shannon BJ, Kahn I, Buckner RL. Parietal lobe contributions to episodic memory retrieval. Trends Cogn Sci. 2005;9(9):445–53.
59. Binder JR, Desai RH, Graves WW, Conant LL. Where is the semantic system? A critical review and meta-analysis of 120 functional neuroimaging studies. Cereb Cortex. 2009;19(12):2767–96.
60. Noonan KA, Jefferies E, Visser M, Lambon Ralph MA. Going beyond inferior prefrontal involvement in semantic control: evidence for the additional contribution of dorsal angular gyrus and posterior middle temporal cortex. J Cogn Neurosci. 2013;25(11):1824–50.
61. Whitney C, Kirk M, O'Sullivan J, Lambon Ralph MA, Jefferies E. The neural organization of semantic control: TMS evidence for a distributed network in left inferior frontal and posterior middle temporal gyrus. Cereb Cortex. 2011;21(5):1066–75.
62. Lambon Ralph MA, Jefferies E, Patterson K, Rogers TT. The neural and computational bases of semantic cognition. Nat Rev Neurosci. 2017;18(1):42–55.
63. Humphreys GF, Lambon Ralph MA, Simons JS. A unifying account of angular gyrus contributions to episodic and semantic cognition. Trends Neurosci. 2021;44(6):452–63.
64. Marini A, Urgesi C. Please get to the point! A cortical correlate of linguistic informativeness. J Cogn Neurosci. 2012;24(11):2211–22.
65. Barnett M, Helphrey J, Childers L. Attention problems and off-topic verbosity among young adult and older adult age cohorts. Appl Neuropsychol Adult. 2022:1–8. https://doi.org/10.1080/23279095.2022.2147009.
66. Galetto V, Andreetta S, Zettin M, Marini A. Patterns of impairment of narrative language in mild traumatic brain injury. J Neurolinguistics. 2013;26(6):649–61.
67. Barker MS, Young B, Robinson GA. Cohesive and coherent connected speech deficits in mild stroke. Brain Lang. 2017;168:23–36.
68. Rogalski Y, Altmann LJP, Plummer-D'Amato P, Behrman AL, Marsiske M. Discourse coherence and cognition after stroke: a dual task study. J Commun Disord. 2010;43(3):212–24.
69. Bartels-Tobin LR, Hinckley JJ. Cognition and discourse production in right hemisphere disorder. J Neurolinguistics. 2005;18(6):461–77.
70. Rogalski Y, Key-DeLyria SE, Hazamy A, Altmann LJP. Global coherence and cognition in Parkinson's disease. J Speech Lang Hear Res. 2022;65(8):2962–77.

Tatiana T. Schnur, Ph.D., is a Professor of Physical Medicine and Rehabilitation at the University of Texas Health Science Center at Houston McGovern Medical School, Houston, Texas. She received a B.A. in cognitive science from the University of Virginia and a Ph.D. in psychology specializing in cognition, brain, and behavior from Harvard University. Subsequently, she received training via a U.S. National Institutes of Health T32 postdoctoral fellowship from the University of Pennsylvania in neurological rehabilitation focusing on language disorders in people with acquired brain disorders resulting from stroke. In her research, Dr. Schnur uses theory-driven hypothesis testing to understand the nature of the brain-behavior basis of language and cognition and resulting deficits from stroke.

Danielle A. Brown, M.S., CCC-SLP, graduated from Rice University, where she studied linguistics and psychology, in 2012. After three years working in the Language and Aphasia Laboratory at the Moss Rehabilitation Research Institute, she attended the University of Arizona where she obtained a master's degree in speech-language pathology. Danielle practiced as a speech-language pathologist for a local school district and the Houston Aphasia Recovery Center in Houston, TX, before joining the Schnur Laboratory. There she investigates the cognitive and linguistic sequelae of stroke with patients recruited from Texas Medical Center-affiliated hospitals.

Kennedy K. Guess, M.A., CCC-SLP, received her master's degree in communication sciences and disorders from the University of Houston. There she completed a master's thesis under Dr. Lynn Maher on aphasia and dialectal code switching. She is a licensed speech-language pathologist and has worked with populations across the life span. She is currently a patient coordinator in the Schnur Laboratory at the University of Texas Health Science Center at Houston investigating deficits following right hemisphere stroke.

Co-speech Gesture Production in Spoken Discourse Among Speakers with Acquired Language Disorders

10

Isobel Chick, Peter Garrard, Laurel J. Buxbaum, and Gabriella Vigliocco

Preview of What Is Currently Known

Gesture production is often impaired in people with acquired language disorders. In left hemisphere stroke, gesture impairments may affect the rate of production, type of gesture produced, and quantity of information transmitted via gesture and speech channels. In right hemisphere stroke and progressive neurological conditions, significantly more research is needed and patterns of co-speech gesture production deficits are not well understood. Certain challenges stand in the way of research progress in this field; it is suggested that making use of a broader range of gesture elicitation tasks and the development of new technology may go some way towards overcoming these obstacles.

Objectives

(a) To provide a classification of co-speech gestures produced by typical and atypical populations.
(b) To outline key features of co-speech gestures produced by patients with acute (stroke) and chronic (dementia and Parkinson's disease) neurological conditions.
(c) To discuss gesture production in clinical populations within existing theoretical models of speech-gesture interaction.
(d) To identify key challenges in gesture studies and make suggestions for future research.

Background

Communication is multimodal: when we talk, we also gesture. These gestures are time-locked to speech, and speakers flexibly distribute information across speech and gesture channels to achieve maximum efficiency in information transmission [1]. Gesture is ubiquitous in human communication and has been shown to support language development in children [2] and language processing in neurologically healthy adults [3], yet surprisingly little is known about gesture production in the presence of acquired language deficits resulting from neurological damage. In this chapter, co-speech gestures are defined, and the features of co-speech gesture production in people with language impairment caused by

I. Chick · G. Vigliocco (✉)
Language and Cognition Lab, University College London, London, UK
e-mail: isobel.chick.21@ucl.ac.uk; g.vigliocco@ucl.ac.uk

P. Garrard
Molecular and Clinical Sciences Research Institute, St George's, University of London, London, UK
e-mail: pgarrard@sgul.ac.uk

L. J. Buxbaum
Moss Rehabilitation Research Institute, Thomas Jefferson University, Philadelphia, PA, USA
e-mail: laurel.buxbaum@jefferson.edu

A. P.-H. Kong (ed.), *Spoken Discourse Impairments in the Neurogenic Populations*,
https://doi.org/10.1007/978-3-031-45190-4_10

stroke are described. The far sparser literature on Alzheimer's disease, primary progressive aphasia, and Parkinson's disease is also reviewed. This is followed by the description of two models of gesture production that account for how speakers can benefit from gesture production. Finally, challenges facing the field of gesture studies are considered.

What Are Co-Speech Gestures?

Although multiple gesture classification systems exist, one of the earliest and most influential attempts at distinguishing co-speech gestures from other communicative hand and body movements was proposed by Kendon [4] and elaborated by McNeill [5], who suggested that such movements comprise a "continuum." This ranges from gesticulations at one end—which are interactional in nature and require the presence of speech to be understood—to sign languages, which are full linguistic systems independent of speech. Co-speech gestures, which Kendon originally termed "language-like gestures," fall somewhere in the middle: they carry semantic content and are fully integrated into utterances, but like gesticulations, their interpretation relies upon the presence of speech. Co-speech gestures differ from *emblems*, which express a conventionalized meaning within a community (such as the "OK" or thumbs-up symbols), and full *pantomimes* (for example, imitating using a hammer), both of which do not require speech to be understood.

While Kendon's continuum is useful in providing a global overview of manual communication, it should be noted that there is often no clear boundary between different gesture categories in everyday communication: a speaker may move their index and middle finger back and forth while talking about cutting a piece of paper (i.e., a language-like gesture) and may then use the same gesture when mimicking the movement of the blades of scissors without speaking (a pantomime gesture).

McNeill subsequently divided Kendon's "language-like" gesture category into four subtypes, termed "speech accompanying" (or co-speech) gestures. These subtypes are iconic, metaphoric, deictic, and beat gestures [5] and have largely been studied in typical populations. *Iconic gestures* represent a concrete referent imagistically by manner of movement or shape, such as depicting "ball" by moving the hands in a circle to mimic its shape or showing the swinging movement of a hammer. *Metaphoric gestures* typically represent abstract concepts, such as moving the index finger upwards while talking about the concept of inflation. Other metaphoric gestures include *number* gestures, which indicate a number on the fingers, and *time* gestures, which use space to differentiate between the past and future, such as using the front of the body to indicate the future and the back to indicate the past [6]. Iconic and metaphoric gestures may be depicted from a character viewpoint, where the speaker depicts an event as though performing it themselves (such as moving the arms through the air as though swimming), or from an observer viewpoint, where the speaker depicts an event as though seeing it from afar (e.g., moving the fingers back and forth to mimic a person running) [5, 6].

In neurologically healthy adults, production of iconic gestures alongside speech facilitates speech comprehension in listeners, and this effect persists across the life span [7]. In connected speech, iconic and metaphoric gestures tend to precede the words they refer to, allowing for prediction of the following word [8]. Iconic and metaphoric gestures may also support speakers in word production; for example, there is evidence that neurologically healthy adults learn novel words faster when they are paired with meaningful gestures, and gestures may also support more effective schematizing of information, particularly spatial information [9, 10].

Deictic gestures are typically points (which include both points produced with the index finger and points produced using the thumb, the whole hand, pointing using an object, etc.) and may refer to concrete visible referents, such as pointing to a house while talking about it or pointing to the self; concrete displaced or absent referents, such as pointing towards the door to indicate where someone has gone; or abstract referents, such as pointing backwards to refer to some time period in the past. Deictic gestures are used to disambiguate speech and to direct the listener's attention to a specific referent [11].

Beats are small, often repetitive up-and-down hand movements that follow the rhythm of speech. Unlike the former three categories of gesture, beats have traditionally been assumed to carry no semantic content. However, more recent studies have suggested that beats may carry spatial information; Yap et al., for example, found that the upwards and downwards timing of beats correlated with spatial semantics in some utterances, such as saying "The ship *sank*" with a time-locked downward beat or "The balloon went *up*" with an upward beat [12]. The communicative purpose of beats is unclear: they may be used for emphasis or to introduce new information [5], as visual markers of lexical stress [13], or to manage the flow of discourse [14]. In people with acquired language impairments, there is some evidence that beats function to regulate the pace of speech and generate rhythm, similar to a metronome [15, 16].

In the context of co-speech gesture production in people with acquired language disorders specifically, it has been argued that additional gesture types exist, used either to compensate for impaired speech production or to facilitate word retrieval [17]. A prime example of this is *letter gestures*, where the speaker traces single letters or strings of letters in the air or on a flat surface and then "reads" the traced word aloud. Indeed, De Beer et al. found that letter gestures were exclusively used by people with poststroke language impairment [17]. A second example is *homophone gestures*, in which the speaker produces a gesture indicating a homophone of the word they want to say, for example by indicating their wedding ring when trying to retrieve the word "ring," as in "I need to ring [telephone] the doctor" [18].

In total, at least 13 different co-speech gesture types have been identified (see Table 10.1): referential; concrete deictic; points to self; iconic observer viewpoint; iconic character viewpoint; pantomime; metaphoric; time; beats; emblems; letter gestures; number gestures; and homophone gestures. It should be noted, however, that there is little agreement on how reliably these categories can be identified and coded, and researchers vary in how they classify gestures.

Table 10.1 Summary of identified gesture types

Gesture type	Description
Referential	Indicates an absent/displaced concrete referent [19]
Concrete deictic	Indicates a present concrete referent [5]
Points to self	Indicates the speaker, typically with a point [6]
Iconic observer viewpoint	Speaker depicts an event as though observing it from a distance, e.g., using fingers to indicate someone running from left to right [5, 6]
Iconic character viewpoint	Speaker depicts an event as though they are performing it themself, such as moving arms as though swimming [5, 6]
Pantomime	Use of the hand/body to enact a part in a narrative; may not require speech to be understood [5]
Metaphoric	Represents a (typically abstract) referent imagistically [5]
Time	Uses space to differentiate the past and future [6]
Beats	Small repetitive movements, may carry spatial content [5, 15, 16]
Emblems	Conventionalized meaning within a community or language group; does not require speech to be understood, e.g., thumbs-up or "OK" symbols [4]
Letter gestures	Traces individual letters or strings [20]
Number gestures	Indicates a number with the fingers [20]
Homophone gestures	Indicates a spoken word that is a homophone to the gestured meaning, e.g., pointing to a wedding ring to indicate a "ring" on the telephone [18]

Note: Adapted from Sekine K, Rose ML. The relationship of aphasia type and gesture production in people with aphasia. Am J Speech Lang Pathol 2013;22(4):662–72

Co-speech Gesture Production in Neurogenic Populations

Having briefly described categories of gestures produced by both neurotypical and language-impaired populations, the focus now turns to the specifics of how people with acquired language impairment caused by acute (poststroke aphasia and right hemisphere damage) and chronic (Alzheimer's disease, primary progressive aphasia, and Parkinson's disease) conditions produce co-speech gestures. Patterns of impairment are discussed, and areas for further research are identified.

Poststroke Aphasia

Left hemisphere stroke typically results in aphasia, a primary language impairment.[1] The majority of research into co-speech gesture production in neurogenic populations is drawn from patients with poststroke aphasia (PWA). Severity of language dysfunction in aphasia varies depending on lesion size and location and often involves both expressive and receptive language abilities [21]. The classical model categorizes aphasia into subtypes depending on the degree of language impairment across three dimensions: fluency of speech, auditory comprehension, and repetition [22, 23]. This yields eight aphasic variants: anomic, conduction, transcortical motor, Broca's, transcortical sensory, Wernicke's, transcortical mixed (also known as isolation aphasia), and global aphasia. The boundaries between variants are not clear cut, and indeed, it is estimated that up to a quarter of PWA may present with an aphasia type that is unclassifiable, although the classical model remains the most commonly used system in English-speaking countries [24].

Most research into co-speech gesture production in PWA is drawn from studies of individuals with (relatively) unimpaired auditory comprehension (i.e., those with anomic, conduction, transcortical motor, and Broca's aphasias under the classical model) or with Wernicke's aphasia. Research into gesture use in PWA with global, isolation/transcortical mixed, and transcortical sensory aphasias is sparse.

Evidence suggests that gestures produced by PWA may vary as a function of aphasia subtype. In a study of narrative production in PWA with non-fluent Broca's and fluent Wernicke's aphasias, Carlomagno and Cristilli found that just as speaking rate differed significantly between PWA groups with Broca's aphasia producing fewer words per minute, gesture rate also varied, although in the opposite direction: the Broca's group produced more gestures per word than the Wernicke's counterparts [25]. However, contrasting results were found by Pritchard et al., who also included PWA with anomic and conduction aphasias as well as Wernicke's and Broca's in their sample, with no difference in gesture rate found between groups [26]. The reason for these differing findings is unclear, although as both studies included very small numbers of Broca's participants (five and three, respectively), further research is required to determine if there is indeed a significant difference in gesture rate between fluent and non-fluent aphasic groups.

Beyond gesture rate, there is some evidence that the relative frequency of gesture types used by PWA differs both from neurologically healthy adults and indeed within people with different aphasic variants. PWA with preserved auditory comprehension and semantic processing (i.e., anomic, conduction, transcortical motor, and Broca's aphasias) have been found to produce more iconic and pantomime gestures than do PWA with other aphasic subtypes. By contrast, PWA with Wernicke's aphasia produce relatively more referential, metaphoric, deictic, and beat gestures. For example, in an early study of gesture production in unstructured discourse in PWA of Wernicke's and Broca's subtypes, Le May et al. found that PWA with Wernicke's aphasia used significantly more metaphoric gestures (referred to as "kinetographs") in unstructured conversation and picture description tasks than Broca's participants, who used significantly more iconic gestures (referred to as "ideographs") [27].

[1] Other less common causes of aphasia include brain tumors and epilepsy. Temporary aphasia can also occur after a transient ischemic attack or "mini-stroke."

Similar results were found by Sekine and Rose in a study of 46 PWA in a story retell task, with Wernicke's participants found to use significantly more metaphoric gestures than PWA with other aphasic subtypes, in particular PWA with Broca's aphasia who used more iconic gestures [6]. Speakers with Wernicke's aphasia have also been found to produce more gestures per minute (though not necessarily per word) than other aphasic groups, but their gestures have been described as vague and difficult for interlocuters to interpret, mirroring characteristics of their speech output [6, 27, 28].

Iconic gesture use in particular has been found to be more common in PWA with anomic and Broca's aphasias during episodes of word-finding difficulty than during fluent connected speech. This could be because gestures may have a facilitatory effect on lexical retrieval (which will be discussed in more detail below) or as a compensatory measure to replace speech [29]. Akhavan et al. demonstrated that in PWA with anomic and Broca's aphasias of varying severity, iconic gesture use was strongly associated with successful word retrieval in a story retell task: 88% of episodes of successful word retrieval were associated with production of an iconic gesture [30]. However, the vast majority of word-finding episodes in the sample remained unresolved, suggesting that even if iconic gestures were used, they were not always facilitatory of lexical retrieval and were sometimes used to replace speech. Indeed, this alternative role for gesture use is supported by evidence that PWA with Broca's and transcortical motor aphasias use co-speech gestures significantly more frequently alongside production of nonwords and word truncations, indicating that in at least some cases, gesture use is a compensatory strategy for impaired speech production [15].

The broad gesture production patterns for different aphasic variants described in the previous paragraphs are summarized in Table 10.2.

Unsurprisingly, because the speech modality is typically impaired in aphasia, evidence suggests that PWA transmit relatively more information via the gesture channel compared with neurologically healthy adults. Rose et al. demon-

Table 10.2 Summary of aphasic subtypes and gesture production characteristics

Aphasia subtype	Key features of gesture production
Anomic	– Gesture production profile broadly similar to neurologically healthy adults but may produce more iconic gestures and beat gestures during episodes of word-finding difficulty [6, 15, 30].
Broca's; conduction	– Produce significantly more iconic gestures than neurologically healthy adults and people with fluent aphasia [25, 27]. – Produce relatively more iconic, pantomime, and deictic gestures than other gesture types [6, 28]. – May produce more iconic gestures and beat gestures during episodes of word-finding difficulty [15, 30]. – May produce gestures slowly and haltingly in line with speech production [31].
Global; transcortical mixed/isolation	– Limited data available, may use emblems more frequently than other gesture types [32].
Transcortical motor	– Gesture production profile broadly similar to neurologically healthy adults [6]. – Produce a high number of semantically rich gestures [6]. – May use beat gestures to get the pace of speech and generate rhythm, particularly during episodes of word-finding difficulty [15].
Transcortical sensory	– Limited data available.
Wernicke's	– Use a more restricted range of gesture types than other aphasic groups [6]. – Gestures may be vague and difficult for interlocuters to interpret [6]. – Use relatively more metaphoric, referential, deictic, and beat gestures and relatively fewer iconic gestures [6, 27]. – Produce fewer iconic gestures per word than PWA with Broca's aphasia [25]. – May produce gestures relatively rapidly in line with speech production [31].

strated that listener comprehension was greater when PWA with conduction, Broca's, transcortical motor, and anomic aphasias combined speech and gesture to transmit messages, compared to when messages were transmitted via speech or gesture alone [33]. For PWA, gestures may carry more of the intended meaning relative to speech than they do for neurologically healthy adults; Pritchard et al. found that in a procedural discourse task, PWA with anomic, conduction, Wernicke's, and Broca's aphasias relied on gestures to convey information absent from speech to a significantly greater degree than neurologically healthy adults, presumably because the speech channel was less available to them, although it was not clear whether gesture usefulness varied between aphasic groups [26]. In turn, interlocuters also rate gestures produced by PWA to be essential to the successful transmission of the message more frequently than they do for neurologically healthy adults [32, 34, 35]. For instance, van Nispen et al. found that on average 22% of co-speech gestures (specifically emblems, deictics, and iconic gestures) produced by PWA with conduction, transcortical motor, Wernicke's, anomic, and Broca's aphasias of varying severity were deemed to be essential for successful communication compared with around 5% for neurologically healthy adults, although sample size for each subtype was small (5–10 per group) [35]. Effective use of the gesture channel does however appear to be of considerable importance in successful communication for at least some PWA.

Limb Apraxia and Communicative Gesture

A key confound in studies of gesture production in PWA after stroke (and indeed, in people with neurological conditions in general) is the presence and severity of upper limb apraxia. Apraxia commonly co-occurs with poststroke aphasia and is characterized by deficits in skilled movements, which cannot otherwise be explained by motor or cognitive deficits [36]. There are, broadly speaking, two major types of limb apraxia characterized by differing underlying mechanisms, lesion profiles, and performance patterns, though the literature is inconsistent. The first type, ideational or conceptual apraxia, reflects loss of conceptual information about actions and manipulable objects. In stroke as well as in the semantic variant of primary progressive aphasia (discussed in more detail below), the disorder most often occurs following damage that includes the left posterior temporal cortex and temporoparietal junction. This region is critical for knowledge of action meaning ("action semantics") and appearance of gestures associated with manipulable objects (e.g., what a "hammering" gesture looks and feels like, or how the hand looks and feels when using scissors). The second type, production or ideomotor apraxia, reflects a deficit in transforming relatively intact action semantic knowledge into a motor plan for positioning the body in space over time. It is most often associated with damage that includes the frontoparietal cortex but spares the temporal lobe [37]. Both subtypes are associated with impaired performance on gesture production tasks and are thus difficult to distinguish behaviorally with most clinical assessment tools, but ideational apraxia is additionally characterized by poor performance on gesture recognition tasks and poor production of both meaningful and meaningless gestures (i.e., meaning does not benefit gesture production). A functional-neuroanatomic framework has not, to our knowledge, been applied in prior studies of communicative gesture in PWA but may be helpful in making sense of at least some of the contradictions in the literature.

Early studies of gesture production in PWA identified impairments in pantomime gesture imitation, meaningless gesture imitation, and tool use, leading to suggestions that gesture production deficits in PWA may be attributable (at least partly) to apraxia [38, 39]. However, these studies did not test the informativeness of gestures produced by individuals with and without apraxia, leaving unresolved the question of whether apraxia influences gestural communication. Other studies have concluded that apraxia may indeed affect the comprehensibility of gestures produced by PWA [40]. For example, Feyereisen et al. reported that although patients with more severe apraxia used the gestural modality to communicate more frequently than patients with less severe apraxia in a referential communication task, their gestures were more difficult for interlocuters to comprehend [41]. Similar results were found by Borod et al., who asked nurses and speech-language pathologists to rate the spontaneous gestural communication of patients with apraxia: the more severe the patient's apraxic deficit, the less effective their use of gestures to communicate [42]. More recently, van Nispen et al. found in a group of PWA that impairments in the production of manipulable object use gestures on an apraxia test were associated with substantial reductions in the informativeness of gestures in conveying information to interlocuters [43]. Hogrefe et el. also demonstrated that impairment on a pantomime to command test strongly predicted comprehensibility of gestures and weakly predicted gesture diversity in a story retell task in individuals with severe aphasia [44].

Taken together, the literature suggests that limb apraxia may be associated with reductions in the communicative content that can be conveyed through the gesture channel. Of interest for future studies will be assessment of whether apraxia profiles (i.e., and in particular, the status of semantic knowledge about actions and manipulable objects) mediate this effect. Based on the prior studies in PWA, it may be the case that patients whose aphasia is associated with damage to the middle and posterior temporal lobe (e.g., Wernicke's) will exhibit conceptual (ideational) apraxia and reduced comprehensibility of the communicative gestures produced, whereas patients with non-fluent aphasias (e.g., Broca's) and relative preservation of the posterior temporal lobe will exhibit production (ideomotor) apraxia and relatively preserved gesture comprehensibility. Additionally of interest will be assessment of whether apraxia profile predicts the ratio of iconic to metaphoric and other gesture types employed by PWA; based on their loss of conceptual knowledge of actions and manipulable objects, it might be predicted that individuals with ideational apraxia may exhibit reductions in at least some types of iconic gestures.

Right Hemisphere Damage (RHD)

As the language and praxic control centers in the brain are usually left lateralized, right hemisphere stroke does not generally cause a primary language or gesture production impairment, but typically results in prosodic and discourse processing deficits in at least 50% of patients [45]. Deficits include monotone speech production, impaired turn-taking, atypical eye-gaze behaviors, and poor comprehension of nonliteral language and emotional prosody [46, 47]. Visuospatial processing deficits are also common [48]. Compared with the literature available on co-speech gesture production in aphasia, far less is known about co-speech gesture production deficits following right hemisphere stroke.

Early case studies suggested that RHD resulted in an "agestural" presentation in which patients were unable to express emotional states through gesture, although imitative pantomime gesture production was spared [49]. More recent studies have concluded that people with RHD produce fewer iconic gestures than neurologically healthy controls, especially in contexts of high emotional content [50–52]. Akbıyık et al. found no difference in overall gesture rates between people with RHD and neurologically healthy controls and indeed found that gesture rate was correlated with overall narrative competence in this group [53]. Interestingly, some studies have found that people with RHD show increased rates of noncommunicative manual behaviors during interaction, such as self-touching, scratching, or grooming [52, 54].

To summarize, patients with RHD demonstrate reduced production of iconic gestures, particularly alongside speech with higher emotional content, while their gesture rate is comparable to that of neurologically healthy adults. Patients with RHD may also produce a greater number of noncommunicative hand movements during speech.

Gesture Production in Chronic Neurogenic Populations

In this section, co-speech gesture production in two other populations of adults with acquired communication impairment will be briefly reviewed: dementia (Alzheimer's disease and primary progressive aphasia) and Parkinson's disease. These conditions are chosen because of their known impact on verbal communication. Compared with research into co-speech gesture production in poststroke aphasia, there have been relatively few studies of co-speech gesture production in progressive neurological conditions.

Gesture Production in Dementia

Communication impairment occurs across a range of dementia subtypes. We have chosen here to focus on two in particular: Alzheimer's disease, the most common form of dementia, and primary progressive aphasia, a presentation of frontotemporal dementia which is characterized (in the early stages) by selective deficits in language processing.

Alzheimer's disease (AD) is a progressive neurological condition in which impairments in memory and learning are the dominant clinical features. Neural degeneration in AD is diffuse but usually starts in mesial temporal regions, accounting for the early memory deficits typical of the condition [55]. In later stages, however, global deficits develop as neural degeneration becomes more widespread. Speech production impairments have been well studied in AD, and in the initial stages, significant word retrieval deficits, circumlocutions, and semantically "empty" speech (i.e., Wernicke's aphasia) are often evident [56, 57]. In late-stage AD, generalized semantic deficits appear and speech production decreases and/or becomes distorted; in the very late stages, people with AD may have minimal or no speech output at all [58].

In contrast to the relatively well-studied speech deficits that occur in AD, gesture production deficits have received less attention. Upper limb apraxia is known to occur early in AD but is particularly evident during late-stage disease [59, 60]. Research into the efficiency of co-speech gesture production in AD is mixed. Overall rates of gesture production have been found to be comparable between people with moderate AD and neurologically healthy adults, but gesture informativeness may be variable [61, 62]. In people with AD, the evidence suggests that gesture production breaks down in parallel with speech, with gestures devoid of semantic content mirroring similarly "empty" speech production [63, 64]. In summary, while overall gesture production frequency is comparable to that of neurologically healthy adults in at least the early-to-moderate stages of AD, production of semantically rich gestures may be impaired alongside the lexico-semantic deficits seen in speech production in this population.

Compared to AD, significantly less is known about gesture production in PPA. PPA is a presentation of frontotemporal dementia in which impairment of language processing is the primary deficit. Currently, three subtypes are recognized: semantic (svPPA), logopenic PPA (lvPPA), and non-fluent (nfvPPA)[2] [65], with a fourth type, mixed PPA, encompassing those whose profiles do not fit readily into any of the aforementioned categories [66]. Because neural degeneration is (initially) localized to the frontal and temporal lobes in PPA, patients may experience minimal or no other symptoms for several years. However, disease progression eventually results in global dementia and, in some cases of lvPPA and nfvPPA, degenerative syndromes involving the motor system such as corticobasal degeneration [67].

To our knowledge, there is to date no comprehensive analysis of co-speech gesture production in any subtype of PPA. In a single case study, Macoir et al. demonstrated that a verb cueing technique utilizing gesture observation improved action naming in an individual with svPPA, with

[2] Note that in the literature, multiple terms are used to refer to each subtype of PPA. svPPA is also known as semantic dementia and PPA-S; lvPPA is also known as logopenic progressive aphasia and PPA-L; nfvPPA is also known as progressive non-fluent aphasia, non-fluent/agrammatic variant PPA, agrammatic PPA, and PPA-G.

the treatment effect lasting for at least four weeks after the intervention. However, the effect of gesture *production* on action naming was not assessed [68].

Limb apraxia is common in PPA, occurring in all three variants, and is associated with decreased volume of the left anterior inferior parietal cortex extending into the posterior superior temporal gyrus [69, 70]. Upper limb apraxia, rigidity, and extrapyramidal features like those seen in corticobasal syndrome and progressive supranuclear palsy have been found in patients with more advanced nfvPPA. In svPPA, loss of semantic knowledge results in progressive lexico-semantic deficits in speech production. A single case study of an individual with svPPA showed evidence of significantly reduced iconic gesture production with predominant use of deictics indicating location, suggesting a gestural presentation similar to that seen in poststroke Wernicke's aphasia [71]. People with svPPA also show increased production of conceptual gesture errors (e.g., vague or unrecognizable gestures), and a recent case series demonstrated that individuals with svPPA—unlike lvPPA and nfvPPA—showed reduced benefits of meaning in gesture imitation accuracy, consistent with conceptual apraxia [72, 73]. In lvPPA, decreased speech output with phonemic paraphasias is common, with co-occurring apraxia and other clinical features reminiscent of AD [67]. Finally, two further case studies showed that two people with lvPPA and mixed PPA, respectively, were able to use gestures as replacements for impaired speech, compensating for word-finding difficulty [74].

Taken together, it may be hypothesized that co-speech gesture production in PPA is impaired along the lines of the deficits seen in speech production, as in some studies of people with AD. However, further research is needed in this population to confirm this.

Gesture Production in Parkinson's Disease

Parkinson's disease (PD) is a progressive neurological condition which is regarded as primarily a disorder of movement, due to the dominance of its three major clinical features: rigidity, tremor, and brady-hypokinesia (slowness and reduced amplitude of movement). Impairments in co-speech gesture production in this population have therefore been assumed to relate to motor deficits. More recently, however, it has been recognized that cognitive deficits are also present in PD, including impairments in memory, executive function, attention, visuospatial processing, and language processing [75, 76]. In particular, processing of action words is impaired in PD, including in early stages of the disease before significant cognitive impairment is present, one explanation for which is that people with PD may have a specific action semantics deficit that contributes to production difficulties for action-related language [77].

There is some evidence that the putative action semantic deficits in patients with PD may differ from that seen in posterior temporal stroke or svPPA, in that PD is associated with abnormalities in motor *simulation* rather than visual semantic feature processing [78]. In one of the few systematic studies of gesture production in PD, Humphries et al. found a difference in the specific type of iconic gestures produced by people with PD compared to neurologically healthy controls: although overall rates of iconic (as well as metaphoric and deictic) gesture production did not differ between groups, people with PD produced more gestures from a character viewpoint (i.e., in which the speaker depicts an event as though they are performing it themselves), compared to healthy controls who described the same event from an observer viewpoint (in which the speaker depicts an event as though observing it from afar) [79]. A possible reason for this finding is that patients with PD have difficulty mentally representing performing actions themselves and need to rely instead on visual information (which largely relates to extra-personal space) to activate motor patterns for gestures [79, 80]. In terms of the rate of gesture production in PD, evidence is mixed, with some studies finding reduced gesture rate per 100 words (taking into account the markedly slower speech production rate in PD) compared with neurologically healthy controls, and others finding no difference [81–83].

To summarize, specific gesture production impairments found in people with PD cannot solely be attributed to motor symptom severity and may instead reflect a more subtle deficit in implicit simulation of motor actions. Reduced gesture rate has been found in this population, along with a tendency towards producing action gestures from a character viewpoint perspective. However, the frequency of production of iconic, metaphoric, and deictic gestures mirrors that produced by neurologically healthy adults overall.

How Are Co-speech Gestures Integrated with Speech?

To account for the characteristics of gesture production in neurogenic populations described above, this section now turns to cognitive models that have been proposed to explain how speech and gestures interact during language production. Two highly influential psycholinguistic models are briefly reviewed: the lexical retrieval hypothesis (LRH) [84] and the information packaging hypothesis [85]. Both models are predicated on the idea that co-speech gestures have a speaker-oriented function: for the LRH, this is related to lexical retrieval, and for the information packaging hypothesis to efficient chunking of information. However, the models differ in the point in time at which they conceive speech and gestures to interact: according to the LRH, speech and gestures interact at later stages of word production, while the information packaging hypothesis assumes interaction from the earliest, conceptual stage.

The Lexical Retrieval Hypothesis (LRH)

The lexical retrieval hypothesis proposes that the function of co-speech gestures (referred to in this model as "lexical gestures") is to facilitate the speaker's lexical retrieval and word production. Word production is hypothesized to be a nonlinear process in which semantic units (concepts), lexical units (words), and phonological structure (phonemes, syllables, etc.) interact multidirectionally. Activation spreads from the semantic level (conceptualization) to the word level (lexical selection) and to the phonological level (phoneme selection), resulting in a state that enables the word to be articulated [86]. According to the LRH, gestures interact with speech after the conceptualization stage and accompany activity at the level of either lexical selection or phoneme selection. Gestures encode spatial representations that may prime word retrieval, at least when the content of speech is spatial in nature. For example, when describing a trip to the seaside, the speaker activates imagistic mental representations of the paths taken during the trip. These mental representations lead to the retrieval and production of gestures that correspond to features of the motion along these paths. In turn, during lexical and phoneme selection, these gestures support the retrieval and articulation of the corresponding words. Constraining a speaker from gesturing should therefore result in dysfluent and anomic speech production, particularly for words with spatial content, because the facilitatory effect of gestures on lexical or phoneme selection is absent [84].

Evidence for the facilitation of word retrieval by gestures in both neurologically healthy adults and adults with acquired language impairment is mixed. In studies of "tip of the tongue" states, where lexical retrieval failure is typically phonological, preventing neurologically healthy adults from gesturing significantly reduces the frequency of successful lexical retrieval [87]; neurologically healthy adults have also been found to produce speech significantly more fluently when they are permitted to gesture, compared with when they are constrained from doing so [84]. However, a more recent study by Kisa et al. in which neurologically healthy adults were prevented from gesturing found no effect of gesture on fluency or word retrieval in a story retell task, for words with either concrete (e.g., "The scuba diver *went down*") or metaphoric (e.g., "My opinion of him *went up*") spatial content [88].

In populations with acquired language impairment, the picture is equally unclear. In broad terms, those with primarily phonological deficits have been found to benefit from production of gestures during word retrieval; for those with language impairment linked to conceptual or lexico-semantic deficits, gesture effects on word retrieval are either absent or inconsistent [89–94]. For example, in a novel word learning paradigm, Kroenke et al. found that successful word retrieval was associated with iconic gesture production in PWA, but only those with phonological deficits benefited. PWA with impaired semantic processing did not [95]. Comparable results were found by Akhavan et al. and Kistner et al., with iconic gestures facilitating word retrieval for PWA with intact semantic processing in both studies, in a story retell task and in spontaneous conversation, respectively [30, 96]. This suggests that where gesture is effective in facilitating lexical retrieval, it does so across communicative contexts. In contrast, Kong et al. reported an association between increased gesture use and episodes of word-finding difficulties in some native Cantonese-speaking PWA, but a minimal facilitatory effect of iconic gestures on lexical retrieval. In fact, iconic gestures were found to play a greater role reinforcing content already present in speech than in facilitating its production [97, 98]. Indeed, where gestures do accompany successful lexical retrieval, this may not be due to the facilitatory effect of the gestures themselves: an alternative hypothesis is that lexical items with stronger conceptual representations simply give rise to both speech and gestures [30].

In summary, it is unclear as to what extent gestures may facilitate lexical retrieval. While it is indeed the case that successful word retrieval may be accompanied by gestures, this is not universal. Particularly in neurogenic populations, alternative functions of gesture, such as its compensatory role in replacing or enhancing verbal information, should be considered alongside the possibility that gestures facilitate word retrieval.

Information Packaging Hypothesis

In contrast with the LRH, the information packaging hypothesis assumes that interaction between speech and gestures occurs from the earliest phase of conceptualization of the message. According to this hypothesis, gestures help speakers to organize or "package" spatial information via "spatio-motoric" thinking, a method of information processing distinct from analytic thinking, in which information is organized hierarchically into words and phrases. Analytic thinking is the mode by which speech is produced, and its templates for speech comprise linguistically specified information, such as semantic and pragmatic features of words and how words can be combined into phrases. In contrast, spatio-motoric thinking, which underlies gesture production, relies on information organized according to action schemas, specifying how the body interacts with the environment, both physical and imaginary. When producing speech and gestures simultaneously, the speaker therefore has access to two modes of information processing, which continuously influence each other during production of the utterance and enable more effective "packaging" or chunking of complex information during communication [85].

Unlike the LRH, the information packaging hypothesis assumes that speech and gesture are separate and independent systems, which continually interact in the service of a common communicative goal. The model is compatible with the production of gestures in the absence of speech, and with incongruities between speech and co-speech gestures, both of which occur in people with acquired communication disorders. For example, in studies of narrative production in people with poststroke language impairment, Dipper et al. and Pritchard et al. both found evidence for a particular gesture-language incongruence in discourse production in PWA: the pairing of "empty" or "light" verbs (i.e., those that contain minimal semantic information) with semantically rich gestures, such as pairing the verb "go" with gestures indicating the manner and direction of movement [26, 99].

To summarize, co-speech gestures are hypothesized to perform speaker-oriented functions during discourse, including aiding lexical retrieval and facilitating effective packaging of communicative information. Both the LRH and the information packaging hypothesis may account for some findings from the neurogenic communication disorder literature. However, the models differ in their respective conceptions of the starting point of gesture integration with speech: in the LRH, in line with gesture's role in facilitating speech production, gestures interact with speech at the level of lexical or phoneme selection, whereas according to the information packaging hypothesis, gestures and speech bidirectionally interact from conceptualization of the message. Further research is required to refine our analyses of the timepoint at which speech and gestures interact, and indeed to determine whether and how this differs between neurologically healthy speakers and those with acquired communication impairments.

Challenges in Researching Co-speech Gesture Production in Neurogenic Populations

Despite the ubiquitous nature of co-speech gesture production, it will be clear from the review above that characterizing features of gesture production in neurogenic populations is challenging, particularly in less common conditions such as PPA. Here, we identify key challenges in conducting gesture research and make suggestions for future progress.

First, constructing appropriate experimental methodologies to capture gestures integrated with speech remains difficult. Neuroimaging techniques such as fMRI are problematic; gesturing inevitably results in movement artifacts which affect data analysis, while attempts to reduce artifacts may result in artificial gesture environments compromising the ecological validity of findings [53]. Consequently, much evidence is based on lesion studies, accounting for the fact that studies involving people with poststroke aphasia dominate the gesture production literature [100]. However, lesions may be large and frequently involve multiple brain regions, making it difficult to identify the precise neuroanatomical networks subserving gesture production. This limitation may be overcome with the use of more recently developed lesion analysis approaches such as support vector regression lesion-symptom mapping, in which behavioral symptoms are related to mapped lesions across the brain, although these analyses require large sample sizes [101].

Second, as mentioned above, limb apraxia remains a major confounding factor in many gesture production studies. Comprehensive assessment of apraxia severity should be incorporated into background testing for research participants from clinical populations and, depending on the research question, may be included in data analysis as a mediating or control variable. Further research into the effect of apraxia profiles on gesture intelligibility, and how apraxia affects production of specific gesture types in clinical populations, would be beneficial.

Task design is an additional confounding factor. That task demands affect gesture production is well known; for example, both neurologically healthy adults and PWA gesture more frequently when producing narratives with spatial content [26, 102], and iconic gestures are more likely to be produced than other gesture types during procedural narratives [103]. Gesture production studies usually elicit gestures using one or at most two tasks, which may or may not involve spontaneous face-to-face interaction. It is unclear whether such studies accurately capture how people with acquired communication disorders gesture in daily life [104]. Ideally, gesture production studies should assess gesture performance across a range of elicitation tasks including naturalistic conversation.

As communication involves at least two people, the use of confederates in study design can also be problematic unless their behaviors are specifically accounted for in data analysis. A speaker will flexibly adapt their communication to the audience, providing more or less information across speech and gesture channels based on the common ground between them [105]. People with acquired neurological conditions also do this: patients with hippocampal amnesia use gestures more frequently when describing procedural narratives to children than to adult listeners, and PWA use more iconic gestures when interacting with unfamiliar listeners than with familiar listeners [96, 106]. Both the confederate and participant may therefore adapt their communication styles to each other, resulting in an artificial interaction. In studies where the researcher is interacting directly with the patient, they will inevitably be familiar with the experimental manipulations and predictions involved and may engage in unintentional "microbehaviors" that influence participant performance [104]. As a result, it may be necessary to elicit gesture production across multiple contexts and with a variety of familiar and unfamiliar interlocuters.

Lastly, gesture coding is typically inconsistent between studies. No single system for coding the form and function of gestures exists, and researchers use varying definitions for gesture types. As a result, conclusions are not necessarily generalizable across studies, particularly if experimental tasks also differ. Using computer software packages and advanced machine learning techniques may help to reduce inconsistency. Programs like ANVIL and ELAN enable detailed frame-by-frame gesture annotation, and tools such as OpenPose employ machine learning to semiautomatically code gestures, reducing the time-consuming task of manual coding [107–109]. Finally, unified gesture coding systems such as the MultiModal MultiDimensional (M3D) labeling system are in development, which can be used to flexibly code gestures across both neurologically healthy adults and patient groups, including traditional categorical coding of gesture types and enabling continuous coding of gesture speed and trajectory [110]. Consistently employing these technologies has the potential to significantly improve our understanding of gesture production in a range of neurogenic populations.

The challenges described above notwithstanding, greater insight into impairment patterns and the neural substrates underlying gesture production could have important benefits for neurorehabilitation. Gesture production is an integral part of certain therapy programs for improving communication in patients with acquired language disorders, such as gestural facilitation of naming, Promoting Aphasics' Communicative Effectiveness (PACE), and Multi-Modality Aphasia Therapy (M-MAT) [92, 111, 112]. In contrast, other therapy programs specifically restrict the use of gesture (e.g., constraint-induced aphasia therapy) [113]. Recent comparative studies suggest that both approaches may be effective in improving communication, in at least some patients [114–116]. However, there remain significant individual differences in treatment response, and there is currently limited understanding of behavioral and lesion markers to identify and predict which patients are likely to derive greater benefit from a particular treatment pathway [116]. Identifying these markers has the potential for significant impact on patient quality of life and should be a primary focus of research moving forward.

Major Takeaways

1. Co-speech gesture production deficits are commonly observed in populations with acquired language impairments.
2. Patterns of impairment are heterogenous and poorly understood, particularly in progressive neurological conditions.
3. Multiple barriers exist in developing a comprehensive understanding of gesture impairments in acquired neurological conditions.
4. Improving experimental design and developing unified gesture coding methods may help to reduce inconsistencies.

References

1. Holler J, & Levinson SC. Multimodal language processing in human communication. trends in cognitive sciences, 2019;23(8):639–652. https://doi.org/10.1016/j.tics.2019.05.006
2. Goldin-Meadow S. How gesture promotes learning throughout childhood. Child Dev Perspect. 2009;3(2):106–11.
3. Holler J, Kendrick KH, Levinson SC. Processing language in face-to-face conversation: questions with gestures get faster responses. Psychon Bull Rev. 2018;25(5):1900–8.
4. Kendon A. Gesticulation and speech: two aspects of the process of utterance. In: Key M, editor. The rela-

tionship of verbal and nonverbal communication. The Hague: Mouton; 1980. p. 207–27.
5. McNeill D. Hand and mind: What gestures reveal about thought. Chicago: University of Chicago Press; 1992.
6. Sekine K, Rose ML. The relationship of aphasia type and gesture production in people with aphasia. Am J Speech Lang Pathol. 2013;22(4):662–72.
7. Dargue N, Sweller N, Jones MP. When our hands help us understand: a meta-analysis into the effects of gesture on comprehension. Psychol Bull. 2019;145(8):765–84. Available from: https://pubmed.ncbi.nlm.nih.gov/31219263/
8. Zhang Y, Frassinelli D, Tuomainen J, Skipper JI, Vigliocco G. More than words: word predictability, prosody, gesture and mouth movements in natural language comprehension. Proc R Soc B. 2021;288:20210500.
9. Hupp JM, Gingras MC. The role of gesture meaningfulness in word learning. Gesture. 2016;15(3):340–56. Available from: https://www.jbe-platform.com/content/journals/10.1075/gest.15.3.04hup
10. Kita S, Alibali MW, Chu M. How do gestures influence thinking and speaking? The gesture-for-conceptualization hypothesis. Psychol Rev. 2017;124(3):245–66.
11. Cochet H, Vauclair J. Deictic gestures and symbolic gestures produced by adults in an experimental context: hand shapes and hand preferences. Laterality. 2014;19(3):278–301.
12. Yap D, Casasanto D. Beat gestures encode spatial semantics. In: 40th Annual Conference of the Cognitive Science Society; 2018.
13. Bosker HR, Peeters D. Beat gestures influence which speech sounds you hear. Proc R Soc B Biol Sci. 2021;288:20202419.
14. Bavelas JB, Chovil N, Lawrie AD, Wade A. Interactive gestures. Discourse Process. 1992;15:469–89.
15. Ferré G. Gesture, prosody and verbal content in non-fluent aphasic speech. Multimodal Commun. 2021;10(1):73–91.
16. Leonard T, Cummins F. The temporal relation between beat gestures and speech. Lang Cogn Process. 2011;26(10):1457–71.
17. de Beer C, de Ruiter JP, Hielscher-Fastabend M, Hogrefe K. The production of gesture and speech by people with aphasia: Influence of communicative constraints. J Speech Lang Hear Res. 2019;62(12):4417–32.
18. Cocks N, Dipper L, Middleton R, Morgan G. What can iconic gestures tell us about the language system? A case of conduction aphasia. Int J Lang Commun Disord. 2011;46(4):423–36.
19. Gullberg M. Handling discourse: gestures, reference tracking, and communication strategies in early L2. Lang Learn. 2006;56(1):155–96.
20. Cicone M, Wapner W, Foldi N, Zurif E, Gardner H. The relation between gesture and language in aphasic communication. Brain Lang. 1979;8(3):324–49.
21. Thye M, Mirman D. Relative contributions of lesion location and lesion size to predictions of varied language deficits in post-stroke aphasia. Neuroimage Clin. 2018;20:1129–38.
22. Goodglass H, Kaplan E. The assessment of aphasia and related disorders. Philadelphia: Lea & Febiger; 1972.
23. Geschwind N. The organization of language and the brain. Science. 1970;170(3961):940–4.
24. Kasselimis DS, Simos PG, Peppas C, Evdokimidis I, Potagas C. The unbridged gap between clinical diagnosis and contemporary research on aphasia: a short discussion on the validity and clinical utility of taxonomic categories. Brain Lang. 2017;164:63–7.
25. Carlomagno S, Cristilli C. Semantic attributes of iconic gestures in fluent and non-fluent aphasic adults. Brain Lang. 2006;99(1–2):104–5.
26. Pritchard M, Dipper L, Morgan G, Cocks N. Language and iconic gesture use in procedural discourse by speakers with aphasia. Aphasiology. 2015;29(7):826–44.
27. le May A, David R, Thomas AP. The use of spontaneous gesture by aphasic patients. Aphasiology. 1988;2(2):137–45.
28. Sekine K, Rose ML, Foster AM, Attard MC, Lanyon LE. Gesture production patterns in aphasic discourse: In-depth description and preliminary predictions. Aphasiology. 2013;27(9):1031–49.
29. Behrmann M, Penn C. Non-verbal communication of aphasic patients. Int J Lang Commun Disord. 1984;19(2):155–68. Available from: https://onlinelibrary.wiley.com/doi/full/10.3109/13682828409007186
30. Akhavan N, Göksun T, Nozari N. Integrity and function of gestures in aphasia. Aphasiology. 2017;32(11):1310–35.
31. McNeill D, Pedelty LL. Right brain and gesture. In: Emmorey K, Reilly J, editors. Language, gesture, and space. New York: Lawrence Erlbaum Associates, Inc; 1995. p. 63–85.
32. de Ruiter J. The production of gesture and speech. In: McNeill D, editor. Language and Gesture. Cambridge: Cambridge University Press; 2000. p. 284–311.
33. Rose ML, Mok Z, Sekine K. Communicative effectiveness of pantomime gesture in people with aphasia. Int J Lang Commun Disord. 2017;52(2):227–37. Available from: https://onlinelibrary.wiley.com/doi/full/10.1111/1460-6984.12268
34. de Ruiter J, de Beer C. A critical evaluation of models of gesture and speech production for understanding gesture in aphasia. Aphasiology. 2013;27(9):1015–30.
35. van Nispen K, van de Sandt-Koenderman M, Sekine K, Krahmer E, Rose ML. Part of the message comes in gesture: how people with aphasia convey information in different gesture types as compared with information in their speech. Aphasiology. 2017;31(9):1078–103.
36. Buxbaum LJ, Randerath J. Limb apraxia and the left parietal lobe. In: Vallar G, Branch Coslett H, edi-

tors. Handbook of Clinical Neurology. Amsterdam: Elsevier BV; 2018. p. 349-63.

37. Buxbaum LJ, Kalénine S. Apraxia: a disorder at the cognitive-motor interface. In: Poeppel M, Mangun R, Gazzaniga D, editors. The cognitive neurosciences. 6th ed. Cambridge: MIT Press; 2020. Available from: http://direct.mit.edu/books/edited-volume/chapter-pdf/2053724/c040700_9780262356176.pdf.
38. Goodglass H, Kaplan E. Disturbance of gesture and pantomime in aphasia. Brain. 1963;86:703–20. Available from: https://academic.oup.com/brain/article/86/4/703/321425
39. Wang L, Goodglass H. Pantomime, praxis, and aphasia. Brain Lang. 1992;42:402–18.
40. Völsch J, Wartenburger I, Stadie N. Do gestures have a hand in verb retrieval? Investigation of iconic and non-iconic gestures in aphasia. Aphasiology. 2021;2022(7):781–804.
41. Feyereisen P, Barter D, Goossens M, Clerebaut N. Gestures and speech in referential communication by aphasic subjects: channel use and efficiency. Aphasiology. 1988;2(1):21–32.
42. Borod JC, Fitzpatrick PM, Helm-Estabrooks N, Goodglass H. The relationship between limb apraxia and the spontaneous use of communicative gesture in aphasia. Brain Cogn. 1989;10(1):121–31.
43. van Nispen K, Mieke WME, van de Sandt-Koenderman E, Krahmer E. The comprehensibility of pantomimes produced by people with aphasia. Int J Lang Commun Disord. 2018;53(1):85–100.
44. Hogrefe K, Ziegler W, Weidinger N, Goldenberg G. Non-verbal communication in severe aphasia: Influence of aphasia, apraxia, or semantic processing? Cortex. 2012;48(8):952–62.
45. Côte H, Payer M, Giroux F, Joanette Y. Towards a description of clinical communication impairment profiles following right-hemisphere damage. Aphasiology. 2010;21(6–8):739–49. Available from: https://www.tandfonline.com/doi/abs/10.1080/02687030701192331
46. Lehman BM. The right hemisphere and disorders of cognition and communication: theory and clinical practice. San Diego: Plural Publishing; 2018.
47. Blake ML, Duffy JR, Myers PS, Tompkins CA. Prevalence and patterns of right hemisphere cognitive/communicative deficits: retrospective data from an inpatient rehabilitation unit. Aphasiology. 2010;16(4–6):537–47. Available from: https://www.tandfonline.com/doi/abs/10.1080/02687030244000194
48. Clough S, Duff MC. The role of gesture in communication and cognition: implications for understanding and treating neurogenic communication disorders. Front Hum Neurosci. 2020;14:323.
49. Ross ED, Mesulam MM. Dominant language functions of the right hemisphere? Prosody and emotional gesturing. Arch Neurol. 1979;36(3):144–8. Available from: https://jamanetwork.com/journals/jamaneurology/fullarticle/577290
50. Hogrefe K, Rein R, Skomroch H, Lausberg H. Co-speech hand movements during narrations: What is the impact of right vs. left hemisphere brain damage? Neuropsychologia. 2016;93:176–88.
51. Hadar U, Burstein A, Krauss R, Soroker N. Ideational gestures and speech in brain-damaged subjects. Lang Cogn Process. 2010;13(1):59–76. Available from: https://www.tandfonline.com/doi/abs/10.1080/016909698386591
52. Cocks N, Hird K, Kirsner K. The relationship between right hemisphere damage and gesture in spontaneous discourse. Aphasiology. 2007;21(3–4):299–319. Available from: https://www.tandfonline.com/doi/abs/10.1080/02687030600911393
53. Akbıyık S, Karaduman A, Göksun T, Chatterjee A. The relationship between co-speech gesture production and macrolinguistic discourse abilities in people with focal brain injury. Neuropsychologia 2018;117:440–53. doi: https://doi.org/10.1016/j.neuropsychologia.2018.06.025.
54. Blonder LX, Burns AF, Bowers D, Moore RW, Heilman KM. Spontaneous gestures following right hemisphere infarct. Neuropsychologia. 1995;33(2):203–13.
55. Mueller KD, Hermann B, Mecollari J, Turkstra LS. Connected speech and language in mild cognitive impairment and Alzheimer's disease: a review of picture description tasks. J Clin Exp Neuropsychol. 2018;40(9):917–39.
56. Nicholas M, Obler LK, Albert ML, Helm-Estabrooks N. Empty speech in Alzheimer's disease and fluent aphasia. J Speech Hear Res. 1985;28(3):405–10.
57. Faber-Langendoen K, Morris JC, Knesevich JW, LaBarge E, Miller JP, Berg L. Aphasia in senile dementia of the Alzheimer type. Ann Neurol. 1988;23(4):365–70. Available from: https://onlinelibrary.wiley.com/doi/full/10.1002/ana.410230409
58. Caramelli P, Mansur LL, Nitrini R. Language and communication disorders in dementia of the Alzheimer type. In: Handbook of Neurolinguistics. New York, NY: Elsevier; 1998. p. 463–73.
59. Rousseaux M, Rénier J, Anicet L, Pasquier F, Mackowiak-Cordoliani MA. Gesture comprehension, knowledge and production in Alzheimer's disease. Eur J Neurol. 2012;19(7):1037–44. Available from: https://onlinelibrary.wiley.com/doi/full/10.1111/j.1468-1331.2012.03674.x
60. Parakh R, Roy E, Koo E, Black S. Pantomime and imitation of limb gestures in relation to the severity of Alzheimer's disease. Brain Cogn 2004;55:272–4.
61. Geladó S, Gómez-Ruiz I, Diéguez-Vide F. Gestures analysis during a picture description task: Capacity to discriminate between healthy controls, mild cognitive impairment, and Alzheimer's disease. J Neurolinguistics. 2022;61:101038.
62. Glosser G, Wiley MJ, Barnoski EJ. Gestural communication in Alzheimer's disease. J Clin Exp Neuropsychol. 2010;20(1):1–13. https://doi.org/10.1076/jcen.20.1.1.1484.

63. Carlomagno S, Pandolfi M, Marini A, di Iasi G, Cristilli C. Coverbal gestures in Alzheimer's type dementia. Cortex. 2005;41(4):535–46.
64. Rousseaux M, Sève A, Vallet M, Pasquier F, Mackowiak-Cordoliani MA. An analysis of communication in conversation in patients with dementia. Neuropsychologia. 2010;48:3884–90.
65. Gorno-Tempini ML, Hillis AE, Weintraub S, Kertesz A, Mendez M, Cappa SF, et al. Classification of primary progressive aphasia and its variants. Neurology. 2011;76(11):1006. Available from: https://pubmed.ncbi.nlm.nih.gov/21325651/
66. Ruksenaite J, Volkmer A, Jiang J, Johnson JC, Marshall CR, Warren JD, et al. Primary progressive aphasia: toward a pathophysiological synthesis. Curr Neurol Neurosci Rep. 2021;21(3):7. https://doi.org/10.1007/s11910-021-01097-z.
67. Harciarek M, Sitek EJ, Kertesz A. The patterns of progression in primary progressive aphasia—implications for assessment and management. Aphasiology. 2014;28(8–9):964–80. https://doi.org/10.1080/02687038.2014.904498.
68. Macoir J, Leroy M, Routhier S, Auclair-Ouellet N, Houde M, Laforce R. Improving verb anomia in the semantic variant of primary progressive aphasia: the effectiveness of a semantic-phonological cueing treatment. Neurocase. 2015;21(4):448–56.
69. Yliranta A, Jehkonen M. Limb and face apraxias in frontotemporal dementia: a systematic scoping review. Cortex. 2020;129:529–47. Available from: https://pubmed.ncbi.nlm.nih.gov/32418629/
70. Nelissen N, Pazzaglia M, Vandenbulcke M, Sunaert S, Fannes K, Dupont P, et al. Gesture discrimination in primary progressive aphasia: the intersection between gesture and language processing pathways. J Neurosci. 2010;30(18):6334.
71. Kindell J, Sage K, Keady J, Wilkinson R. Adapting to conversation with semantic dementia: using enactment as a compensatory strategy in everyday social interaction. Int J Lang Commun Disord. 2013;48(5):497–507.
72. Dresang HC, Williamson R, Kim H, Hillis AE, Buxbaum LJ. Gesture profiles distinguish primary progressive aphasia variants. bioRxiv : the preprint server for biology, 2023.01.19.524719. https://doi.org/10.1101/2023.01.19.524719
73. Baumard J, Lesourd M, Remigereau C, Merck C, Jarry C, Etcharry-Bouyx F, et al. The – weak – role of memory in tool use: evidence from neurodegenerative diseases. Neuropsychologia. 2019;129:117–32.
74. Volkmer A, Mistry S, Thompson D, Warren JD, Beeke S. Collaborative turn-construction practices of people with primary progressive aphasia and their family conversation partners. Journal of Interactional Research in Communication Disorders, 2023;14(3):456–85. https://doi.org/10.1558/jircd.25504
75. Verbaan D, Marinus J, Visser M, van Rooden SM, Stiggelbout AM, Middelkoop HA, et al. Cognitive impairment in Parkinson's disease. J Neurol Neurosurg Psychiatry. 2007;78:1182–7. Available from: www.jnnp.com
76. Raskin SA, Sliwinski M, Borod JC. Clustering strategies on tasks of verbal fluency in Parkinson's disease. Neuropsychologia. 1992;30(1):95–9. Available from: https://pubmed.ncbi.nlm.nih.gov/1738474/
77. Bocanegra Y, García AM, Pineda D, Buriticá O, Villegas A, Lopera F, et al. Syntax, action verbs, action semantics, and object semantics in Parkinson's disease: dissociability, progression, and executive influences. Cortex. 2015;69:237–54.
78. Klostermann F, Wyrobnik M, Boll M, Ehlen F, Tiedt HO. Tracing embodied word production in persons with Parkinson's disease in distinct motor conditions. Sci Rep. 2022;12:16669. https://doi.org/10.1038/s41598-022-21106-6.
79. Humphries S, Holler J, Crawford TJ, Herrera E, Poliakoff E. A third-person perspective on co-speech action gestures in Parkinson's disease. Cortex. 2016;78:44–54.
80. Humphries S, Holler J, Crawford T, Poliakoff E. Cospeech gestures are a window into the effects of Parkinson's disease on action representations. J Exp Psychol Gen. 2021;150(8):1581–97. https://doi.org/10.1037/xge0001002.supp.
81. Saatci Yurtsever S, Öztop Çakmak Ö, Yapıcı Eser H, Ertan S, Demir-Lira E, Göksun T. Production and comprehension of co-speech gestures in Parkinson's disease. Neuropsychologia. 2021;163:108061.
82. Cleary RA, Poliakoff E, Galpin A, Dick JPR, Holler J. An investigation of co-speech gesture production during action description in Parkinson's disease. Parkinsonism Relat Disord. 2011;17(10):753–6.
83. Poliakoff E, Marciniak M, Bettis A, Humphries S. Speaking with your hands in Parkinson's: Investigating the rate and precision of co-speech gestures. In: MDS Virtual Congress 2021; 2021. p. 1122. Available from: https://www.mdsabstracts.org/abstract/speaking-with-your-hands-in-parkinsons-investigating-the-rate-and-precision-of-co-speech-gestures/.
84. Rauscher FH, Krauss RM, Chen Y. Gesture, speech, and lexical access: the role of lexical movements in speech production. Psychol Sci. 1996;7(4):226–31.
85. Kita S. How representational gestures help speaking. In: McNeill D, editor. Language and Gesture. Cambridge: Cambridge University Press; 2000. p. 162-85.
86. Dell GS, Chang F, Griffin ZM. Connectionist models of language production: lexical access and grammatical encoding. Cogn Sci. 1999;23(4):517–42.
87. Frick-Horbury D, Guttentag RE. The effects of restricting hand gesture production on lexical retrieval and free recall. Am J Psychol. 1998;111(1):43–62.
88. Kısa YD, Goldin-Meadow S, Casasanto D. Do gestures really facilitate speech production? J Exp Psychol Gen. 2021;151(6):1252–71.
89. Bonifazi S, Tomaiuolo F, Altoè G, Ceravolo M, Provinciali L, Marangolo P. Action observation as a useful approach for enhancing recovery of verb production: new evidence from aphasia of innovative low-cost interventions in language rehabilitation. Eur J Phys Rehabil Med. 2013;49(4):473–81.

90. Boo M, Rose ML. The efficacy of repetition, semantic, and gesture treatments for verb retrieval and use in Broca's aphasia. Aphasiology. 2010;25(2): 154–75.
91. Raymer AM, Singletary F, Rodriguez A, Ciampitti M, Heilman KM, Rothi LJG. Effects of gesture+verbal treatment for noun and verb retrieval in aphasia. J Int Neuropsychol Soc. 2006;12(6):867–82. Available from: https://www.cambridge.org/core/journals/journal-of-the-international-neuropsychological-society/article/abs/effects-of-gestureverbal-treatment-for-noun-and-verb-retrieval-in-aphasia/CC7F4968B259441581B6EC774DD91EA7
92. Raymer AM, McHose B, Smith KG, Iman L, Ambrose A, Casselton C. Contrasting effects of errorless naming treatment and gestural facilitation for word retrieval in aphasia. Neuropsychol Rehabil. 2012;22(2):235–66.
93. Rose M, Douglas J, Matyas T. The comparative effectiveness of gesture and verbal treatments for a specific phonologic naming impairment. Aphasiology. 2010;16(10):1001–30.
94. Rose M, Sussmilch G. The effects of semantic and gesture treatments on verb retrieval and verb use in aphasia. Aphasiology. 2008;22(7–8):691–706.
95. Kroenke KM, Kraft I, Regenbrecht F, Obrig H. Lexical learning in mild aphasia: gesture benefit depends on patholinguistic profile and lesion pattern. Cortex. 2013;49(10):2637–49.
96. Kistner J, Dipper LT, Marshall J. The use and function of gestures in word-finding difficulties in aphasia. Aphasiology. 2019;33(11):1372–92.
97. Pak-Hin Kong A, Law SP, Ching-Yin Kwan C, Lai C, Lam V, et al. A coding system with independent annotations of gesture forms and functions during verbal communication: development of a database of speech and GEsture (DoSaGE). J Nonverbal Behav. 2015;39:93–111.
98. Kong APH, Law SP, Chak GWC. A comparison of coverbal gesture use in oral discourse among speakers with fluent and nonfluent aphasia. J Speech Lang Hear Res. 2017;60(7):2031–46.
99. Dipper L, Pritchard M, Morgan G, Cocks N. The language-gesture connection: evidence from aphasia. Clin Linguist Phon. 2015;29(8–10):748–63. https://doi.org/10.3109/02699206.2015.1036462.
100. Emmorey K, Ozyurek A. Language in our hands: neural underpinnings of sign language and co-speech gesture. In: Gazzaniga M, Mangun, G, editors. The cognitive neurosciences. Cambridge, Mass.: MIT Press; 2014. p. 656–66.
101. Zhang Y, Kimberg DY, Coslett HB, Schwartz MF, Wang Z. Multivariate lesion-symptom mapping using support vector regression. Hum Brain Mapp. 2014;35(12):5861–76.
102. Kita S, Lausberg H. Generation of co-speech gestures based on spatial imagery from the right-hemisphere: evidence from split-brain patients. Cortex. 2008;44(2):131–9. Available from: https://pubmed.ncbi.nlm.nih.gov/18387542/
103. Stark BC, Cofoid C. Task-specific iconic gesturing during spoken discourse in aphasia. Am J Speech Lang Pathol. 2021:1–18.
104. Stark BC, Clough S, Duff M. Suggestions for improving the investigation of gesture in aphasia. J Speech Lang Hear Res. 2021;64(10):4004.
105. Doedens WJ, Meteyard L. Measures of functional, real-world communication for aphasia: a critical review. Aphasiology. 2020;34(4):492–514.
106. Clough S, Hilverman C, Brown-Schmidt S, Duff MC. Evidence of audience design in amnesia: adaptation in gesture but not speech. Brain Sci. 2022;12(8):1082. Available from: https://www.mdpi.com/2076-3425/12/8/1082/htm
107. Kipp M. ANVIL: A generic annotation tool for multimodal dialogue. In: EUROSPEECH 2001 Scandinavia, 7th European Conference on Speech Communication and Technology. International Speech Communication Association; 2001. p. 1367–70.
108. Lausberg H, Sloetjes H. Coding gestural behavior with the NEUROGES-ELAN system. Behav Res Methods. 2009;41(3):841–9.
109. Ienaga N, Cravotta A, Terayama K, Scotney BW, Saito H, Busà MG. Semi-automation of gesture annotation by machine learning and human collaboration. Lang Resour Eval. 2022;56(3):673–700. Available from: https://link.springer.com/article/10.1007/s10579-022-09586-4
110. Rohrer PL, Vilà-Giménez I, Florit-Pons J, Gurrado G, Gibert NE, Ren P, et al. The MultiModal MultiDimensional (M3D) labeling system. OSF. 2020; Available from: https://osf.io/ankdx/
111. Davis GA. PACE revisited. Aphasiology. 2011;19(1):21–38. Available from: https://www.tandfonline.com/doi/abs/10.1080/02687030444000598
112. Rose ML. Releasing the constraints on aphasia therapy: the positive impact of gesture and multimodality treatments. Am J Speech Lang Pathol. 2013;22(2) https://doi.org/10.1044/1058-0360%282012/12-0091%29.
113. Pulvermüller F, Neininger B, Elbert T, Mohr B, Rockstroh B, Koebbel P, et al. Constraint-induced therapy of chronic aphasia after stroke. Stroke. 2001;32(7):1621–6. https://doi.org/10.1161/01.STR.32.7.1621.
114. Attard M, Rose ML, Lanyon L. The comparative effects of multi-modality aphasia therapy and constraint-induced aphasia therapy-plus for severe chronic Broca's aphasia: an in-depth pilot study. Aphasiology. 2013;27(1):80–111.
115. Pierce JE, Menahemi-Falkov M, O'Halloran R, Togher L, Rose ML. Constraint and multimodal approaches to therapy for chronic aphasia: a systematic review and meta-analysis. Neuropsychol Rehabil. 2017;29(7):1005–41. https://doi.org/10.1080/09602011.2017.1365730.
116. Rose ML, Nickels L, Copland D, Togher L, Godecke E, Meinzer M, et al. Results of the COMPARE trial of constraint-induced or multimodality aphasia therapy compared with usual care in chronic post-stroke aphasia. J Neurol Neurosurg Psychiatry. 2022:1–9.

Isobel Chick, M.Sc., qualified as a speech and language therapist at the University of Reading before specializing in adult and pediatric neurorehabilitation in clinical practice. She previously worked at the Acquired Brain and Communication Disorders Lab at the University of Reading and is currently a doctoral researcher at the Language and Cognition Lab at University College London.

Peter Garrard, Ph.D., qualified in medicine at Bristol University in 1990. He trained in general medicine, specializing in neurology and completing a Ph.D. in cognitive neuroscience during a clinical training fellowship at the University of Cambridge. He has been fully accredited in neurology since 2000. He held senior clinical academic positions at University College London and the University of Southampton, before moving to St. George's, where he is currently Professor of Neurology, in 2011.

Laurel J. Buxbaum, Psy.D., directs the Cognition and Action Laboratory at Moss Rehabilitation Research Institute and is Professor of Rehabilitation Medicine at Thomas Jefferson University. She has served as Associate Editor of the journals *Cognition, Cortex*, and *Journal of Neuropsychology*. She is the recipient of the International Neuropsychological Society's *Arthur Benton Mid-Career Award*, the Widener University Graduate *Award for Excellence in Professional Psychology*, the American Society of Neurorehabilitation's *Kenneth Viste Award*, and the British Neuropsychological Society's *Freda Newcombe Prize*. Her laboratory focuses on the cognitive neuroscience of skilled action and tool representations, as well as relationships between action and language.

Gabriella Vigliocco, Ph.D., is Professor of the Psychology of Language at University College London. She received her Ph.D. from the University of Trieste and previously worked at the University of Wisconsin and the Max Planck Institute for Psycholinguistics. Her work has been supported by major funders, and she has published broadly in cognitive science and neuroscience. Her research aims to understand the cognitive and neurobiological foundations of human communication. She currently investigates how children, adults, and people with aphasia use language in social interaction, focusing on how verbal and nonverbal elements of communication come together in language development and use.

11 Discourse Production in Multilingual People with Aphasia

Mira Goral

Preview of What Is Currently Known
Assessing communication abilities and impairment in multilingual people with aphasia is challenging. Multilingual people with aphasia can have comparable or differential abilities in their different languages. Multilingual people with aphasia, like typical multilingual speakers, often mix elements from all their languages in a single discourse. Various approaches to the analysis of discourse production in aphasia have been used in the literature.

Objectives
(a) To present challenges associated with assessing multilingual people with aphasia.
(b) To discuss discourse production as an alternative measure for assessing language and communication of multilingual people with aphasia.
(c) To highlight challenges associated with the analysis of discourse production of multilingual people with aphasia.
(d) To discuss language mixing as a typical phenomenon in discourse in multilingual people with aphasia.

M. Goral (✉)
Department of Speech-Language-Hearing Sciences, Lehman College, The City University of New York, Bronx, New York, USA
e-mail: MIRA.GORAL@lehman.cuny.edu

Introduction

Multilingual people who acquire aphasia due to brain damage challenge monolingual-based clinical practices and scientific investigations. In this chapter, the characteristics of discourse production in multilingual people with aphasia (MPWA) and the value of using discourse production in the assessment of their languages will be discussed. It will start with a brief overview of the manifestation of aphasia in multilingual people, followed by a discussion of the challenges of assessing language and communication impairments in multiple languages. A brief introduction to discourse analysis as a measure that captures communication strengths and weaknesses in aphasia in multilingual people will then be given, summarizing results from recent studies. After arguing for the usefulness of assessing discourse production in all languages relevant to the person with aphasia, the chapter will conclude with avenues for future study.

Aphasia

Aphasia is an acquired language disorder, resulting from brain damage due to stroke, tumor, or degenerative disease. The profile of the acquired impairment varies across individuals in terms of severity and scope. For example, people with mild aphasia can engage in meaningful commu-

A. P.-H. Kong (ed.), *Spoken Discourse Impairments in the Neurogenic Populations*,
https://doi.org/10.1007/978-3-031-45190-4_11

nicative exchanges despite their word-finding difficulty and reduced ability to comprehend multiple-person conversations, whereas people with severe aphasia can struggle to produce simple phrases and sentences, experience notable word-finding difficulties, and have difficulties comprehending spoken language and engaging in a conversation. Different aphasia profiles are associated with differential or comparable difficulty in language production versus language comprehension, and in the degree to which the linguistic impairment hinders functional communication [1].

When aphasia is experienced by multilingual people—individuals who use more than one language to communicate—it can affect all of their languages. Research reports on multilingual people who have aphasia demonstrate that in many, albeit not all cases, parallel impairments are evident in the languages of the multilingual person [2–4]. A couple of definitions are in order here. The term multilingualism encompasses people who have high proficiency in both or all their languages, as well as those who have different levels of proficiency in one—their dominant language—than in the other language(s) they use. Some multilingual people acquire all their languages simultaneously, from an early age, and for some—as in sequential multilingualism—there is one first language, the one acquired from birth, and other languages are learned in later childhood or in adulthood [5]. According to Grosjean, multilingual people are those who use more than one language to communicate, regardless of their proficiency levels [6].

The term parallel impairments refers to the relationship between the impairment observed post-onset relative to the abilities (reported) pre-onset [3, 7]. The literature has seen a lively discussion regarding the question of whether parallel levels of impairments and recovery in aphasia are the norm rather than the exception, and, when non-parallel patterns are observed, what variables determine which language will be better spared and better recovered [2, 8]. At least three factors often interact here—the age (and manner) of the language learning, the proficiency achieved in each language, and the degree that each language is used throughout the life of the individual and at the time of the aphasia onset [7]. For example, many people with aphasia demonstrate better post-onset abilities in their earlier acquired language(s) [8, 9], but if a later learned language becomes the one most used post-onset, its performance can surpass that of an early acquired one [10, 11]. Furthermore, languages that are not used much post-onset may undergo attrition which will compound the effects of the aphasia [12].

Critical to this line of research is the method in which the abilities of each language are assessed. Assessment in MPWA is challenging not only for theoretically driven investigations but also in the clinic. Challenges include potential confounds associated with the procedure of administrating the assessment (e.g., establishing a language mode, administering the assessment by monolingual vs. multilingual examiners) and those associated with using comparable tests in all the languages assessed [13].

Assuring comparable materials across languages has been an ongoing effort in the field. One of the most used assessment tests designed specifically for assessing MPWA is the Bilingual Aphasia Test (BAT) [14]. The BAT, a comprehensive assessment of word, sentence, and paragraph level production and comprehension tasks is available in over 70 languages. The different language versions are constructed to be comparable in the range of abilities they test and in levels of difficulty within the subtests. However, the validity of the BAT and all its versions has not been established and the contribution of proficiency versus aphasia to the observed performance in each language is difficult to disentangle [15, 16]. Furthermore, certain aspects of syntax and morphology, verb retrieval, and detailed analysis of connected language production are not sufficiently included in the test [17, 18]. Another available tool is the Comprehensive Aphasia Test (CAT), which was developed in English while taking into account psycholinguistic and psychometrics properties. The CAT has been adapted to multiple additional languages, taking into account language-specific characteristics [19, 20]. Here, too, careful construction of the different language versions of the test is a strength, but these versions were developed and normative data were collected by and large from monolingual speakers of each language. Multilingual individuals' familiarity with specific items, picture stimuli, and structures is difficult to establish. Furthermore, the functional communication consequences are difficult to appraise on the basis of the standardized assessment, a challenge for many aphasia batteries and tests.

Indeed, a key question in the presence of aphasia is the degree to which the linguistic deficits affect daily communication. People with aphasia experience difficulty using language to tell their stories and engage in meaningful conversations. This difficulty is related to the degree of the aphasia severity and to the specific aphasia profile, and varies across individuals. The use of discourse—language beyond single words and sentences—is fundamental to communication: We tell each other what happened to us, what we saw or heard happened to others, what we plan to do in the future, etc. Effective, informative discourse contains well-formed sentences that are organized in a coherent manner and are tied to each other. Impairments of any number of linguistic aspects will contribute to difficulty communicating via discourse production.

Discourse Production in Aphasia

The ubiquitous word-level measures and interventions in aphasia, while informative, have their limits. In assessment, performance at the word level and at the discourse level do not always align, with some persons with aphasia (PWA) performing better at single-word retrieval tasks and others at connected language production tasks [21]. Moreover, generalization from single word performance to discourse level performance following intervention has proven difficult to achieve [22, 23]. If the goal is to understand discourse-level impairment and to affect discourse-level improvement, discourse needs to be targeted directly.

Impairments of discourse production in aphasia may include reduced overall output, reduced variety of words used, incomplete or ungrammatical sentences, reduced cohesion and coherence, reduced complexity, and presence of dysfluencies, including pausing, rephrasing, and abandoned utterances [24, 25]. Increased attention has been given in the aphasia literature to the analysis of discourse and the specific outcome measures used [25–30]. As these review papers reveal, great variability characterizes the measures reported across studies that focus on discourse production. For example, in their review, Bryant et al. [24] found a variety of elicitation methods and of linguistic analysis measures. The review, which included 175 studies, found over 50 different individual measures and little agreement across studies. Several recent studies have attempted to provide psychometric information and validation to a subset of such outcome measures [25, 31]. The measures that have received much attention as well as validation span microanalyses of words and sentences and macroanalyses of coherence and content. These include, for example, lexical measures (e.g., lexical diversity), syntactic measures (e.g., sentence complexity and grammaticality), coherence measures (e.g., local and global coherence), measures of productivity (e.g., total number of words and total number of content units), and measures of dysfluency (e.g., pauses, reformulations, and mazes) [24, 32–34].

Scholars have recognized not only the importance of measuring discourse-level performance in aphasia but also of targeting it directly in aphasia treatment. As well, the use of discourse production as a measure of treatment outcome has become more common as researchers and clinicians have emphasized the importance of aphasia treatment generalization to functional language outcomes. A recent review of discourse-level aphasia treatment demonstrates the plethora of studies that have employed discourse-based treatment and discourse-based measurements [28]. At the focus of the review was script training—an intervention that comprises repeated production of discourse tailored to the interest, needs, and level of impairment of the individual [35].

Whereas the analysis of discourse in aphasia has been explored primarily in English, additional languages have been investigated, including Cantonese [36], Japanese [37], Norwegian, and Italian, among others [29, 38]. Cross-linguistic differences can affect the analyses of specific micro- and macrostructures of discourse, as languages vary in how, for example, they mark cohesion between sentences, their use of verb morphology, and in their anaphora use. For PWA who are users of more than one language, assessing discourse performance in all languages, for the purpose of assessing aphasia severity as well as for the purpose of measuring treatment generalization within- and across-languages, is critical, although challenging. The next section will discuss in detail the study of discourse production in MPWA.

Eliciting and Analyzing Discourse Production in MPWA

In addition to selecting the outcome measures which best reflect the degree of impaired and spared communication abilities in aphasia, three considerations unique to the discourse produced in the multiple languages of MPWA need attention. One is the common practice of multilingual people to mix elements from more than one language in their language production; another is the presence of cross-linguistic influences; and, finally, the challenge of dissociating characteristics of the discourse production that are related to the aphasia versus to language proficiency levels prior to and following the aphasia onset. These considerations are addressed through examples from the literature. The relatively few existing studies that focus on discourse production in MPWA illustrate these three considerations and demonstrate the importance of including discourse production as a measure of communication abilities in aphasia and as an outcome measure to evaluate treatment efficacy [32, 39–41].

Consider the study of Neumann et al. [39], which analyzed several aspects of discourse production in each of the two languages of their bilingual participant. Neumann and colleagues elicited narratives from a Yiddish-English bilingual participant with moderate stroke-induced non-fluent aphasia and focused their analysis on sentence grammaticality and complexity, the use of discourse markers, and language mixing. The narratives were elicited in each language separately, using cue words (e.g., "custom," "accident"). The authors found that the participant produced longer narratives in his first language (L1, Yiddish) than in his early acquired second language (L2, English), and that more of his sentences were grammatical in L1 than in L2. This was consistent with his better performance in L1 on several of the BAT subtests (e.g., following complex commands; derivational morphology). In contrast, language mixing was more frequent during narrative production in L1 than in L2, contrary to the authors' prediction. The direction of language mixing observed, however, is consistent with the participant's report of using primarily English since the aphasia onset. The study demonstrates the importance of examining frequency and direction of language mixing in connected language production and the potential dissociation between measures of specific linguistic impairments and communication abilities. The topic of language mixing is addressed further below.

Another study that demonstrates the unique contribution of analyzing discourse reports on a bilingual participant with progressive aphasia [18]. The authors elicited and analyzed data from an English-Norwegian bilingual person with the logopenic variant of primary progress aphasia (PPA). The connected language production was elicited with a picture sequence description task (from the BAT), an autobiographical interview, and during small talk before and after the formal testing tasks in each language. The authors noted the participant's ability to engage in conversation, especially in his L1, despite marked word finding difficulties observed during picture naming. The difference between the single word tasks and the connect language production was especially true for the conversation assessment, during which the interlocutor could play an active part in the communication exchange. Of note, in most studies that report on discourse production in MPWA, elicited narratives—monologues—are utilized. Monologues may be easier to score than dialogues on a variety of linguistic measures, but dialogues may be more reflective of real-life communication [42, 43]. A recent review of the use of conversation as an outcome measure in aphasia revealed great variability in the way conversations with PWA were analyzed [44].

Several studies in the growing literature on treatment effects following intervention with MPWA included in their outcome measures elicited language production [32, 38, 40, 45]. For example, three studies, each reporting on treatment-related changes in a multilingual person, focused on the connected language production measures and demonstrated the contribution of measuring discourse production to language intervention outcomes in aphasia [32, 40, 45]. In one, Lerman et al. [40] used a comprehensive battery of tests at the word, sentence, and discourse levels to examine language production in their Hebrew-English speaking participant with mild-moderate non-fluent stroke-induced aphasia. The participant was assessed in each language and then administered 36 hours of intervention in his L2 English, targeting his word retrieval and sentence production. Following intervention, the authors observed improved performance in the treated language, English, on measures of word retrieval including object and action picture naming and sentence generation. Improved performance was noted in the untreated language, L1 Hebrew, only in the discourse measures (picture sequence description, elicited narratives). The study demonstrates that skipping the discourse-level measures would have resulted in a partially inaccurate profile of the treatment outcomes.

A similar conclusion was reached by Altman et al. [32] who studied a Hebrew-English-French trilingual person with mild aphasia. Here, too, intervention was administered in L2 English, and assessment was conducted in all three languages with a variety of measures. Whereas minimal change was observed in the participant's L1 on several tasks following treatment in L2, discourse analysis revealed positive response to treatment in L1 as well. The importance of including discourse measures may be especially true for the less-impaired language in MPWA. In a treatment study that focused on discourse-level treatment, Grasso and colleagues [45] administered a computerized version of script training in each of the two languages of a Spanish-English bilingual person with stroke-induced aphasia. The authors measured accuracy of script words, grammatical errors, speech rate, and intelligibility in trained and untrained scripts and found improvement in all measures in the trained scripts in each language, and little generalization to untrained scripts. They also found improvement of performance on the trained scripts when tested in the non-treated language (cross-language generalization).

In the studies described above, discourse was used as an outcome measure and the productions obtained by the participants were coded for a number of variables. In some studies, language mixing was also coded (e.g., counting the number of words produced in the non-target language [35]). The topic of language mixing has been at the core of several investigations with MPWA [46, 47]. One recent study specifically examined language mixing in discourse production in MPWA [46]. The participants, 11 multilingual individuals of varied language background and aphasia severity, each produced discourse in response to picture sequences and narrative prompts. The authors found that the frequency of language mixing was related to the severity of the aphasia generally as well as to the degree of relative impairment in each of the languages of the participants. Namely, greater language mixing was observed for individuals with more severe compared to milder aphasia, and mixing elements from a less impaired language was more common than mixing elements from the more impaired language. The more common mixed word type was nouns (e.g., using the English word "airplane" while telling a story in Spanish), as has been found for neurotypical multilingual speakers and for PWA in earlier studies [48, 49]. Other common word types include verbs (e.g., using "argue" in English while describing a picture in Hebrew) and discourse markers (such as "so").

Typically, analyses of discourse produced by MPWA treat each language, elicited separately, as the target language. Words and phrases from the non-target language are not counted toward correct content units, or in measures of sentence completeness and discourse coherence. Counting the relevant content and function words in each language separately likely results in more impaired performance as compared to when counting all elements from either language [50]. Considering elements from all language is akin to the conceptual scoring reported for bilingual children, who typically score better when words they demonstrated knowing in any one of their languages are counted toward their vocabulary knowledge [51]. Moreover, many multilingual speakers habitually mix elements from their complete linguistic repertoire rather than use only one language when speaking to interlocutors who use the same languages. Therefore, it may be that not only scoring, but also eliciting mixed language discourse during testing—approximating what is common for the MPWA in their daily communicative interactions—may be a more ecologically valid approach than eliciting discourse in each language separately [52].

One study with MPWA directly compared the discourse production elicited when the participants were told they were telling the story to a monolingual person and when they were told they were speaking with a bilingual person [49]. The findings suggest that the MPWA were sensitive to the communicative situation, and mixed their languages more when it was pragmatically appropriate than when they were attempting to speak to a monolingual interlocutor. The study did not find that the narratives produced in the bilingual conditions were superior to those produced in the monolingual condition in terms of measures such as total number of words produced, number of dysfluencies, and coherence.

Two related phenomena that can affect the analysis of discourse data are cross-linguistic influences in the production of MPWA, and aspects of the discourse that may be attributed to a less than complete mastery of the language rather than to the aphasia. Both are rather difficult to identify when measuring lexical diversity, grammaticality, and dysfluency measures of the connected language production. For example, sentences with verb agreement errors are common in the production of both people with aphasia and second language users. As well, word-finding difficulties during connected language production are a hallmark in aphasia but are also typical of second language users and of language attrition, and what may be coded as semantic paraphasia could also be word choice influenced by the multilingual's other language [12, 41]. Existing measures of discourse for aphasia do not include those aspects of analysis needed for MPWA.

Future Directions: Discourse Analysis as an Alternative to Standardized Testing in MPWA

With increasing attention to ecologically valid assessment and intervention in aphasia and to PWA's wellbeing, the need to assess all the languages that are relevant to an MPWA is no longer controversial. To overcome many of the challenges associated with the administration of standardized tests to assess MPWA's multiple languages, and to examine functional aspects of communication, discourse production measures emerge as an excellent choice. Validation studies for a number of the outcome measures that can be extracted from discourse production help make the process of discourse analysis increasingly more standardized. Additional research studies are needed to assure that these measures can be used comparably across multiple languages.

Phenomena that are specific to the discourse production of MPWA include language mixing, that is, the use of elements from the complete linguistic repertoire of the multilingual person rather than from one language at a time [53]. Conceptualizing language mixing as the norm is at the core of the translanguaging approach to multilingualism, which encourages multilingual people to use their complete linguistic repertoire in various communication situations. Similarly, for multilingual people with aphasia who communicate with other multilingual people, there is little reason to restrict discourse production to one language or to separate the languages in the analysis. Studies that examine assessment and treatment procedures that encourage the use of multiple languages by MPWA are needed, to establish administration and analysis protocols. Additionally, multilingual people experience cross-language influences that can affect how they use each of their languages and can mistakenly be taken as errors if considered from a monolingual-centric view.

Finally, pre-onset language proficiencies can affect all aspects of language abilities as observed post the aphasia onset and can be challenging to dissociate [12]. This is true for all levels of language production, including discourse. Taking into account a detailed language background history from MPWA can help disentangle the influence of pre-onset proficiency levels and of the acquired aphasia on performance. Additional research studies will help generate strategies for dissociating proficiency-related versus aphasia-related aspects of performance in aphasia. Finally, further research studies that examine discourse production of MPWA in naturalistic settings while language mixing is not discouraged will help generate ecologically valid data on mixing phenomena in MPWA.

Major Takeaways

1. Assessing conversation abilities and impairments in multilingual people with aphasia is a viable alternative to standardized testing.
2. Considering responses in all languages rather than separately in each language is helpful in assessing communication abilities in multilingual people with aphasia.
3. Translanguaging can be a useful framework in eliciting and analyzing discourse production in multilingual people with aphasia.
4. Multilingualism-related phenomena include language mixing, cross-linguistic influences, and pre-onset proficiency-related performance differences.

References

1. Papathanasiou I, Coppens P. Aphasia and related neurogenic communication disorders. 3rd ed. Burlington: Jones & Bartlett Learning; 2021.
2. Albert ML, Obler LK. The bilingual brain: neuropsychological and neurolinguistic aspects of bilingualism. New York: Academic Press; 1978.
3. Gray T, Kiran S. A theoretical account of lexical and semantic naming deficits in bilingual aphasia. J Speech Lang Hear Res. 2013;56(4):1314–27. https://doi.org/10.1044/1092-4388(2012/12-0091).
4. Paradis M. Bilingual and polyglot aphasia. In: Berndt RS, editor. Handbook of neuropsychology. 2nd ed. Amsterdam: Elsevier Science; 2001. p. 69–91.
5. Grosjean F. Bilingual: life and reality. Cambridge: Harvard University Press; 2012.
6. Grosjean F. The mysteries of bilingualism: unresolved issues. Hoboken: Wiley; 2022.
7. Lerman A, Goral M, Obler LK. The complex relationship between pre-stroke and post-stroke language abilities in multilingual aphasia. Aphasiology. 2020;34(11):1319–40. https://doi.org/10.1080/02687038.2019.1673303.
8. Kuzmina E, Goral M, Norvik M, Weekes B. What influences language impairment in bilingual aphasia? A meta-analytic review. Front Psychol. 2019;10:445. https://doi.org/10.3389/fpsyg.2019.00445.
9. Goral M. What can aphasia tell us about how the first-acquired language is instantiated in the brain? Languages. 2022;7(4):283. https://doi.org/10.3390/languages7040283.
10. Peñaloza C. The influence of prestroke proficiency on poststroke lexical-semantic performance in bilingual aphasia. Aphasiology. 2020;34(10):1223–40. https://doi.org/10.1080/02687038.2019.1666082.
11. Goral M, Naghibolhosseini M, Conner PS. Asymmetric inhibitory treatment effects in multilingual aphasia. Cogn Neuropsychol. 2013;30(7–8):564–77. https://doi.org/10.1080/02643294.2013.878692.
12. Lerman A, Goral M, Obler LK. Rehabilitating an attrited language in a bilingual person with aphasia. Clin Linguist Phon. 2022;37:272. https://doi.org/10.1080/02699206.2022.2052966.
13. Norvik M, Goral M. Assessment challenges in acquired aphasia in multilingual individuals. In: Røyneland U, Blackwood R, editors. Multilingualism across the lifespan. London: Routledge; 2021. p. 189–208.
14. Paradis M, Libben G. The assessment of bilingual aphasia. Hillsdale: Lawrence Erlbaum Associates; 1987.
15. Lee S, Faroqi-Shah Y. Performance of Korean-English bilinguals on an adaptation of the screening bilingual aphasia test. Int J Lang Commun Disord. 2021;56(4):719–38. https://doi.org/10.1111/1460-6984.12623.

16. Muñoz ML, Marquardt TP. The performance of neurologically normal bilingual speakers of Spanish and English on the short version of the bilingual aphasia test. Aphasiology. 2008;22(1):1–17. https://doi.org/10.1080/02687030600670742.
17. Knoph M. Language assessment of a Farsi-Norwegian bilingual speaker with aphasia. Clin Linguist Phon. 2011;25(6–7):530–9. https://doi.org/10.3109/02699206.2011.563900.
18. Lind M, Simonsen HG, Ribu IS, Svendsen BA, Svennevig J, de Bot K. Lexical access in a bilingual speaker with dementia: changes over time. Clin Linguist Phon. 2018;32:353–77. https://doi.org/10.1080/02699206.2017.1381168.
19. Fyndanis V, Lind M, Varlokosta S, Kambanaros M, Soroli E, Ceder K, Grohmann KK, Rofes A, et al. Cross-linguistic adaptations of the comprehensive aphasia test: challenges and solutions. Clin Linguist Phon. 2017;31(7–9):697–710. https://doi.org/10.1080/02699206.2017.1310299.
20. Swinburn K, Porter G, Howard D. Comprehensive aphasia test. 2nd ed. New York: Routledge; 2022.
21. Kavé G, Goral M. Do age-related word retrieval difficulties appear (or disappear) in connected speech? Neuropsychol Dev Cogn B Aging Neuropsychol Cogn. 2017;24(5):508–27. https://doi.org/10.1080/13825585.2016.1226249.
22. Best W, Greenwood A, Grassly J, Herbert R, Hickin J, Howard D. Aphasia rehabilitation: does generalisation from anomia therapy occur and is it predictable? A case series study. Cortex. 2013;49(9):2345–57. https://doi.org/10.1016/j.cortex.2013.01.005.
23. Webster J, Whitworth A, Morris J. Is it time to stop "fishing"? A review of generalisation following aphasia intervention. Aphasiology. 2015;29(11):1240–64. https://doi.org/10.1080/02687038.2015.1027169.
24. Bryant L, Ferguson A, Spencer E. Linguistic analysis of discourse in aphasia: a review of the literature. Clin Linguist Phon. 2016;30:489–518. https://doi.org/10.3109/02699206.2016.1145740.
25. Pritchard M, Hilari K, Cocks N, Dipper L. Psychometric properties of discourse measures in aphasia: acceptability, reliability, and validity. Int J Lang Commun Disord. 2018;53(6):1078–93. https://doi.org/10.1111/1460-6984.12420.
26. Armstrong E. Aphasic discourse analysis: the story so far. Aphasiology. 2000;14:875–92. https://doi.org/10.1080/02687030050127685.
27. Dipper LT, Marshall J, Boyle M, Botting N, Hersh D, Pritchard M, Cruice M. Treatment for improving discourse in aphasia: a systematic review and synthesis of the evidence base. Aphasiology. 2021;35(9):1125–67. https://doi.org/10.1080/02687038.2020.1765305.
28. Hubbard HI, Nelson LA, Richardson JD. Can script training improve narrative and conversation in aphasia across etiology? Semin Speech Lang. 2020;41(1):99–124. https://doi.org/10.1055/s-0039-3401030.
29. Linnik A, Bastiaanse R, Höhle B. Discourse production in aphasia: a current review of theoretical and methodological challenges. Aphasiology. 2016;30:765–800. https://doi.org/10.1080/02687038.2015.1113489.
30. Marini A, Andreetta S, Del Tin S, Carlomagno S. A multi-level approach to the analysis of narrative language in aphasia. Aphasiology. 2011;25:1372–92. https://doi.org/10.1080/02687038.2011.584690.
31. Stark BC, Dutta M, Murray LL, Bryant L, Fromm D, MacWhinney B, et al. Standardizing assessment of spoken discourse in aphasia: a working group with deliverables. Am J Speech Lang Pathol. 2021;30:491–502. https://doi.org/10.1044/2020_AJSLP-19-00093.
32. Altman C, Goral M, Levy ES. Integrated narrative analysis in multilingual aphasia: the relationship among narrative structure, grammaticality and fluency. Aphasiology. 2012;26:1029–52. https://doi.org/10.1080/02687038.2012.686103.
33. Rochon E, Saffran EM, Berndt RS, Schwartz MF. Quantitative analysis of aphasic sentence production: further development and new data. Brain Lang. 2000;72:193–218. https://doi.org/10.1006/brln.1999.2285.
34. Stark BC, Bryant L, Themistocleous C, den Ouden DB, Roberts AC. Best practice guidelines for reporting spoken discourse in aphasia and neurogenic communication disorders. Aphasiology. 2022;37:761. https://doi.org/10.1080/02687038.2022.2039372.
35. Cherney LR, Halper AS, Kaye RC. Computer-based script training for aphasia: emerging themes from post-treatment interviews. J Commun Disord. 2011;44(4):493–501. https://doi.org/10.1016/j.jcomdis.2011.04.002.
36. Kong A. The main concept analysis in Cantonese aphasic oral discourse: external validation and monitoring chronic aphasia. J Speech Lang Hear Res. 2011;54:148–59. https://doi.org/10.1044/1092-4388(2010/09-0240).
37. Yazu H, Kong A, Yoshihata H, Okubo K. Adaptation and validation of the main concept analysis of spoken discourse by native Japanese adults. Clin Linguist Phon. 2022;36(1):17–33. https://doi.org/10.1080/02699206.2021.1915385.
38. Knoph M, Gram Simonsen H, Lind M. Cross-linguistic transfer effects of verb-production therapy in two cases of multilingual aphasia. Aphasiology. 2017;31:1482–509. https://doi.org/10.1080/02687038.2017.1358447.
39. Neumann Y, Walters J, Altman C. Codeswitching and discourse markers in the narratives of a bilingual speaker with aphasia. Aphasiology. 2017;31:221–40. https://doi.org/10.1080/02687038.2016.1184222.
40. Lerman A, Edmonds L, Goral M. Cross-language generalisation in bilingual aphasia: what are we missing when we do not analyse discourse? Aphasiology. 2019;33(9):1154–62. https://doi.org/10.1080/02687038.2018.1538493.
41. Conner PS, Goral M, Anema I, Borodkin K, Haendler Y, Knoph M, Mustelier C, Paluska E, Melnikova Y, Moeyaert M. The role of language proficiency and

linguistic distance in cross-linguistic treatment effects in aphasia. Clin Linguist Phon. 2018;32(8):739–57. https://doi.org/10.1080/02699206.2018.1435723.
42. Perkins L. Applying conversation analysis to aphasia: clinical implications and analytic issues. Eur J Disord Commun. 1995;30(3):372–83. https://doi.org/10.3109/13682829509021449.
43. Beeke S, Maxim J, Wilkinson R. Using conversation analysis to assess and treat people with aphasia. Semin Speech Lang. 2007;28(2):136–47. https://doi.org/10.1055/s-2007-970571.
44. Azios JH, Archer B, Simmons-Mackie N, Raymer A, Carragher M, Shashikanth S, Gulick E. Conversation as an outcome of aphasia treatment: a systematic scoping review. Am J Speech Lang Pathol. 2022;31(6):2920–42. https://doi.org/10.1044/2022_AJSLP-22-00011.
45. Grasso SM, Cruz DF, Benavidez R, Peña ED, Henry ML. Video-implemented script training in a bilingual Spanish–English speaker with aphasia. J Speech Lang Hear Res. 2019;62(7):2295–316. https://doi.org/10.1044/2018_JSLHR-L-18-0048.
46. Goral M, Norvik M, Jensen B. Variation in codeswitching in multilingual aphasia. Clin Linguist Phon. 2019;33:915–29. https://doi.org/10.1080/02699206.2019.1584646.
47. Fyndanis V, Lehtonen M. Cognitive control and pathological language mixing in aphasia. In: Røyneland U, Blackwood R, editors. Multilingualism across the lifespan. London: Routledge; 2021. p. 209–30.
48. Muñoz ML, Marquardt TP, Copeland G. A comparison of the codeswitching patterns of aphasic and neurologically normal bilingual speakers of English and Spanish. Brain Lang. 1999;66(2):249–74. https://doi.org/10.1006/brln.1998.2021.
49. Paplikar A. Language-mixing in discourse in bilingual individuals with non-fluent aphasia. 2016.
50. Schultz F, Antolovic K, Hejazi Z, Goral M. Using a translanguaging framework to examine language production in a trilingual person with aphasia. Poster presented at the workshop on multilingual acquisition, processing and use, London. 2022.
51. Gibson TA, Peña ED, Bedore LM, McCarter KS. A longitudinal investigation of the semantic receptive-expressive gap in Spanish-English bilingual children. Int J Biling Educ Biling. 2022;25(3):819–33. https://doi.org/10.1080/13670050.2020.1721427.
52. Goral M. Intervention choices and considerations for multilingual people with aphasia. Invited talk at the 16th annual Eleanor M. Saffran conference, Philadelphia. 2022.
53. Otheguy R, García O, Reid W. Clarifying translanguaging and deconstructing named languages: a perspective from linguistics. Appl Linguist Rev. 2015;6(3):281–307. https://doi.org/10.1515/applirev-2015-0014.

Mira Goral is a Professor of Speech-Language-Hearing Sciences at Lehman College and the Graduate Center of The City University of New York (CUNY). She completed her B.A. in Linguistics at Tel Aviv University and her Ph.D. in Neurolinguistics at the Graduate Center, CUNY. She has co-edited three books and has published in the areas of bilingualism, multilingualism, aphasia, dementia, language attrition, and language and cognition in older adulthood.

Part II

Current Methods and Technology in Neurogenic Disordered Discourse Elicitation, Processing, and Analysis

Clinically Feasible Analysis of Discourse: Current State and Looking Forward

12

Sarah Grace H. Dalton and Jessica D. Richardson

Preview of What Is Currently Known
It has long been acknowledged that there is a mismatch between the outcomes that individuals with aphasia desire, and the outcomes most commonly targeted in research and therapy. Discourse ability better matches the desired outcomes of people with aphasia to re-engage in meaningful conversation and relationships. However, several barriers exist to implementing discourse analysis in clinical practice including lack of time for training and implementation and lack of psychometrically validated measures. Researchers have begun to address these barriers, and there are now several measures that may be clinically feasible.

Objectives
(a) To provide an overview of potentially transcriptionless discourse analysis measures.
(b) To highlight psychometric data for the reviewed measures.
(c) To provide an overview of potential uses of measures in stroke-induced aphasia.
(d) To provide an overview of potential uses of measures in progressive aphasia.

S. G. H. Dalton (✉)
Department of Speech Pathology and Audiology, Marquette University, Milwaukee, WI, USA
e-mail: sarahgrace.dalton@marquette.edu

J. D. Richardson
Department of Speech and Hearing Sciences, University of New Mexico, Albuquerque, NM, USA

Background

Boyle [1] outlined a procedure (see Table 1 in Boyle [1]) by which clinicians could more effectively determine the most appropriate methods, procedures, and analyses to use when measuring their clients' discourse. She asserts that one must have a clear goal for their analyses, and that they must be aware of both the strengths and weaknesses of various measures to utilize them appropriately. This chapter will serve as a resource that will help to answer one of the questions Boyle poses in her procedure, namely "Can you implement the outcome measure in your workplace?" by addressing a major consideration for clinical utility—transcription of discourse [1].

Transcription allows for the precise and thorough quantification of discourse behaviors of interest and is therefore attractive to many, especially within the research community. However, transcription is generally not clinically feasible, given high productivity requirements and caseloads in many clinical settings. Therefore, discourse measures that can be analyzed with no or minimal transcription will be the focus of this chapter. For each measure, key research evidence, including availability of materials, training, and psychometric data for both stable and progressive aphasia will be highlighted. More complex measures available at more advanced levels of transcription, which may be valuable in specific settings or under unique circumstances

A. P.-H. Kong (ed.), *Spoken Discourse Impairments in the Neurogenic Populations*,
https://doi.org/10.1007/978-3-031-45190-4_12

will also be *briefly* reviewed. Finally, a discussion with some recent advances that should facilitate increased utilization of discourse analysis in clinical settings is given, with a highlight on what problems still need to be addressed in order to truly make clinical discourse analysis feasible at all levels.

No Transcription

The least effortful option to analyze a discourse sample is to use measures that do not require transcription. This option is often preferred in clinical practice due to limited time for assessment and clinical documentation.

Perceptual Measures

Recent surveys indicate that most speech-language pathologists (SLPs) who conduct discourse assessment rely on their perceptions to determine the quality of discourse production [2–4]. Some SLPs use formal, standardized scales while others rely on informal impressions. In this section, research findings regarding perceptual measures, in particular listener judgments or ratings will be reviewed. In our opinion, these are ecologically valid discourse measures since communication partners' perceptions of an individual's language will affect if/how they engage. Similarly, if communication partners do not perceive changes in communication following therapy, we must consider whether we are targeting the most appropriate behaviors. Given such ecological validity, there is a large body of work on this topic. While it is outside the scope of the chapter to systematically review it, key studies to illustrate potential uses of listener judgments in clinical practice will be highlighted. Discussion of rating scales such as those available on aphasia assessments (e.g., Western Aphasia Battery [WAB-R] [5]) are not included since readers may be more familiar with these scales.

Listener Judgments of Discourse

Many studies using listener judgments of discourse are descriptive in nature [6–15]. These studies have typically investigated differences in listener judgments between healthy controls and persons with aphasia (PWAs) [6–8] or between different groups of PWAs [9, 10]. Listeners have been asked to rate aspects such as content and clarity of procedural [7] and narrative [8] discourse; coherence and clarity of personal narratives [12]; or ease of understanding, speaker enjoyment, believability, and whether the story was interesting [6]. Ulatowska, Olness, and colleagues have examined differences in discourse production between African American individuals with and without aphasia [13], between African American and Caucasian individuals [14], and have examined relationships between discourse production and performance on standardized aphasia assessments for African Americans with aphasia [15]. Across these different types of investigations, listener judgments have demonstrated good sensitivity, consistently identifying differences between controls and PWAs, different features of aphasia, and dialectal differences in discourse and its relationship to standardized testing.

Several studies have used listener judgments to identify potential changes in response to treatment [16–20]. The rationale for this is that listener perceptions of change should have good ecological validity—if a potential communication partner rates post-treatment discourse samples higher than pre-treatment samples they may be more likely to engage in conversation with the individual with aphasia or may find communication easier. Hickey and Rondeau [19] demonstrated that individuals with varying levels of knowledge of aphasia are sensitive to changes in discourse following treatment, and that raters with no experience or knowledge of aphasia had lower initial ratings than those with more experience, but that post-treatment ratings were similar to those with more experience. From this, the authors suggest that studies of social validity may have greater power when inexperienced raters are used. Cupit and colleagues [18] demonstrated that changes in ratings for both naive and experienced raters were only present in individuals who had completed therapy, further highlighting the validity of listener ratings for evaluating treatment change. Ratings used in these studies are similar to those used in descriptive studies (e.g., coherence, informativeness, clarity).

Qualitative Ratings of Discourse in Primary Progressive Aphasia (PPA)

In comparison to the body of literature on listener ratings in stroke-induced aphasia, there is relatively little research on perceptual and/or listener ratings in primary progressive aphasia (PPA). Pattee and colleagues [21] investigated the impact of two augmentative and alternative communication interventions (AAC; American Sign Language and speech generating device use) on discourse informativeness. They demonstrated that inexperienced raters who read transcripts of discourse samples rated almost all post-treatment samples as more informative than pre-treatment samples, across both conditions. Similarly, Rebstock and Wallace [22] demonstrated that listeners were better able to identify communicative attempts following a treatment which included semantic feature analysis and multimodal communication strategies. Qualitative ratings of listener perceptions may be a powerful method for ensuring that treatment targets functional communication outcomes, which is particularly critical for this population of individuals with progressive language impairment. Additional research is needed to determine the validity of listener judgments (and perceptual ratings) for persons with PPA (PwPPAs).

General Considerations

A common characteristic of studies for listener ratings is the varying methodology and focus of ratings. Many of the studies do not provide the rating response form for replication or use by other clinicians and researchers. More recently, the Discourse Rating Scale for Aphasia (DRSA) [23] was created to elicit listener ratings of discourse-specific behaviors. It includes items related to high-level discourse features such as completeness and relevance, as well as items seen on other perceptual ratings scales, such as grammar, word-finding difficulties, and paraphasias. A unique characteristic of the DRSA is that there are two versions available, one for the listener, and one for the individual with aphasia. Navarro [23] reports good construct validity of the DRSA, with correlations observed between the DRSA and several standardized aphasia assessments. However, the DRSA currently has limited psychometric data available with respect to reliability or validity (other than construct validity) and could benefit from expansion to include additional macrostructural ratings.

Perceptual and listener ratings provide a reference or metric of discourse abilities that can be easily communicated with clinicians, patients, and other support communities. These analyses generally have good face and ecological validity, but the limited scope of rating scales and listener judgments may lead to a lack of specificity or detail needed for treatment planning, goal setting, and prognosis. For example, two individuals could receive low informativeness ratings, but severe non-fluent aphasia limits verbal output in one individual, while logorrhea and semantic jargon render the discourse incomprehensible in the other individual. On a rating scale these individuals might present similarly but would require significantly different management. Careful consideration of the information needed from the discourse analysis should inform selection of perceptual rating scales or features for listener judgments. Further information regarding the psychometrics of specific, standardized rating scales are needed to increase the utility of this analytic approach.

Finally, considerations should be given to the method of rating. The studies discussed above use a variety of rating measures, from discrete Likert scales (i.e., rating 1–5, with no midpoints) to visual analog and anchor-based measures (i.e., marking a line with or without endpoints such as 1–100 or "clear"–"unclear"), where generally an example is provided, and then all other ratings are completed in relation to that example (either better than or worse than). It is important to consider the strengths and weaknesses of various rating methodologies when choosing how individuals will record their ratings.

Quantitative Measures

Core Lexicon Analysis

The core lexicon analysis (CoreLex) [24, 25] developed out of investigations aimed at understanding the vocabulary used by PWAs, and how that is compared to peers without language impairments [26–29]. A core lexicon is the set of lexical items most frequently used by healthy controls when producing a structured discourse (e.g., story retell, picture scene/sequence description, procedure) [25, 30]. CoreLex measures the typicality of words used to produce a structured discourse task, in comparison to the word choice of adults without language impairment, providing insights into lexical retrieval (including for specific parts of speech). Some CoreLex checklists have been developed with both content (noun, verb, adjective, adverb) and function (pronouns, determiners, prepositions, etc.) lexemes in a single list [30], while other checklists have been developed for specific parts of speech separately [31]. A recent compendium of CoreLex checklists was published [24] detailing methods of development, elicitation procedures, stimuli, full checklists, and available psychometrics for all available CoreLex lists.

A major benefit of CoreLex is its simple scoring, with one point given for each lexical item on the checklist (regardless of how many times an item is produced). Importantly, CoreLex checklists require that the individual produce the specific lexical item, rather than a semantically similar concept (so if "run" is a CoreLex item, a production of "jog" or "sprint" would not receive credit). Inflected forms of a CoreLex item do receive credit since they are the same lexeme (e.g., run, runs, running, ran or she, her, hers). In addition, for CoreLex checklists that combine content and function lexemes, the part of speech of a produced lexeme is not important. For example, if the lexeme "dress" were on a CoreLex checklist, then for productions such as "she wore a beautiful *dress*," and "she *dressed* up to go to the ball," either could receive credit.

Regardless of the specific formulation, studies of CoreLex have demonstrated its high inter-rater and intra-rater reliability [32]. It also has good ability to distinguish between PWAs and healthy controls [30, 33, 34] and between different subtypes of aphasia [30, 31, 34]; it also correlates with other microlinguistic [32], macrolinguistic [32], and hybrid [30] discourse measures. With respect to clinical applicability, there is preliminary evidence that CoreLex is sensitive to changes in response to treatment [33, 35] and in recovery from acute to chronic stages [36]. Finally, automated analysis of CoreLex is available for the AphasiaBank stimuli [37], and original [38] and modern [39] Cookie Theft images using the AphasiaBank's Computerized Language ANalysis (CLAN) [40] program. However, this automated analysis does require transcription, so it may not be most time effective unless additional quantitative analyses are planned.

CoreLex may provide a rough estimate of grammatical adequacy since some checklists include both content and function lexemes. However, given its relative simplicity and word-level analysis, CoreLex should not be over-interpreted with respect to high-level discourse behaviors such as informativeness, coherence, or organization. This simple, checklist-based scoring system should enable clinicians and researchers to use CoreLex in "real time," or from an audio- or video-recording. However, studies to date have primarily relied upon previously transcribed discourse samples, so the accuracy and reliability of implementing CoreLex without transcription is unknown at this time.

Content Units

Yorkston and Beukelman [41] developed the content unit (CU) analysis to quantify the informativeness of discourse samples. Using the Cookie Theft image [38], Yorkston and Beukelman created a list of words and phrases produced by at least one (out of 78) healthy controls when describing the image [41]. Single words were identified when a word was produced in multiple contexts while phrases were groupings of words that were *always* produced as a unit. In addition, acceptable alternatives for some CUs were identified as they were judged by the authors to communicate the same concept. In this manner, 57 CUs were identified. French and English CU lists for the Bank Theft image from the Protocole Montreal-Toulouse d'Examen Linguistique de l'Aphasie (MT-86) [42, 43] have also been developed, along with new derived measures—number of different CUs and number of different CUs divided by the length of the sample [44]. These studies and others also found that CUs are sensitive to differences between healthy controls speakers and PWAs, as well as to differences due to aphasia severity [41, 44, 45], but may not be sensitive to changes due to spontaneous recovery [44]. These studies also demonstrated good test-retest and inter-rater reliability. Finally, CUs are sensitive to changes in response to a variety of interventions, ranging from AAC [46], to app-based [47], to intensive therapy [48].

More recently, Berube and colleagues [39] developed an updated, or "modern" Cookie Theft image, which includes representation of diverse races and ethnicities and less rigid gender roles. Berube and colleagues also changed the elicitation prompt in order to elicit a longer discourse sample. An updated list of CUs was developed to reflect these changes, with a total of 96 CUs identified. In addition, Berube and colleagues separated their CUs into those that appear on the left and right sides of the image, to better extend the utility of the measure for individuals with right hemisphere damage [49]. Research using this updated stimulus demonstrates that CUs produced shortly after a stroke can predict long-term recovery, identify differences between left and right hemisphere stroke [50], and are associated with lesion site, lesion size, and other language measures [50, 51]. Finally, an adaptation for use with semi-structured discourse tasks (e.g., public speaking) has recently been made available [52].

Information Units

McNeil, Doyle, and colleagues developed the Information Unit (IU) [53] in association with their Story Retell Procedure (SRP) [54]. Similar to the measures above, IUs represent a closed set of words and phrases needed to (re)tell a minimally informative story. Essentially, IUs are defined as content relevant words except articles, conjunctions, and auxiliary verbs (see Appendix A for full definition) [53]. Importantly, good inter-rater reliability [55], concurrent reliability, and known group validity has been established for %IUs and %IUs/min [53, 56, 57]. Georgeadis and colleagues [58] demonstrated the validity of conducting the SRP protocol through videoconferencing. No significant differences were found between the face-to-face and telerehabilitation settings for PWAs. Finally, IUs are sensitive to change in response to completion of an intensive comprehensive aphasia program [59]; however, this study only included military members (active duty or retired) and the sample was 92% male, so caution must be used when applying to non-military and female individuals.

A unique aspect of IUs is that four equivalent forms of the SRP have been validated [54, 60], which decreases concerns about learning effects on repeated assessment. Each form of the SRP consists of three stories, with stimuli taken from the 2 practice and 10 test items of the Discourse Comprehension Test (DCT) [61]. While the DCT is no longer in print, the SRP materials (checklists and stimuli) are available at: https://computerizedrevisedtokentest.com/story-retell-procedure/.

Quantitative Measures in PPA

Both CUs and CoreLex have been used to investigate discourse production in PwPPAs. Both measures are sensitive to differences between healthy controls and PwPPAs [33, 62] while CUs are also sensitive to differences between PPA subtypes [62] and have been used to track longitudinal change in an individual with logopenic variant PPA [63]. Of note, Gallée and colleagues developed new CU lists (with some modifications) for the WAB-R picnic scene, further expanding the utility of this approach. The new CU lists are reported in Table 2 of the article [62]. At this time, there are no psychometric data available for either measure in this population.

General Considerations

For the three quantitative analyses discussed above, checklist scoring procedures increase clinical feasibility and yield high scoring reliability. Although not fully discussed (but see IUs discussion above), derived efficiency scores, either production over time (e.g., CoreLex/min) or per word (e.g., CUs/total words), can be calculated for each measure. For clinical feasibility, we recommend using derived efficiency scores over time since timing the discourse sample is far easier than counting total number of words, unique words, etc. Derived efficiency scores have good sensitivity to group differences, and potentially to treatment response [33].

Since these measures do not provide information about the organization and structure of discourse per se, it is possible that an individual could receive a high score on one of these measures while not actually attempting to produce a discourse (e.g., simply producing a list of words related to the stimulus with no attempt to produce sentences). However, in our experience, even severe non-fluent PWAs will often use extralinguistic and paralinguistic channels to construct a discourse (e.g., varying prosody, repeating words for emphasis, supplementing spoken words with gestures). The CoreLex analysis attempts to guard against this concern by including both content (nouns, verbs, adjectives, adverbs) and function (e.g., determiners, prepositions, pronouns, copulas) words in the checklists. This allows an examiner to make some quantitative observations regarding the grammaticality of the discourse sample by comparing the number of content vs. function words produced. However, individuals could have very disorganized or poorly sequenced discourse samples but remain on topic; scores on these measures would not be sensitive to such disruptions. On the other hand, research on all three measures has demonstrated that they are related to high-level discourse behaviors suggesting they may be fast and efficient ways to estimate discourse performance and more functional communication abilities.

Finally, since CoreLex checklists only include the most frequently produced lexemes it is most accurately conceptualized as a measure of word retrieval *typicality*. It may not fully reflect informativeness since synonyms or semantically related lexemes are not scored. In contrast, both CU and IU accept alternative lexemes, making them a more direct measure of informativeness. A new related measure, "content word fluency," was first reported by Alyahya and colleagues [64]. While CoreLex, CUs and IUs score a single point per item on their checklists, the content word fluency scores one point for every production of each word on the checklist. For example, if an individual produced the following when asked how to make a peanut butter and jelly sandwich:

> *Well first you gotta get out your ingredients. You'll need the peanut butter, the jelly—I like blackberry best—the bread, a knife, and either a plate or a paper towel. So first get two slices of bread and put them on the paper towel. Then, open up the peanut butter and spread it on one side of both slices of bread. That part's super important, cause you don't want soggy bread from the jelly. Then open up the jelly and spread it on top of the peanut butter. Next you gotta put the two pieces of bread together, peanut butter and jelly sides together. Then if you want you can cut it in half and eat and enjoy!*

Using CoreLex scoring rules, the individual might score one point for each of these CoreLex items: you, get, the, a, peanut, butter, jelly, bread, knife, and, plate, slice, two, spread, put, together, cut, eat. This yields a CoreLex score of 23. In contrast, the content word fluency scoring system would give 5 points for "bread," 4 points for "jelly," 2 points for "put," etc. This is an important distinction since an informative and understandable discourse will require repetition of specific content words. However, future research on content word fluency is needed before recommending it for clinical use.

Orthographic Transcription

The next level of transcript complexity, orthographic transcription, faithfully represents the words produced in a discourse sample, without concern for detailed coding of errors, parts of speech, or other features. Oftentimes filled pauses and partial word productions are included in the transcript. Some orthographic transcripts may use widely recognized codes such as "xxx" to indicate unintelligible speech, or "." to indicate informal utterance boundaries for simplicity or to increase readability. Phonological paraphasias and neologistic productions are often represented with an approximate orthographic spelling, rather than close phonetic transcription. While this is a relatively simple transcription procedure, it opens the door to more detailed quantitative discourse analysis, in addition to the analysis options discussed in the previous section.

Word-Level Measures

Informativeness

Many of the discourse measures compatible with completing only orthographic transcription are measures of informativeness. These are primarily word-level measures that count unique, informative words that are related to the task. In addition, word-level analyses that rely on frequency counts or percentages of words or word types can be calculated (e.g., number/percent word classes). If the duration of the discourse sample is recorded, measures of how efficiently an individual produces the discourse or behavior of interest are available (e.g., words per minute).

Correct Information Units

The correct information unit (CIU) [65] is perhaps the most utilized informativeness measure in aphasia. Due to the large body of research, key psychometrics and data needed for clinical implementation along with examples for use will be highlighted here.

CIUs are single words that are "accurate, relevant, and informative relative to the eliciting stimulus" but that do not have to be grammatically correct (pg. 340) [65]. This initial study reported the total number of CIUs, percent CIUs (%CIUs), and CIUs per minute (CIUs/min) produced by healthy controls and PWAs, with significant differences between groups observed on all measures. Nicholas and Brookshire also provided scoring rules and examples (see Appendix B in the article [65]) to aid in accurate and reliable application of CIUs by others. Multiple studies have reported good intra-rater [65–70] and inter-rater reliability [65–73] although others report lower inter-rater [74] and test-retest [67] reliability.

Boyle [66] reported that test-retest reliability for total CIUs was high enough to be used in group studies but may not be stable as a treatment outcome measure for individual clients. In contrast, CIUs/min was reported to have adequate stability for both group results and individual treatment outcome use, and Boyle [66] reports that changes of 12 or more CIUs/min are likely attributable to treatment effects rather than random variability. Interpretation of the results for %CIUs is less straightforward due to the presence of an outlier who significantly affected reliability. Ultimately, %CIUs may be appropriate for group results, but Boyle urged users to exercise caution given the presence of the outlier, suggesting that some PWAs might not be stable on this measure. In their review, Pritchard and colleagues [75] suggest that CIUs demonstrate good validity in that it measures what it intends to measure (i.e., content validity) and is sensitive to differences between PWAs and healthy controls [65], as well as to differences between discourse genres (i.e., construct or known groups validity) [71]. Studies have also identified differences in response to various treatments [20, 70, 71, 76] and suggest that CIUs may be sensitive to aphasia severity [72].

Use in PPA

As stated above, relatively little research on the discourse abilities of PwPPAs has been conducted. Of that body, a fair amount has used CIUs, mirroring its popularity in stable, stroke-induced aphasia. One of the earliest investigations demonstrated that various discourse measures, including %CIUs, are sensitive to changes over time [77]. Interestingly, the authors found that different discourse measures did not decline in tandem. Instead, they observed initial output deficits (decreased speech rate followed by decreased MLU) before finally observing content-based deficits as measured by %CIUs.

This highlights the importance of considering which discourse domains are assessed when monitoring change over time or measuring treatment outcomes. PwPPAs have a lower proportion of CIUs during picture description than both healthy adults and individuals with mild cognitive impairment, but not lower than individuals with Alzheimer's dementia [78]. Additionally, proportion CIU was not sensitive to differences across PPA variants in this investigation.

Beales and colleagues [79] reported that %CIUs have moderate to good reliability and CIUs/min have good to excellent reliability across three discourse genres (everyday monologue, narrative, and picture description). This is a critical investigation since much of the PPA treatment literature focuses on measuring generalization to discourse as a secondary treatment outcome. A review of lexical retrieval treatments in PwPPAs reported mixed support for generalization to discourse [80]. Since that review, one study has demonstrated increased %CIUs [81], one reported no changes [82], and one reported a mixed response following lexical retrieval treatment [83].

Moving the focus beyond lexical retrieval, Rogalski and Edmonds reported increased %CIUs (from below the normal range pre-treatment into the normal range post-treatment) following Attentive Reading and Constrained Summary [84]. Finally, Whitworth and colleagues reported improved %CIUs and CIUs/min following a discourse level treatment although participants varied with respect to significant differences across the variables and across time-points (immediately following and 4 weeks after treatment) [85].

General Considerations

As discussed above with CoreLex, CU, and IU, derived efficiency scores have demonstrated good stability and sensitivity. It is recommended here that efficiency over time may be a simple calculation for practicing SLPs to use. Unlike CU, IU, and CoreLex analyses, CIU analysis is not constrained to specific stimuli with pre-specified lists. This flexibility allows an examiner to select topics amongst several discourse genres so that the sample elicited is most appropriate for an individual client. There is also emerging evidence that CIUs can be reliably scored in conversation (the gold standard for functional outcomes measurement), albeit with some modifications to the original protocol [86, 87]. An additional strength of CIUs compared to the others is that the entire discourse sample is used, rather than a small subset. On the other hand, CIUs can take *much* longer to score than CUs, IUs, and CoreLex, especially for longer discourse samples, individuals with hyperfluency, or those with milder deficits.

Although not discussed in depth, the lexical information unit (LIU) [88] is similar to CIU, but with more restrictive criteria for included material. LIUs exclude words and phrases produced in utterances that are not grammatical and/or that have some pragmatic concern, or words that are errored (e.g., phonological paraphasias). It is believed that the more restrictive definition for LIUs would require both utterance segmentation and detailed error coding to score reliably, which limits clinical feasibility.

Proposition-Level Measures

Proposition-level informativeness measures provide a better understanding of how individuals chain together individual concepts (e.g., words and clauses) into a larger message.

Main Concept Analysis

The main concept analysis (MCA) was initially created by Nicholas and Brookshire [89] in order to measure informativeness that was closely related to the discourse macrostructure, or expression of the main ideas and overall gist, of the discourse. As such, MCA is generally classified as a hybrid analysis that quantifies both microlinguistic and macrolinguistic aspects of the discourse [90]. Nicholas and Brookshire provide scoring rules in Appendix A of their article along with a list of main concepts (MCs) and scoring examples for the Cookie Theft stimulus [38] in Appendix B [89]. In this initial study, MCs were determined by a group of 10 SLPs for

8 stimuli, where concepts used by 7 out of 10 SLPs were considered the MCs. The only instructions SLPs were given were to focus on the main ideas or gist of the story, and that MCs should have one and only one main verb. The original MCA evaluated "...presence, completeness, and accuracy... (p. 146)" [89] of each main concept. "Essential elements" were identified which had to be produced for an MC to be determined "complete," and the information in the utterance had to be correct in the context of the stimulus presented in order to be judged "accurate." MCs did not have to be produced with the same words, or in the same format as the MCs, as long as the concept was adequately communicated. For example, an acceptable production of the MC "The woman is doing dishes" could be "The maid is cleaning the plate." Several codes were used to identify the possible range of presence, accuracy, and completeness:

- Absent (AB): MCs that were not produced in the discourse sample.
- Accurate/Complete (AC): MCs which were produced with all essential elements and all elements were correct.
- Accurate/Incomplete (AI): MCs which were produced with one or more essential elements missing, but all elements that were produced were correct.
- Inaccurate/Complete (IC): MCs which were produced with all essential elements, but one or more elements were incorrect.
- Inaccurate/Incomplete (II): MCs which were missing one or more essential elements and one or more of the essential elements that was produced was incorrect.

After analyzing the data, Nicholas and Brookshire combined the IC and II codes due to poor reliability identifying inaccurate/incomplete MCs. Finally, Nicholas and Brookshire reported good inter-rater, intra-rater, and test-retest reliability (after combining the IC and II codes). MCA was also sensitive to changes between healthy controls and PWAs, particularly with respect to errors, and control speakers rarely produced errored MCs, while PWAs regularly produced MCs that were incomplete and/or inaccurate.

Kong and colleagues have extended the utility of MCA by developing MC lists for Cantonese [91, 92], Japanese [93], Korean [94], Taiwanese Mandarin [95], English [96], Spanish [97], Dutch [98], and Irish-English [99] speakers. Each of these articles utilizes the same set of discourse stimuli (which can be obtained from Dr. Anthony Kong or through the published tool that contains standard scoring sheets in English and Chinese) [100] and elicitation procedures, and methods for identifying main concepts. Each article publishes the MCA checklist developed for the language, normative data from a sample of healthy control speakers, and a comparison of PWAs to the norms. For US-based SLPs, this body of work may provide access to standardized, norm-referenced discourse analysis for clients who are bilingual or multilingual, or who do not speak English. However, it is important to note that these investigations have also demonstrated that dialect can impact the form in which an MC is produced and whether a concept rises to the level of an MC [97], so care must be taken when comparing client performance to normative data.

Main concept checklists have also been developed by Richardson and Dalton [101, 102] for the semi-spontaneous discourse tasks included in the AphasiaBank protocol. In their studies, MCs were determined by first identifying the relevant concepts for each task produced by 92 healthy control speakers included in the AphasiaBank database. The relevant concepts that were produced by 33% of the control speakers were then included on the MC checklists. (Developed also were shorter checklists containing MCs that corresponded to 50% and 66% thresholds.) In contrast to previous coding and scoring systems [89, 91], authors did not combine IC and II codes into a single code, nor did they assign an equal score to those codes, to guard against a scoring bias where semantic paraphasias and phonological paraphasias were not treated similarly. Normative data for the 92 original healthy controls are available in the original checklist development manuscripts [101, 102]. Normative data for an expanded healthy control dataset (N = 145) as well as for 238 PWAs are available in a follow-up manuscript that provides descriptive and comparative statistical information for both groups [103], and for aphasia subtypes for the overall MC score as well as for each MC code. Dalton and Richardson [103] showed that MCA was sensitive to differences between healthy controls and PWAs, even for persons with latent aphasia, but that sensitivity differed by aphasia subtype, with greatest sensitivity for persons with Broca's and Wernicke's aphasia.

Several additional investigations have relied upon the Richardson and Dalton procedures to develop MCs for additional stimuli [104–106]. Currently, Kurland and colleagues [104] are developing the "Brief Assessment of Transactional Success" (BATS) which will include MC checklists from 16 audio and/or video samples with normative data and alternative productions for scoring. While these checklists are not currently available, we encourage readers to keep an eye out for these materials in the future. Doyle, McNeil, and colleagues analyzed a similar measure which they referred to as percent story propositions [53, 54, 60, 107]. Although it is unclear how story propositions were identified, they contained essential elements similar to Nicholas and Brookshire, and could be scored across the spectrum of presence, accuracy, and completeness. Finally, Stark [108] reported on the utility of an MCA-like proposition analysis for tracking longitudinal change during Cinderella story retelling in an individual with chronic aphasia. She reported that this proposition analysis was sensitive to tracking change over time. While Stark provides the list of propositions used in her analysis, the story propositions reported by Doyle, McNeil, and colleagues are not available publicly as of now.

MCA has demonstrated good intra- and inter-rater reliability [89]. Test-retest reliability is also good, with stability sufficient for use at the group level [66]. As described above, numerous studies have demonstrated MCAs sensitivity to differences between healthy controls and PWAs [94, 103]. MCA is also sensitive to differences between healthy controls and individuals with latent aphasia, who generally cannot be identified on standardized assessments due to their lack of sensitivity to these mild but functionally debilitating deficits [103, 109]. MCA has good construct validity, correlating with other discourse measures and standardized test performance [30, 110, 111]. Additionally, MCA has good ecological validity, as demonstrated by strong positive correlations with listener judgments of improved communication [7, 18]. Finally, MCA is appropriate for monitoring treatment outcomes [18, 108, 112–114].

Main Event Analysis

Capilouto and colleagues' Main Event Analysis (MEA) was informed by Nicholas and Brookshire's MCA but sought to encode relationships between various concepts where appropriate. To this end, a main event (ME) allows more than one main verb [115]. ME lists are available for several stimuli published by Nicholas and Brookshire [65]. Normative performance as measured by the proportion of MEs produced out of all possible MEs is available for younger and older adults [115]. Importantly, MEA scoring is binary, corresponding to Nicholas and Brookshires "AC" and "AB" scoring codes. Studies using MEA report good inter-rater [116–118] and intra-rater reliability [117]. MEA is sensitive to changes related to healthy aging [115, 117] and to differences in performance between PWAs and healthy controls [116]. Finally, significant differences on ME performance have been reported between discourse samples elicited using the instructions to "talk about what is going on…" versus "tell me a story with a beginning, middle, and end" as well as between single picture and picture sequence tasks—highlighting the importance of both the task instructions used and the discourse tasks/genres selected when assessing a client's communication.

Thematic Unit Analysis

A related measure to both MCA and MEA, the concept of thematic units (TUs) was reported by Gleason and colleagues and defined as a basic idea related to the story [28]. This is a rather vague definition but when reviewing the list of TUs reported by Gleason and colleagues, it is clear that their themes do not meet the definition of main concepts or main events. Unfortunately, while Gleason's article includes the TU lists for their tasks, the elicitation images are not available, which greatly limits utilization applicability. More recently Marini and colleagues [88, 119, 120] developed an analysis they referred to as thematic units as well. Upon careful review of their and other articles [121–126], it appears that this analysis is closer to Gleason's "target lexemes" [28] or the CoreLex and CIU analyses reported above (sections "Core Lexicon Analysis" and "Correct Information Units") than a proposition-level analysis.

Use in PPA

MCA is the primary proposition-level discourse analysis used with PwPPAs to date. PwPPAs produce fewer AC main concepts and are less efficient in their accurate and complete MC production compared to healthy controls [33]. MCA has demonstrated sensitivity for treatment-related changes in response to group therapy [127]. Given this promising result, further research is needed to investigate the psychometric properties of MCA in this population. Richardson and colleagues created the Main Concept, Sequencing, and Story Grammar (MSSG) analysis, to better evaluate MCs along with other aspects of discourse macrostructure [128, 129]. Research is currently ongoing with this measure in PwPPAs. Readers are recommended to continue to Chap. 13 for additional information on MSSG and other macrostructural analyses.

General Considerations

MCA and MEA can provide richer insight into an individual's discourse abilities than is possible with single-word measures. These analyses are a hybrid between microlinguistic and macrolinguistic analysis, and therefore have some of the strengths of both. In particular, the MCA coding and scoring system allows for description of both accuracy and completeness. This may allow for better individualization of treatment planning, as the approach for an individual with limited but accurate output would differ from one whose output is sometimes inaccurate but relatively complete or someone who is highly verbose, inaccurate, and incomplete. Additionally, proposition-level analyses help guard against high scores for individuals who are simply listing items rather than truly producing a discourse. MCA and MEA both have good reliability and validity, and evidence suggests MCA may be sensitive to and appropriate for measuring treatment outcomes. In addition, it may be possible to score MCA without orthographic transcription (either online or from a video- or audio-recording) given the availability of detailed checklists and scoring rules. However, it is important to note that while we expect these measures can be reliably scored without utterance segmentation (or possibly transcription), only one study has investigated this directly [130]. Armstrong and colleagues reported no significant differences between variables scored with a transcript vs. scored directly from a video-recording; this is promising but more research is needed. Therefore, caution should be used, especially in terms of scoring reliability for these measures when scoring without utterance segmentation.

Transcription + Segmentation

Once a discourse sample has been orthographically transcribed, the next step is to segment into utterances. There are two major utterance segmentation systems: c-units (or communication units) [131] and t-units (or terminable units) [132]. Both c-units and t-units have the same base definition, which is that an utterance includes an independent clause along with any subordinate clauses or other modifiers. For both c-units and t-units, if a potential utterance could be divided without any loss of meaning then it should be considered two (or more) utterances. For example, "The girl was at the table," "While the girl was at the table the boy played," and "The girl was happy because she got a kitten for her birthday" would all be considered a single c-unit or t-unit. In contrast, something like "the girl colored a picture and then she hung it on the refrigerator" would be considered two utterances in both systems: (1) "The girl colored a picture." (2) "And then she hung it on the refrigerator."

The major difference between t-units and c-units is how occurrences such as incomplete or abandoned utterances, responses to "wh-" questions that do not require complete independent clauses, etc., are handled. While c-units would include all of the above examples as utterances to be analyzed, t-units limit utterances to only complete independent clauses along with any subordinate or dependent clauses. When deciding upon a segmentation definition, it is important to consider the focus of the desired discourse analysis. C-units may be more appropriate if the goal is to understand aspects of errored productions, or if the interest is in overall communicativeness. In contrast, if the goal is to carefully analyze only accurate and complete utterances, t-units may be more appropriate.

Adding segmentation to basic orthographic transcription changes the scope of information that can be revealed through discourse analysis. With no or only orthographic transcription, analyses are limited to primarily microlinguistic information, with perhaps the exception of the proposition-level informativeness measures. Segmenting utterances allow for investigation of macrolinguistic or macrostructural measures such as story grammar [133], story goodness index [134], or MSSG [128, 129]. (Macrostructural measures are reviewed in greater detail in Chap. 13).

Web-Based Scoring of CoreLex and MCA

It is generally recognized that the wide availability of technology and the advancements in computing power will need to be leveraged to improve the feasibility of discourse analysis in clinical settings. In this section, one way in which researchers can leverage technology to improve the feasibility of currently available measures will be briefly described.

While both CoreLex and MCA checklists and training materials were designed for clinical feasibility and to reduce the need for close transcription of discourse samples, hand-scoring of checklists can still be time-intensive, particularly for discourse stimuli that elicit longer samples (e.g., the Cinderella story) and include more CoreLex lexemes and main concepts. To address this challenge, researchers have developed two companion web applications specifically for clinical use [135–137] from open-source software [138, 139].

While the apps do require orthographic transcription input, they are able to quickly parse the transcripts and greatly simplify scoring. For both apps, after clicking "get started," an initial page where clinicians can select the discourse stimulus to be scored, and input the duration of the sample, client/participant ID, and notes (e.g., departures from the procedure, testing conditions that might affect performance or normative comparison) is displayed (Fig. 12.1). On the next page, the transcript is entered for analysis. After completing the scoring, a results page presents the individual's performance; comparisons to healthy control and PWAs normative samples; and plots of individual performance against the norms. If duration was entered on the first page, efficiency

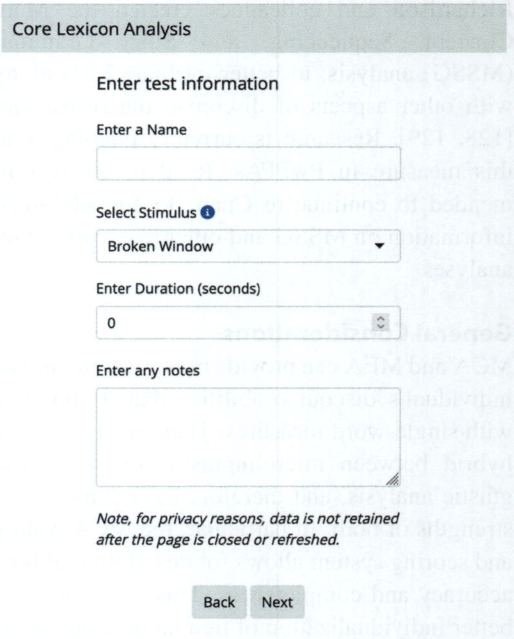

Fig. 12.1 CoreLex app page for entering client ID and other details [136]

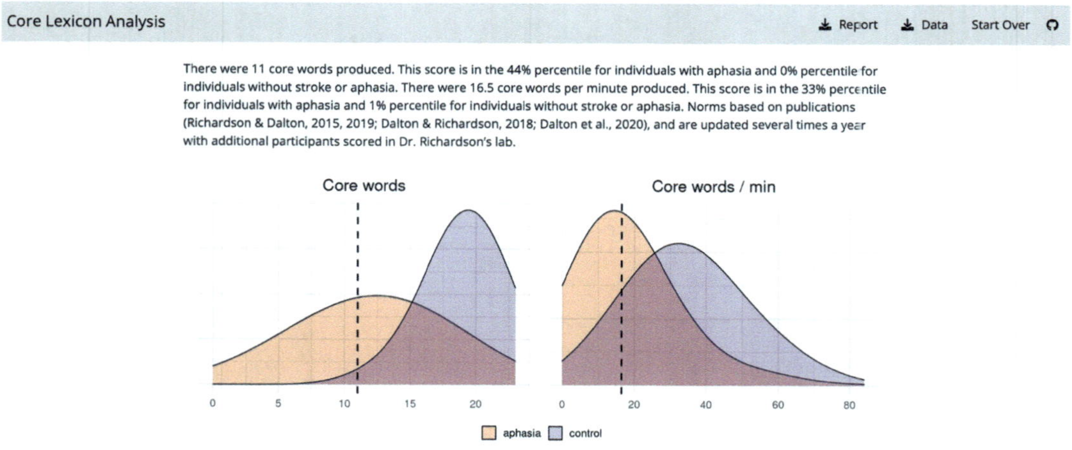

Fig. 12.2 Example results page after scoring CoreLex via the app [136]

results are also available (Fig. 12.2). Finally, a written report and the analysis can be downloaded to include in a patient record or to use as a support when explaining assessment results.

The CoreLex application leverages R's natural language processing tools to identify lexemes from orthographic transcripts and matches these lexemes with the Corelex checklists. After the transcript has been parsed, all lexemes are automatically and displayed in a checklist format next to the transcribed sample. This allows for quick scanning of the transcript and identified items to make sure no errors have been made. After verifying and accepting the analysis, the scoring page presents the results as described above.

Given the greater complexity of MCA, several training modules have been developed that provide immediate feedback on transcription and scoring accuracy with explanations for correct responses (See Fig. 12.3). After selecting the discourse stimulus to be scored and entering the transcript, the MCA app presents each main concept for the stimulus one by one, along with the transcript (Fig. 12.4). The utterance corresponding to a main concept can be highlighted and then the scorer will be prompted to determine for each essential element within an MC whether it is accurate, inaccurate, or absent. Once completed, the app advances to the next MC until all MCs have been scored. The results page presents the information described above, with the addition that MC scores are available using both Richardson and Dalton and Kong and colleagues' scoring systems for greater flexibility. However, normative comparisons are only available for the Richardson and Dalton scoring system.

In the future, it is our hope that these web apps will be paired with automated transcription procedures as discussed in the following section, which would further reduce the time needed to score.

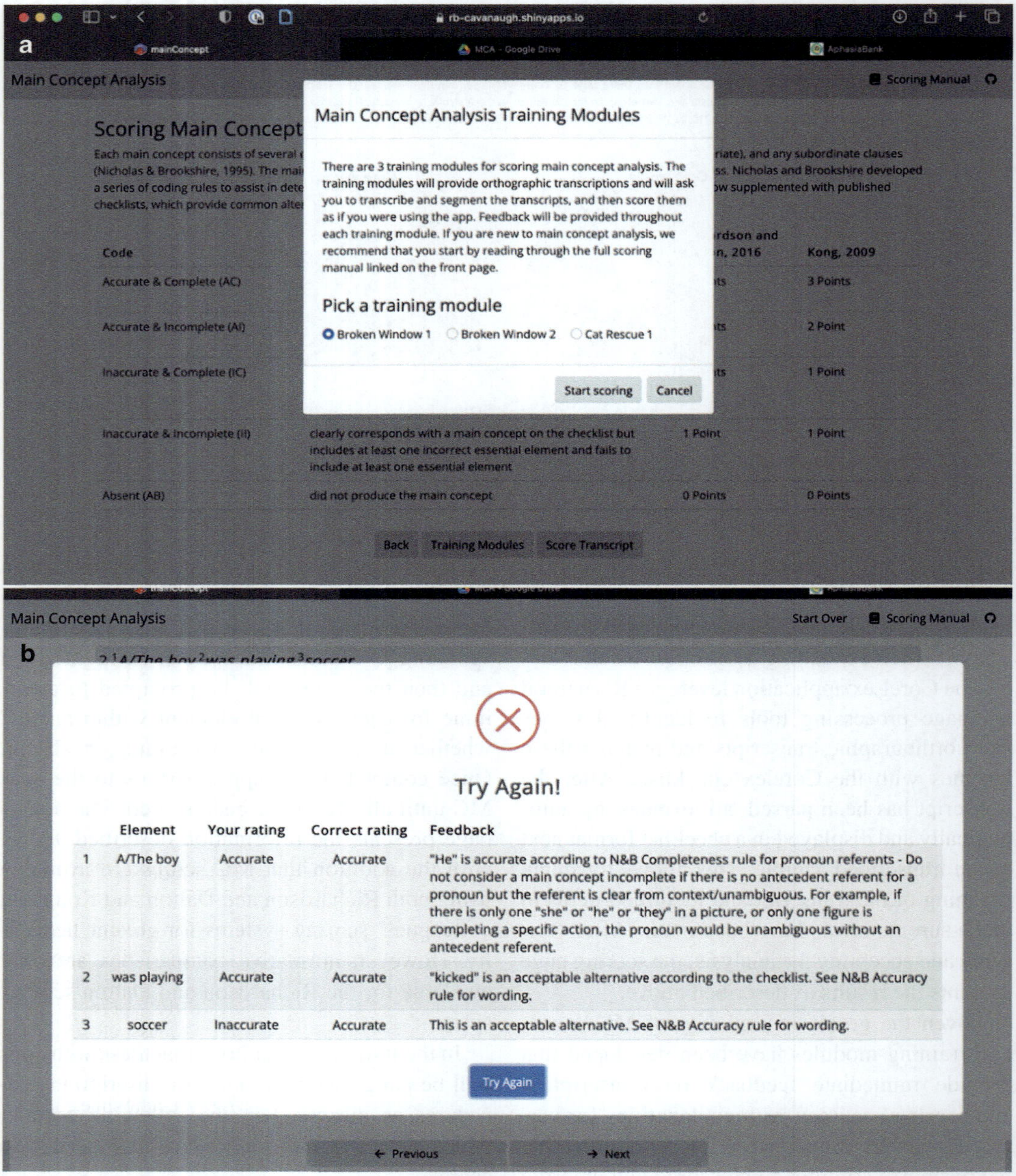

Fig. 12.3 (**a**) Entry page into MCA training where you can select amongst three modules; (**b**) Example of feedback provided following incorrect score in MCA training module [137]

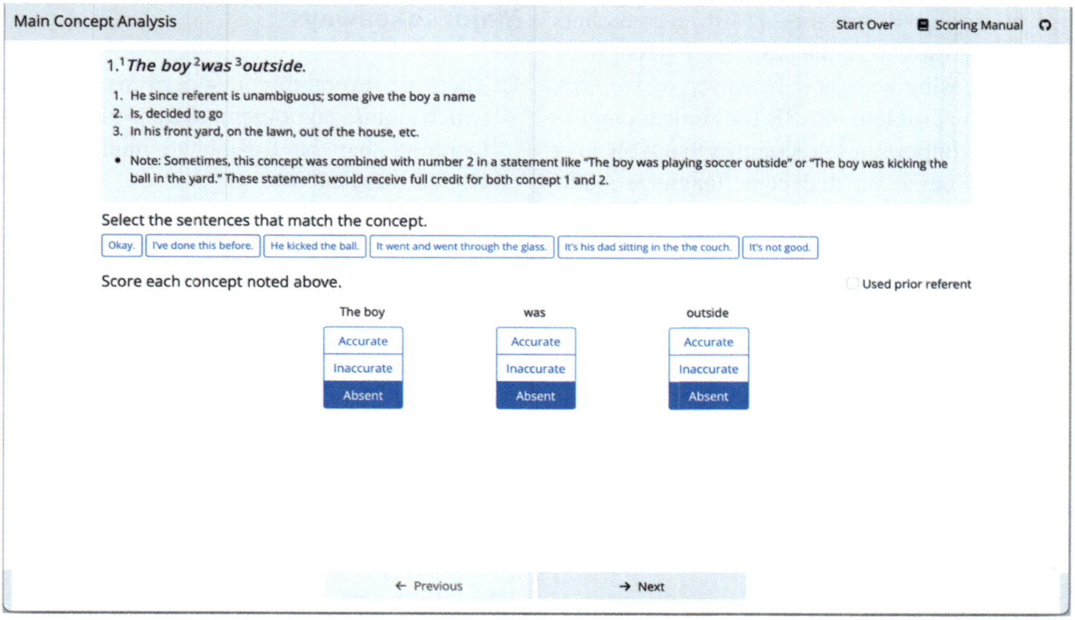

Fig. 12.4 Example of MCA scoring page with the MC, alternatives and scoring notes, utterance options, and breakdown of essential elements [137]

Future Needs

While time is not the only barrier to clinical implementation of discourse, it is perhaps the most intractable. Issues of limited training, availability of normative data, and concerns about insurance reimbursement have and are being addressed. However, until either practice requirements such as high productivity numbers and high caseloads change (unlikely without extensive advocacy at state and federal levels) or a radical change in the time required for transcription is achieved, clinical implementation of discourse analysis will likely remain limited, despite clinicians' and clients' desires.

Automatic speech recognition (ASR) to automate transcription of discourse has long been seen as the future of transcription-based discourse analysis [140]. While significant advancements have been made in the accuracy of automated transcription for individuals with intact language, several issues are unresolved for individuals with disordered speech. First, the artificial intelligence programs used for ASR are trained on samples of individuals with intact language. However, PWAs commonly make language errors that are unpredictable, which AI struggles to correctly parse. In addition, aphasia commonly co-occurs with apraxia and dysarthria, which degrade the quality of speech input into transcription software. This combination of unpredictable language errors and reduced speech intelligibility present significant difficulties and result in relatively errorful transcripts. For example, a recent investigation reported that the word recognition rate of discourse was only 69%, and word error rate 39% when analyzing samples from 70 individuals (10 control; 11 logopenic variant PPA; 25 semantic variant PPA; 14 non-fluent variant PPA; 10 behavioral variant fronto-temporal dementia) [141]. Interestingly, despite the poor accuracy of the transcription, statistical analyses using the automatic transcription were still somewhat sensitive to group differences [140]. Researchers continue efforts to refine ASR for PWAs [142], with increasing accuracy. However, as we seek to solve the problem of ASR for clinical populations, it is important to recognize that ASR may be biased based on dialect or language status [143]. It is critical that clinicians remember any ASR system is only as good as the data it is trained on, and that currently available databases for sourcing training data lack racial and ethnic diversity and may not have adequate representation of various dialects. This is a focus area for future growth by AphasiaBank and other databases, and we encourage researchers and clinicians who have access to more diverse patient populations to contribute samples to support these initiatives.

Summary

As we conclude our discussion of clinically feasible discourse analysis, it is important to highlight that while researchers have hypothesized that the various measured reviewed above can be reliably used without or with minimal transcription, only a very few studies have used the measures in this fashion (often because additional discourse measures that did require transcription were also being evaluated). To our knowledge, there have been no direct comparisons between accuracy and reliability of transcription-based and non-transcription-based implementation of these measures, which is a critical gap that must be addressed.

In our estimation, the future of clinical implementation of discourse will require a two-pronged approach where there is continued work to develop non-transcription-based or minimally transcription-based measures in conjunction with continued improvement of automatics speech recognition technologies to eventually eliminate or significantly reduce the time needed for accurate transcription of discourse samples. Fortunately, this area of practice is receiving more and more attention, and we are hopeful that advances will occur rapidly.

Major Takeaways

1. There are several discourse analysis measures which require no or minimal transcription and therefore may be feasible to implement in clinical practice.
2. Perceptual ratings of discourse have excellent ecological validity and may be a quick and informative way to identify changes in discourse.
3. Checklists for word-level analysis of multiple discourse stimuli are widely available, some with normative data for reference.
4. Proposition-level analyses may provide richer insights into discourse performance than word level measures and could possibly be implemented without orthographic transcription.

Acknowledgments As always, we are grateful for persons with aphasia who share their time and their stories with us so we can learn more about discourse and life participation. We thank the creators of AphasiaBank for developing the rich repository and for the many labs that so generously contribute to the database. We would also like to thank Dr. Rob Cavanaugh for his work developing the web-based MCA and CoreLex scoring apps.

References

1. Boyle M. Choosing discourse outcome measures to assess clinical change. Semin Speech Lang. 2019;41(1):1–9.
2. Bryant L, Spencer E, Ferguson A. Clinical use of linguistic discourse analysis for the assessment of language in aphasia. Aphasiology. 2016;31(10):1105–26.
3. Stark BC, Dutta M, Murray LL, Fromm D, Bryant L, Harmon TG, Ramage AE, Roberts AC. Spoken discourse assessment and analysis in aphasia: an international survey of current practices. J Speech Lang Hear Res. 2021;64(11):4366–89.
4. Cruice M, Botting N, Marshall J, Boyle M, Hersh D, Pritchard M, Dipper L. UK speech and language therapists' views and reported practices of discourse analysis in aphasia rehabilitation. Int J Lang Commun Disord. 2020;55(3):417–42.
5. Kertesz A. Western aphasia battery—revised. Pearson; 2006.
6. Behrns I, Wengelin Å, Broberg M, Hartelius L. A comparison between written and spoken narratives in aphasia. Clin Linguist Phon. 2009;23(7):507–28.

7. Ulatowska HK, Doyel AW, Stern RF, Haynes SM, North AJ. Production of procedural discourse in aphasia. Brain Lang. 1983;18(2):315–41.
8. Ulatowska H, North AJ, Macaluso-Haynes S, Doyel AW, Freedman-Stern R. Production of narrative discourse in aphasia. Brain Lang. 1983;19(2):317–34.
9. Kong AP-H, Wong CW-Y. An integrative analysis of spontaneous storytelling discourse in aphasia: relationship with listeners' rating and prediction of severity and fluency status of aphasia. Am J Speech Lang Pathol. 2018;27(4):1491–505.
10. Park H, Rogalski Y, Rodriguez AD, Zlatar Z, Benjamin M, Harnish S, Bennett J, Rosenbek JC, Crosson B, Reilly J. Perceptual cues used by listeners to discriminate fluent from nonfluent narrative discourse. Aphasiology. 2011;25(9):998–1015.
11. Webster J, Morris J. Communicative informativeness in aphasia: investigating the relationship between linguistic and perceptual measures. Am J Speech Lang Pathol. 2019;28(3):1115–26.
12. Ulatowska HK, Reyes B, Santos TO, Garst D, Vernon J, McArthur J. Personal narratives in aphasia: understanding narrative competence. Top Stroke Rehabil. 2013;20(1):36–43.
13. Ulatowska HK, Olness GS, Wertz RT, Thompson JL, Keebler MW, Hill CL, Auther LL. Comparison of language impairment, functional communication, and discourse measures in African-American aphasic and normal adults. Aphasiology. 2001;15(10–11):1007–16.
14. Olness GS, Ulatowska HK, Wertz RT, Thompson JL, Auther LL. Discourse elicitation with pictorial stimuli in African Americans and Caucasians with and without aphasia. Aphasiology. 2002;16(4–6):623–33.
15. Ulatowska H, Streit Olness G, Wertz R, Samson A, Keebler M, Goins K. Relationship between discourse and Western aphasia battery performance in African Americans with aphasia. Aphasiology. 2003;17(5):511–21.
16. Ross KB, Wertz RT. Comparison of impairment and disability measures for assessing severity of, and improvement in, aphasia. Aphasiology. 1999;13(2):113–24.
17. Ballard KJ, Thompson CK. Treatment and generalization of complex sentence production in agrammatism. J Speech Lang Hear Res. 1999;42(3):690–707.
18. Cupit J, Rochon E, Leonard C, Laird L. Social validation as a measure of improvement after aphasia treatment: its usefulness and influencing factors. Aphasiology. 2010;24(11):1486–500.
19. Hickey E, Rondeau G. Social validation in aphasiology: does judges' knowledge of aphasiology matter? Aphasiology. 2005;19(3–5):389–98.
20. Jacobs BJ. Social validity of changes in informativeness and efficiency of aphasic discourse following linguistic specific treatment (LST). Brain Lang. 2001;78(1):115–27.
21. Pattee C, Von Berg S, Ghezzi P. Effects of alternative communication on the communicative effectiveness of an individual with a progressive language disorder. Int J Rehabil Res. 2006;29(2):151–3.
22. Rebstock AM, Wallace SE. Effects of a combined semantic feature analysis and multimodal treatment for primary progressive aphasia: pilot study. Commun Disord Q. 2018;41(2):71–85.
23. Navarro J. Using discourse rating scales to measure effectiveness of treatment in people with aphasia [thesis]. 2020;1–60.
24. Dalton SG, Kim H, Richardson JD, Wright HH. A compendium of core lexicon checklists. Semin Speech Lang. 2019;41(1):45–60.
25. Kim H, Wright HH. A tutorial on core lexicon: development, use, and application. Semin Speech Lang. 2019;41(1):20–31.
26. MacWhinney B, Fromm D, Holland A, Forbes M, Wright H. Automated analysis of the Cinderella story. Aphasiology. 2010;24(6–8):856–68.
27. Fromm D, Forbes M, Holland A, MacWhinney B. PWAs and PBJs: language for describing a simple procedure. Paper presented at: clinical aphasiology conference. 2013 May. Tucson.
28. Gleason JB, Goodglass H, Obler L, Green E, Hyde MR, Weintraub S. Narrative strategies of aphasic and normal-speaking subjects. J Speech Lang Hear Res. 1980;23(2):370–82.
29. MacWhinney B, Fromm D. AphasiaBank as BigData. Semin Speech Lang. 2016;37(1):10–22.
30. Dalton SG, Richardson JD. Core-lexicon and main-concept production during picture-sequence description in adults without brain damage and adults with aphasia. Am J Speech Lang Pathol. 2015;24(4):S923–38.
31. Kim H, Kintz S, Zelnosky K, Wright HH. Measuring word retrieval in narrative discourse: core lexicon in aphasia. Int J Lang Commun Disord. 2019;54(1):62–78.
32. Kim H, Wright HH. Concurrent validity and reliability of the core lexicon measure as a measure of word retrieval ability in aphasia narratives. Am J Speech Lang Pathol. 2020;29(1):101–10.
33. Dalton SG, Hubbard HI, Richardson JD. Moving toward non-transcription based discourse analysis in stable and progressive aphasia. Semin Speech Lang. 2019;41(1):32–44.
34. Kim H, Kintz S, Wright HH. Development of a measure of function word use in narrative discourse: core lexicon analysis in aphasia. Int J Lang Commun Disord. 2020;56(1):6–19.
35. DeDe G, Hoover E. Measuring change at the discourse-level following conversation treatment. Top Lang Disord. 2021;41(1):5–26.
36. Kim H, Berube S, Hillis AE. Core lexicon in aphasia: a longitudinal study. Aphasiology. 2023;37(10):1679–91.
37. Dalton SG, Stark BC, Fromm D, Apple K, MacWhinney B, Rensch A, Rowedder M. Validation of an automated procedure for calculating core lexicon from transcripts. J Speech Lang Hear Res. 2022;65(8):2996–3003.
38. Goodglass H, Kaplan E, Weintraub S. BDAE: the Boston diagnostic aphasia examination. Philadelphia: Lippincott Williams & Wilkins; 2001.

39. Berube S, Nonnemacher J, Demsky C, Glenn S, Saxena S, Wright A, Tippett DC, Hillis AE. Stealing cookies in the twenty-first century: measures of spoken narrative in healthy versus speakers with aphasia. Am J Speech Lang Pathol. 2019;28(1S):321–9.
40. MacWhinney B, Fromm D, Forbes M, Holland A. AphasiaBank: methods for studying discourse. Aphasiology. 2011;25(11):1286–307.
41. Yorkston KM, Beukelman DR. An analysis of connected speech samples of aphasic and normal speakers. J Speech Hear Disord. 1980;45(1):27–36.
42. Nespoulous JL, Joanette Y, Lecours AR. Protocole Montreal-Toulouse d'examen linguistique de l'aphasie (MT-86). Isbergues: Ortho Edition; 1986.
43. Nespoulous JL, Lecours AR, Lafond D, Joanette Y, Lemay A, Puel M, Cot F, Rascol A. Protocole Montre ́al-Toulouse d'examen linguistique de l'aphasie, MT 86, Module standard initial. Montreal: Ortho Edition; 1992.
44. Larfeuil C, Dorze GL. An analysis of the word-finding difficulties and of the content of the content of the discourse of recent and chronic aphasic speakers. Aphasiology. 1997;11(8):783–811.
45. Craig HK, Hinckley JJ, Winkelseth M, Carry L, Walley J, Bardach L, Higman B, Hilfinger P, Schall C, Sheimo D. Quantifying connected speech samples of adults with chronic aphasia. Aphasiology. 1993;7(2):155–63.
46. Hux K, Buechter M, Wallace S, Weissling K. Using visual scene displays to create a shared communication space for a person with aphasia. Aphasiology. 2010;24(5):643–60.
47. Stark BC, Warburton EA. Improved language in chronic aphasia after self-delivered iPad speech therapy. Neuropsychol Rehabil. 2016;28(5):818–31.
48. Hinckley JJ, Craig HK. Influence of rate of treatment on the naming abilities of adults with chronic aphasia. Aphasiology. 1998;12(11):989–1006.
49. Berube SK, Goldberg E, Sheppard SM, Durfee AZ, Ubellacker D, Walker A, Stein CM, Hillis AE. An analysis of right hemisphere stroke discourse in the modern Cookie theft picture. Am J Speech Lang Pathol. 2022;31(5S):2301–12.
50. Agis D, Goggins MB, Oishi K, Oishi K, Davis C, Wright A, Kim EH, Sebastian R, Tippett DC, Faria A, Hillis AE. Picturing the size and site of stroke with an expanded National Institutes of Health Stroke Scale. Stroke. 2016;47(6):1459–65.
51. Keator LM, Faria AV, Kim KT, Saxena S, Wright AE, Sheppard SM, Breining BL, Goldberg E, Tippett DC, Meier E, Hillis AE. An efficient bedside measure yields prognostic implications for language recovery in acute stroke patients. Cogn Behav Neurol. 2020;33(3):192–200.
52. McCann CM, Plourde J, Moore C, Purdy SC. Linguistic analysis in public speaking: evidence from a gavel club for people with aphasia. Clin Linguist Phon. 2020;35(8):793–808.
53. McNeil MR, Doyle PJ, Fossett TR, Park GH, Goda AJ. Reliability and concurrent validity of the information unit scoring metric for the story retelling procedure. Aphasiology. 2001;15(10–11):991–1006.
54. Doyle PJ, McNeil MR, Park G, Goda A, Rubenstein E, Spencer K, Carroll B, Lustig A, Szwarc L. Linguistic validation of four parallel forms of a story retelling procedure. Aphasiology. 2000;14(5–6):537–49.
55. Hula W, McNeil M, Doyle P, Rubinsky H, Fossett T. The inter-rater reliability of the story retell procedure. Aphasiology. 2003;17(5):523–8.
56. Brodsky MB, McNeil MR, Doyle PJ, Fossett TR, Timm NH, Park GH. Auditory serial position effects in story retelling for non-brain-injured participants and persons with aphasia. J Speech Lang Hear Res. 2003;46(5):1124–37.
57. McNeil MR, Doyle PJ, Park GH, Fossett TRD, Brodsky MB. Increasing the sensitivity of the story retell procedure for the discrimination of normal elderly subjects from persons with aphasia. Aphasiology. 2002;16(8):815–22.
58. Georgeadis A, Brennan D, Barker L, Baron C. Telerehabilitation and its effect on story retelling by adults with neurogenic communication disorders. Aphasiology. 2004;18(5–7):639–52.
59. Winans-Mitrik RL, Hula WD, Dickey MW, Schumacher JG, Swoyer B, Doyle PJ. Description of an intensive residential aphasia treatment program: rationale, clinical processes, and outcomes. Am J Speech Lang Pathol. 2014;23(2):S330.
60. McNeil MR, Sung JE, Yang D, Pratt SR, Fossett TR, Doyle PJ, Pavelko S. Comparing connected language elicitation procedures in persons with aphasia: concurrent validation of the story retell procedure. Aphasiology. 2007;21(6–8):775–90.
61. Brookshire RH, Nicholas LE. Discourse comprehension test. Communication Skill Builders; 1993.
62. Gallée J, Cordella C, Fedorenko E, Hochberg D, Touroutoglou A, Quimby M, Dickerson BC. Breakdowns in informativeness of naturalistic speech production in primary progressive aphasia. Brain Sci. 2021;11(2):130.
63. Hilger A, Ramsberger G, Gilley P, Menn L, Kong A. Analysing speech problems in a longitudinal case study of logopenic variant PPA. Aphasiology. 2014;28(7):840–61.
64. Alyahya RS, Conroy P, Halai AD, Lambon Ralph MA. An efficient, accurate and clinically-applicable index of content word fluency in aphasia. Aphasiology. 2021;36(8):921–39.
65. Nicholas LE, Brookshire RH. A system for quantifying the informativeness and efficiency of the connected speech of adults with aphasia. J Speech Lang Hear Res. 1993;36(2):338–50.
66. Boyle M. Test–retest stability of word retrieval in aphasic discourse. J Speech Lang Hear Res. 2014;57(3):966–78.
67. Cameron RM, Wambaugh JL, Mauszycki SC. Individual variability on discourse measures over repeated sampling times in persons with aphasia. Aphasiology. 2010;24(6–8):671–84.

68. Murray LL, Holland AL, Beeson PM. Spoken language of individuals with mild fluent aphasia under focused and divided-attention conditions. J Speech Lang Hear Res. 1998;41(1):213–27.
69. Murray L, Ballard K, Karcher L. Linguistic specific treatment: just for Broca's aphasia? Aphasiology. 2004;18(9):785–809.
70. Murray L, Timberlake A, Eberle R. Treatment of underlying forms in a discourse context. Aphasiology. 2007;21(2):139–63.
71. Altmann LJ, Hazamy AA, Carvajal PJ, Benjamin M, Rosenbek JC, Crosson B. Delayed stimulus-specific improvements in discourse following anomia treatment using an intentional gesture. J Speech Lang Hear Res. 2014;57(2):439–54.
72. Gordon JK. Measuring the lexical semantics of picture description in aphasia. Aphasiology. 2008;22(7–8):839–52.
73. Murray LL, Karcher L. A treatment for written verb retrieval and sentence construction skills. Aphasiology. 2000;14(5–6):585–602.
74. Kendall DL, Rosenbek JC, Heilman KM, Conway T, Klenberg K, Gonzalez Rothi LJ, Nadeau SE. Phoneme-based rehabilitation of anomia in aphasia. Brain Lang. 2008;105(1):1–17.
75. Pritchard M, Hilari K, Cocks N, Dipper L. Reviewing the quality of discourse information measures in aphasia. Int J Lang Commun Disord. 2017;52(6):689–732.
76. Wambaugh JL, Wright S, Mauszycki SC, Nessler C, Bailey D. Combined aphasia and apraxia of speech treatment (CAAST): systematic replications in the development of a novel treatment. Int J Speech Lang Pathol. 2017;20(2):247–61.
77. Rogers MA, Alarcon NB. Dissolution of spoken language in primary progressive aphasia. Aphasiology. 1998;12(7–8):635–50.
78. Faroqi-Shah Y, Gehman M. The role of processing speed and cognitive control on word retrieval in aging and aphasia. J Speech Lang Hear Res. 2021;64(3):949–64.
79. Beales A, Whitworth A, Cartwright J, Panegyres PK, Kane RT. Determining stability in connected speech in primary progressive aphasia and Alzheimer's disease. Int J Speech Lang Pathol. 2018;20(3):361–70.
80. Beales A, Whitworth A, Cartwright J. A review of lexical retrieval intervention in primary progressive aphasia and Alzheimer's disease: mechanisms of change, generalisation, and cognition. Aphasiology. 2018;32(11):1360–87.
81. Paek EJ, Murray LL, Newman SD. Effects of concurrent action and object naming treatment on naming skills and functional brain activation patterns in primary progressive aphasia: an fMRI study with a case-series design. Brain Lang. 2021;218:104950.
82. Croot K, Taylor C, Abel S, Jones K, Krein L, Hameister I, Nickels L. Measuring gains in connected speech following treatment for word retrieval: a study with two participants with primary progressive aphasia. Aphasiology. 2014;29(11):1265–88.
83. Kim M. Effect of lexical retrieval cascade treatment on naming and discourse of individuals with logopenic variant of primary progressive aphasia (lvPPA). Clin Arch Commun Disord. 2017;2(3):197–208.
84. Rogalski Y, Edmonds LA. Attentive reading and constrained summarisation (ARCS) treatment in primary progressive aphasia: a case study. Aphasiology. 2008;22(7–8):763–75.
85. Whitworth A, Cartwright J, Beales A, Leitão S, Panegyres PK, Kane R. Taking words to a new level: a preliminary investigation of discourse intervention in primary progressive aphasia. Aphasiology. 2017;32(11):1284–309.
86. Leaman MC, Edmonds LA. Revisiting the correct information unit: measuring informativeness in unstructured conversations in people with aphasia. Am J Speech Lang Pathol. 2019;28(3):1099–114.
87. Leaman MC, Edmonds LA. Assessing language in unstructured conversation in people with aphasia: methods, psychometric integrity, normative data, and comparison to a structured narrative task. J Speech Lang Hear Res. 2021;64(11):4344–65.
88. Marini A, Andreetta S, del Tin S, Carlomagno S. A multi-level approach to the analysis of narrative language in aphasia. Aphasiology. 2011;25(11):1372–92.
89. Nicholas LE, Brookshire RH. Comprehension of spoken narrative discourse by adults with aphasia, right-hemisphere brain damage, or traumatic brain injury. Am J Speech Lang Pathol. 1995;4(3):69–81.
90. Armstrong E. Aphasic discourse analysis: the story so far. Aphasiology. 2000;14(9):875–92.
91. Kong AP-H. The use of main concept analysis to measure discourse production in Cantonese-speaking persons with aphasia: a preliminary report. J Commun Disord. 2009;42(6):442–64.
92. Kong AP-H. The main concept analysis in Cantonese aphasic oral discourse: external validation and monitoring chronic aphasia. J Speech Lang Hear Res. 2011;54(1):148–59.
93. Yazu H, Kong AP-H, Yoshihata H, Okubo K. Adaptation and validation of the main concept analysis of spoken discourse by native Japanese adults. Clin Linguist Phon. 2021;36(1):17–33.
94. Kong AP-H. Main concept analysis for acquired deficits of spoken narratives: preliminary data on inter-rater agreement and potential application to the Korean-speaking population. Clin Arch Commun Disord. 2018;3(1):14–21.
95. Kong AP, Yeh CC. A Taiwanese Mandarin main concept analysis (TM-MCA) for quantification of aphasic oral discourse. Int J Lang Commun Disord. 2015;50(5):580–92.
96. Kong AP-H, Whiteside J, Bargmann P. The main concept analysis: validation and sensitivity in differentiating discourse produced by unimpaired English

speakers from individuals with aphasia and dementia of Alzheimer type. Logoped Phoniatr Vocol. 2015;41(3):129–41.
97. Kong AP. Dialectally-sensitive norms of the Spanish version of main concept analysis (Span-MCA) for quantifying neurogenically impaired spoken discourse. Rev Invest Logoped. 2021;11(2):e69932.
98. Criel Y, Deleu M, De Groote E, Bockstael A, Kong AP-H, De Letter M. The Dutch main concept analysis: translation and establishment of normative data. Am J Speech Lang Pathol. 2021;30(4):1750–66.
99. Kong AP-H, Ross A, Pettigrew C. A main concept analysis for aphasic discourse in Irish-English speakers. J Clin Speech Lang Stud. 2012;19(1):19–43.
100. Kong AP-H. The Main Concept Analysis (MCA) for oral discourse production. Hong Kong: The Commercial Press (H.K.) Limited. 2016.
101. Richardson JD, Dalton SG. Main concepts for three different discourse tasks in a large non-clinical sample. Aphasiology. 2015;30(1):45–73.
102. Richardson JD, Dalton SG. Main concepts for two picture description tasks: an addition to Richardson and Dalton, 2016. Aphasiology. 2019;34(1):119–36.
103. Dalton SG, Richardson JD. A large-scale comparison of main concept production between persons with aphasia and persons without brain injury. Am J Speech Lang Pathol. 2019;28(1S):293–320.
104. Kurland J, Liu A, Stokes P. Phase I test development for a brief assessment of transactional success in aphasia: methods and preliminary findings of main concepts in non-aphasic participants. Aphasiology. 2021;37(1):39–68.
105. Hameister I, Nickels L. The cat in the tree—using picture descriptions to inform our understanding of conceptualisation in aphasia. Lang Cogn Neurosci. 2018;33(10):1296–314.
106. Rivera A, Hirst J, Edmonds LA. Evaluation of language predictors of main concept production in Spanish/English bilingual discourse using Nicholas and Brookshire stimuli. Am J Speech Lang Pathol. 2018;27(1):52–70.
107. Doyles PJ, McNeil MR, Spencer KA, Goda AJ, Cottrell K, Lustig AP. The effects of concurrent picture presentations on retelling of orally presented stories by adults with aphasia. Aphasiology. 1998;12(7–8):561–74.
108. Stark JA. Content analysis of the fairy tale Cinderella–a longitudinal single-case study of narrative production: “from rags to riches”. Aphasiology. 2010;24(6–8):709–24.
109. Fromm D, Forbes M, Holland A, Dalton SG, Richardson J, MacWhinney B. Discourse characteristics in aphasia beyond the western aphasia battery cutoff. Am J Speech Lang Pathol. 2017;26(3):762–8.
110. Richardson JD, Hudspeth Dalton SG, Fromm D, Forbes M, Holland A, MacWhinney B. The relationship between confrontation naming and story gist production in aphasia. Am J Speech Lang Pathol. 2018;27(1S):406–22.
111. Doyle PJ, Goda AJ, Spencer KA. The communicative informativeness and efficiency of connected discourse by adults with aphasia under structured and conversational sampling conditions. Am J Speech Lang Pathol. 1995;4(4):130–4.
112. Albright E, Purves B. Exploring sentence Shaper™: treatment and augmentative possibilities. Aphasiology. 2008;22(7–8):741–52.
113. Avent J, Austermann S. Reciprocal scaffolding: a context for communication treatment in aphasia. Aphasiology. 2003;17(4):397–404.
114. Coelho CA, McHugh RE, Boyle M. Semantic feature analysis as a treatment for aphasic dysnomia: a replication. Aphasiology. 2000;14(2):133–42.
115. Capilouto GJ, Wright HH, Wagovich SA. CIU and main event analyses of the structured discourse of older and younger adults. J Commun Disord. 2005;38(6):431–44.
116. Capilouto GJ, Wright HH, Wagovich SA. Reliability of main event measurement in the discourse of individuals with aphasia. Aphasiology. 2006;20(2–4):205–16.
117. Capilouto GJ, Wright HH, Maddy KMC. Microlinguistic processes that contribute to the ability to relay main events: influence of age. Neuropsychol Dev Cogn B Aging Neuropsychol Cogn. 2015;23(4):445–63.
118. Kong AP, Linnik A, Law SP, Shum WW. Measuring discourse coherence in anomic aphasia using rhetorical structure theory. Int J Speech Lang Pathol. 2018;20(4):406–21.
119. Marini A, Carlomagno S, Caltagirone C, Nocentini U. The role played by the right hemisphere in the organization of complex textual structures. Brain Lang. 2005;93(1):46–54.
120. Andreetta S, Cantagallo A, Marini A. Narrative discourse in anomic aphasia. Neuropsychologia. 2012;50(8):1787–93.
121. Brisebois A, Brambati SM, Désilets-Barnabé M, Boucher J, García AO, Rochon E, Leonard C, Desautels A, Marcotte K. The importance of thematic informativeness in narrative discourse recovery in acute post-stroke aphasia. Aphasiology. 2019;34(4):472–91.
122. Brisebois A, Brambati SM, Boucher J, Rochon E, Leonard C, Désilets-Barnabé M, Desautels A, Marcotte K. A longitudinal study of narrative discourse in post-stroke aphasia. Aphasiology. 2021;36(7):805–30.
123. Henderson A, Kim H, Kintz S, Frisco N, Wright H. Working memory in aphasia: considering discourse processing and treatment implications. Semin Speech Lang. 2017;38(1):40–51.
124. Kim H, Kintz S, Zelnosky K, Wright HH. Measuring word retrieval in narrative discourse: core lexicon in aphasia. Int J Lang Commun Disord. 2018;54(1):62–78.
125. Kintz S, Wright HH. Discourse measurement in aphasia research. Aphasiology. 2017;32(4):472–4.
126. Marcotte K, Lachance A, Brisebois A, Mazzocca P, Désilets-Barnabé M, Desjardins N, Brambati SM. Validation of videoconference administration of picture description from the western aphasia bat-

tery–revised in neurotypical Canadian French speakers. Am J Speech Lang Pathol. 2022;31(6):2825–34.
127. Duhigg CC, Strawn A, Uffer JQ, Hubbard HI, Adams J, Richardson JD. Combined computerized and virtual group treatment for persons with primary progressive aphasia. Poster session presented at: Academy of Aphasia; 2022; Virtual.
128. Greenslade KJ, Stuart JE, Richardson JD, Dalton SG, Ramage AE. Macrostructural analyses of Cinderella narratives in a large nonclinical sample. Am J Speech Lang Pathol. 2020;29(4):1923–36.
129. Richardson JD, Dalton SG, Greenslade KJ, Jacks A, Haley KL, Adams J. Main concept, sequencing, and story grammar analyses of Cinderella narratives in a large sample of persons with aphasia. Brain Sci. 2021;11(1):110.
130. Armstrong L, Brady M, Mackenzie C, Norrie J. Transcription-less analysis of aphasic discourse: a clinician's dream or a possibility? Aphasiology. 2007;21(3–4):355–74.
131. Miller J, Iglesias A. Systematic analysis of language transcripts (SALT). Research version. 2008.
132. Hunt KW. Grammatical structures written at three grade levels. NCTE research report no. 3. [Internet]. ERIC. 1964 [cited 2023 Jan 27]. https://eric.ed.gov/?id=ED113735
133. Ulatowska HK, North AJ, Macaluso-Haynes S. Production of narrative and procedural discourse in aphasia. Brain Lang. 1981;13(2):345–71.
134. Lê K, Coelho C, Mozeiko J, Krueger F, Grafman J. Measuring goodness of story narratives: implications for traumatic brain injury. Aphasiology. 2011;25(6–7):748–60.
135. Cavanaugh R, Dalton SG, Richardson JD. Technical session ASHA 2022. In: Novel web applications to facilitate discourse analysis in everyday clinical practice.
136. Cavanaugh R, Dalton SG, Richardson J. coreLexicon: an open-source web-app for scoring core lexicon analysis. R package version 0.0.1.0000. 2021. https://github.com/aphasia-apps/coreLexicon
137. Cavanaugh R, Richardson J, Dalton SG. mainConcept: an open-source web-app for scoring main concept analysis. R package version 0.0.1.0000. 2021. https://github.com/aphasia-apps/mainConcept
138. R Core Team. R: a language and environment for statistical computing. Version 4.0.3 [software]. R Foundation for Statistical Computing. 2020. https://www.r-project.org/
139. Chang W, Cheng J, Allaire J, Sievert C, Schloerke B, Xie Y, Allen J, McPherson J, Dipert A, Borges B. Shiny: web application framework for r [manual]. 2020. https://CRAN.R-project.org/package=shiny
140. MacWhinney B. From CHILDES to TalkBank. In: Research on child language acquisition. Somerville: Cascadilla; 2001. p. 17–34.
141. Jarrold W, Rofes A, Wilson S, Pressman P, Stabler E, Gorno-Tempini M. A "verbal thermometer" for assessing neurodegenerative disease: automated measurement of pronoun and verb ratio from speech. In: 42nd annual international conference of the IEEE Engineering in Medicine & Biology Society (EMBC). 2020 July 20. IEEE. pp. 5831–5837.
142. Torre IG, Romero M, Álvarez A. Improving aphasic speech recognition by using novel semi-supervised learning methods on AphasiaBank for English and Spanish. Appl Sci. 2021;11(19):8872.
143. Martin JL, Wright KE. Bias in automatic speech recognition: the case of African-American language. Appl Linguist. 2023;44:613–30.

Additional Resources

Articles

Dipper L, Marshall J, Boyle M, Hersh D, Botting N, Cruice M. Creating a theoretical framework to underpin discourse assessment and intervention in aphasia. Brain Sci. 2021;11(2):183. https://doi.org/10.3390/brainsci11020183.
Linnik A, Bastiaanse R, Höhle B. Discourse production in aphasia: a current review of theoretical and methodological challenges. Aphasiology. 2016;30(7):765–800. https://doi.org/10.1080/02687038.2015.1113489.
Pritchard M, Hilari K, Cocks N, Dipper L. Reviewing the quality of discourse information measures in aphasia. Int J Lang Commun Disord. 2017;52(6):689–732. https://doi.org/10.1111/1460-6984.12318.
Aphasiology, Issue 11—Discourse in Aphasia.

Books/Book Chapters

Coelho C, Cherney LR, Shadden BB, editors. Discourse analysis in adults with and without communication disorders: a resource for clinicians and researchers. Plural Publishing; 2022.

Online Resources

AphasiaBank Database. https://aphasia.talkbank.org. Discourse topic webpage. https://aphasia.talkbank.org/discourse/
FOQUSAphasia. https://foqusaphasia.com
CoreLex Web App. https://aphasia-apps.shinyapps.io/coreLexicon/
MCA Web App. https://rb-cavanaugh.shinyapps.io/mainConcept/
LUNA. https://blogs.city.ac.uk/luna/

C-Star lecture series. https://cstar.sc.edu/lecture-series/. Lucy Bryant. "Implementing spoken discourse analysis in clinical aphasia practice: a virtual future". Gayle DeDe. "Conversation treatment for people with aphasia: a randomized controlled trial"

Publisher's website for the MT-86. https://www.orthoedition.com/evaluations/mt-81*

SRP materials (checklists and audio files) are available from the computerized revised token test website. https://computerizedrevisedtokentest.com/story-retell-procedure/*

*Inclusion of this website should not be considered an endorsement for use of this assessment.

Sarah Grace H. Dalton is an Assistant Professor at Marquette University in the Department of Speech Pathology and Audiology. She directs the Building Rehabilitation Advances in Neuroscience (BRAiN Lab) where her research focuses on improving the lives of persons living with aphasia by improving assessment and treatment methods.

Jessica D. Richardson is an Associate Professor at The University of New Mexico in the Department of Speech and Hearing Sciences and the Center for Brain Recovery and Repair. She directs the Brain Scouts Lab where her research focuses on improving the lives of persons living with aphasia, due to stable or progressive causes, and of their care partners.

13 Assessing Impaired Macrostructures in Discourse Production of Persons with Aphasia

Jessica D. Richardson, Sarah Grace H. Dalton, and Kathryn J. Greenslade

Preview of What Is Currently Known
Utilization of discourse macrostructures allows language users to organize and reduce complex information into socially acceptable communication packages via organization of local microstructures. Until recently, discourse macrostructure had been viewed as relatively intact in persons with aphasia (PWAs) but, as this chapter highlights, PWAs differ from controls at many levels of macrostructural analysis—propositions, story grammar, sequencing, and more—even persons with latent aphasia. Discourse macrostructures are not preserved in PWAs and the presence and impact of such deficits should be a clinical and research focus. Translation of the theoretical construct of macrostructures into clinical use has not been straightforward, and there are varied definitions and measures throughout the aphasia literature. What follows is a presentation and discussion of some of the most commonly used measures that meet the following criteria: available and accessible procedural information; available and accessible normative reference data; and demonstrated promise for detection and other management (e.g., tracking recovery, response to treatment). With these criteria in place, a resource of macrostructural analysis tools that clinicians can access and use in the real world is presented in this chapter.

Objectives
(a) To define discourse macrostructure.
(b) To give examples of ways to measure discourse macrostructures.
(c) To list and describe several different approaches for measuring narrative discourse macrostructures.
(d) To describe macrostructural deficits in persons with aphasia.
(e) To locate resources needed for administering selected macrostructural analyses.

J. D. Richardson (✉)
Department of Speech and Hearing Sciences, University of New Mexico, Albuquerque, NM, USA

S. G. H. Dalton
Department of Speech Pathology and Audiology, Marquette University, Milwaukee, WI, USA
e-mail: sarahgrace.dalton@marquette.edu

K. J. Greenslade
Department of Communication Sciences and Disorders, University of New Hampshire, Durham, NH, USA
e-mail: kathryn.greenslade@unh.edu

Macrostructures

The word "macro" indicates examination of something on a large scale. "Structure," in the context of discourse, refers to the aggregate of coherently linked concepts, and the linguistic elements used to express those concepts. Using discourse macrostructures allows language users to organize, shorten, and simplify information into

A. P.-H. Kong (ed.), *Spoken Discourse Impairments in the Neurogenic Populations*,
https://doi.org/10.1007/978-3-031-45190-4_13

a socially acceptable form, communicated via context-dependent, locally organized microstructures, including "words, phrases, clauses, sentences, and connections between sentences" ([1], p. 29). Macrostructures are dictated by superstructures, which are socio-culturally conventionalized "schematic forms that [organize] the global meaning of a text" ([1], p. 108). Van Dijk [1] introduced several types of superstructures, including narrative, arguments, scholarly papers, and newspaper articles, with important differences in elements. For example, while narratives and arguments both require settings, narratives feature episodes with sub-structures, while arguments feature premises (including facts with backing) and conclusions. Further, subtypes of narrative superstructures vary enough in their elements enough to warrant distinct analyses: story grammar analysis for fictional stories, which identifies initiating events, reactions, plans, attempts, and direct consequences as compared to high point analysis for personal anecdotes, which identifies complicating actions, a high point, and resolution with evaluations interspersed throughout [2]. As another example, scientific publications follow a superstructure that defines a problem (background, aims, hypotheses) and solution (methods, results, discussion) [1].

Descriptions of discourse macrostructures draw on both structuralist and functionalist theoretical perspectives, including examination of suprasentential aspects of discourse alongside semantic units (from words and above) and context of use. Translation of the theoretical construct of macrostructures into clinical use has been less straightforward; operationalization has led to a substantial variability in definitions and measures throughout the aphasia literature. Further, until fairly recently macrostructure had been viewed as relatively intact in persons with aphasia (PWAs) [3, 4]. Therefore, a focus on developing standardized, psychometrically sound macrostructural measures traditionally has not been a priority.

What follows is a discussion of commonly used, research-supported measures for PWAs that also meet the following criteria: available and accessible procedural information; available and accessible normative reference data; and demonstrated promise for detection and other management (e.g., tracking recovery, response to treatment). Additionally, as story grammar is the most commonly used and well-understood macrostructural analysis, the focus of this chapter is limited to monologic, semi-spontaneous spoken language tasks elicited via picture description and story retelling, excluding personal stories and expository/procedural discourse. Guided by these criteria, a toolbox of macrostructural analyses that clinicians can access and use in the real world is presented. Below, selected measures are briefly described, with information from highlighted research articles to introduce the measure and/or allow for replication. For each article, resources related to assessment fidelity (e.g., materials, elicitation, and coding/scoring procedures) and normative references, along with a summary of findings, are provided. By integrating this information with knowledge of a client's abilities/needs, clinicians can select the most appropriate and/or feasible measures, and then use provided guidance to obtain the necessary resources for optimal administration and interpretation.

Proposition Analysis

The term "proposition" has been used to refer to concepts, sentences, statements, word-level meanings, that-clauses, fact concepts, text base, and/or conceptual chunks [5–8]. The words, phrases, and sentences used when expressing propositions have been categorized as discourse microstructure, [6, 8] but the examination of the relevance of propositions has been categorized as discourse macrostructure [1, 6, 8]. Proposition-level measures of correctness or completeness relate to both microstructure and macrostructure since incorrect and/or incomplete essential (compared to a standard) concepts generally reduce overall narrative coherence [5, 6, 8, 9] and expression of topic "gist" [1]. One of the most well-known and supported measures is main concept analysis (MCA) [10, 11]. Briefly, a main concept

(MC) list for a discourse task, developed from healthy control samples, includes a closed list of propositions constituting the "outline of the gist or essential information" for the task ([11], p. 148). Each MC consists of conceptual elements considered to be essential. A coding system is applied to determine the accuracy and completeness of a proposition that matches an MC [10–14]. MCA thus informs whether speakers are able to accurately and completely communicate concepts considered to be essential for expressing the overall *gist* of a discourse about which speakers share knowledge [10, 11], a critical component of macrostructural analysis. For a more in-depth discussion of this and other proposition-level analyses, see Chap. 12 [15] in this volume.

Story Grammar Analysis

Story grammar measures are commonly used to examine macrostructures [16] and have been lauded for their psychometric strengths [17]. In general, story grammar analyses examine how well a narrator meets organizational expectations related to the logical and/or linear sequencing of events, characters, and relationships between events and characters to facilitate listeners' ability to follow a story [18–23]. Other terms for story grammar in the literature are "discourse grammar," "linguistic framework," and "narrative superstructure" [24, 25]. Various measures are presented below to provide descriptions of resources to facilitate utilization by readers. While studies below often investigated additional measures alongside story grammar, the discussion here is restricted to story grammar.

Ulatowska et al. [24]

Ulatowska et al. [24] investigated "superstructure" via story grammar analysis of picture sequence description and story retelling in PWAs and healthy controls.

Materials

For picture sequence description, authors used the "Cat Story," a 5-frame picture sequence, which is included as Fig. 1 in Ulatowska et al. ([24], p. 350) For story retelling, authors used the "Rooster Story," a 6-sentence short story found in Ulatowska et al. ([24], p. 350)

Elicitation Procedures

Few details regarding elicitation were provided. Discourse and other cognitive-linguistic measures were administered in the participants' home by speech-language pathologists and/or psychologists. Authors stated they elicited the "Cat Story" "with the help of sequence pictures" ([24], p. 349). and that the participants retold the "Rooster Story" "immediately following the examiner's reading of the story" ([24], p. 349).

Coding/Scoring Procedures

Discourse samples were audio-recorded and transcribed verbatim. False starts and repetitions were removed from transcriptions. Discourse was segmented into T-units, as defined by Hunt [26]. In terms of story grammar, authors marked the occurrence of the following superstructural elements identified by Labov [27], which are briefly described ([24], p. 350–1): (1) abstract, (2) setting (e.g., time, location, participants, background), (3) complicating action, (4) evaluation, (5) resolution, and (6) coda. The authors note that these elements make up an episode, and that clauses within an episode or narrative are usually temporally sequenced. Per the results section, some elements are essential (settings, complicating actions, and resolutions), and others are optional (abstract, introducers, codas). Evaluations were described as "a necessary condition of acceptable narrative" ([24], p. 355), but were not included as an essential element in the reporting or tables.

Participants for Reference

See Table 1 in Ulatowska et al. ([24], p. 349). This study included 10 PWAs (8 male) between the ages of 54–70 ($M = 60.2$) with 10–18 years of education (M = 13.4). Participants ranged from 6 to 103 months post onset (MPO) (M = 23.6). Seven were characterized as having mild aphasia, three as having mild-moderate aphasia. Ten healthy controls were matched for sex, age (range 54–71, M = 58.7), and education (range 12–20, M = 14.4).

Summary of Findings

Narratives of PWAs generally contained the essential elements required to meet criterion for complete episodes (i.e., setting, complicating event, and resolution); more variability was observed with optional elements (e.g., abstracts, evaluation, codas). Specifically, authors commented on significantly reduced evaluations produced by PWAs compared to controls. The sequencing of story grammar elements was reported to be preserved for all narratives according to subjective ratings of content. While story grammar and sequencing variables did not differ significantly between mildly impaired PWAs and controls, results for the "Cat Story" showed significant differences between these groups for number of clauses (just not for the *essential* story grammar elements), number of clauses containing evaluations, content, and clarity.

Ulatowska et al. [25]

Ulatowska et al. [25] investigated "superstructure" via story grammar analysis of picture sequence description and story retelling in PWAs and healthy controls. Materials and procedures are similar to Ulatowska et al. [24] with some minor differences.

Materials

See section "Materials" above.

Elicitation Procedures

See section "Elicitation Procedures" above, with the exception that only speech-language pathologists administered the discourse tasks.

Coding/Scoring Procedures

See section "Coding/Scoring Procedures" above. As with Ulatowska et al. [24], evaluation was excluded from both essential and optional lists. Instead, it was reported separately. The article's Appendix ([25], p. 333) includes helpful scoring examples potentially useful for training.

Participants for Reference

See Table 1 in Ulatowska et al. ([25], p. 320). This study included 15 PWAs (10 or 12 males; unclear due to mathematical error in manuscript) between the ages of 24–71 (M = 50.4) with between 10 and 17 years of education (M = 13.4). Participants ranged from 2 to 220 MPO (M = 49.4). All were characterized as having moderate aphasia. Fifteen healthy controls were matched for sex, age (range 18–73, M = 50.8), and education (range 10–17, M = 13.3).

Summary of Findings

Significant between-group differences were reported, with moderately impaired PWAs having fewer optional and essential components (i.e., setting, resolution) and thus fewer overall complete episodes. Despite these differences, the authors concluded that participants demonstrated preserved narrative structure.

Coelho et al. [28]

Coelho et al. [28] conducted a longitudinal study throughout the first year of recovery for a person with mild fluent aphasia.

Materials

Authors used a 19-frame picture story of "The Bear and The Fly," with pictures from the commercially available book of the same name by Winter [29].

Elicitation Procedures

Few details regarding elicitation were provided. Authors elicited "The Bear and The Fly Story" after showing the picture story on a projector screen (8 × 10 in.) and then asking the participants to retell the story.

Coding/Scoring Procedures

Discourse samples were audio-recorded and transcribed verbatim. Discourse was segmented into T-units, as defined by Hunt [30]. Following Stein and Glenn's [19] story grammar framework, authors identified and counted three essential episodic components: (1) "initiating event that causes a character to formulate a goal-directed behavioral sequence"; (2) attempt/action; and (3) "direct consequence marking attainment or non-attainment of the goal" ([28], p. 147). Complete episodes contained all three essential components.

Participants for Reference

This study included a 55-year-old male PWA with 12 years of education. The investigators followed him from 1 to 12 MPO and he was characterized as having mild anomic aphasia. Three healthy controls (all male) with a mean age of 56 years (no other details provided) were enrolled for comparison. Relevant comparison data are found on pages 150 and 151 of the article [28].

Summary of Findings

Despite gains in PICA (Porch Index of Communicative Ability) [31] scores (from 71st percentile to 93rd percentile) over time, story grammar performance did not improve. Whereas controls generated 4–5 episodes in their retells, the PWA never generated more than 2 episodes over 12 months of tracking. The discrepancy in recovery trajectory between overall communication abilities and story grammar was inconsistent with previous reports of mildly impaired PWAs and indicated the need for more research.

Coelho et al. [32]

Coelho et al. [32] conducted a discourse study in a larger sample of healthy controls and in persons with closed head injury who were presumably non-aphasic, as "they had achieved fluent conversation and did not demonstrate significant deficits on traditional clinical language tests" and scored above 93 on the Western Aphasia Battery, where 93.8 and above is considered not aphasic [33]. (Please make note, however, that there is emerging research [14] on latent aphasia that includes people who score above this cutoff.) While not promoted as a study of PWAs, we focus here on relevant details related to the methods and the control sample for potential comparison to PWAs.

Materials

For story retelling, authors again used a 19-frame picture story of "The Bear and The Fly" [29]. For story generation, authors used the picture scene titled "Runaway" by Norman Rockwell [34], which can be located via an internet search with relevant keywords (e.g., title, artist).

Elicitation Procedures

Authors provided elicitation details in the manuscript ([32], p. 502–503) and on TBI Bank in the Coelho Corpus [35]. For "The Bear and The Fly," authors showed the picture story on a projector screen (23 × 30.5 cm) and then instructed participants to "Tell me that story." For the "Runaway" story, authors presented the picture scene and instructed participants to "Tell me a story about what you think is happening in this picture." Participants were allowed to view the picture throughout the story generation. For both tasks, once a participant stopped telling the story, the assessor waited 10 s, asked "Is that the end of the story?", and then moved on to the next task following participant affirmation.

Coding/Scoring Procedures

Discourse samples were audio-recorded and transcribed verbatim. Discourse was segmented into T-units, as defined by Liles [36]. Authors refer readers to another Coelho article [20] for more details regarding discourse analysis procedures, and we incorporate relevant information here. Following Stein and Glenn's [19] story grammar framework, authors identified and counted three essential episodic components: (1) "initiating event that prompts a character to formulate a goal-directed behavior"; (2) attempt/action; and (3) "direct consequence marking attainment or nonattainment of the goal" ([20], p. 1238). Complete episodes contained all three essential components; incomplete episodes contained two out of three essential components. Two story grammar measures were analyzed: (1) number of total episodes—"number of complete and incomplete episodes," a measure of "content organization" ([32], p. 504); and (2) proportion of T-units contained within episode structure (T-units in episode structure/total T-units) ([32], p. 504), a measure of one's ability to "use story grammar as an organizational plan for language" ([20], p. 1238). Table 3 in Coelho [20] includes helpful descriptions and scoring examples potentially useful for training.

Participants for Reference

This study included 32 persons with CHI and 43 matched controls without brain injury ([32], p. 502). Controls (30 males) were predominantly Caucasian/White between the ages of 16–63 ($M = 31.9$) with between 11 and 24 years of education ($M = 15.3$) and representing three SES (Hollingshead) categories (Professional, Skilled, Unskilled Workers).

Summary of Findings

Authors sought to combine conversational and narrative measures to classify groups (neither of which included persons with a clinical diagnosis of aphasia). One story grammar measure—proportion of T-units within episode structure—correlated moderately with the discriminant function analysis and was the strongest contributor to discrimination between groups; however, the group discrimination relying on narrative measures alone was not significant. When authors combined narrative measures with conversational measures (not described above), group discrimination improved and was significant.

Whitworth and colleagues [37, 38]

Whitworth and colleagues [37, 38] investigated story grammar outcomes (under the heading of "coherence") following a novel discourse treatment NARNIA, *N*ovel *A*pproach to *R*eal-life communication: *N*arrative *I*ntervention in *A*phasia.

Materials

The Curtin University Discourse Protocol (CUDP) [39] was used for discourse-level tasks, which include an event recount, a procedure, giving an option, and telling a story. In keeping with this chapter's focus, the details presented here will focus on the Cinderella story retelling. No physical materials beyond the CUDP instructions were used.

Elicitation Procedures

After several other discourse tasks, the clinician transitions with "*Now we are going to change to something different. Can you tell me the story of Cinderella?*". (Clinicians have the option to stop the retelling after 5 min.)

Coding/Scoring Procedures

Discourse samples were audio-recorded and transcribed. Discourse was segmented into C-units, as defined by Loban [40] and entered into Systematic Analysis of Language Transcripts (SALT) [41]. Note that while SALT can be used to automate aspects of this analysis (e.g., counting story grammar codes), it is not essential. Each C-unit was assigned a story grammar (coherence) code: (1) orientation of character (OC), (2) orientation to location (OL), (3) orientation to time (OT), (4) orientation other (OO), (5) initiating event (IE), (6) response/plan (Res), (7) Events (E), (8) Evaluative comment (EC), (9) conclusion (Conc), or (10) end marker (End). Comments about the task that did not contribute to the story (e.g., "that was easy/hard") were excluded. These codes overlap somewhat with Stein and Glenn [19] and are from an instructional program in Australia for writing informational texts [42].

Codes were tallied under main categories of (1) beginning/orientation (OC, OL, OT, OO), (2) middle/body (IE, Res, E), and (3) end/conclusion (EC, Conc). See the following for additional guidance, descriptions, and examples potentially useful for training: Whitworth et al. [38] Table 1

(p. 1349) and Appendix 1 (pp. 1378–1381); and Whitworth et al. [39] Table 1 (p. 460) and Appendices (pp. 477–481).

Participants for Reference

See Table 2 (p. 1357) and Appendix 2 (p. 1382) in Whitworth et al. [38] for PWAs. The study of response to NARNIA involved 14 PWAs (8 males) between the ages of 37 and 87 ($M = 59$); years of education were not provided but occupations were described. Participants ranged from 2 to 166 MPO ($M = 32$). Seven were characterized as having mild aphasia and seven as having moderate aphasia. (Authors provide a similar breakdown on those participants assigned to the NARNIA condition and those assigned to Usual Care (UC).) See Table 2 Whitworth et al. [39] for healthy controls. Thirty healthy controls (15 male) were enrolled between the ages of 20 and 89; additional age descriptives are included in Table 2 [39] by age bin. Neither education nor occupation are reported.

Summary of Findings

Focusing on the Cinderella narrative, PWAs in both NARNIA and UC groups demonstrated numerical improvements in story grammar for the three categories (beginning/orientation, middle/body, end/conclusion). The largest effect size was observed in the middle/body category for the NARNIA group ($p = 0.055$, $d = 1.069$), but the only statistically significant improvement was in the middle/body category for the UC group ($p = 0.009$, $d = 0.665$). More notable changes in content organization were observed with the other discourse genres assessed in the study.

Sequencing Analysis

Narratives that have meaningful conditional relationships between propositions (e.g., one event or component, expressed in a proposition, allows or requires another event) are coherent narratives [1]. Therefore, thorough macrostructural analysis should extend beyond counting of essential components and consider the sequencing of those components. Persons with linguistic and/or cognitive deficits often produce narratives with essential concepts that match up to essential story grammar components but present them out of sequence and/or with revisions and backtracking, which negatively impacts coherence and overall communication.

Manning and Franklin [43]

Manning and Franklin [43] conducted a narrative analysis of previously collected data [44, 45] to explore cognitive influences on narrative breakdowns. Though authors investigated several variables related to story grammar, not all were described sufficiently for replication. Discussion in this chapter is restricted to the well-described sequencing, or temporal, variables.

Materials

Picture cards depicting the Cinderella story (source of pictures not reported).

Elicitation Procedures

Authors cite their usage of Quantitative Production Analysis (QPA) procedures for their elicitation [46]. If this is the case, cards are only to be used when participants say they do not know the story; if a review of cards occurs, then during the review of cards, the examinee and clinician can discuss the pictures. However, authors stated that all participants viewed the Cinderella story picture cards and were provided brief descriptions. Following the review, the cards were removed and participants were asked to retell the story in their own words. Clinician dialogue during the retelling was kept to a minimum and any comments were limited to encouragement to continue/complete the task [46].

Coding/Scoring Procedures

Narrative samples were first "cleaned" (e.g., neologisms, fillers, and repairs deleted); cleaning instructions are located in their Appendix A. Samples were then segmented into communication units (C-units) following guidelines from Saffran et al. [46] and SALT Software [41]. With reference to Langacker [47], C-units were then further segmented into attentional frames (AFs), which are usually chunks of information separated by intonational changes (i.e., intonational groups), and often correspond to clauses [48, 49]. Additional helpful segmenting details are in Appendix A of Manning and Franklin [43] and Appendix A of Saffran et al. [46].

Cognitive grammar framework analysis was then conducted on segmented data within an Excel spreadsheet. We focus here on the order of temporal events for the Cinderella story, reported via their temporal sequencing error variable—the percentage of AFs with temporal sequence errors. An AF was determined to have an error if the information was not provided in "logical temporal order" and disrupted the "flow of temporal information" ([43], p. 423). No further guidance (e.g., suggested order of events) for making error judgments was provided.

Participants for Reference

This study included narrative samples from 22 PWAs (10 males) between the ages of 40–80 ($M = 60.64$). PWAs ranged from approximately 7 to 120 MPO. Sixteen PWAs were characterized as non-fluent, six as fluent. Cognition was reported to be within normal limits; aphasia severity was not reported. Ten healthy controls (2 males) between the ages of 32–80 ($M = 53.1$) were included for comparison. Years of education were not reported for PWAs or controls.

Summary of Findings

As a group, PWAs made significantly more temporal sequencing errors than controls; this difference held for both fluent and non-fluent PWAs but there were no significant differences between the aphasic groups. Authors plotted temporal sequencing errors by noun naming scores with the following results: no PWAs demonstrated both noun naming and temporal sequencing WNL; 11 PWAs demonstrated both impaired noun naming and temporal sequencing; 8 PWAs demonstrated noun naming WNL but impaired temporal sequencing; and 3 PWAs demonstrated impaired noun naming but temporal sequencing WNL. Temporal sequencing was obviously different from controls according to these results, but authors found no significant correlations between temporal sequencing and noun naming, cognitive performance, or other microstructural variables under investigation.

Multidimensional Macrostructural Analyses

Kong and Reres [50]

Leveraging the AphasiaBank database, Kong and Reres [50] developed a brief discourse assessment titled Narrative Assessment Profile (NAP) intended to characterize main concepts, story grammar, core lexical usage, and sequencing. While normative healthy control data are not fully available, the protocol is adequately described and normative information for a small sample of PWAs was provided.

Materials

Authors relied upon AphasiaBank transcripts for the following: Refused Umbrella (6-frame picture sequence), Cinderella (story retelling following perusal of wordless picture book), and Peanut Butter and Jelly (procedural description). Materials for these tasks, including elicitation procedures, are included on the AphasiaBank website.

Elicitation Procedures

Standardized elicitation details are in the Kong and Reres manuscript ([50], p. 176) and listed in further detail on AphasiaBank.

Coding/Scoring Procedures

Transcripts and video recordings of discourse samples were available from AphasiaBank; refer to their manuals for transcription details. Authors stated they orthographically transcribed (presumably from the videos) the discourse samples of PWA collected for this study; further segmentation was not described. The following variables were calculated for events: (1) e.total (total of all attempted events, correct and incorrect), (2) e.matched (total target events attempted), (3) e.missed (total target events absent), (4) e.irrelevant (total non-target and irrelevant events), and (5) e.extra (presumably = e.total – e.matched – e.irrelevant). Authors list target events in their Appendix A. For sequencing of events, it appears that each transition between target events (e.g., event 1 to event 2) was given a point value when presented in correct sequence, and then tallied to obtain s.total, which corresponds to the percentage of correct transitions/total transitions produced. Authors provide information needed for scoring sequencing in their Appendix C. While not directly related to macrostructure, the presence or absence of lexical targets (with synonyms or alternative forms allowed) were tallied for each task (i.pb&j, i.umbr, i.cind) and totaled (i. total) (akin to Core Lexicon [15]). Target lexical items are provided in their Appendix B. The methods section ([50], pp. 174–176) contains additional helpful details for coding and scoring [50].

Participants for Reference

See Table 1 in Kong and Reres [50]. This study included 12 PWAs (6 males) between the ages of 29;9–73;6 ($M = 54$) with between 12 and 16 years of education ($M = 13.8$). Participants ranged from 12 to 272 MPO ($M = 64.08$). (Occupations are reported for most participants; group-level race/ethnicity data are also provided.) Six PWAs had mild aphasia, five moderate aphasia, and one severe aphasia according to WAB AQ scores; nine were non-fluent, three fluent. Ten healthy controls between the ages of 36;8–81;5 ($M = 66$) with between 12 and 20 years of education ($M - 15.1$) (occupations reported) were used for test development (e.g., identification of target events).

Summary of Findings

Seven out of ten healthy controls produced each target event (21 total across tasks) and target lexical items (283 total across tasks) listed in their Appendices A and B; nine out of ten healthy controls produced target events in the sequences presented in their Appendix C. PWAs produced an average of 11.92 (of 21) target events and an average of 23.17 (of 283) target lexical items. Slightly over half of target events produced were presented in the correct order. Results for additional variables are reported in Table 2 and are also reported separately for fluent ($N = 3$) and non-fluent ($N = 9$) aphasic profiles. Authors report correlations (in their Table 4) between NAP discourse variables and performance on other standardized batteries.

Greenslade et al. [51]

Recognizing the strong psychometrics and rich procedural knowledge of both main concept analysis (MCA) and story grammar component coding, Greenslade and colleagues [51] complemented it with easy-to-obtain sequencing information to develop the standardized and norm-referenced multilevel analytic approach called Main Concept, Sequencing, and Story Grammar Analyses, or MSSG. Richardson and colleagues [52] then applied this approach in the largest study of story grammar in PWAs to date.

Materials

Authors relied upon AphasiaBank transcripts for the Cinderella retells; standardized AphasiaBank instructions have participants review the Cinderella picture book by Grimes [53] with the words covered prior to attempting the storytelling. Materials for these tasks, including elicitation procedures, are included on the AphasiaBank website.

Elicitation Procedures

Standardized elicitation details are in the manuscript [52] and listed in further detail on AphasiaBank. Briefly, following review of the aforementioned picture book, participants were instructed: "Now tell me as much of the story of Cinderella as you can. You can use any details you know about the story, as well as the pictures you just looked at."

Coding/Scoring Procedures

Coding and scoring procedures are described fully in MSSG manuscripts [51, 52] and links to additional online (and regularly updated) resources are listed at the end of this manuscript.

Transcripts were in CHAT (Codes for Human Analysis of Transcripts) form [54] or were orthographic transcriptions; line numbers were added to all transcripts. (Note: this analysis can be conducted without reliance on CHAT transcription format.)

Main concept analysis (MCA) is the first step of MSSG analyses and is described in more detail in Chap. 12 [15] in this volume. Cinderella transcripts were scored for MCs using standardized checklists and scoring procedures [10, 11, 13, 14]. Briefly, a main concept (MC) consists of one main verb and its constituent arguments, as well as prepositional phrases and/or subordinate clauses that operate on the main verb, as appropriate [10, 11]. Each participant's transcript was scored for the presence or absence of MCs. Missing MCs were coded as absent (AB); present MCs could be assigned one of four codes based upon the accuracy and completeness of the essential elements within each MC—(1) accurate/complete (AC), (2) accurate/incomplete (AI), (3) inaccurate/complete (IC), and (4) inaccurate/incomplete (II). MC codes were transformed to numeric scores with the following formula [14]: *MC composite score* = (#AC × 3) + (#AI × 2) + (#IC × 2) + (#II × 1).

Sequencing is the next part of MSSG analyses (though it can be conducted before or after the story grammar analysis in practice) and relies upon the line numbers added to the transcripts. Detailed information regarding acceptable sequencing of MCs is located in the manuscripts [51, 52] and online resources. Correctly sequenced MCs were assigned three points. Incorrectly sequenced MCs that were signaled as being out of sequence by the speaker (e.g., "I forgot to mention…," use of temporal terms) were assigned two points. Incorrectly sequenced MCs unaccompanied by signaling were assigned 1 point. Absent MCs were assigned a sequencing score of 0. Points for all MCs were tallied for the *sequencing* score.

A combined *main concept + sequencing (MC + Sequencing)* score was calculated by adding the MC and sequencing scores for each concept.

The final MSSG analysis, story grammar (SG) analysis, yields several variables. Twenty-eight of the 34 Cinderella MCs were pre-assigned one of six story grammar component codes: (1) setting, (2) initiating event, (3) attempt, (4) direct consequence, (5) mental state (i.e., internal response, plan, or reaction), and (6) conclusion. The remaining six MCs were assigned coding options since the order of their production, neighboring MCs, or specific formulation determined their story grammar component. Each MC that received a code other than AB (absent) also received 1 point for the corresponding component (with one exception, see original resources). Points for all MCs were totaled for an *essential story grammar components* score, which tallies recognizable attempts at essential concepts/story grammar components and is comparable to previously reported MC Attempts [14, 55].

Twenty-four of the 27 Cinderella MCs existing within the episodic structure (i.e., MCs between the pre-assigned "setting" and "conclusion" codes) were pre-assigned an episode number (one through five); the remaining 3 MCs were assigned episode options. Within each episode, 1 point was given for the presence of each required episodic SG component (i.e., initiating event, attempt, and direct consequence). These points were then tallied for the *total episodic components* score.

Episodes were deemed complex episodes if they contained at least two required episodic SG components (i.e., initiating event, attempt, direct consequence). Each complex episode received 1 point while episodes including no or only 1 episodic SG component received 0 points. Points were totaled across episodes for the *episodic complexity* score.

Authors also presented an *MSSG classification* that was inspired by the Story Goodness Index, [56, 57] where the *MC + Sequencing* dimension (x-axis) was plotted against their *total episodic components* dimension (y-axis). The MSSG classification facilitates straightforward visualization of the relationship between participants' ability to tell accurate, complete, and logically sequenced stories (MC + Sequencing) and

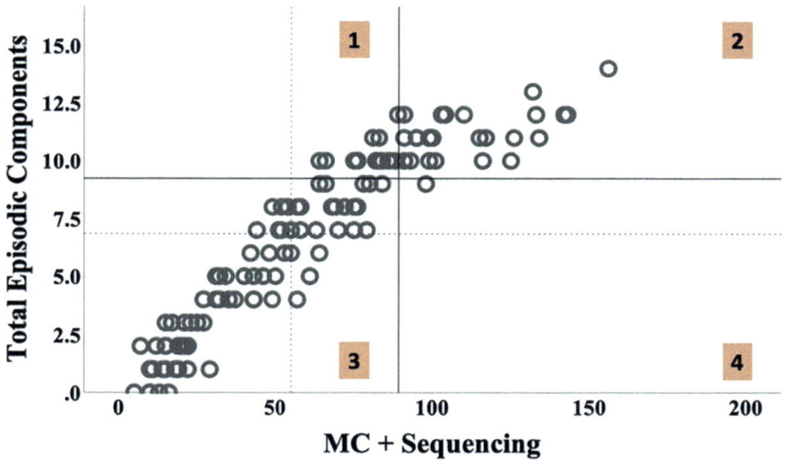

Note. MSSG classification quadrants are defined by cutoff points at 1 SD (solid line) and 2 SD (dotted line) below the mean. Quadrant 2 contains the highest scores for both dimensions, Quadrant 3 contains the lowest scores for both dimensions. Quadrant 4 contains high sequenced content and low overall episodic structure.

Fig. 13.1 Sample MSSG classification plot

their ability to maintain overall episodic structure (total episodic components) by dividing into four quadrants determined by normative (standard deviation) cutoffs shown below (see Fig. 13.1).

Resources with guidance, descriptions, and other examples useful for training include: rules for MC coding in Nicholas and Brookshire [11]; MC checklists in Richardson and Dalton [13] and MSSG procedures in Greenslade et al. [51]; MC and MSSG online manuals located in additional resources; and normative and comparative information for PWAs and healthy controls in Richardson and Dalton [13], Dalton and Richardson [14], Greenslade et al. [51], and Richardson et al. [52].

Participants for Reference

See Table 1 in Richardson et al. [52] This study included 370 PWAs (219 males) between the ages of 25–90;7 (M = 62) with between 7 and 25 years of education (M = 15.4). MPO was not reported. Aphasia subtypes included the following: 122 anomic, 85 Broca, 67 conduction, 4 global, 54 latent (or not aphasic by WAB; NABW), 12 transcortical motor, 2 transcortical sensory, and 24 Wernicke. (Descriptives are also broken down by aphasia subtype). Fifty-three PWAs had latent aphasia, 127 mild aphasia, 133 moderate aphasia, 41 severe aphasia, and 10 very severe aphasia according to WAB AQ scores; five were unclassified. One-hundred and ten healthy controls (45 males) between the ages of 20–89;5 (M = 58.3) with between 11 and 23 years of education (M = 15.8) were included for comparison. Group-level race/ethnicity data are also reported (Greenslade et al. [51] also reports on a sample of 92 healthy controls.).

Summary of Findings

Statistically and practically significant differences between PWAs and healthy controls were reported for all MSSG variables. These differences were observed not only at the omnibus group level (PWAs vs. controls) but also for each aphasia subtype, notable even for persons with latent or very mild aphasia who scored as NABW. Medium to large effect sizes for nearly all MSSG variables and aphasia subtypes supported the practical significance of this multilevel analytic approach. Authors demonstrated on a large scale, and with a wide range of aphasia subtypes and severity, that narrative macrostructure is not as well-preserved as previously believed and that it should receive more focus in both assessment and treatment.

Macrostructure Rating Scales

There are several reports using rating scales of macrostructure, with rating bins defined well-enough for good reliability. While not suitable as standalone measures, such scales may be useful for communicating about discourse status and treatment targets with clients and their families and may also hold some promise for tracking recovery.

Bottenberg and colleagues [58, 59]

Bottenberg and colleagues [58, 59] examined "narrative level" according to Applebee's [60] 6-level rating system for narrative structure and connections in PWAs and healthy controls.

Materials

Three sets of stimuli were used (toy dolls, picture scene, picture sequence), only one of which is readily available—a picture scene titled "Looking Out to Sea" by Norman Rockwell [61], which can be located via an internet search with relevant keywords (e.g., title, artist). Only the procedures and findings for the available stimulus, referred to as "Rockwell" in the manuscript, are discussed here.

Elicitation Procedures

Few details regarding elicitation were provided. Participants were shown the pictured scene and instructed to "*Tell me a story about* ______." where perhaps they inserted "this picture," "this scene," or the title of the print into the blank.

Coding/Scoring Procedures

Discourse samples were audio-recorded and transcribed. Authors analyzed for narrative level, use of logical connectives, and cohesive harmony; only narrative level is discussed here because of its potential for replicability and its similarity to other macrostructural measures, such as story grammar, discussed in this chapter. Applebee [60] developed a 6-level rating system, where the lowest rating is a 1 for "heaps," or unlinked mentions of characters and/or actions; the highest rating is a 6 for "narrative" which contains a central theme, a forward momentum, and climax. Intermediate ratings (numbered 2–5) include simple sequences, primitive narratives, unfocused chains, and focused chains [59]. The Rockwell discourse sample was assigned a rating between 1 and 6. Additional scoring examples potentially useful for training are found in original Applebee [60] and Hedberg and Stoel-Gammon [62].

Participants for Reference

See Table 1 in Bottenberg et al. ([58], p. 242). This study included 10 PWAs (9 males) between the ages of 36 and 71 (M = 57) with between 9 and 18 years of education (M = 13.6). Participants ranged from 2 to −96 MPO (M = 30.2). Nine were characterized as having mild aphasia and one as having moderate aphasia, according to the PICA [31]. Ten healthy controls were matched for sex, age (range 34–74, M = 61), and education (range 10–17, M = 12.7).

Summary of Findings

Narrative level (collapsing across all three samples) differed significantly between PWAs and controls, and PWAs were more variable overall. Looking at the "Rockwell" data specifically, narrative level ratings for PWAs (range 1–4, M = 2.7) were significantly lower than controls (range 3–5, M = 3.7).

Bottenberg and Colleagues [63]

Bottenberg and colleagues [63] also applied a different 8-level rating system based on Stein and Glenn [19] and Hedberg and Stoel-Gammon [62] to study "overall organization or suprastructure" ([63], p. 204) of discourse in PWAs.

Materials

Three picture stimuli were used—the Cookie Theft picture [64] and two-colored picture sequences showing a fire scene and the Kennedy assassination. Only procedures and findings for the readily available stimulus, referred to as "Cookie Theft" in the manuscript, is discussed here.

Elicitation Procedures

Authors provided elicitation details in the manuscript ([63], p. 204). Authors presented the Cookie Theft picture and instructed the participant to "Look at [the picture] and tell me the best story you can." Minimal prompts to continue or to indicate attention were provided (e.g., "hmmm," head nod). If the participant paused for >20 s, the assessor asked "Can you tell me more?" or "Is that all?". Sampling was completed following participant indication (verbal or nonverbal).

Coding/Scoring Procedures

Discourse samples were audio-recorded and transcribed; unintelligible words were transcribed phonetically or marked "unintelligible." The following were marked in the sample according to conventions outlined by Hedberg and Stoel-Gammon [62]: revisions, self-corrections, false starts, perseverations, stereotypic comments, asides (though it is unclear if this is critical for the rating system below, or only needed for other analyses included in the study). Discourse was segmented into T-units, as defined by Hunt [30]. Authors applied a different 8-level rating system based on Stein and Glenn [19], Hedberg and Stoel-Gammon [62], and McCabe and Peterson [2]. Of the 8 levels, the lowest rating is a 0 for "unrelated statements" and the highest rating is a 7 for "interactive episode," which involves at least two characters whose goals and actions influence one another. Intermediate ratings (numbered 1–6) include descriptive sentences, action sequences, reactive sequences, abbreviated episodes, completed episodes, or compound/complex episodes. Additional scoring examples useful for training are found in Hedberg and Stoel-Gammon [62].

Participants for Reference

See Table 1 in Bottenberg et al. [63] This study included 12 PWAs (7 males) between the ages of 38–65 (M = 50;6) with between 11 and 20 years of education (M = 13.9). Participants ranged from 3 to 282 MPO (M = 71.91). Inclusion criteria required they be considered mild-moderately impaired according to PICA scores.

Summary of Findings

While the study focus was to determine the impact of varied story elicitation stimuli on a wide range of discourse variables, authors noted that most participants produced complete stories for all stimuli under investigation, with mean story grammar level ratings that ranged from 4 to 4.5 (4 = abbreviated episodes, 5 = completed episodes); however, no ratings of 7 (highest rating, interactive episode) were observed in their sample. In Table 3 ([63], p. 206), authors show findings by stimuli, and Cookie Theft stories received the lowest ratings: M = 4.0 (SD = 1.38; range 1–6).

Summary

Macrostructures clearly are not preserved in PWAs as a group and the presence and impact of such deficits has been overlooked until fairly recently. In this chapter, several tools for macrostructural analysis that identify strengths and weaknesses to guide treatment and management have been identified. Though admittedly biased, we feel that the most sound and operationalized approach described in this chapter is the MSSG analyses. However, it is limited to the Cinderella story retelling, and should likely be accompanied by other stimuli and associated analyses for optimal well-rounded assessment.

Other recently introduced measures that, with additional development and/or operationalization, show promise for contributing to our knowledge of macrostructural deficits in PWAs. For example, Hameister and Nickels [65] determined the median MC order (i.e., which MC was most commonly presented first, second, etc.) for the "Cat in the Tree" (or "Cat Rescue") picture scene and introduced a Difference-in-Order ratio (DiO ratio) to express the difference between the expected versus produced order of MCs. There are also other recently introduced and promising temporal and efficiency measures. DeDe and Salis [66] examined the Cinderella story retelling in persons with mild and latent aphasia, focusing on temporal speech production variables (e.g., pauses, mazes, speech rate, repetitions, revisions) and discourse organization variables (e.g., percentage of formulation time for utterances that continue episodes, episode omission, episode recurrence). They found that the temporal measures sensitively characterized differences between controls and people with latent aphasia and advocated for the inclusion of temporal information to discourse assessment to increase sensitivity. Expanding derived efficiency measures, such as MC/min [67], to MSSG analyses or similar, would require very little additional effort (e.g., timing the narrative, simple calculation) and may provide additional valuable information that can be targeted to improve overall communication.

Finally, though not featured in this chapter, coherence measures can be used to provide additional information about one's effective presence and usage of macrostructures [1]. Of particular interest is how PWAs are able to convey the main ideas of a narrative in a coherent fashion, so that consecutive utterances are related to each other (local coherence) and to the overarching topic (global coherence) [1, 3, 68, 69]. There are well-known 5-point rating scales for local and global coherence [3, 69, 70] with well-defined rating descriptions, as well as the 4-point global coherence rating scale [71, 72]. More recently, Linnik and colleagues [73] introduced a coherence rating system that involves four aspects—informativeness, clarity, understandability, and connectedness.

As emphasized throughout, readers should not rely solely on this chapter as the training resource or manual to implement a featured measure, rather readers should use this chapter as a navigation resource to locate the resources needed to conduct their selected analyses with the greatest fidelity and precision. Even though our focus was on the strongest and most well-described measures involving monologic story retelling, if readers dive into even a subset of the resources referenced, they will discover a rich literature full of additional and acceptable approaches.

Major Takeaways

1. Proposition-level measures of correctness or completeness relate to both microstructure and macrostructure since incorrect and/or incomplete relevant (or essential, compared to a standard) concepts generally reduce overall narrative coherence and expression of topic "gist."
2. Story grammar analyses examine how well a narrator meets organizational expectations related to the logical and/or linear sequencing of events, characters, and relationships between events and characters to facilitate listeners' ability to follow a story.
3. Thorough macrostructural analysis should extend beyond counting essential story grammar components and consider the sequencing of those components.
4. The brief Narrative Assessment Profile (NAP) is intended to characterize main concepts, story grammar, core lexical usage, and sequencing.
5. Main Concept, Sequencing, and Story Grammar, or MSSG, analysis is a standardized, norm-referenced multilevel analytic approach that incorporates the coding of main concepts (MCs), sequencing, and story grammar components.

Acknowledgments As always, we are grateful for persons with aphasia who share their time and their stories with us so we can learn more about discourse and life participation. We thank the creators of AphasiaBank for developing the rich repository and for the many labs that so generously contribute to the database.

References

1. Van Dijk TA. Macrostructures: an interdisciplinary study of global structures in discourse, interaction, and cognition. Hillsdale: Erlbaum; 1980.
2. Peterson C, McCabe A. Developmental psycholinguistics: three ways of looking at a child's narrative. Springer Science and Business Media; 2013.
3. Glosser G, Deser T. Patterns of discourse production among neurological patients with fluent language disorders. Brain Lang. 1991;40(1):67–88.
4. Olness G. Narrative structure in aphasia: impact of task and aphasia severity. 2016.
5. Frederiksen CH, Bracewell RJ, Breuleux A, Renaud A. The cognitive representation and processing of discourse: function and dysfunction. In: Joannette Y, editor. Discourse ability and brain damage. New York: Springer; 1990. p. 69–110.
6. Kintsch W, Van Dijk TA. Toward a model of text comprehension and production. Psychol Rev. 1978;85(5):363.
7. Van Dijk T. Discourse, context and cognition. Discourse Stud. 2006;8(1):159–77.
8. Van Dijk TA. Discourse and knowledge: a sociocognitive approach. Cambridge University Press; 2014.
9. Brandão L, Castelló FG, Van Dijk TA, Parente MA, Peña-Casanova J. Cognition and discourse production in Alzheimer's disease: using informative prompts. Psychol Neurosci. 2009;2:147–55.
10. Nicholas LE, Brookshire RH. A system for scoring main concepts in the discourse of non-brain-damaged and aphasic speakers. Clin Aphasiol Conf. 1993;21:87–99.
11. Nicholas LE, Brookshire RH. Presence, completeness, and accuracy of main concepts in the connected speech of non-brain-damaged adults and adults with aphasia. J Speech Lang Hear Res. 1995;38(1):145–56.
12. Kong AP, Whiteside J, Bargmann P. The main concept analysis: validation and sensitivity in differentiating discourse produced by unimpaired English speakers from individuals with aphasia and dementia of Alzheimer type. Logoped Phoniatr Vocol. 2016;41(3):129–41.
13. Richardson JD, Dalton SG. Main concepts for three different discourse tasks in a large non-clinical sample. Aphasiology. 2016;30(1):45–73.
14. Dalton SG, Richardson JD. A large-scale comparison of main concept production between persons with aphasia and persons without brain injury. Am J Speech Lang Pathol. 2019;28(1S):293–320.
15. Dalton SG, Richardson JD, Cavanaugh R. Clinically feasible discourse analysis: current state and looking forward. In: Kong A, editor. Spoken discourse impairments in the neurogenic populations.
16. Dipper L, Marshall J, Boyle M, Botting N, Hersh D, Pritchard M, et al. Treatment for improving discourse in aphasia: a systematic review and synthesis of the evidence base. Aphasiology. 2021;35(9):1125–67.
17. Pritchard M, Hilari K, Cocks N, Dipper L. Psychometric properties of discourse measures in aphasia: acceptability, reliability, and validity. Int J Lang Commun Disord. 2018;53(6):1078–93.
18. Rumelhart DE. On evaluating story grammars. Cogn Sci. 1980;4:313–6.
19. Stein NL, Glenn CG. An analysis of story comprehension in elementary school children. In: Freedle RO, editor. New directions in discourse processing. New York: Ablex; 1979. p. 53–120.
20. Coelho CA. Story narratives of adults with closed head injury and non-brain-injured adults: influence of socioeconomic status, elicitation task, and executive functioning. J Speech Lang Hear Res. 2002;45:1232–48.
21. Mozeiko J, Le K, Coelho C, Krueger F, Grafman J. The relationship of story grammar and executive function following TBI. Aphasiology. 2011;25(6–7):826–35.
22. Cannizzaro MS, Coelho CA. Analysis of narrative discourse structure as an ecologically relevant measure of executive function in adults. J Psycholinguist Res. 2013;42(6):527–49.
23. Richardson JD, Hudspeth SG. Story grammar analysis in persons with mild aphasia. 2014.
24. Ulatowska HK, North AJ, Macaluso-Haynes S. Production of narrative and procedural discourse in aphasia. Brain Lang. 1981;13(2):345–71.
25. Ulatowska HK, Freedman-Stern R, Doyel AW, Macaluso-Haynes S, North AJ. Production of narrative discourse in aphasia. Brain Lang. 1983;19(2):317–34.
26. Hunt KW. Grammatical structures written at three grade levels. NCTE research report no. 3. 1965.
27. Labov W. The transformation of experience in narrative syntax. In: Language in the inner city; 1972. p. 354–396.
28. Coelho CA, Liles BZ, Duffy RJ, Clarkson JV, Elia D. Longitudinal assessment of narrative discourse in a mildly aphasic adult. Clin Aphasiol. 1994;22:145–55.
29. Winter P. The bear & the fly. New York: Crown Publishers; 1976.
30. Hunt KW. Syntactic maturity in schoolchildren and adults. Monogr Soc Res Child Dev. 1970;35(1):1–61.
31. Porch B. Porch index of communicative ability. 1967.
32. Coelho C, Youse K, Le K, Feinn R. Narrative and conversational discourse of adults with closed head injuries and non-brain-injured adults: a discriminant analysis. Aphasiology. 2003;17(5):499–510.
33. Kertesz A. Western aphasia battery test manual: Psychological Corporation; 1982.
34. Rockwell N. The runaway: cover illustration for the Saturday evening post. 1958.
35. Coelho Corpus on TBIBank [Internet]. https://tbi.talkbank.org/access/English/Coelho.html
36. Liles BZ. Cohesion in the narratives of normal and language-disordered children. J Speech Lang Hear Res. 1985;28(1):123–33.
37. Whitworth A. Using narrative as a bridge: linking language processing models with real-life communication. Semin Speech Lang. 2010;31(1):64–75.

38. Whitworth A, Leitao S, Cartwright J, Webster J, Hankey GJ, Zach J, et al. NARNIA: a new twist to an old tale. A pilot RCT to evaluate a multilevel approach to improving discourse in aphasia. Aphasiology. 2015;29(11):1345–82.
39. Whitworth A, Claessen M, Leitao S, Webster J. Beyond narrative: is there an implicit structure to the way in which adults organize their discourse? Clin Linguist Phon. 2015;29(6):455–81.
40. Loban W. Language development: kindergarten through grade twelve. NCTE Committee on Research Report No. 18. 1976.
41. Miller J, Iglesias A. Systematic analysis of language transcripts (SALT). Research version. 2008;16.
42. Ministry of Education, Western Australia. First steps series: teaching children how to write informational texts. Perth: Ministry of Education; 1992.
43. Manning M, Franklin S. Cognitive grammar and aphasic discourse. Clin Linguist Phon. 2016;30(6):417–32.
44. Webster JM. A semantic and syntactic analysis of aphasic speech (Doctoral dissertation, Newcastle University). 1999.
45. Bird H, Franklin S. Cinderella revisited: a comparison of fluent and non-fluent aphasic speech. J Neurolinguistics. 1996;9(3):187–206.
46. Saffran EM, Berndt RS, Schwartz MF. The quantitative analysis of agrammatic production: procedure and data. Brain Lang. 1989;37(3):440–79.
47. Langacker RW. Cognitive grammar: a basic introduction. New York: Oxford University Press; 2008.
48. Chafe W. Discourse, consciousness, and time: the flow and displacement of conscious experience in speaking and writing. Chicago: University of Chicago Press; 1994.
49. Langacker RW. Discourse in cognitive grammar. Cogn Linguistics. 2001;12:143–88.
50. Kong AP, Reres A, Kong AP, Reres A. Proposing a quick, objective, comprehensive analysis of impaired spoken discourse in post-stroke aphasia. Clin Arch Commun Disord. 2021;6(3):172–86.
51. Greenslade KJ, Stuart JE, Richardson JD, Dalton SG, Ramage AE. Macrostructural analyses of Cinderella narratives in a large nonclinical sample. Am J Speech Lang Pathol. 2020;29(4):1923–36.
52. Richardson JD, Dalton SG, Greenslade KJ, Jacks A, Haley KL, Adams J. Main concept, sequencing, and story grammar analyses of Cinderella narratives in a large sample of persons with aphasia. Brain Sci. 2021;11(1):110.
53. Lewis Z. Walt Disney's Cinderella. Random House Disney; 1995.
54. MacWhinney B. Tools for analyzing talk part 1: the chat transcription format. Carnegie [Google Scholar]. 2017.
55. Dalton SG, Richardson JD. Core-lexicon and main-concept production during picture-sequence description in adults without brain damage and adults with aphasia. Am J Speech Lang Pathol. 2015;24(4):S923–38.
56. Le K, Coelho C, Mozeiko J, Krueger F, Grafman J. Measuring goodness of story narratives: implications for traumatic brain injury. Aphasiology. 2011;25(6–7):748–60.
57. Coelho C, Lê K, Mozeiko J, Tyler E, Krueger F, Grafman J. Characterizing discourse deficits following penetrating head injury. A preliminary model. Am J Speech Lang Pathol. 2013;22:S438–48.
58. Bottenberg D, Lemme M, Hedberg N. Analysis of oral narratives of normal and aphasic adults. Clin Aphasiol. 1985;15:241–7.
59. Lemme ML, Hedberg NL, Bottenberg DE. Cohesion in narratives of aphasic adults. Clinical aphasiology: proceedings of the conference 1984. BRK Publishers; 1984. p. 215–222.
60. Applebee AN. The child's concept of story: ages two to seventeen. Chicago: University of Chicago Press; 1978.
61. Rockwell N. Looking out to sea. 1927.
62. Hedberg NL, Stoel-Gammon C. Narrative analysis: clinical procedures. Top Lang Disord. 1986;7(1):58–69.
63. Bottenberg D, Lemme M, Hedberg N. Effect of story content on narrative discourse of aphasic adults. Clin Aphasiol. 1987;17:202–9.
64. Goodglass H, Kaplan E. The assessment of aphasia and related disorders. 1972.
65. Hameister I, Nickels L. The cat in the tree–using picture descriptions to inform our understanding of conceptualisation in aphasia. Lang Cogn Neurosci. 2018;33(10):1296–314.
66. DeDe G, Salis C. Temporal and episodic analyses of the story of Cinderella in latent aphasia. Am J Speech Lang Pathol. 2020;29(1S):449–62.
67. Dalton SG, Hubbard HI, Richardson JD. Moving toward non-transcription based discourse analysis in stable and progressive aphasia. Semin Speech Lang. 2020;41(1):32–44.
68. Richards JC, Schmidt RW. Longman dictionary of language teaching and applied linguistics. Routledge; 2013.
69. Van Leer E, Turkstra L. The effect of elicitation task on discourse coherence and cohesion in adolescents with brain injury. J Commun Disord. 1999;32(5):327–49.
70. Coelho C, Flewellyn L. Longitudinal assessment of coherence in an adult with fluent aphasia: a follow-up study. Aphasiology. 2003;17(2):173–82.
71. Wright HH, Koutsoftas A, Fergadiotis G, Capilouto G. Coherence in stories told by adults with aphasia. Procedia Soc Behav Sci. 2010;6:111–2.
72. Fergadiotis G, Wright HH. Global discourse coherence in normal and aphasic discourse. Trends Exp Psycholinguistics. 2011.
73. Linnik A, Bastiaanse R, Stede M, Khudyakova M. Linguistic mechanisms of coherence in aphasic and non-aphasic discourse. Aphasiology. 2022;36(2):123–46.

Additional Resources

Articles

Dalton SG, Hubbard HI, Richardson JD. Moving toward non-transcription based discourse analysis in stable and progressive aphasia. Semin Speech Lang. 2020;41(1):32–44. Thieme Medical Publishers.

Linnik A, Bastiaanse R, Höhle B. Discourse production in aphasia: a current review of theoretical and methodological challenges. Aphasiology. 2016;30(7):765–800.

Books/Book Chapters

Coelho C, Cherney LR, Shadden BB, editors. Discourse analysis in adults with and without communication disorders: a resource for clinicians and researchers. Plural Publishing; 2022.

Online Resources

Main concept training materials. https://drive.google.com/drive/folders/1bxazjgQWx-WD8ELTJjwBm_5IToRpgQhQ?usp=share_link

Main concept, sequencing, and story grammar analyses (MSSG) training materials. https://drive.google.com/drive/folders/1U4yq_MbXL34ZBoxSDS3VjOt1xi4_kazs?usp=share_link

Main Concept Github app—Cavanaugh R, Richardson J, Dalton SG. mainConcept: an open-source web-app for scoring main concept analysis. R package version 0.0.1.0000. 2021. https://github.com/aphasia-apps/mainConcept

AphasiaBank. https://aphasia.talkbank.org/

FOQUSAphasia. https://www.foqusaphasia.com/

Jessica D. Richardson is an Associate Professor at The University of New Mexico in the Department of Speech and Hearing Sciences and the Center for Brain Recovery and Repair. She directs the Brain Scouts Lab where her research focuses on improving the lives of persons living with aphasia, due to stable or progressive causes, and of their care partners.

Sarah Grace Dalton is an Assistant Professor at Marquette University in the Department of Speech Pathology and Audiology. She directs the Building Rehabilitation Advances in Neuroscience (BRAiN Lab) where her research focuses on improving the lives of persons living with aphasia by improving assessment and treatment methods.

Kathryn J. Greenslade is an Assistant Professor in the Department of Communication Sciences and Disorders and Director of the Social Communication Intervention and Assessment Lab (SoCIALab) at The University of New Hampshire. Her research focuses on ways to assess and support social communication across neurodiverse populations.

Assessing Discourse Ability in Adults with Traumatic Brain Injury

14

Jennifer Mozeiko, Louisa Suting, and André Lindsey

Preview of What Is Currently Known

In 2005, the Academy of Neurologic Communication Disorders and Sciences [1] issued a report highlighting the need for functional, reliable, and feasible assessment tools specific to traumatic brain injury (TBI). Evidence points to an increasing adoption of discourse analysis [2] among speech-language pathologists (SLPs). There has been extensive research on non-standardized assessment since that time but, as of 2014, only 10% of SLPs working with people with acquired cognitive communicative deficits following TBI reported the use of discourse analysis or other functional performance [3]. The utility of discourse analysis in this population was becoming increasingly compelling [4] but the translation of research knowledge to clinical practice remained elusive. This was likely due to time constraints of SLPs and a lack of consensus on technique. A standardized, norm referenced measure of narrative discourse production and comprehension was available to assess children between the ages of 5 and 12 years of age (Test of Narrative Language) [5], but nothing similar had been available for adults.

Objectives

(a) To present and discuss the utility of discourse analysis as an assessment measure.
(b) To describe advantages and disadvantages of discourse assessment compared to other methods.
(c) To enumerate several approaches to the assessment of discourse.
(d) To explain whether recent technological advancements are enough to overcome barriers to use.

Introduction

Following brain injury, psychosocial deficits may be subtle and yet damaging to the maintenance of relationships critical to having a good quality of life. Evidence that conversational discourse ability has been significantly correlated with psychosocial skills makes clear that discourse skills must be addressed directly in rehabilitation [6]. However, methodological challenges in both the assessment and rehabilitation of discourse continue to be pervasive.

In this chapter, the advantages and disadvantages of discourse analysis will be discussed, followed by how technological advances have

J. Mozeiko (✉) · L. Suting
Department of Speech, Language and Hearing Sciences, University of Connecticut, Storrs, CT, USA
e-mail: jennifer.mozeiko@uconn.edu; louisa.suting@uconn.edu

A. Lindsey
School of Education, Nevada State University, Henderson, NV, USA
e-mail: andre.lindsey@nevadastate.edu

A. P.-H. Kong (ed.), *Spoken Discourse Impairments in the Neurogenic Populations*,
https://doi.org/10.1007/978-3-031-45190-4_14

influenced its adoption. The standardized and non-standardized assessments of social and cognitive skills that have been published since the year 2000 will also be described and summarized. The five standardized tests target an adult population with an acquired brain injury and include an assessment of discourse production, comprehension, or both. Non-standardized assessment consists of descriptive reports from SLPs, rating scales (also outlined here), and discourse analyses.

The Advantages of Discourse Analysis

Discourse analysis is an underutilized tool that can be a valuable addition to any clinician's toolbox, particularly benefiting those treating individuals with neurological disorders such as TBI. One of the key benefits of discourse analysis is that it directly reflects how people typically engage with one another. Individuals across all cultures converse and story-tell. Discourse analysis utilizes this cross-cultural method of social engagement to elicit and identify potential deficits. Furthermore, discourse analysis provides clinicians with a glimpse of other deficits that may be present in different areas of cognition, while also capturing the interaction between communication and cognitive processing. Language assessments such as aphasia batteries most thoroughly examine word- and sentence-level comprehension and production addressing the prominent levels of impairment of that disorder. Word- and sentence-level deficits are not the prominent area of concern following TBI, however. Deficits at the discourse level are more common [1, 7]. Discourse analysis is a tool that is sensitive to changes precipitated by TBI and can be utilized to capture structural, pragmatic, and psychosocial changes resulting from injury, enabling clinicians to characterize and address areas of concern [1, 7].

An additional benefit of discourse analysis is that it is cost-effective unlike many standardized tests. Monitoring narrative organization, structure, and content production does not require a comparative normed sample though this would be ideal. Clinicians can elicit a language sample, record it, and manually score it for all of the aforementioned variables of interest. This means that discourse analysis can be feasibly done without purchasing expensive tests or software making it an option for most clinicians. Furthermore, training for discourse analysis can be completed relatively quickly and can be designed so that it is integrated into graduate coursework.

For clinicians who prefer standardized assessments, there has been an increase in the number of tests that use discourse to evaluate communicative competence and/or cognitive-linguistic functioning (see section "Standardized Assessment Tools"). These assessments provide an efficient means of assessing functional communication performance. Collectively, both informal and formal measures of discourse analysis can be utilized to gauge an individual's performance throughout their time in rehabilitative care.

One major advantage of discourse assessments is that they engage multiple cognitive faculties [8–10]. Many clinicians may not initially assess memory and executive functions during their evaluation, particularly if their assessments are part of a routine protocol. Decreased critical content production and/or poor organization revealed during discourse analysis lends support for further cognitive assessment. The more complex nature of discourse, relative to naming and word retrieval tasks, results in a more in-depth grasp of cognitive-communicative performance.

Challenges of Discourse Analysis

Time is one of the most significant barriers to widespread use of discourse analysis as an assessment tool. Historically, in-depth language transcriptions have been a laborious process. Clinicians had to elicit a sample, record it, manually transcribe it, and then score it. Clinicians working in adult neurogenic care settings performing language analyses are likely more accustomed to more succinct visual description tasks such as the *Cookie Theft* from the Boston

Diagnostic Aphasia Battery [11] and the *Picnic Scene* from the Western Aphasia Battery [12]. These images are utilized to elicit utterances enabling a relatively quick assessment of semantic and syntactic production. Unfortunately, as previously noted, these are not areas commonly impaired following TBI. Discourse analysis better captures the interplay between language and other domains of cognition, but it is more complex and more time consuming. Presenting a visual story and having the client/patient retell it is more time consuming than a picture description task, but it enables a more thorough assessment of cognitive-communicative function. Notably, many of the newer discourse assessments capture pragmatic function without assessing linguistic structure. Therefore, clinicians noticing deficits in narrative organization and/or content production will need to perform a more time intensive structural discourse analysis to better gauge performance.

In addition to barriers posed by eliciting utterances and transcribing them, scoring also poses a challenge for most clinicians who are likely unfamiliar with the methods currently in use. Micro- and macrolinguistic analyses typically entail some level of training. There is a need for online assessment to increase efficiency and reduce the learning curve currently required to identify impaired communicative function based on discourse performance. Researchers have been developing assessments intended to be more rapidly scored (e.g., [13, 14] easing the burden faced by clinicians. Additionally, freely available language analysis tools such as Coh-Metrix may enable clinicians to rapidly identify micro-and macro-linguistics deficits [15]. Further research is still needed to validate assessments and get them to a point of routine clinical use.

Another potential issue in the interpretation of discourse analysis is that identification of deficits is not necessarily indicative of how clinicians should begin treatment. Memory, attention, and several differing executive functions play a role in discourse processes [9, 16–18]. Currently, there is only a small body of research examining discourse interventions for individuals who have sustained a TBI. Steel and colleagues [19] performed a recent literature review and found only six intervention studies aimed at treating narrative discourse. Metacognitive instruction was a component of each of these interventions with most studies primarily targeting intervention towards understanding narrative structure and production. Discourse analysis can be used to successfully identify deficits, but there needs to be further understanding for how various executive functions differentially influence treatment targets and accommodations. A systematic review by Lê and colleagues [20] revealed that current treatment approaches for discourse are most beneficial for individuals with mild-to-moderate TBI. They suggest that assessment may identify impairments, but further work is needed to support remediation.

During assessment, clinicians must be cognizant of potential cultural and gender differences that can influence how stories are told. For example, individuals of Asian descent including Asian Americans frequently provide less detail when recalling autobiographical information relative to individuals of European descent including European Americans [21]. Similar differences have also been noted in Western and Asian literature [22]. Additionally, there are gender differences in the stories of individuals of European and Asian descent and in stories of individuals of African American descent with women providing longer narratives with more details [21, 23]. Clinically, this suggests that assessing accuracy of content production using conversation or narratives regarding autobiographical events may be complicated if asking a spouse to validate a response given that female spouses may provide more details than male counterparts. These issues may be circumvented by providing specific instructions guiding an individual to retell a narrative in complete detail, but research is needed to ensure this solution. More research is needed to ensure that sex, gender, and cultural differences do not invalidate results or lead to incorrect interpretations of performance.

A critical barrier to routine use of discourse analysis is lack of education and awareness. Researchers note that many SLPs lack confidence with respect to intervention practices regarding cognitive-communication disorders (CCDs) [24]. Knowledge of the CCDs is critical to rehabilitative care, setting the foundation for any assessment or treatment performed. Clinicians are more likely to utilize discourse assessments if they have in-depth understanding of what they are investigating and the potential ramifications of letting the disorder go untreated.

There is still work to be done before discourse analysis is used consistently as a component of TBI assessment. Increased knowledge of CCDs and the development and distribution of low-cost time-efficient assessments sensitive to changes in discourse processing are initial hurdles impeding implementation. Discourse analysis can be a component of TBI assessment protocols. Additional education and research are needed to help establish its place in the clinic.

Use of Technology in Discourse Assessment

Advances in technology have the potential to reduce the amount of time devoted to transcribing discourse samples and leading to increased use of discourse analysis in clinical practice [25]. The first step in discourse analysis is data collection and transcription. As previously noted, these processes are each time consuming and may deter a clinician from use despite its high sensitivity and potential importance in both assessment, prognosis, and treatment of cognitive communication disorders post-traumatic brain injury. Technology has the potential to ease this burden. Recent literature has shown how the process of recording, transcribing, and analyzing discourse has been made simpler and more streamlined; however, no one protocol has yet emerged as standard practice.

Recording Discourse

Many technological devices (phones, tablets, computers) are suitable for recording an audio or video discourse sample with no need for additional microphones or expensive recording equipment. Even relatively short files, however, tend to take up a large digital space and so secure storage will need to be carefully planned as will the length of time the files are kept prior to deletion. Concerns about adhering to patient privacy laws may be enough to deter clinicians from recording in the first place as was suggested in a recent survey of SLPs from Australia, the USA, the UK, and New Zealand [2].

Most descriptions of recording samples are those done in a research or clinical environment [26], but some recent collections have been from the home environment in an attempt to improve ecological validity [27, 28]. The home recordings were completed with individuals with aphasia, and it remains to be seen if those with TBI would manage the recording device as successfully. When recording the language of someone with a language disorder, the individual may feel they are in a test-taking mode and are more attentive to their language production than usual, resulting in a better-than-normal sample. This same feeling could also elicit a stress reaction in some which would negatively impact discourse production. Therefore, recordings should include a period of habituation to the device where there is opening and closing material not included in the final analysis [6]. For example, Coelho and Youse recorded 15-min conversations of individuals who had sustained a TBI and compared them to conversations with employees in the same setting [29]. To account for an initial period of self-consciousness about being recorded, the researchers only analyzed the middle 6 min hypothesizing that it was likely the most natural part of the conversation. There is evidence that these shorter recordings do not result in the above-described hyper awareness that negatively impacts conversational behavior, but this is difficult to assess [30].

Transcription of Discourse

Transcription may be the most time-intensive aspect of the process, with reports that it can take up to 3 h to *transcribe and analyze* just 15 min of discourse [7]. The transcription process alone will vary greatly depending on the severity of the individual's deficits and the rate of speech among other variables. Unintelligible words and phrases may be listened to repeatedly until understood and faster production rates may mean more stops and starts in the transcription process. Automated speech recognition (ASR) has the potential to aid this process if speech is unaffected but dysarthria reduces their accuracy [31]. These programs have improved rapidly and are now standard on smartphones. Research examining child language sample transcriptions revealed that Google Cloud Speech (a voice recognition software) was significantly more accurate at real-time transcriptions relative to SLPs and trained transcribers [7]. Recent work looking at ASR for individuals with aphasia suggests that despite being less accurate than human transcription, it could have an important role in making discourse analysis more clinically feasible [7]. Concerns regarding accuracy, cost, and privacy need to be addressed by developers and medical facilities before the software can be utilized more routinely.

Analysis of Discourse

Latent Semantic Analysis (LSA) software such as the commercially available package Systematic Analysis of Language Transcripts (SALT; [32]) and the Child Language Data Exchange System (CHILDES; [31]) software program CLAN [33] are flexible programs that can facilitate the analysis process, but research does not reflect widespread adoption.

Technology in use with other clinical population may offer potential benefits. For example, Automated Language Environment Analysis (LENA; [34]) is a technology that has been used to study the word gap in children of lower socioeconomic status. LENA consists of a small recording device that can be worn by the participant of interest, and it will record for as long as 18 h. This ensures collection of a highly naturalistic discourse sample. LENA includes automated processing of the data yielding word counts, the number of turns between the device wearer and the communication partner, the amount of silence in the recording, as well as the amount of electronic time. This technology has recently been utilized with individuals with aphasia [28], but data are preliminary and accuracy has not yet been confirmed.

Approaches to Discourse Analysis

There are several approaches to discourse production and comprehension analysis. These are included within standardized tests of social and cognitive functioning and may also be done using rating scales, in which the perception of the person with the TBI or a conversational partner makes judgments about various discourse forms. Discourse can also be sampled without scales or standardized tests, but this requires understanding the different types of discourse that might be elicited (i.e., narrative, procedural, conversational) and various ways to analyze and interpret each. These are outlined in detail in a recent review by Steel and Togher [2], and readers are directed to this comprehensive resource for review. The section below includes selected samples to provide the reader with a high-level overview.

Standardized Assessment Tools

In recent years, there has been some development in the standardized assessments that measure social and cognitive functions that are frequently impacted by TBI or other acquired neurological conditions. A brief overview is provided of these standardized assessment tools in Table 14.1 and described below.

The **Assessment Battery of Communication** (ABaCo) [35], originating from Cognitive Pragmatic Theory [39, 40], provides a comprehensive assessment of the pragmatic abilities of people with TBI or other acquired neurological conditions. The ABaCo utilizes videotaped scenes and the examiner's prompts to assess the five scales outlined in Table 14.1. Each scale is divided into comprehension and production

Table 14.1 Standardized assessments of TBI

Tests	Tasks	Potential clinical use	Discourse measures
Assessment Battery of Communication (ABaCo) [35]	It consists of five evaluation scales to measure a wide range of communication skills: • Linguistic • Extralinguistic • Paralinguistic • Context • Conversational	• Guide individualizing rehabilitation planning • Use as outcome measure • Measure recovery	*Conversational scale*: • The examiner has four short conversations with the participants, each lasting between 5–6 min and focused on a simple topic (such as hobbies or favorite television shows) • The clinician uses the scales to rate various aspects of the conversation
Functional Assessment of Verbal Reasoning and Executive Strategies (FAVRES) [36]	Made up of four tasks based on common daily activities: • Planning an event • Scheduling a workday • Deciding on a gift • Building a case to solve a common problem	• Guide rehabilitation programs • Evaluate skills for return to work	*Discourse task:* • Each task requires the participants to produce written rationale explaining why they chose a specific answer • Discourse is evaluated through post-hoc discussion evaluating the written discourse (Task 4: Building a Case) • This takes approximately 15 min to complete
Montreal Evaluation of Communication (MEC) [37]	It consists of nine tasks that assess four communicative processes: • Discourse • Pragmatic • Lexical-semantic • Prosodic	• Estimate prognosis • Use as outcome measure of intervention programs • Guide individualizing rehabilitation planning	*Conversational discourse sub-test:* • It involves having a 10-min spontaneous conversation with the examiner on two different topics • A checklist is rated following this discussion
Assessment of Pragmatic Abilities and Cognitive Substrates (APAC) [38]	It consists of three major parts: • Non-literal information processing in real news stories rated with comprehension questions • Autobiographical narratives production • Picture descriptions rated with discourse checklists	• Evaluate an individual's pragmatic abilities and deficits following brain injury • Guide individualizing rehabilitation planning	*Narrative task:* • The aim is to assess the participant's ability to comprehend the main aspects of a narrative text and discourse • This task consists of six stories and two non-literal expressions • These stories are read to the participants at a normal rate, and several question items are administered following each story • It takes about 10 min to complete

tasks. The linguistic scale assesses the comprehension and production of communication acts such as questions, requests, commands, assertions, and identification and production of emotive content. The extralinguistic scale assesses the use and understanding of communication acts expressed through the gesture modality only; however, the paralinguistic scale assesses communication acts through gestures, facial expressions, and prosody. The context scale assesses the adequacy or inadequacy of communicative acts with respect to discourse norms and social norms. Finally, the conversation scale assesses social communicative functions like turn-taking and topic management. Administration of the full battery takes approximately 90 min. However, the battery is modular, and each scale may be administered separately during customized clinical sessions to facilitate clinical use.

The **Functional Assessment of Verbal Reasoning and Executive Strategies** (FAVRES; [36]) was designed to evaluate high-level cognitive-communication skills (complex communication, verbal reasoning, and executive functions). The FAVRES is specifically intended for individuals with an acquired brain injury. It includes four functional tasks that simulate activity-based encounters in daily life. These tasks require decision-making, reasoning, and filtering out unimportant information. In addition, they present a novel problem in a meaningful context, such as work, school, family, or social settings. The FAVRES tasks are measured in terms of the individual's efficiency, accuracy, and quality of the rationale provided. Higher scores on FAVRES tasks have been associated with positive outcomes such as being able to return to work and ongoing employment in persons with mild to severe TBI [41–43]. The FAVRES appears to be a promising assessment tool for predicting employment success following traumatic brain injury [42].

The **Montreal Evaluation of Communication** (MEC or D-MEC) [37] is a standardized test that examines social communication deficits with pragmatic components of language such as discourse, lexico-semantic processes, metaphor and pragmatic inference, and prosody in individuals with non-aphasic communication disorders. It is designed to be administered in an acute care setting. Performance is evaluated based on 17 different communication behaviors and two conversation topics that necessitate a topic shift. The MEC checklist includes measures that assess the capacity for self-correction, imprecise expression of ideas, and inappropriate remarks. Studies have shown that better conversational discourse performance, as measured by D-MEC, has been associated with better global outcomes and lower disability ratings. Therefore, conversational discourse impairment could be identified early in acute care with the D-MEC, allowing for early identification and intervention [44]. This tool may also aid in measuring pragmatic recovery, as few TBI assessment tools are used during the acute recovery stages. However, administering this instrument takes a significant amount of time. It typically lasts an hour and a half and requires two 45-minute sessions, which may fatigue patients with moderate-severe injuries. To overcome this drawback, the Montreal Communication Evaluation Brief Battery- MEC B was created. The MEC B contains an entirely new set of tasks for each category and includes tasks measuring reading and writing. It takes 25–40 min to administer and has shown satisfactory reliability and validity. Clinicians can use it to plan rehabilitation programs and as an outcome measure for intervention programs [45].

The most recently developed norm-referenced tool is called the **Assessment of Pragmatic Abilities and Cognitive Substrates** (APACS) [38] was designed to evaluate pragmatic abilities in people who have acquired communicative deficits. Discourse and non-literal language are the two main areas of focus for APACS. Tasks require description, interview, narrative, humor, and figurative language, and it results in three composite scores: a total APACS score and pragmatic comprehension and pragmatic production scores. Administration of the full battery takes approximately 35–40 min. Tasks involve semi-structured interviews of autobiographical topics and photographic picture descriptions rated with discourse checklists, comprehension of non-literal information in real news articles, multiple choice sentence matching tasks, story completion tasks, and verbal explanation tasks.

Rating Scales

Clinicians may opt to utilize various rating scales to quantify social communication deficits in individuals with TBI in conjunction with or as an alternative to standardized testing. Typically, these tools are brief and user-friendly. The clinical feasibility and practicality of using some of these rating scales are discussed in detail in the following section.

The **La Trobe Communication Questionnaire** (LCQ) [46] is a pragmatic scale designed to measure perceived communicative ability. The self-rating scales that quantify the perception of change in communication post-TBI are completed by both the individual with TBI and a communication partner. Many recent studies have used the LCQ to quantify the perspectives of people most familiar with post-injury changes of individuals with TBI [47–49]. However, for the LCQ to be effective, the person with TBI and their familiar communication partner must be able to identify and recognize communication impairments. It might not be as helpful at the beginning of recovery, especially in a hospital setting [48], since changes in communication may become more apparent as the individual with TBI resumes social and work-related activities [50, 51].

The **Pragmatic Profile of Impairment in Communication** (PPIC) [52] is a pragmatic communication behavioral rating scale used to measure functional or social communication after TBI. It has good inter-rater reliability, high internal consistency, and good concurrent validity [48]. PPIC is a clinician-rated assessment with two scoring systems: individual behaviors and a feature summary scale. Studies have used this scale as a primary outcome measure in the remediation of social communication impairments [47, 53] and as a measure of recovery from video-recorded conversation samples [48, 54]. The PPIC administration necessitates the use of videotaped interactions, making it less suitable for use in hospitals. However, the inclusion of severity ratings and frequency ratings of behaviors make this a helpful instrument for measuring changes [2].

The **Adapted Kagan Scale** [55] is made up of the Adapted Measure of Participation in Conversation (MPC) scale and the Adapted Measure of Support in Conversation (MSC) scale. The MPC is used to assess the level of participation of the individual with TBI in a conversation, whereas the MSC quantifies the ability of the communication partner to acknowledge their partner's competence. This is one of the few scales that measure the collaborative aspects of the conversation by assessing the participation of both the individual with TBI and their communication partner. Several recent studies have used this scale as an informative outcome measure for the communication partner training intervention after TBI and in group-based communication skills treatment [42, 49, 50, 56, 57]. Clinicians can use this scale to identify and prioritize areas that the communication partner should focus on to facilitate joint conversations. For example, instead of concentrating on the underlying cause of the impairment in social communication, this tool makes it possible to examine the conversation as a mutual activity. The Adapted Kagan Scales have been used to explore the effects of joint video self-modeling to improve self-regulation, provide individuals with TBI and communication partners with more insight into maladaptive behaviors, and improve communication interactions [49].

The **Pragmatic Rating Scale** (PRS) [51, 58] consists of 16 items divided into three subscales: "nonverbal communication" encompassing extralingual aspects (e.g., eye contact, body language, gesture), "propositional communication" refers to parts of information conveyed by the speaker (e.g., verbosity, initiation, clarity, cohesion), and "interactional communication" refers to the reciprocal give-and-take conversation between individuals (e.g., repair, feedback, responsiveness). It is recommended that ratings be applied to a dyadic conversation approximately 10 min in length. PRS has high clinical feasibility, and clinicians can quickly learn it and score it while observing or collecting conversational samples [58].

Global Impression Scales (GIS) [59] rate the overall impression of the conversation, taking into account the skills of the person with acquired brain injury and their communication partner. It has four scales which are scored on a non-point Likert scale: appropriateness (e.g., relevance, suitability, and aptness of the conversation), effortfulness (e.g., degree of difficulty and amount of work required to initiate and maintain the conversation), interestingness (e.g., the degree to which the individual can engage, hold the attention of, and stimulate a spontaneous response) and rewardingness (the degree of gratification or enjoyment to be derived from the interaction. This scale has been demonstrated as a sensitive outcome measure in clinical trials [57]. GIS can be used in goal setting, monitoring progress, and evaluating outcomes for social communication interventions.

In addition to traditional standardized tests and rating scales, recent years have seen the development of easy-to-use screening tools that can help caregivers and non-specialists characterize cognitive and communication difficulties in individuals with acquired brain injury. **Cognitive-Communication Checklist for Acquired Brain Injury (CCCABI)** [60] is one such tool that consists of a one-page checklist of 45 potential areas of cognitive and communication difficulties, including daily communications (such as those with family, community, and workplace) and specific functional difficulties (such as discourse, reading comprehension, and written expression). This tool has been found useful not only by caregivers but also by SLPs who can use it to track communication difficulties over a period of recovery. This tool is available for free online at http://www.ccdpublishing.com/cccabi.aspx.

Discourse Tasks and Measures

Historically, researchers studying discourse and TBI have not used formal standardized measures of assessment. They have instead studied monologic discourse (e.g., descriptive, narrative, procedural) and conversational discourse. Several tasks are used to elicit monologic discourse. For example, participants may be asked to detail a procedure (e.g., how to make a sandwich), describe a picture, discuss a personal event, generate a story (given a single image or sequence of pictures), or expository task (producing a verbal or written argument). Analysis of monologic tasks can provide information on the amount and complexity of verbal output and examine the organizational and conceptual aspects of spoken discourse [1, 2, 61]. It includes the analysis of microlinguistic/within-sentence measures (e.g., words, T-units, or C-units per narrative), microstructural/across-sentence measures (e.g., cohesion and cohesive adequacy), macrostructural measures (global and local coherence), and superstructural measures (e.g., story grammar and story completeness) [7].

Of note discourse analysis is not confined to these measures. For example, Jones and Turkstra took a non-traditional approach to studying monologic discourse [61]. In their study, they examined storytelling performance in people with TBI with a focus on the manner of narrative performance. They used the Charismatic Leadership Communication Scale (CLCS) to rate 1-min video samples of narrative discourse. The listeners rated the samples based on their interest in engaging in a conversation with the speaker. The authors reported that a person's charisma is influenced by non-verbal behaviors like gesture and speech rate, as it was this that appeared to determine how interested listeners were in conversing with that person. This strategy provides a more global view of discourse among adults with TBI [2].

At the conversational level, interactive aspects of communication can be evaluated, such as the patient's awareness of the communication partner (pragmatic aspects of communication). This can provide quantifiable measures of family perception of improvements over time. The conversational discourse elicitation task typically involves the SLP or someone previously unknown to the person with TBI engaging in conversation with the individual with TBI [2]. Prompts used to engage in conversation include various contexts such as informal conversation (e.g., about any mutual interests), purposeful conversation (e.g., joint discussion about planning an activity), or problem-solving tasks (e.g., discussion about the function of an unfamiliar topic). These conversations are then typically analyzed using rating scales outlined in the sections above [47, 62]. The differing elicitation prompts can help uncover various communication deficits within spoken discourse [62].

In addition to the prompts used to elicit discourse samples, there is a growing interest in the role a communication partner may play in the elicitation of discourse samples. In recent studies on conversational discourse exchanges, discourse samples are elicited between the person with a TBI and familiar communication partners (rather than unfamiliar partners) [2, 63–65]. This change in format was done to address the issue of power balance and roles within traditional discourse elicitation contexts [2]. These tasks try to engage both the individual with TBI and the communication partner, equalizing the dynamics of interactions [2]. Effects of such elicitation methods were examined by Jogensen and Togher, who studied the discourse samples generated by the retelling of a video segment watched together by an individual with TBI and their familiar communication partner [64]. Kilov and colleagues examined discourse participation and performance in a shared problem-solving task involving a person with TBI and a friend together trying to determine the function of an unfamiliar object [63]. Both studies found that familiarity with communication partners affected the qualitative content of the discourse samples, which could help in understanding the difficulties faced by the participants in real-life interactions. These tasks may demonstrate the impact of the power and familiarity of communication partners on the discourse of people with TBI.

The contribution of communication partners with respect to discourse performance is a growing area of interest for researchers studying discourse performance. Studies have analyzed conversations with friends following TBI using Exchange Structure Analysis (ESA) [66] to describe the contributions of communication partners within a conversation [65, 67] and as an outcome measure for communication partner training [67]. ESA is a discourse analysis tool that encapsulates the dynamic nature of interaction while emphasizing the subtle influences of power and familiarity on an interaction, including the relationship between speakers, the discourse task, and the mode of communication. Specifically, it analyzes communication exchanges by classifying turns of speech or "moves" according to their function(s), such as statements (giving information), questions (demanding information), offers (giving service), and commands (demanding service). The results of such analysis can help a clinician use relevant contexts to guide therapy and educate a person with TBI and their communication partner to facilitate better communication by highlighting specific areas of improvement.

Topic analysis is one of the more notable areas of concern for persons with TBI who present with discourse deficits. It is used to examine the patterns and problems in topic management. Mentis and Prutting used topic analysis to examine the monologues and conversations of people with TBI [68]. During topic analysis, language samples (conversation and/or monologues) are video recorded, transcribed, and analyzed. Topic analysis includes topic introduction and maintenance. Topic introductions indicate the extent to which the speaker initiates topics for discussion and how the topics are introduced (such as novel topic initiation and topic shifts). Topic maintenance refers to a speaker's ability to express content related to a topic of a conversation or the test prompts and provide transitional cues to the listener as they change topic of the conversation. They are coded using the total number of turns per topic, the number of words per turn, and shifts in each conversation. Topic analysis has been applied to examine the nature and patterns of topics in conversational discourse and changes occurring in these topic choices over 3–6 months post-injury in individuals with TBI [69]. Brassel and colleagues identified three main conversational themes (impacts of injury, drive towards returning to life pre-injury, and connecting with people outside rehabilitation settings). The authors observed that the nature of topics related to these themes changed 6 months post-injury; and the participants engaged more frequently in conversations related to their family and friends [68].

In order to assess readiness to return to work following a TBI, researchers have been using a standardized elicitation procedure called the Functional Workplace Elicitation Protocol [43, 70] using the Voicemail Elicitation Task (VET). VET is a standardized computerized language elicitation procedure that utilizes voicemail message scenarios to elicit language samples in different conditions. Each scenario requires participants to provide a message that conveys new information and makes a request (e.g., requesting time off work to attend a family event). Scenarios are thematically related to workplace events, such as leaving a voicemail for a coworker, with the four voicemail recipient conditions based on status (superior, subordinate, or colleague) and different levels of familiarity (friends or new coworkers). Analysis of the use of politeness-marker production is central to the VET. Politeness-markers include modal verbs and adjuncts such as "would," "could," "just," "possibly," "probably," and so on. VET is sensitive to performance and able to discriminate between individuals with TBI who are stably employed and those whose employment is unstable. Individuals with TBI who have unstable employment histories produced fewer politeness-markers than their stably employed peers [43, 71]. The VET is also sensitive to change as a result of interventions. For example, participants who received computer-based workplace communication training, demonstrated an increase in trained and untrained politeness-marker use [72]. This platform holds promise as a functional clinical discourse assessment tool that can be used to identify persons at risk for social communication-related job instability after TBI. Further, it facilitates the tracking of progress during and following intervention.

Summary

Advantages of discourse analysis outweigh the challenges and should be included in every assessment of individuals with TBI. This is because it provides very specific and functional targets for rehabilitation and is easily used to measure progress over time. What an individual *says* is often how they are perceived. Values, morals, ideas, and intelligence are often conveyed verbally, and so even subtle discourse deficits can contribute to shrinking social networks and reduced quality of life. Clinicians are encouraged to make use of the tools that are readily available if they are not confident with non-standardized means. Standardized tests and checklists are easy ways to introduce discourse analysis into their repertoire. In the meantime, we urge the field to better train clinicians. It is the job of clinical supervisors, faculty instructors, and also of colleagues to ensure that new clinicians are prepared to become proficient with discourse analysis from the start.

Major Takeaways

1. Discourse can be a cost-effective method of examining the cognitive-communicative functioning of individuals who have sustained brain injuries. Increased training is needed so that more clinicians are proficient in utilizing this valuable clinical tool.
2. Technological advancements may require basic technology skills and privacy knowledge, perhaps adding to the uncertainty felt by those considering the implementation of discourse assessment for the first time. However, these advancements reduce the total time needed for this type of analysis and make adoption of these techniques clinically feasible.
3. Discourse analysis is now included in some standardized tests developed for TBI. Some of these are norm referenced. These subtests are described and are one solution to a clinician's lack of confidence in conducting discourse assessment.
4. Rating scales are an alternative to standardized testing of discourse, relying on the perception of the SLP, the family member, or the individual with TBI.
5. Discourse assessment can be conducted without any pre-packaged materials but in order to do so successfully, the administering clinician will require some advanced training.

References

1. Coelho C, Ylvisaker M, Turkstra LS. Nonstandardized assessment approaches for individuals with traumatic brain injuries. In: Semin Speech Lang [Internet]. 2005 [cited 2015 Feb 1]. p. 223–41.
2. Steel J, Togher L. Social communication assessment after traumatic brain injury: a narrative review of innovations in pragmatic and discourse assessment methods. Brain Inj. 2019;33(1):48–61.
3. Frith M, Togher L, Ferguson A, Levick W, Docking K. Assessment practices of speech-language pathologists for cognitive communication disorders following traumatic brain injury in adults: an international survey. Brain Inj. 2014;28(13–14):1657–66.
4. Myers JR, Solomon NP, Lange RT, French LM, Lippa SM, Brickell TA, et al. Analysis of discourse production to assess cognitive communication deficits following mild traumatic brain injury with and without posttraumatic stress. Am J Speech Lang Pathol. 2022;31(1):84–98.
5. Gillam RB, Pearson NA. Test of narrative language: examiner's manual. Pro-ed; 2004.
6. Snow PC, Douglas JM. Subject review: conceptual and methodological challenges in discourse assessment with TBI speakers: towards an understanding. Brain Inj. 2000;14(5):397–415.
7. Coelho CA. Management of discourse deficits following traumatic brain injury: progress, caveats, and needs. Semin Speech Lang. 2007;28(2):122–135. Copyright© 2007 by Thieme Medical Publishers, Inc., New York, NY, USA.
8. Marini A, Andreetta S, del Tin S, Carlomagno S. A multi-level approach to the analysis of narrative language in aphasia. Aphasiology. 2011;25(11):1372–92.
9. Lindsey A, Mozeiko J, Krueger F, Grafman J, Coelho C. Changes in discourse structure over time following traumatic brain injury. Neuropsychologia. 2018;119:308–19.
10. VanSolkema M, McCann C, Barker-Collo S, Foster A. Attention and communication following TBI: making the connection through a meta-narrative systematic review. Neuropsychol Rev. 2020;30(3):345–61.
11. Goodglass H, Kaplan E, Weintraub S. BDAE: the Boston diagnostic aphasia examination. 2001.
12. Kertesz A. Western aphasia battery-revised (WAB-R). Austin. 2006.
13. Le K, Coelho C, Mozeiko J, Krueger F, Grafman J. Measuring goodness of story narratives: implications for traumatic brain injury. Aphasiology. 2011;25(6–7):748–60.
14. Lindsey A, Hurley E, Mozeiko J, Coelho C. Follow-up on the story goodness index for characterizing discourse deficits following traumatic brain injury. Am J Speech Lang Pathol. 2019;28(1S):330–40.
15. Graesser AC, McNamara DS, Louwerse MM, Cai Z. Coh-Metrix: analysis of text on cohesion and language. Behav Res Methods Instrum Comput. 2004;36(2):193–202.
16. Marini A, Zettin M, Galetto V. Cognitive correlates of narrative impairment in moderate traumatic brain injury. Neuropsychologia. 2014;64:282–8.
17. Galetto V, Andreetta S, Zettin M, Marini A. Patterns of impairment of narrative language in mild traumatic brain injury. J Neurolinguistics. 2013;26(6):649–61.
18. Mozeiko J, Le K, Coelho C, Krueger F, Grafman J. The relationship of story grammar and executive function following TBI. Aphasiology. 2011;25(6–7):826–35.
19. Steel J, Elbourn E, Togher L. Narrative discourse intervention after traumatic brain injury: a systematic review of the literature. Top Lang Disord. 2021;41(1):47–72.
20. Lê K, Coelho C, Fiszdon J. Systematic review of discourse and social communication interventions in traumatic brain injury. Am J Speech Lang Pathol. 2022;31(2):991–1022.
21. Wang Q. Once upon a time: explaining cultural differences in episodic specificity: culture and episodic specificity. Soc Personal Psychol Compass. 2009;3(4):413–32.
22. Wang Q, Yang JCI. Culture and storytelling in literature. Narrat Inq [Internet]. 2022 25 [cited 2022 Sep 9]. http://www.jbe-platform.com/content/journals/10.1075/ni.21093.wan
23. Bradford WA. Gender differences in the narrative productions of African American adults. Am J Speech Lang Pathol. 2019;28(2):623–38.
24. Morrow EL, Turkstra LS, Duff MC. Confidence and training of speech-language pathologists in cognitive-communication disorders: time to rethink graduate education models? Am J Speech Lang Pathol. 2021;30(2S):986–92.
25. Fox CB, Israelsen-Augenstein M, Jones S, Gillam SL. An evaluation of expedited transcription methods for school-age children's narrative language: automatic speech recognition and real-time transcription. J Speech Lang Hear Res. 2021;64(9):3533–48.
26. King KA, Hough MS, Walker MM, Rastatter M, Holbert D. Mild traumatic brain injury: effects on naming in word retrieval and discourse. Brain Inj. 2006;20(7):725–32.
27. Arnett S, Mozeiko J. Evaluating the accuracy of self-ratings of language in adults with aphasia and non-brain injured adults: a pilot study. Semin Speech Lang. 2022;43:378.
28. Suting LB, Mozeiko J. Analysis of real-world language use in a person with Wernicke's aphasia. Perspect ASHA Spec Interest Groups. 2021;6(3):553–65.
29. Coelho CA, Youse KM, Le KN. Conversational discourse in closed-head-injured and non-brain-injured adults. Aphasiology. 2002;16(4–6):659–72.
30. Wiemann JM. Effects of laboratory videotaping procedures on selected conversation behaviors. Hum Commun Res. 1981;7(4):302–11.
31. MacWhinney B. The CHILDES system. Am J Speech Lang Pathol. 1996;5(1):5–14.
32. Mengistu KT, Rudzicz F. Comparing humans and automatic speech recognition systems in recognizing

dysarthric speech. In: Canadian conference on artificial intelligence. Springer; 2011. p. 291–300.
33. Jacks A, Haley KL, Bishop G, Harmon TG. Automated speech recognition in adult stroke survivors: comparing human and computer transcriptions. Folia Phoniatr Logop. 2019;71(5–6):286–96.
34. Greenwood CR, Schnitz AG, Irvin D, Tsai SF, Carta JJ. Automated language environment analysis: a research synthesis. Am J Speech Lang Pathol. 2018;27(2):853–67.
35. Angeleri R, Bosco FM, Zettin M, Sacco K, Colle L, Bara BG. Communicative impairment in traumatic brain injury: a complete pragmatic assessment. Brain Lang. 2008;107(3):229–45.
36. MacDonald S. Functional assessment of verbal reasoning and executive strategies (FAVRES). Guelp: Clinical Publishing; 2005.
37. Joanette Y, Ska B, Côté H. In: Édition O, editor. Protocole Montréal d'Évaluation de la Communication. Isbergues: France; 2004.
38. Arcara G, Bambini V. A test for the assessment of pragmatic abilities and cognitive substrates (APACS): normative data and psychometric properties. Front Psychol. 2016;7:70.
39. Bara BG. Cognitive pragmatics. Cambridge: MIT Press; 2010.
40. Airenti G. Conversation and behavior games in the pragmatics of dialogue. Cogn Sci. 1993;17(2):197–256.
41. Isaki E, Turkstra L. Communication abilities and work re-entry following traumatic brain injury. Brain Inj. 2000;14(5):441–53.
42. Rietdijk R, Simpson G, Togher L, Power E, Gillett L. An exploratory prospective study of the association between communication skills and employment outcomes after severe traumatic brain injury. Brain Inj. 2013;27(7–8):812–8.
43. Meulenbroek PA, Togher L, Turkstra, L. Functional workplace communication elicitation for persons with traumatic brain injury. In: Clinical aphasiology conference. Tucson, AZ; 2013.
44. LeBlanc J, de Guise E, Champoux MC, Couturier C, Lamoureux J, Marcoux J, et al. Acute evaluation of conversational discourse skills in traumatic brain injury. Int J Speech Lang Pathol. 2014;16(6):582–93.
45. Casarin FS, Pagliarin KC, Altmann RF, de Mattos Pimenta Parente MA, Ferré P, Côté H, et al. Montreal communication evaluation brief battery—MEC B: reliability and validity. Codas. 2020;32(1):e20180306.
46. Douglas JM, O'Flaherty CA, Snow PC. Measuring perception of communicative ability: the development and evaluation of the La Trobe communication questionnaire. Aphasiology. 2000;14(3):251–68.
47. Finch E, Cornwell P, Copley A, Doig E, Fleming J. Remediation of social communication impairments following traumatic brain injury using metacognitive strategy intervention: a pilot study. Brain Inj. 2017;31(13–14):1830–9.
48. Steel J, Ferguson A, Spencer E, Togher L. Social communication assessment during post-traumatic amnesia and the post-acute period after traumatic brain injury. Brain Inj. 2017;31(10):1320–30.
49. Hoepner JK, Olson SE. Joint video self-modeling as a conversational intervention for an individual with traumatic brain injury and his everyday partner: a pilot investigation. Clin Arch Commun Disord. 2018;3(1):22–41.
50. Behn N, Togher L, Power E, Heard R. Evaluating communication training for paid carers of people with traumatic brain injury. Brain Inj. 2012;26(13–14):1702–15.
51. MacLennan DL, Cornis-Pop M, Picon-Nieto L, Sigford B. The prevalence of pragmatic communication impairments in traumatic brain injury. In: National Brain Injury Association Conference. Minneapolis, MN; 2002.
52. Linscott RJ, Knight RG, Godfrey HPD. The profile of functional impairment in communication (PFIC): a measure of communication impairment for clinical use. Brain Inj. 1996;10(6):397–412.
53. Dahlberg CA, Cusick CP, Hawley LA, Newman JK, Morey CE, Harrison-Felix CL, et al. Treatment efficacy of social communication skills training after traumatic brain injury: a randomized treatment and deferred treatment controlled trial. Arch Phys Med Rehabil. 2007;88(12):1561–73.
54. Braden C, Hawley L, Newman J, Morey C, Gerber D, Harrison-Felix C. Social communication skills group treatment: a feasibility study for persons with traumatic brain injury and comorbid conditions. Brain Inj. 2010;24(11):1298–310.
55. Togher L, Power E, Tate R, McDonald S, Rietdijk R. Measuring the social interactions of people with traumatic brain injury and their communication partners: the adapted Kagan scales. Aphasiology. 2010;24(6–8):914–27.
56. Mann K, Power E, Barnes S, Togher L. Questioning in conversations before and after communication partner training for individuals with traumatic brain injury. Aphasiology. 2015;29(9):1082–109.
57. Behn N, Marshall J, Togher L, Cruice M. Feasibility and initial efficacy of project-based treatment for people with ABI. Int J Lang Commun Disord. 2019;54(3):465–78.
58. Iwashita H, Sohlberg MM. Measuring conversations after acquired brain injury in 30 minutes or less: a comparison of two pragmatic rating scales. Brain Inj. 2019;33(9):1219–33.
59. Bond F, Godfrey H. Conversation with traumatically brain injured individuals: a controlled study of behavioural changes and their impact. Brain Inj. 1997;11(5):319–30.
60. MacDonald S. The cognitive-communication checklist for acquired brain injury: a means of identifying, recording, and tracking communication impairments. Am J Speech Lang Pathol. 2021;30(3):1074–89.
61. Jones CA, Turkstra LS. Selling the story: narratives and charisma in adults with TBI. Brain Inj. 2011;25(9):844–57.

62. Tu LV, Togher L, Power E. The impact of communication partner and discourse task on a person with traumatic brain injury: the use of multiple perspectives. Brain Inj. 2011;25(6):560–80.
63. Kilov AM, Togher L, Grant S. Problem solving with friends: discourse participation and performance of individuals with and without traumatic brain injury. Aphasiology. 2009;23(5):584–605.
64. Jorgensen M, Togher L. Narrative after traumatic brain injury: a comparison of monologic and jointly-produced discourse. Brain Inj. 2009;23(9):727–40.
65. Bogart E, Togher L, Power E, Docking K. Casual conversations between individuals with traumatic brain injury and their friends. Brain Inj. 2012;26(3):221–33.
66. Halliday MAK. In: Arnold E, editor. An introduction to functional grammar. 2nd ed. London; 1994.
67. Sim P, Power E, Togher L. Describing conversations between individuals with traumatic brain injury (TBI) and communication partners following communication partner training: using exchange structure analysis. Brain Inj. 2013;27(6):717–42.
68. Mentis M, Prutting CA. Analysis of topic as illustrated in a head-injured and a normal adult. J Speech Lang Hear Res. 1991;34(3):583–95.
69. Brassel S, Kenny B, Power E, Elbourn E, McDonald S, Tate R, et al. Conversational topics discussed by individuals with severe traumatic brain injury and their communication partners during sub-acute recovery. Brain Inj. 2016;30(11):1329–42.
70. Meulenbroek P, Turkstra LS. Job stability in skilled work and communication ability after moderate–severe traumatic brain injury. Disabil Rehabil. 2016;38(5):452–61.
71. Meulenbroek P, Cherney LR. The voicemail elicitation task: functional workplace language assessment for persons with traumatic brain injury. J Speech Lang Hear Res. 2019;62(9):3367–80.
72. Meulenbroek P, Cherney LR. Computer-based workplace communication training in persons with traumatic brain injury: the work-related communication program. J Commun Disord. 2021;91:106104.

Jennifer Mozeiko is a speech-language pathologist, Associate Professor, and researcher directing the Aphasia Rehab Lab at the University of Connecticut. After earning her B.A., she worked at the Harvard School of Public Health, taught English in Hong Kong, and then returned to Boston where she worked in e-commerce for several years before pursuing her interest in language disorders following brain injury. Her research is focused on improving treatment and the quality of life of people with acquired brain injury. Dr. Mozeiko has been recognized as a Tavistock Distinguished Scholar.

Louisa Suting is a doctoral student in the Department of Speech, Language, and Hearing Sciences at the University of Connecticut. Her primary focus revolves around enhancing the treatment outcomes for individuals with acquired brain injury. Her research work encompasses the development of ecologically valid measures to assess language recovery and exploring objective biomarkers for tailoring personalized treatments for individuals impacted by acquired brain injury.

André Lindsey is an Assistant Professor at Nevada State University. He has worked clinically remediating a variety of neurogenic impairments in both short- and long-term rehabilitation settings. He studies how linguistic processing interacts with memory and executive functions. His research examines compensatory techniques and methods of cognitive rehabilitation for individuals with traumatic brain injury.

Assessing Discourse Ability in Adults with Right Hemisphere Damage

15

Melissa Johnson and Jessie Preston

Preview of What Is Currently Known

People with right hemisphere brain damage (RHD) are a heterogeneous group with a range of impairments in discourse (e.g., topic maintenance, tangentiality) that fall under the umbrella of pragmatics. Tools for the assessment of discourse and pragmatics for individuals with RHD are limited in comparison with other populations served by speech-language pathologists (SLPs). While there are standardized assessments available, many focus solely on cognitive deficits associated with RHD. Furthermore, SLPs are not consistently relying on formal measures to assess discourse and pragmatics in the RHD population resulting in clients failing to receive adequate education and treatment in this area. Recently, efforts have been made to close this gap, enhancing the tools available to SLPs working with the RHD population.

Objectives

(a) To discuss the role of speech-language pathologists (SLPs) in the assessment of discourse in people with right hemisphere brain damage (RHD).
(b) To discuss the challenges and barriers SLPs face in the assessment of discourse in people with RHD.
(c) To describe apragmatism and its components (linguistic, paralinguistic, extralinguistic) as it presents in the discourse of individuals with RHD.
(d) To explain the RHDBank as a resource for understanding and assessing discourse in people with RHD across the continuum of care.
(e) To present various options for analyzing and interpreting discourse samples.

Introduction

People with right hemisphere brain damage (RHD) are a heterogeneous group with few as yet identifiable patterns of deficits across subsets of the population [1, 2]. Estimates of the prevalence of cognitive-communication deficits in this population range from 50 to 80% [3]. Assessment of the cognitive and communication strengths and challenges of people with RHD has historically been hampered by the existence of very few standardized assessment tools targeted for this population [4]. Furthermore, those assessments that do exist typically evaluate the cognitive sequelae following RHD, with much less focus on changes in communication [5]. In fact, in 2020, Ramsey and Blake found that 80% of speech-language pathologists (SLPs) surveyed did not assess some of the hallmark features of RHD (anosognosia, aprosodia, and pragmatics) at all, or if they did

M. Johnson (✉) · J. Preston
Communication Sciences and Disorders Department, Nazareth University, Rochester, NY, USA
e-mail: mjohnso2@naz.edu; jpresto8@naz.edu

A. P.-H. Kong (ed.), *Spoken Discourse Impairments in the Neurogenic Populations*, https://doi.org/10.1007/978-3-031-45190-4_15

so, it was through observation alone [5]. This might be acceptable if observation was sufficient to accurately identify these communication changes. However, Lehman Blake [6], in a 2006 study, found that only one-third of SLPs were "highly accurate" (i.e., at least 70% accurate; p. 261) at differentiating the discourse of healthy older adults from those with RHD. This was despite the fact that these were experienced SLPs and that the speaker groups were significantly different from each other in terms of tangentiality and egocentrism, two frequently occurring characteristics of RHD. It is not known how many of the participants with RHD who were categorized as healthy older adults in this study did not, in fact, have any communication impairments, as not every person with a right hemisphere brain injury will present with deficits. Nonetheless, as a profession, we should not be satisfied with 70% accuracy by one-third of practicing SLPs. Further, it is known that adults with RHD can experience negative changes in their social relationships [7] and the ability to participate in their previous vocational or avocational pursuits [3]. We also know that people with RHD are often under-referred, under-assessed, under-treated, and/or lost to follow-up unless they have more severe or more obvious cognitive impairments, such as left-side inattention (left neglect) or aprosodia (impaired prosody) [2, 8]. Thus, the potential to miss potentially life-altering communication impairments makes it imperative that we work to improve our assessment capabilities with this population.

It can be argued that an important contributing factor to this assessment problem is a knowledge gap in the field of speech-language pathology as it relates to the communication strengths and impairments of people with RHD [9]. To help address this, Minga and colleagues [10] proposed the term "apragmatism" to describe the challenges people with RHD can present with in their discourse production and comprehension (see Chap. 5 for a detailed review). They defined this term as, "a disorder in conveying and/or comprehending meaning or intent through linguistic, paralinguistic, and/or extralinguistic modes of context-dependent communication" (p. 6). Linguistic aspects of apragmatism encompass anything related to the words or syntactic structures used to convey meaning and intent. This can include, for example, difficulty understanding abstract language such as metaphors or idioms [11], difficulty integrating and interpreting complex information [12], reduced use of question-asking [13], being verbose or having a paucity of output [6], demonstrating poor cohesion (e.g., unclear pronoun referents) of discourse [14], or having difficulty maintaining topic [15]. Paralinguistic aspects of apragmatism in RHD relate to the production and comprehension of prosodic features of discourse [16]. Prosody can convey linguistic information, such as the yes/no question form (e.g., "Do you like sushi?") or the word the speaker wishes to stress in a sentence (e.g., "What are YOU doing here?" vs. "What are you doing HERE?"), as well as emotional content (e.g., sarcasm, mood). Receptive emotional aprosodia has been associated with RHD although more research is needed in this area, as well as in regard to the expressive aspects of aprosodia [14]. Extralinguistic aspects of apragmatism include use and interpretation of behaviors such as eye contact, gestures, and facial expression, all of which can be reduced in people with RHD [10].

Apragmatism, by its very nature, occurs in the context of communication with another person through various forms of discourse. There are a variety of subtypes of discourse depending on the purpose and the context in which they are produced. As has been described elsewhere in this text, there are monologic (e.g., story narratives and procedural discourse) and dialogic forms of discourse (i.e., conversation). Conversation is the most common form of discourse used by most people in their daily lives [17].

Discourse assessment and interpretation in the RHD population present challenges to the practicing clinician. While clinicians may feel confident in their ability to detect discourse changes in people with RHD [5], the sometimes subtle nature of discourse impairments post-RHD can make it difficult to differentiate between a true disorder or deficit and a difference that was present premorbidly. Furthermore, cultural and linguistic differences impacting communication are additional variables for clinicians to consider when assessing individuals. For example, during an initial encounter with a new conversation partner, individuals with RHD asked fewer questions than a control group [18]. However, BLACK healthy control participants also asked fewer questions than WHITE healthy participants [19]. Moreover, since most conversation partners were young white women, the impact of age and race differences on question asking may have played an important role in the number of questions asked. Thus, cultural differences between the individual and the clinician must be considered to ensure that the clinician does not incorrectly assume that an observed discourse characteristic is related to the individual's injury rather than to a cultural difference.

It is important for SLPs, as experts in communication, to serve as the primary interprofessional team members in assessing and treating any discourse impairments in clients with RHD. In addition, SLPs should actively educate other members of the team, including clients and their families, regarding these impairments. In order for SLPs to be successful in this role, valid and reliable diagnostic tools must be available.

RHDBank

SLPs have long known that standardized assessment measures can never paint the full picture of a client's abilities [20, 21]. Nonetheless, such tools can provide important information and help discern which behaviors deviate from the norm. Of the tools available to assess people with RHD, many are not psychometrically strong [22], and most clinicians have not adopted them for regular use in assessing this population [5]. These assessments are also limiting in that most do not assess discourse and, if they do, they do not thoroughly address all components of apragmatism as it manifests in the discourse of individuals with RHD. In addition, standardized assessments administered in a clinical setting may not reflect the "real life" functional ability of an individual [21]. For example, individuals may present with more challenges when completing a functional task than when these skills are assessed using a standardized measure in the clinical setting.

Given the shortage of standardized tools and their inherent limitations, using formal, but non-standardized measures is a reasonable and beneficial option. It is important to emphasize that "standardized" is not the only kind of "formal" assessment; similarly, "non-standardized" is not synonymous with "informal" assessment. According to Coelho and colleagues [23], "a formal assessment tool [is] one that has systematically applied procedures, whereas an informal assessment lacks defined procedures. In this sense, the broad category of formal measures includes…systematic assessments such as functional behavior assessment" (p. 224).

Beginning in 2015, new tools have been in development that can help address this need for formal assessment measures. Specifically, the RHDBank (a division of TalkBank; https://rhd.talkbank.org/), the RHDBank protocol, and the RHDBank Grand Rounds provide valuable information and guidance to aid SLPs in systematically assessing discourse in this population. Similar to other corpora of TalkBank (e.g., AphasiaBank, TBIBank), RHDBank is a shared database of multimedia interactions for the study of communication in people with RHD. Interested researchers and clinicians can easily access the password-protected database by sending an email to macw@cmu.edu. In fact, as of 2021, at least 90 such interested parties have accessed the database [9].

RHDBank Protocol

A standard RHDBank protocol for collecting discourse data was developed to allow researchers and clinicians to study and compare participants' samples that were collected at disparate times and locations. The protocol was developed using parts of the established AphasiaBank protocol and adding specific tasks that were thought to be sensitive to the RHD discourse impairments [9]. The RHDBank protocol and stimuli can all be accessed freely online without the need for a password. We suggest that collecting and analyzing data using this protocol can be a powerful tool in the assessment of discourse in people with RHD. The various components of the protocol and how they can be used will be described herein.

The RHDBank protocol includes a variety of discourse genres, with scripted administration instructions to ensure consistency, including (1) narrative discourse, or storytelling, which is elicited in response to an illustrated Cinderella storybook and in response to the "Cat Rescue" picture [24]; (2) procedural discourse, which is obtained by asking participants to describe how to make a peanut and jelly sandwich; (3) picture description of the "Cookie Theft" picture [25]; and, (4) "free speech" samples during which the participant is asked to describe their current communication abilities and to share their stroke story. In addition, the RHDBank includes a novel question elicitation task. While questions are often a part of conversational exchange, question asking is elicited intentionally in the RHDBank protocol by asking participants with RHD to look at pictures of unfamiliar objects and to generate three questions that would help them to identify the object. In one study, people with RHD asked questions that focused more on relatively unimportant details than did the healthy adults, making their question-asking less efficient and effective at accomplishing the purpose of the task [13].

Finally, dialogic discourse is elicited by asking participants to engage in a "first-encounter conversation" with an unfamiliar partner [26] (https://rhd.talkbank.org/protocol/investigator-rhd/encounter.html). To our knowledge, there have not been any published studies analyzing these first-encounter conversations in people with RHD. However, they have the potential to be rich sources of data for research and clinical practice.

To facilitate accurate assessment and to allow for valid and reliable inter- and intra-client comparisons, the manner of data collection must also be standard. As such, it is recommended that all data collection be video-recorded in a quiet, well-lit room, with minimal visual distractors. Care should be taken to avoid backlighting, to ensure that clients' faces are well-lit, and that faces are not blocked by hats or hair, which would make it difficult to assess clients' facial expressions, an important aspect of extralinguistic communication. It is also important to monitor the time allocated for each task. Some people with RHD can be very verbose, while others say very little. The RHDBank protocol provides guidance as to the time allotted for each task, as well as a script to be used if the full time has elapsed.

A critical consideration in using the RHDBank protocol for assessment is that the clinician administers the tasks consistently and with fidelity. For example, if a clinician chooses to administer a discourse task but does not wish to impose the time limit in an effort to measure a given client's verbosity, it would be important for the clinician to do so in the post-therapy assessment, as well, to ensure that the two samples can be reliably compared. In addition, a clinician may wish to set "rules" for their data analysis. In a recent sample collected by one of this chapter's authors, the participant immediately revised many of his questions (e.g., "What about kids? Brothers or sisters?"). It was decided that this would count as one yes/no question, as his intent was to ask his conversation partner about her siblings. Of course, other clinicians or researchers might have approached this differently. In any case, the important point for clinical assessment is that the clinician documents these choices to ensure that the same decisions are made at the next point of data collection so that the samples can be compared.

In addition to the discourse tasks, a variety of supplemental tasks have been included in the RHDBank protocol to assist in the identification and understanding of the contributions of various cognitive processes to the production of discourse in people with RHD [21]. These include the Apples Test [27] to assess hemispatial neglect, an indented paragraph reading task [26] to assess for neglect dyslexia, and the *Cognitive-Linguistic Quick Test* (CLQT) [28] to assess various cognitive domains. In addition, the *Communication Participation Item Bank* (CPIB) [29] was included to facilitate insight into the perceived impact of discourse impairments on the lives of people with RHD. As anosognosia (i.e., limited awareness of deficits) is often associated with RHD, the CPIB could also be administered to a close support person (e.g., spouse, adult child) to help gauge differences in the perception of communication changes on life participation.

For students or others who are new or less familiar with the discourse of people with RHD, the RHDBank website has a link to the "RHDBank Grand Rounds," a curated sample of videos, case descriptions, definitions, and suggested activities, which can be used to gain understanding and competency in assessing and interpreting discourse in people with RHD.

Measuring Discourse

Once discourse samples have been collected, clinicians must decide how to analyze them and how to use and interpret the information they glean. Part of this depends on the ultimate use of the assessment data, such as to inform treatment planning, to communicate with insurers and other providers, or for client and family education, among other purposes. The procedures described herein include some suggestions, but the ultimate decision regarding how to measure discourse data will be driven by the clinician and the purposes of the assessment. For some measures, a written transcript of the client's discourse will be sufficient. For others, a review of the video-recording will be necessary. Transcripts can be orthographic and can include various features including length of pause time (if applicable), backchannels (i.e., utterances a person makes to signal attention, agreement, etc., such as, "Yeah," "Really," "Huh,"), use of gestures, facial expressions, and any other features of particular interest to the clinician.

Transcripts that are uploaded to the RHDBank have been transcribed using the Codes for the Human Analysis of Transcripts (CHAT) format. Transcripts that are in this format can be readily analyzed using the software Computerized Language ANalysis (CLAN), which is freely available (see https://www.talkbank.org/). Tutorials and manuals are also available on the website for free download. While there is a learning curve to using these platforms, they can be powerful tools for analyzing discourse samples with a few simple keystrokes. Without the use of CLAN, counting variables of interest in a client's discourse can be completed manually. However, this need not be a major deterrent as the clinician will be analyzing one transcript at a time to show baseline status or to monitor progress.

There is evidence that question-asking is reduced in some people with RHD [13]. Thus, for a client with RHD, their first encounter conversation could also be analyzed for the number and types of questions asked. In addition, the number of topic shifts, the number of interruptions, or the number of turns per participant could be tallied. For example, participant #nazareth03a spent 2 min of his 5-min first-encounter conversation describing some of his favorite books without allowing time or conversational space for his conversation partner to comment (https://rhd.talkbank.org/). A potential goal for this client might be to increase conversational turn-taking. By using the standard protocol of the first-encounter conversation, progress monitoring could be achieved by counting the number of pre- and post-treatment conversational turns in such a conversation. For those using CHAT and CLAN, clinicians can code any number of behaviors using the format [+ (variable)] at the end of utterances of interest. Then, a simple frequency count can be coded in CLAN to determine the number of times the code appeared.

Global Coherence

Coherence in discourse is a measure of how well utterances hang together, or adhere to the topic at hand, and can be divided into local and global forms. Global coherence (GC) can be defined as the degree to which specific utterances relate to the overarching topic [30] and is a reflection of the speaker's ability to maintain a logical connection to the topic [31], whereas local coherence (LC) refers to the connection of one utterance to the previous one [30, 32]. Depending on the nature of the client's discourse, measurement of either or both forms may be beneficial. Utterances can be rated for GC using the 4-Point Global Coherence Rating Scale [31]. The scale has also been adapted to rate conversational discourse [17].

Little is known about the LC and GC characteristics of people with RHD. However, a few small, preliminary, unpublished studies using RHDBank data have shown that RHD is related to poorer GC in narrative, procedural, and conversational discourse [33–36] (see RHDBank https://rhd.talkbank.org/posters/ for poster presentations on this topic).

Main Concept Analysis

Main concept analysis (MCA) measures how well a speaker adheres to the gist of a story and provides the listener with its essential elements. Richardson and Dalton [37] analyzed AphasiaBank transcripts from healthy controls of the *Cinderella* story narrative, the *Broken Window* story sequence (task not included in the RHDBank), and the peanut butter and jelly procedural discourse task. For each task, they generated three lists of concepts that were mentioned by at least 33%, 50%, and 66% of the sample; these were determined to be the main concepts. To conduct an MCA, the examiner first decides which of these lists of main concepts to use to measure the novel sample against. It can be argued that, since tangentiality is a hallmark feature of many people with RHD, evaluating the sample against the 50% or 66% lists is more clinically meaningful. If measuring against the 33% list, only one-third of the normative sample mentioned that concept, meaning that it is somewhat less essential, and may be considered somewhat tangential. Conducting MCA, then, requires reviewing a sample narrative and determining which of the main concepts were included in the sample. Then, each main concept that is mentioned is scored as to whether it is accurate and/or complete. Any main concepts that are not mentioned are scored zero; utterances that do not mention any of the concepts are not scored. A total score can be derived and compared against the possible maximum score for that task and/or against a previously rated sample from the same participant. Thus, an MCA can identify tangentiality in a person with RHD who mentions many non-essential elements, (e.g., see the procedural discourse sample in the RHDBank for participant #nazareth05a or the *Cinderella* story narrative from participant #nazareth03a) and omits elements that are mentioned by most people who tell this story.

Interpreting Discourse Measures

For both GC and MCA, there are, as of yet, no norms against which to compare a given person's discourse sample. This is a limiting factor in determining whether or not the person's discourse deviates from that of healthy controls and is an important direction for future research. However, the current lack of norms does not mean that these measures are not of value. In combination with clinical observation, and interviewing the client and their family, these scores can be an important way to quantify discourse changes from a person's pre-stroke baseline. In addition, these scores can be used as a benchmark against which progress in therapy can be measured. For example, a treatment goal could be established to improve topic maintenance and adherence to the purpose of a given interaction, then main concept and GC analyses could be performed, demonstrating any improvement in these skills.

Discourse Assessment Across the Continuum of Care

Across the continuum of care, discourse assessment in the RHD population is often overlooked. Early on in recovery during the acute care stay, formal or standardized assessment is not always feasible. Individuals may be in this setting for a short period of time, be too critically ill to participate in a lengthy assessment, or the focus of the SLP's intervention may be in other areas (e.g., swallowing). There is an understandable focus on deficits that directly impact an individual's medical stability and safety during this time [38]. Once an individual enters the acute rehabilitation phase of recovery, the SLP's focus may be on cognition, as the overall goal during this stage of recovery is working towards a safe discharge home [39]. Given that individuals with RHD may present with left hemispatial neglect, anosognosia, and/or executive dysfunction [22] which are correlated with independence and safety [40–42], the SLP may focus on these skills at the expense of discourse and pragmatics.

Despite these considerations, assessing discourse in this population from the beginning of the recovery process is crucial. If SLPs reliably and routinely identify and assess for these impairments from the onset, there is a lower likelihood that any pragmatics deficits will be missed and that the clients will be discharged without education or intervention in this area. It is known that if pragmatics deficits exist, they can be detrimental to a person's quality of life, relationships, vocational and avocational pursuits, community reintegration, and independence [7, 43]. Thus, when pragmatics impairments are not addressed early on in recovery, individuals will be discharged without education regarding discourse impairments and without a recommendation that discourse and pragmatics be treatment priorities. This is a tremendous disservice; providing individuals with RHD and their loved ones with the information needed to understand and manage discourse/pragmatics changes is critical.

As the experts in communication, SLPs need tools to assess these impairments so that they can better serve this population. As soon as possible in a client's recovery, standardized and formal assessments, as well as informal, functional, and dynamic assessments of discourse and pragmatics should be undertaken [23]. The RHDBank protocol is a formal tool with tasks that are simple enough to administer at the bedside, in a clinical setting, or in the client's home. Documenting findings throughout the continuum of care facilitates a smoother transition from one professional to the next and reduces the likelihood that discourse assessment and treatment will be overlooked and that clients will be lost to follow-up.

During the acute care phase after a right hemisphere stroke or injury, discourse can be elicited at the bedside to provide the SLP with objective information and, at a minimum, a baseline to compare to at a later date. During the acute rehabilitation phase of recovery, more in-depth assessment and intensive treatment can begin. Clients typically receive daily therapy, so time spent with the SLP is sufficiently long to delve deeply into a patient's discourse and pragmatics. This is an excellent time to complete the RHDBank protocol in its entirety, perhaps using GC and/or MCA, among other measures to directly assess the linguistic, paralinguistic, and extralinguistic components of apragmatism.

There is evidence that, for the acquired brain injury population, once an individual returns home and begins to integrate back into the community, they may report more awareness of their deficits [44]. Although there is limited research on this in the RHD population, the same may be true as individuals work to adjust to their "new normal." In one poignant example, the wife of a 55-year-old man with RHD stated the following [43]:

> *His speech was always clear, and he could understand what he heard and read and could write but his communication was completely different—does that make sense? He would just go quiet in a group of people, he cannot participate ... he doesn't seem able to come up with new topics. A lack of communication about stroke, and what changes, and what they can and can't offer was a significant problem for me as a family member* (p. 129).

In addition, there is evidence that the emotional state of individuals with right hemisphere stroke tends to decline after around 6 months post-stroke [45]. This reinforces the importance of assessing and treating discourse impairments throughout the continuum of care. In addition, SLPs can take time to complete family/caregiver surveys or interviews along with continuing to employ formal and informal measures to assess and treat all components of apragmatism as the client and family's adjustment proceeds.

There is also a unique opportunity in the home setting to observe and assess individuals in their natural environment and routine. For example, a variation on the "first encounter" conversation task from the RHDBank protocol can be incorporated into the clinician's first visit with the client. By slightly modifying the instructions, the clinician can tell the client that they would like to get to know each other during the first 5 min of their time together. This is a realistic and functional way to take objective data on, for example, how many and what types of questions the individual asks, and whether or not the client is verbose or tangential. A similar scenario can then be set up with another novel conversation partner after a period of therapy has been completed to gauge progress. This further highlights the importance of documentation of discourse impairments along the continuum of care, ensuring that the next professional is able to take advantage of opportunities for functional assessment of these skills starting with their first encounter with the patient.

As with any communication deficit, discourse assessment results cannot be viewed in isolation. When interpreting discourse with this population, it is important to also assess an individual's cognitive skills to examine any interaction between cognitive impairments and discourse production. Individuals with RHD commonly have difficulty with attention, executive functions, and awareness of their deficits [22]. The implications for treatment of this intersection of cognition and discourse must also be considered. For example, it is known that, in healthy adults, executive function is correlated with the structure of narrative discourse [46]. Other connections between cognition and discourse are also likely [47]. For instance, an individual who has difficulty with topic maintenance may have a co-occurring attention impairment that is impacting this skill. Alternatively, an individual who has anosognosia may have a difficult time recognizing the impact of their impaired discourse on their communication partners and, therefore, may not be able to fully embrace treatment approaches or compensatory strategies. While a full exploration of these cognitive contributors to discourse impairments is not possible within the confines of this chapter, the SLP must endeavor to tease these pieces apart to interpret assessment findings and formulate a treatment plan.

Conclusion

As described above, it is in the production and comprehension of discourse where the apragmatic deficits associated with RHD can best be evaluated. The three components of apragmatism (i.e., linguistic, paralinguistic, extralinguistic) offer a useful scaffold upon which to examine the assessment of discourse in this population.

As readers peruse this text, several chapters on treating disordered discourse across various populations (i.e., aphasia, primary progressive aphasia, traumatic brain injury, dementia) can be found, but such a chapter dedicated to treating disordered discourse in people with RHD is currently absent. That is because the field of speech-language pathology has not yet developed the evidence-based tools to do so. It is our hope that, as we refine our ability to assess discourse objectively and in a standard manner, we will be able to conduct the types of rigorous, clinically relevant research studies that will allow us to generate and evaluate treatment approaches in this population.

To be sure, there is much work still to be done in this area. However, the tools described in this chapter provide some immediate options for clinicians and researchers interested in understanding discourse in people with RHD. This overview of assessment of discourse in people with RHD can be considered something of a call to action for the field of speech-language pathology. Let us continue to advance our understanding of discourse in this population so that we can provide them with the same critical support, education, and evidence-based treatment approaches that we provide to our clients and patients with disordered discourse resulting from other etiologies.

Major Takeaways

1. Assessment of individuals with RHD is challenging for SLPs due to limited availability of resources, and knowledge gaps in the field.
2. Apragmatism in individuals with RHD can result in a negative impact on social relationships and interactions.

3. Discourse is often overlooked in the assessment of individuals with RHD resulting in under-treatment of pragmatics deficits.
4. The RHDBank provides a formal protocol that can be modified for use to assess discourse across the continuum of care.
5. There are multiple options for analyzing and interpreting discourse samples to identify elements of apragmatism (linguistic, paralinguistic, extralinguistic).

Acknowledgments The authors would like to thank Margaret Blake, Ph.D., CCC-SLP for her review of this chapter and for her suggestions. We would also like to thank Dr. Davida Fromm and Dr. Brian MacWhinney for their expertise in establishing and maintaining the RHDBank and for their assistance in data analysis. Most importantly, we would like to thank the RHDBank participants for their willingness to tell their stories so we can learn from them and strive to better serve them and other right hemisphere stroke survivors with a deeper understanding of the communication changes they have experienced.

References

1. Sheppard SM, Stockbridge MD, Keator LM, Murray LL, Blake ML. The company prosodic deficits keep following right hemisphere stroke: a systematic review. J Int Neuropsych Soc. 2022;28:1–16. https://doi.org/10.1017/S1355617721001302.
2. Blake ML, Duffy JR, Tompkins CA, Myers PS. Right hemisphere syndrome is in the eye of the beholder. Aphasiology. 2003;17:423–32. https://doi.org/10.1080/02687030344000120.
3. Tompkins CA. Rehabilitation for cognitive-communication disorders in right hemisphere brain damage. Arch Phys Med Rehabil. 2012;93:S61–9. https://doi.org/10.1016/j.apmr.2011.10.015.
4. Minga J, Stockbridge MD, Durfee A, Johnson M. Clinical guidelines for eliciting discourse using the RHDBank protocol. Am J Speech Lang Pathol. 2022;31:1949–62. https://doi.org/10.1044/2022_ajslp-22-00097.
5. Ramsey A, Blake ML. Speech-language pathology practices for adults with right hemisphere stroke: what are we missing? Am J Speech Lang Pathol. 2020;29:741–59. https://doi.org/10.1044/2020_AJSLP-19-00082.
6. Lehman BM. Clinical relevance of discourse characteristics after right hemisphere brain damage. Am J Speech Lang Pathol. 2006;15:255–67. https://doi.org/10.1044/1058-0360(2006/024).
7. Hewetson R, Cornwell P, Shum DHK. Relationship and social network change in people with impaired social cognition post right hemisphere stroke. Am J Speech Lang Pathol. 2021;30:962–73. https://doi.org/10.1044/2020_ajslp-20-00047.
8. Cherney LR. Unilateral neglect: a disorder of attention. Semin Speech Lang. 2002;23(2):117–28. https://doi.org/10.1055/s-2002-24988.
9. Minga J, Johnson M, Blake ML, Fromm D, MacWhinney B. Making sense of right hemisphere discourse using RHDBank. Top Lang Disord. 2021;41:99–122. https://doi.org/10.1097/tld.0000000000000244.
10. Minga J, Sheppard S, Johnson M, Hewetson R, Cornwell P, Blake ML. Apragmatism: the renewal of a label for communication disorders associated with right hemisphere brain damage. Int J Lang Commun Disord. 2023;58:651. https://doi.org/10.1111/1460-6984.12807
11. Brownell HH, Simpson TL, Bihrle AM, Potter HH, Gardner H. Appreciation of metaphoric alternative word meanings by left and right brain-damaged patients. Neuropsychologia. 1990;28:375–83. https://doi.org/10.1016/0028-3932(90)90063-t.
12. Myers P. Profiles of communication deficits in patients with right cerebral hemisphere damage: implications for diagnosis and treatment. Aphasiology. 2005;19:1147–60. https://doi.org/10.1080/02687030500331585.
13. Minga J, Fromm D, Williams-DeVane C, MacWhinney B. Question use in adults with right-hemisphere brain damage. J Speech Lang Hear Res. 2020;63:738–48. https://doi.org/10.1044/2019_jslhr-19-00063.
14. Stockbridge MD, Berube S, Goldberg E, Suarez A, Mace R, Ubellacker D, et al. Differences in linguistic cohesion within the first year following right- and left-hemisphere lesions. Aphasiology. 2021;35:357–71. https://doi.org/10.1080/02687038.2019.1693026.
15. Brady M, Mackenzie C, Armstrong L. Topic use following right hemisphere brain damage during three semi-structured conversational discourse samples. Aphasiology. 2003;17:881–904. https://doi.org/10.1080/02687030344000292.
16. Stockbridge MD, Sheppard SM, Keator LM, Murray LL, Lehman BM. Aprosodia subsequent to right hemisphere brain damage: a systematic review and meta-analysis. J Int Neuropsychol Soc. 2022;28:709–35. https://doi.org/10.1017/s1355617721000825.
17. Leaman MC, Edmonds LA. Measuring global coherence in people with aphasia during unstructured conversation. Am J Speech Lang Pathol. 2021;30:359–75. https://doi.org/10.1044/2020_ajslp-19-00104.
18. Minga J, Fromm D, Jacks A, Stockbridge MD, Nelthropp J, MacWhinney B. The effects of right hemisphere brain damage on question-asking in conversation. J Speech Lang Hear Res. 2022;65:727–37. https://doi.org/10.1044/2021_jslhr-21-00309.
19. Fannin D, Elleby J, Tackett M, Minga J. Intersectionality of race and question-asking in women after right hemisphere brain damage. J Speech Lang Hear Res. 2023;66:314–24. https://doi.org/10.1044/2022_jslhr-22-00327.

20. Wilson BA. Goal planning rather than neuropsychological tests should be used to structure and evaluate cognitive rehabilitation. Brain Impair. 2003;4:25–30. https://doi.org/10.1375/brim.4.1.25.27030.
21. LeBlanc JM, Hayden ME, Paulman RG. A comparison of neuropsychological and situational assessment for predicting employability after closed head injury. J Head Trauma Rehabil. 2000;15:1022–40. https://doi.org/10.1097/00001199-200008000-00005.
22. Blake ML. The right hemisphere and disorders of cognition and communication: theory and clinical practice. San Diego: Plural Publishing; 2017.
23. Coelho C, Ylvisaker M, Turkstra LS. Nonstandardized assessment approaches for individuals with traumatic brain injuries. Semin Speech Lang. 2005;26:223–41. https://doi.org/10.1055/s-2005-922102.
24. Nicholas LE, Brookshire RH. A system for quantifying the informativeness and efficiency of the connected speech of adults with aphasia. J Speech Hear Res. 1993;36:338–50. https://doi.org/10.1044/jshr.3602.338.
25. Goodglass H, Kaplan E. The assessment of aphasia and related disorders. 3rd ed. Philadelphia: Lea & Febiger; 1983.
26. Kennedy MRT, Strand EA, Burton W, Peterson. Analysis of first-encounter conversations of right-hemisphere-damaged adults. Clin Aphasiology. 1994;22:67–80.
27. Bickerton WL, Samson D, Williamson J, Humphreys GW. Separating forms of neglect using the Apples test: validation and functional prediction in chronic and acute stroke. Neuropsychology. 2011;25:567–80. https://doi.org/10.1037/a0023501.
28. Helm-Estabrooks N. Cognitive linguistic quick test. San Antonio: Pearson Assessment; 2001.
29. Baylor C, Yorkston K, Eadie T, Kim J, Chung H, Amtmann D. The Communicative Participation Item Bank (CPIB): item bank calibration and development of a disorder-generic short form. J Speech Lang Hear Res. 2013;56:1190–208. https://doi.org/10.1044/1092-4388(2012/12-0140).
30. Glosser G, Deser T. Patterns of discourse production among neurological patients with fluent language disorders. Brain Lang. 1991;40:67–88. https://doi.org/10.1016/0093-934x(91)90117-j.
31. Harris Wright H, Capilouto GJ. Considering a multi-level approach to understanding maintenance of global coherence in adults with aphasia. Aphasiology. 2012;26:656–72. https://doi.org/10.1080/02687038.2012.676855.
32. Van Leer E, Turkstra L. The effect of elicitation task on discourse coherence and cohesion in adolescents with brain injury. J Commun Disord. 1999;32:327–49. https://doi.org/10.1016/s0021-9924(99)00008-8.
33. Cator J, Johnson M, Fromm D, MacWhinney B. Global coherence of story narratives in right hemisphere brain damage (RHD). Poster session presented at: American Speech-Language-Hearing Association Annual Convention; 2017 November 16–18; Los Angeles, CA.
34. Johnson M, Costley C, Randolph E, Fromm D, MacWhinney B. Peanut butter and princesses: analyzing discourse in people with right hemisphere brain damage (RHD). Poster session presented at: American Speech-Language-Hearing Association Annual Convention; 2021 November 18–20; Washington, DC.
35. Johnson J, Costley C, Fox K, Fromm D. Let's chat: conversational analysis in people with right hemisphere brain damage (RHD). Poster session presented at: American Speech-Language-Hearing Association Annual Convention; 2022 November 17–19; New Orleans, LA.
36. Johnson M, Randolph E, Fromm D, MacWhinney B. Comparisons of narrative discourse in right hemisphere brain damage (RHD), aphasia and healthy adults. Poster session presented at: American Speech-Language-Hearing Association Annual Convention; 2019 November 14–16; Orlando, FL.
37. Richardson JD, Dalton SG. Main concepts for three different discourse tasks in a large non-clinical sample. Aphasiology. 2016;30:45–73. https://doi.org/10.1080/02687038.2015.1057891.
38. Vogel AP, Maruff P, Morgan AT. Evaluation of communication assessment practices during the acute stages post stroke. J Eval Clin Pract. 2010;16:1183–8. https://doi.org/10.1111/j.1365-2753.2009.01291.x.
39. Morrow EL, Hereford AP, Covington NV, Duff MC. Traumatic brain injury in the acute care setting: assessment and management practices of speech-language pathologists. Brain Inj. 2020;34:1590–609. https://doi.org/10.1080/02699052.2020.1766114.
40. Cherney LR, Halper AS, Kwasnica CM, Harvey RL, Zhang M. Recovery of functional status after right hemisphere stroke: relationship with unilateral neglect. Arch Phys Med Rehabil. 2001;82:322–8. https://doi.org/10.1053/apmr.2001.21511.
41. Jehkonen M, Ahonen J, Dastidar P, Koivisto A, Laippala P, Vilkki J, et al. Predictors of discharge to home during the first year after right hemisphere stroke. Acta Neurol Scand. 2001;104:136–41. https://doi.org/10.1034/j.1600-0404.2001.00025.x.
42. Vossel S, Weiss PH, Eschenbeck P, Fink GR. Anosognosia, neglect, extinction and lesion site predict impairment of daily living after right-hemispheric stroke. Cortex. 2013;49:1782–9. https://doi.org/10.1016/j.cortex.2012.12.011.
43. Hewetson R. Social participation following right hemisphere stroke: influence of a cognitive-communication disorder. [Dissertation]. Queensland: Griffith University; 2018. https://doi.org/10.25904/1912/1712.
44. Turner B, Fleming J, Ownsworth T, Cornwell P. Perceptions of recovery during the early transition phase from hospital to home following acquired brain injury: a journey of discovery. Neuropsychol Rehabil. 2011;21:64–91. https://doi.org/10.1080/09602011.2010.527747.
45. Nelson LD, Cicchetti D, Satz P, Sowa M, Mitrushina M. Emotional sequelae of stroke: a longitudinal

perspective. J Clin Exp Neuropsychol. 1994;16:796–806. https://doi.org/10.1080/01688639408402693.
46. Cannizzaro MS, Coelho CA. Analysis of narrative discourse structure as an ecologically relevant measure of executive function in adults. J Psycholinguist Res. 2013;42:527–49. https://doi.org/10.1007/s10936-012-9231-5.
47. Wright HH, Capilouto GJ, Srinivasan C, Fergadiotis G. Story processing ability in cognitively healthy younger and older adults. J Speech Lang Hear Res. 2011;54:900–17. https://doi.org/10.1044/1092-4388(2010/09-0253).

Additional Resources

Online Resources

RHDBank website. https://rhd.talkbank.org/
"Right hemisphere brain damage" website. https://www.righthemisphere.org/
The American-Speech-Language-Hearing Association (ASHA) website. https://www.asha.org/public/speech/disorders/right-hemisphere-brain-damage

Melissa Johnson is an Associate Professor at Nazareth University in Rochester, NY where she teaches and provides clinical education in the area of neurogenic communication disorders. Her research interests are in understanding the impacts of right hemisphere brain damage on cognitive-communication abilities, especially in the area of apragmatism, as well as co-delivered music and speech therapy for people with aphasia. She is a co-developer of the RHDBank, a founding member of the International Right Hemisphere Collaborative, and a co-developer of the educational website, https://www.right-hemisphere.org/.

Jessie Preston is a Clinical Assistant Professor and manager of the Neurogenic Communication and Cognition Clinic at Nazareth University in Rochester, New York. Jessie teaches and provides clinical education related to assessment and treatment of neurogenic communication disorders. Her clinical interests include interprofessional work and using a collaborative approach for the treatment of adults, in particular with a diagnosis of aphasia, right hemisphere brain damage, and Parkinson's disease.

... 15. Gambiarte, M., ... discourse structure ...

16. Wright, H. H., ...
... doi.org/10.1044/ ...

Additional Resources

Online Resources

... Right hemisphere brain damage ...

The American Speech-Language-Hearing Association (ASHA) website ...

Automatic Assessment of Speech and Language Impairment in Natural Speech

16

Ying Qin and Tan Lee

Preview of What Is Currently Known
Artificial intelligence (AI) has become the most influential technology that leads to revolutionary changes to modern society in many aspects. As one of the key areas of AI, speech and language technologies are applied widely to human–computer communication and interaction. Apart from the well-known speech-to-text and text-to-speech functions, state-of-the-art speech and language technologies can be used to extract and analyze non-verbal and paralinguistic information in human speech, and hence facilitate automatic assessment of speech and language disorders. The major technical challenges are due to the lack of annotated data of disordered speech and the impact of language specificity.

Objectives
(a) To define automatic assessment of speech and language impairment in natural speech.
(b) To elaborate the motivations of automatic assessment.
(c) To introduce state-of-the-art methods and systems of automatic speech and language assessment.
(d) To discuss the challenges, and pros and cons of existing approaches.

Introduction

Speech is a preferred and natural modality of communication for human beings. Along the speech communication pathway, there are many imperfections that may obstruct the information flow. Impairments on speech and language abilities are affecting the daily life of a large population worldwide. Speech impairment deteriorates a person's ability to produce accurate and natural speech in the desired manner. The aspects concerned may involve speech sound articulation, speech fluency, and/or voice quality. Commonly known types of speech disorders include voice disorder, apraxia, dysarthria, and stuttering. Language impairment refers to impaired comprehension and/or use of spoken, written, and/or other symbol systems. Individuals with expressive language disorders exhibit difficulties in producing language, for example, speaking and/or writing. Speech and language impairment may occur independently, or a person may suffer from both at the same time.

Y. Qin
Institute of Information Science in School of Computer and Information Technology, Beijing Jiaotong University,
Beijing, People's Republic of China
e-mail: yingqin@bjtu.edu.cn

T. Lee (✉)
Department of Electronic Engineering, The Chinese University of Hong Kong,
Hong Kong, Hong Kong SAR
e-mail: tanlee@ee.cuhk.edu.hk

A. P.-H. Kong (ed.), *Spoken Discourse Impairments in the Neurogenic Populations*,
https://doi.org/10.1007/978-3-031-45190-4_16

The discussion in this chapter is focused on speech and language impairment manifested in spoken discourse. Specifically, the target spoken discourses contain spontaneous speech elicited by narrative tasks, for example, picture description, storytelling, and monologue. This type of speech is differentiated from that produced by reading speech materials of designated content. Depending on the cause of disorder or disease, the symptoms of impairment may vary greatly, from voice abnormalities and articulation distortions or errors to speech disfluency, inappropriate intonation, word retrieval difficulties, and nonsensical speech.

Analysis of spoken discourse is an essential component of the clinical assessment process for diagnosing and evaluating the type and severity of speech and language impairment. The assessment is carried out by trained speech-language pathologists (SLP) with pertinent clinical, linguistic, and cultural background. The subjectivity and possible bias in perceptual judgement have long been a major concern. The reliability and accuracy of assessment results depend greatly on the SLP's professional knowledge and experience. Manual transcription of spontaneous discourse is very time-consuming, thus limiting the efficacy of subjective evaluation. Given the significant manpower shortage of SLPs, many patients may not be able to receive timely diagnosis and treatment. Computer-assisted automatic assessment is believed to be an effective means to address the above issues. Automatic assessment enables objective evaluation of speech and language with consistent standards. It makes diagnosis and treatment of speech impairment more efficient and less costly. In a multi-lingual society like Luxembourg City, New York, Hong Kong, and Singapore, where the inhabitants speak many different languages and dialects, automatic assessment systems can help overcome the language and culture barriers. The development of computer-based assessment technology does not aim at creating robots to replace human SLPs with fully automated diagnosis and treatment services. The goal is to assist the SLPs to improve both accuracy and efficiency of work by automating tedious and error-prone processes of data analysis and providing objective and reproducible evidence.

Automatic assessment of speech and language impairment refers to the computational process of deriving and analyzing symptoms-related speech features from acoustic signals. The design of an automatic assessment system involves the use of signal processing algorithms, spoken language technology, machine learning (ML), and deep learning models. In accordance with different goals of assessment, the system is made to perform a task of detection, classification, or regression on input speech. One simple example is to detect the existence of impairment, i.e., to determine if the speech is from an impaired speaker or an unimpaired one. The system can also be designed to predict a categorical label or numerical score that indicates the severity of an impairment, which is realized by classification model or regression model, respectively.

In this chapter, two mainstream approaches to automatic assessment of speech and language impairments in continuous speech are described. They are namely the two-step approach and the end-to-end approach as illustrated in Fig. 16.1. In the two-step approach, text and acoustic features for characterizing speech and language impairment are extracted. By leveraging state-of-the-art automatic speech recognition (ASR) systems, a wide variety of features can be computed at different linguistic and acoustic levels. In the second step, an independent classification or regression model trained with selected features is used to give the assessment result. In the end-to-end approach, a sophisticated deep neural network (DNN) model is built to generate assessment result directly from raw speech and/or text input. The end-to-end model is trained to learn by itself useful features that are related to the assessment goal. Simply speaking, feature extraction and classification/regression are carried out in an integrated manner by a single DNN model.

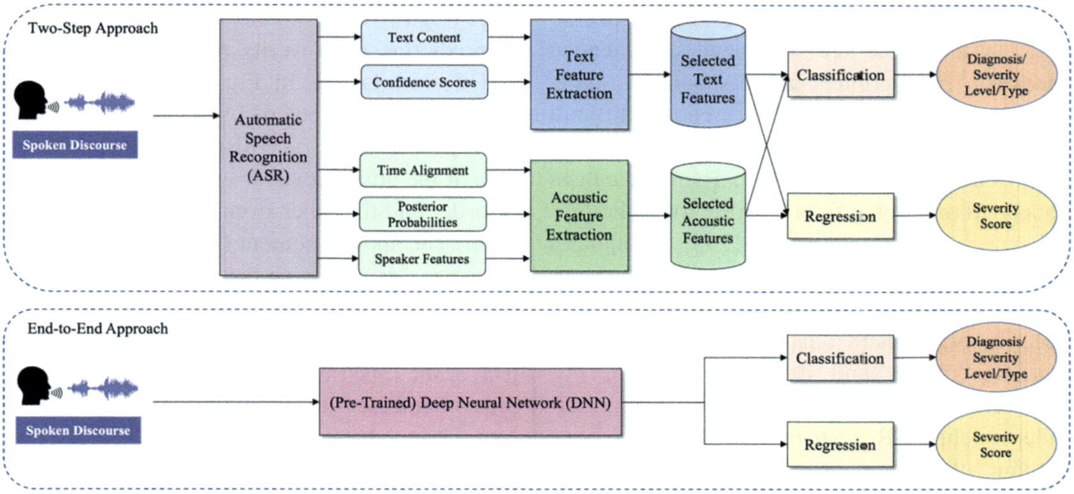

Fig. 16.1 The two-step approach and the end-to-end approach to automatic assessment of speech and language impairment in spoken discourse

Two-Step Approach

The core components of a two-step assessment system are feature extraction and classification/regression model. The most crucial task is how to identify and compute useful features that can quantify impairments in speech. Speech impairment is analyzed primarily on the acoustic aspect, for example, voice quality, articulation, and fluency. Language impairment is characterized based on linguistic content and properties, for example, vocabulary, word usage, and grammar. In conventional speech and language assessment, SLPs listen to the elicited speech, measure its fluency, and grade the speech content subjectively. Examples of commonly used criteria for scoring are "effortful and hesitant," "frequent paraphasia," "some response (to the task)," and "incomplete description" [1]. It is a great challenge to transform such descriptive know-hows to computational processes by which numerical or symbolic features are obtained efficiently from speech signals.

An efficient and useful assessment system is desired to have the following capabilities. First, it should be able to operate automatically without requiring human adjustment and tuning. Second, different dimensions of speech and language impairment should be covered. Acoustic features characterizing speech impairment are derived from audio recordings. Text-based linguistic features capturing language impairment are extracted from speech transcription. Speech impairment is reflected mostly by the acoustic signal. Linguistic features for characterizing vocabulary and content-related language impairment are extracted from transcribed text content. For spontaneous speech in natural spoken discourses, an ASR system is used to generate text transcription automatically and time alignment of input speech to support subsequent steps of feature extraction. The performance of ASR, i.e., accuracy of recognition, has a significant impact on the efficacy of extracted features, particularly the linguistic features. General-purpose ASR systems perform very well in typical applications of human–computer interaction where the input speech is clearly articulated by co-operative speakers. For highly ungrammatical spontaneous speech recorded in heterogeneous acoustic environment, it would be unrealistic to expect an error-free text transcription from the ASR system. It is preferred to develop application-specific ASR systems that are optimized on intended speaker population and disorder type. Pathological speech data are scarce and difficult to collect, making the data-hungry deep learning approach to ASR less effective. There have been concerted research efforts on ASR for pathological speech, such as dysarthria [2–4] and aphasia [5–7]. Commonly used techniques for developing domain-specific ASR include speaker adaptation [2, 3], domain adaptation [7], multi-task learning [5, 6], and data augmentation [4]. Speaker adaptation aims at tuning a speaker-independent ASR system trained with a large amount of normal speech to suit a specific impaired speaker. The data requirement for adaptation is significantly lower than training a speaker-dependent ASR system. Domain adaptation and multi-task learning approaches facilitate the use of out-of-domain training data, for example, speech from unimpaired speakers or speech data with similar impairment symptoms, to improve the recognition accuracy. In domain adaptation, a generic ASR system is first trained with out-of-domain data. Subsequently, a relatively small amount of impaired speech is used to adjust the generic system. In multi-task learning, the primary ASR task is achieved with impaired speech, while ASR on out-of-domain data are treated as secondary tasks. Data augmentation is a straightforward way to increase the amount of task-related training data. For example, speech from healthy speakers can be modified into impaired speech via perturbation of speech spectrum, pitch, and tempo.

As shown in Fig. 16.1, a multitude of information can be obtained from the ASR system to characterize different aspects of speech. In addition to the word sequence that best matches input speech, the ASR system can produce rich representations of speech, including alternative word hypotheses, confidence scores on hypothesized phonemes and words, start and end time of phoneme and word units, and occurrences and locations of silent pauses. Text features computed from such rich representations have been shown to be robust to speech recognition errors [6]. Acoustic posterior probabilities and speaker features (e.g., i-vectors) were shown to be effective in predicting the severity of voice disorder [8] and dysarthria [9]. In Fig. 16.2, the posterior probabilities computed over vowel segments from people with voice disorder are plotted [8]. One of the utterances is from a subject with mild disorder and the other from one with severe disorder. The spoken content (in the form of phone sequences) is shown on the top of each plot. The vertical dashed lines indicate the time boundaries of syllables. For the utterance from the mild subject, at the time interval when a specific vowel is present and recognized, the respective posteriors have large values, i.e., close to 1. The posteriors of other phones approach 0. On the contrary, the vowels' posteriors in the severe utterance fluctuate significantly. Even for a correctly recognized vowel, the corresponding posterior values could be much lower than 1. The examples demonstrate the effectiveness of using ASR posterior features to detect and quantify voice disorder in natural speech.

Supra-segmental temporal features, such as pause duration and speaking rate, can be derived from time alignment of recognized words, phones, silence intervals, and other sound events that are generated as part of the ASR output. For automatic speech assessment in people with aphasia [6], a set of duration features, for example, "average duration of silence segment" and "nonspeech-to-speech duration ratio," were extracted from ASR time alignment. They showed high correlations with the Aphasia Quotient (AQ) of the Western Aphasia Battery. In parallel with ASR, other short-term or long-term acoustic features, for example, spectral, cepstral, and temporal features, can be computed directly from the acoustic signal.

Based on the text output of ASR, text features can be derived to reflect the characteristics of speech impairment in the linguistic aspect. There are two main types of text features, namely statistics-based features and neural network learned features. Statistics-based text features are designed by leveraging knowledge acquired in clinical practice. Examples of statistics-based features include vocabulary richness, for example, type-token ratio, occurrence statistics of

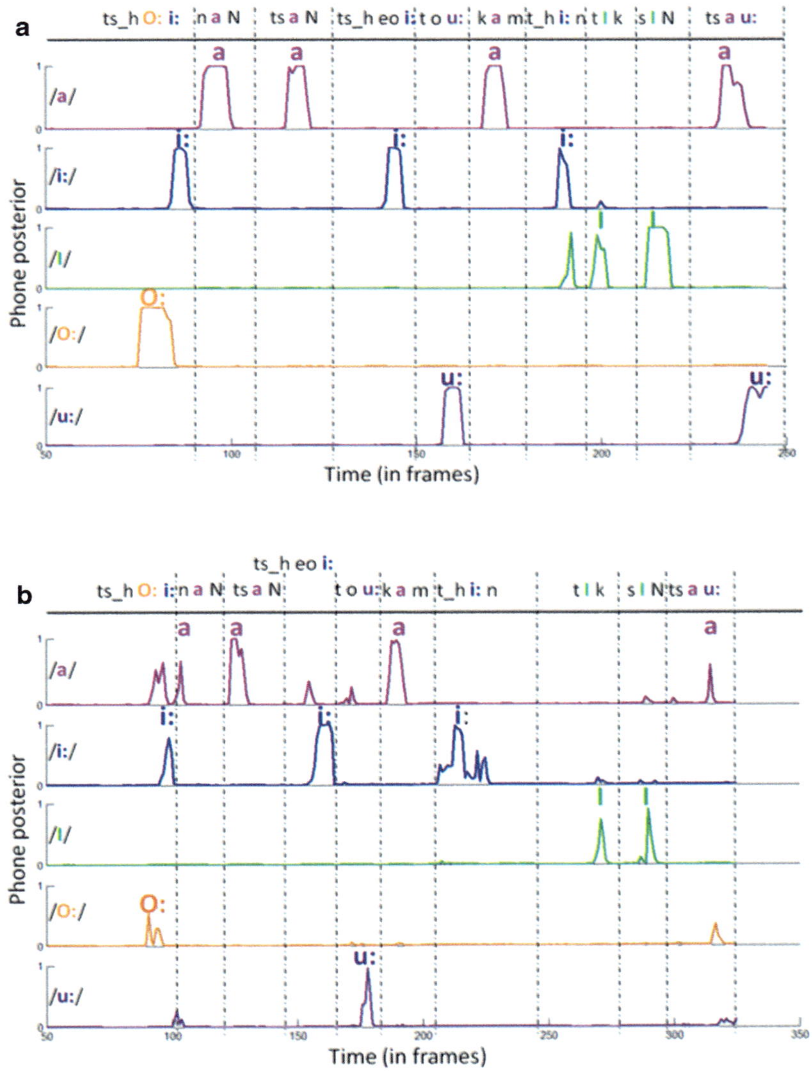

Fig. 16.2 Plots of frame-level phone posteriors on five selected vowels in example utterances from speakers with (**a**) mild voice disorder and (**b**) severe voice disorder [8]

semantic word categories, designated grammatical constituents, and LIWC (Linguistic Inquiry and Word Count) word categories. Text features learned by neural network models have gained tremendous success in recent years. Word embedding approaches, for example, Word2Vec [6] and GloVe [10], were investigated on modeling transcription of narrative speech from impaired speakers.

Figure 16.3a, b show examples of discourse-level vector representations from people with aphasia and normal speakers [6], respectively. The vector representations are derived from syllable-level embeddings learned using the Word2Vec model. The high-dimensional vectors are projected to two-dimensional feature space for visualization purpose. Different colors are used to represent the seven different narrative tasks. It is obviously seen that, for spoken discourse produced by unimpaired speaker, discourse-level vectors computed on different narrative tasks can be clearly separated from each other. Whilst for impaired speech, there is a noticeable degree of overlap among discourse-level vectors. This is related to the fact that speech from impaired speakers contains very few task-

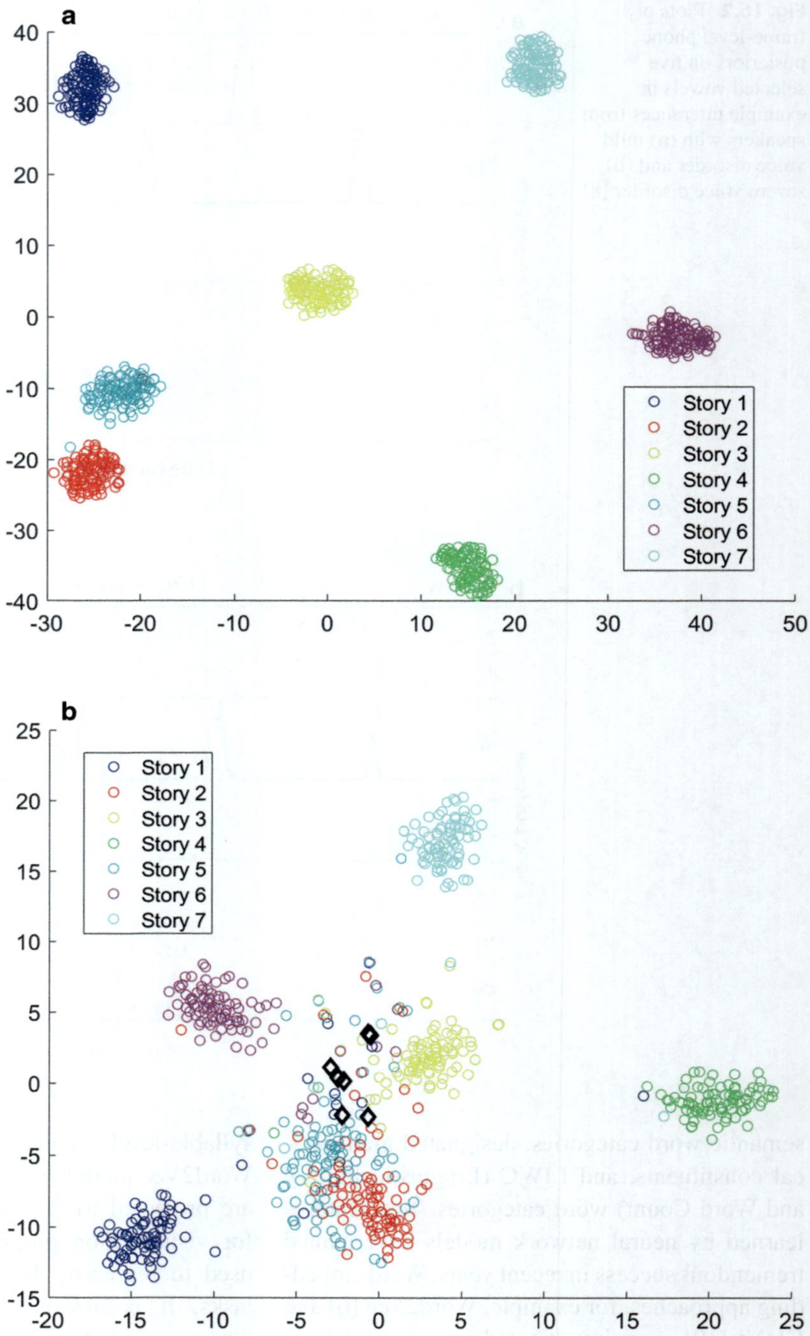

Fig. 16.3 Two-dimensional visualization of discourse-level vectors based on (**a**) manual transcription of unimpaired speech, (**b**) manual transcription of impaired speech. Different colors illustrate different topics of narrative tasks. The black diamond symbols in (**b**) mark the discourse-level vectors from a specific speaker, who was diagnosed as Broca's aphasia with AQ value of 42.0 [6]

specific content words. Specifically, the discourse-level vector representations obtained from an impaired speaker with Broca's aphasia (AQ: 42.0 out of 100), which are marked by black diamonds in Fig. 16.2b, can be hardly separated. Speech from this speaker contains almost only non-content words. Text features that capture such discrepancy between impaired and normal speakers are extracted for the purpose of detecting language impairment. In [6], it was shown that rich representations of ASR outputs could mitigate the impact of ASR errors on text feature extraction.

Pre-trained language models such as BERT and BERT-like models have pushed further the capabilities of data-driven language models. With relatively small amount of domain-specific data, these models can be fine-tuned to accomplish various downstream tasks, including extraction of impairment-related text features. In [11, 12], word embeddings derived from BERT-like models were applied to automatic assessment of Alzheimer's Disease (AD) and showed better performance than Word2Vec.

Given a large collection of text and acoustic features, effective methods of feature selection are needed. Correlation analysis can be carried out between the candidate features and ground-truth labels, for example, neuropsychology test scores. As a result, a low-dimension feature representation is constructed as the input to a classification model for detecting the existence of impairment or determining type/severity level, or a regression model for predicting severity score. Commonly used machine learning models for classification and regression include multi-layer perceptron, support vector machine, random forest, etc.

End-to-End Approach

Two-step approaches are knowledge driven, with powerful machine learning models performing classification or regression tasks with hand-drafted speech and language features. These features are designed and selected based on expert knowledge. Their coverage and scope are limited by human knowledge. There may exist useful impairment-related characteristics in raw speech data not being captured by these features. In addition, feature design and modeling are dealt with separately. Compared with two-step approaches, end-to-end approaches aim at establishing a mapping directly from impaired speech to assessment result. With proper design of neural network models, detection, classification, or regression of impaired speech are made more efficient without explicit feature extraction and feature selection. In this way, feature design and assessment model can be jointly optimized in neural network model training, and feature extraction is fully data-driven without human effort.

Existing end-to-end approaches to speech and language assessment are divided into text-based end-to-end assessment, and speech-based end-to-end assessment. Text-based systems extract impairment-related features from transcription of input speech for assessment purpose. Strictly speaking, they are not in the full "end-to-end" manner as an ASR system is needed to generate transcription from input speech. Convolutional Neural Network (CNN) [13] and pre-trained BERT-like models [14] were adopted to develop text-based end-to-end assessment systems for aphasia and AD, respectively. To alleviate the effect of ASR errors, rich representations of ASR output such as confusion network and confidence scores were incorporated into end-to-end assessment models [13, 14].

Speech-based end-to-end approaches are exemplified as shown in Fig. 16.4. It is a real "end-to-end" approach, which derives assessment result from raw speech. Previous studies used waveform or spectrogram of impaired utterances as input to CNNs. The CNNs generate assessment results for people with AD [16] and people with aphasia [17], respectively. Lacking impaired speech data for model training is a major obstacle to the development of speech-based end-to-end assessment system. Recently, self-supervised pre-training models such as wav-2vec have demonstrated good success in ASR and other speech signal processing applications. After self-supervised learning based on a large amount of task-independent speech, pre-trained models can learn much prior knowledge of acoustic and semantic information that can be transferred to downstream tasks. Pre-trained models have led to extensive research on end-to-end assessment for pathological speech. Wav2vec2.0 models based on an additional ASR pre-training were applied to downstream assessment task for people with AD [15] and showed superior performance than CNNs on the same

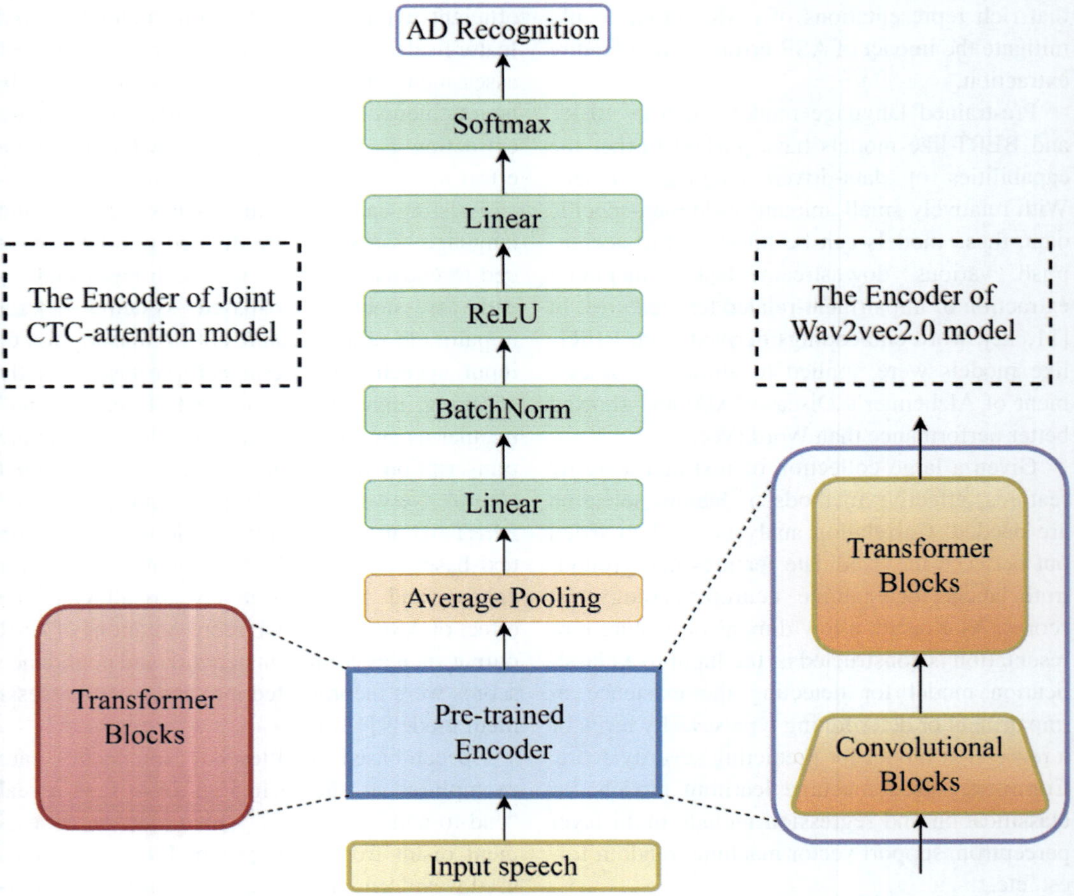

Fig. 16.4 The end-to-end AD recognition model that leverages the pre-trained wav2vec2.0 (right) [15]

task. The right-hand side of Fig. 16.4 illustrates the architecture of end-to-end AD recognition model that leverages the pre-trained wav2vec2.0.

Despite the demonstrated successes, end-to-end assessment approaches are criticized of being "black box." Features learned by neural networks could not be related to clinical observations and the assessment results may not be convincing and useful from clinical or pathological perspectives. Some efforts have been made to explore the explanation of features learned by neural networks. The Class Activation Mapping (CAM) method [17] was used to visualize and interpret features that were implicitly learned by the CNN model. Given a 15-s speech segment from a speaker with aphasia scoring 74.2/100 in AQ, Fig. 16.5 shows the utterance-level (3-s) scores and CAM visualization generated by the CNN model. In Fig. 16.5a, lower utterance-level score represents the utterance contributing more to the class of low AQ. In Fig. 16.5b, blue areas indicate regions having negative influence on the class of high AQ, while red color means the CNN model tend to classify the utterance as high AQ. Silence parts are highlighted as negative in blue, while speech parts are as positive activation in red. Utterances with longer pauses tend to have lower classification scores from CNN model. In addition, the magnitudes of positive activation (red) are found to be higher at the transition regions between speech parts and silence parts. Thus, speakers who have high speaking rate with many transitions in their speech have a higher probability to be classified as high AQ class. These observations confirm that the CNN model can learn

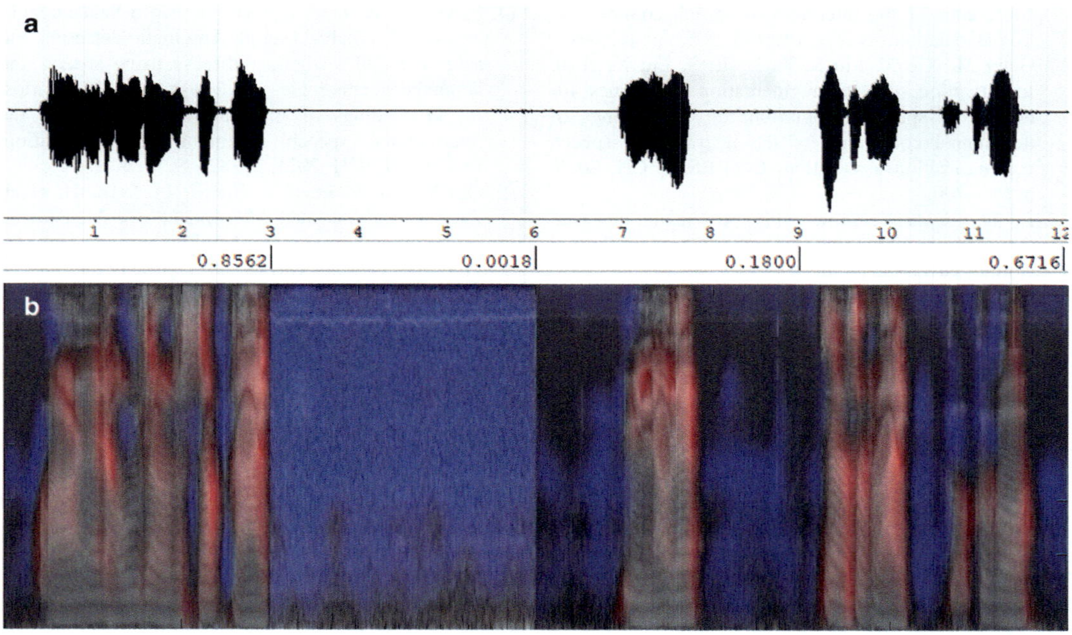

Fig. 16.5 Utterance-level scores and CAM visualization of the same speech segment from a speaker with aphasia scoring 74.2/100 in AQ. The positive and negative activations for high AQ class are highlighted in red and blue colors, respectively [17]

impairment-related features that are similar to human-designed features such as duration of silence segments and speaking rate.

End-to-end approach provides a promising way to efficiently process speech data and implicitly learn task-specific features from speech data. While it is believed that the attempt to applying end-to-end model to automatic assessment is meaningful, there is a long way to go before meaningful practical applications can be developed. Close collaboration and interaction between SLPs and speech engineers beyond merely data exchange are needed.

Major Takeaways

1. Machine Learning (ML) techniques can be used to "mine" high-dimensional sets of features from language to find those associated with a disease state.
2. ML models can be evaluated using different performance metrics, and it is important to understand how these are calculated to ensure effective reporting for a dataset.
3. There are a myriad of features that can be computed from a speech sample, providing information about different linguistic domains—which of these are of interest will depend on the question at hand.
4. There are some brilliant open-source ML and NLP (natural language processing) tools, as well as resources to learn to use them, but users should take care to understand how features are calculated when using "off-the-shelf" tools.
5. It is important to be aware of wider issues regarding how research using ML techniques, and speech, can impact society.

References

1. Kertesz A. Western aphasia battery—Revised. PsychCorp; 2007.
2. Sriranjani R, Ramasubba Reddy M, Umesh S. Improved acoustic modeling for automatic dysarthric speech recognition. In: 2015 21st national conference on communications, NCC 2015. 2015. p. 1–6.
3. Kim MJ, Yoo J, Kim H. Dysarthric speech recognition using dysarthria-severity-dependent and speaker-adaptive models. In: Proceedings of the annual

conference of the international speech communication association, INTERSPEECH. 2013. p. 3622–6.
4. Geng M, Xie X, Liu S, Yu J, Hu S, Liu X, et al. Investigation of data augmentation techniques for disordered speech recognition. In: Proceedings of the annual conference of the international speech communication association, INTERSPEECH. 2020. p. 696–700.
5. Le D, Licata K, Mower PE. Automatic quantitative analysis of spontaneous aphasic speech. Speech Comm. 2018;100:1–12.
6. Qin Y, Lee T, Kong APH. Automatic assessment of speech impairment in Cantonese-speaking people with aphasia. IEEE J Select Topics Signal Process. 2020;14(2):331–45.
7. Le D, Provost EM. Improving automatic recognition of aphasic speech with AphasiaBank. In: Proceedings of the annual conference of the international speech communication association, INTERSPEECH. 2016. p. 2681–5.
8. Liu Y, Lee T, Law T, Lee KYS. Acoustical assessment of voice disorder with continuous speech using ASR posterior features. IEEE/ACM Trans Audio Speech Lang Process. 2019;27(6):1047–59.
9. Laaridh I, Kheder W ben, Fredouille C, Meunier C. Automatic prediction of speech evaluation metrics for dysarthric speech. In: Proceedings of the annual conference of the international speech communication association, INTERSPEECH. 2017. p. 1834–8.
10. Mirheidari B, Blackburn D, Walker T, Venneri A, Reuber M, Christensen H. Detecting signs of dementia using word vector representations. In: Proceedings of the annual conference of the international speech communication association, INTERSPEECH. 2018. p. 1893–7.
11. Syed MSS, Syed ZS, Lech M, Pirogova E. Automated screening for Alzheimer's dementia through spontaneous speech. In: Proceedings of the annual conference of the international speech communication association, INTERSPEECH. 2020. p. 2222–6.
12. Pompili A, Rolland T, Abad A. The INESC-ID multi-modal system for the ADReSS 2020 challenge. In: Proceedings of the annual conference of the international speech communication association, INTERSPEECH. 2020. p. 2202–2206.
13. Qin Y, Lee T, Kong APH. Automatic assessment of language impairment based on raw ASR output. In: Proceedings of the annual conference of the international speech communication association, INTERSPEECH. 2019. p. 3078–82.
14. Pappagari R, Cho J, Joshi S, Moro-Velazquez L, Zelasko P, Villalba J, et al. Automatic detection and assessment of Alzheimer disease using speech and language technologies in low-resource scenarios. In: Proceedings of the annual conference of the international speech communication association, INTERSPEECH. 2021. p. 3825–9.
15. Qin Y, Liu W, Peng Z, Ng SI, Li J, Hu H, et al. Exploiting pre-trained ASR models for Alzheimer's disease recognition through spontaneous speech. In: Proceedings of NCMMSC. 2021. p. 917–28.
16. Cummins N, Pan Y, Ren Z, Fritsch J, Nallanthighal VS, Christensen H, et al. A comparison of acoustic and linguistics methodologies for Alzheimer's dementia recognition. In: Proceedings of the annual conference of the international speech communication association, INTERSPEECH. 2020. p. 2182–6.
17. Qin Y, Wu Y, Lee T, Kong APH. An end-to-end approach to automatic speech assessment for Cantonese-speaking people with aphasia. J Signal Process Syst. 2020;92(8):819–30.

Ying Qin is a Lecturer in the Institute of Information Science, School of Computer and Information Technology at Beijing Jiaotong University. She received her Ph.D. degree in Electronic Engineering, Department of Electronic Engineering, The Chinese University of Hong Kong. Her research interests mainly focus on automatic speech assessment, automatic speech recognition, and machine learning with applications on pathological speech.

Tan Lee is a Professor at the Department of Electronic Engineering, The Chinese University of Hong Kong. His research interests include speech and audio signal processing, spoken language technology, deep learning models for speech and language, paralinguistics in speech, and neurological basis of speech and language. Prof. Lee's recent work is focused on applying signal processing and machine learning methods to the classification and generation of atypical speech in challenging communication scenarios across different speaker populations. Prof. Lee was an Associate Editor for the IEEE/ACM Transactions on Audio, Speech, and Language Processing, an Area Chair of the Technical Programme Committees of INTERSPEECH 2014, 2016, and 2018, and the General Co-Chair of ISCSLP 2018 and 2021. He was the Vice Chair of ISCA Special Interest Group on Chinese Spoken Language Processing.

Machine Learning, Features, and Computational Approaches to Discourse Analysis

17

Natasha Clarke and Peter Garrard

Preview of What Is Currently Known

Neurogenic diseases can give rise to a wide variety of linguistic changes, which computational approaches have been harnessed to identify and classify. In particular, natural language processing (NLP) is a powerful set of techniques that can be used to quantify semantic, syntactic and lexical features of discourse, while machine learning (ML) tools can be used to make classifications and predictions based on these features. The approaches have furthered our understanding of how discourse changes in the face of neurological disorders, especially dementia, and the extent to which they may serve as "digital biomarkers" of disease. NLP and ML continue to provide novel insights and find new applications as technological advances lead to improvements in the speed and accuracy of these computational tools.

Objectives

(a) To present core concepts of machine learning (ML) algorithms and pitfalls when training models
(b) To explain how ML can be used to classify groups
(c) To review common metrics for reporting ML performance and how they are calculated
(d) To present key preprocessing steps in analysis of transcribed speech
(e) To summarize lexical, syntactic, entropic, and word-embedding features that can be calculated from speech
(f) To review different categories of discourse and how these are operationalized in research settings
(g) To describe some of the current tools available for computation of features and conducting ML studies
(h) To discuss current wider issues facing the field, including bias in data, trust in ML, and regulation

Introduction

In Shakespeare's *Twelfth Night*, Feste disguises himself as a priest, while *As You Like It* has Rosalind pretending to be a boy pretending to be Rosalind. Even more confusing has been the debate over the identity of Shakespeare himself, in which one side has argued that the true author used the name as a disguise, and that "Shakespeare of Stratford" was someone else entirely. The debate began on the basis of historical records, but later adopted quantitative linguistic methods,

N. Clarke
Centre de recherche de l'Institut universitaire de gériatrie de Montréal, Montreal, Canada

P. Garrard (✉)
Molecular and Clinical Sciences Research Institute, St George's University of London, London, UK
e-mail: pgarrard@sgul.ac.uk

A. P.-H. Kong (ed.), *Spoken Discourse Impairments in the Neurogenic Populations*,
https://doi.org/10.1007/978-3-031-45190-4_17

comparing the size of Shakespeare's (or "Shakespeare's") vocabulary with those of his contemporaries. The digital revolution changed the terms of the debate entirely by allowing larger quantities of machine-readable texts to be rapidly analyzed and painstaking counting of individual word types to be replaced by the rapid calculation of novel textual metrics.

It was soon realized that the same set of techniques could be harnessed to study the language of people with neurological impairment. One of the most celebrated studies focused on Iris Murdoch, the prolific twentieth century novelist who was diagnosed with Alzheimer's disease in her mid 70 s, but whose written vocabulary was becoming depleted even before symptoms emerged [1]. Subsequent developments in the use of connected speech as a disease biomarker include the incorporation of machine learning (ML) into the analytical armamentarium.

Core Principles of Machine Learning

ML refers to a powerful set of computational techniques that are able to automatically recognize patterns in data. Given a dataset of individuals, each with a corresponding *N*-dimensional vector of phenotypic features and associated values (*X*), different types of algorithm can be used to find patterns associated with group membership, latent variables, and continuous outcomes.

Supervised and Unsupervised Learning

When the ground-truth associated with each individual in the dataset is known (e.g., presence or absence of disease, sometimes referred to as the class label), supervised learning algorithms can be used to predict this "target" (*y*). Binary classification tasks are most common, comparing a group with a known-diagnosis to a suitable control group usually composed of neurotypical, healthy persons, but multiclass classification, for example, comparing groups with different diseases or at different stages in a disease, can also be employed. An algorithm or set of algorithms can be used to inductively associate aberrant feature values with group membership via an iterative process: each instance is classified as belonging to a group, with weights assigned to each feature. The power of these combined weights to predict labels of unseen instances is tested, and weights updated according to performance when compared to the ground-truth label, until optimal performance is achieved. The same logic applies in regression tasks, in which the aim is to find an equation that enables a set of features to predict the value of an unknown, continuous variable.

Common algorithms used in classification tasks include the following:

(i) Decision trees, which can be thought of as akin to a flowchart with a series of decisions made leading to classification output.
(ii) Logistic regression, in which a threshold is applied to the output of a regression algorithm in order to assign group membership.
(iii) Distance-based maximum-margin classifiers such as support vector machines [2].

The majority of ML studies utilizing discourse features adopt a supervised approach since commonly ground-truth labels are known [3]. Unsupervised learning, by contrast, requires no ground-truth to be associated with each feature vector. Rather, an algorithm is used to find any latent patterns or structure underlying the data. For example, clustering algorithms aim to group X so that similarity of features within each cluster is maximized, but between different clusters is minimized.

Feature Importance as a Window on Disease

Once an algorithm has been trained the weights that have come to be associated with each feature can be examined, providing data-driven insights into discourse impairments that characterize a disease [4]. This is particularly useful as a method to search or "mine" high-dimensional data, which is difficult using univariate statistics [5]. However, some ML approaches resemble "black boxes," offering no insights into the basis on which a decision was reached [6]. This is particularly true of deep learning (also referred to as neural networks), a subset of ML algorithms that comprise multiple interconnected representational layers that encode complex interactions among features [2]. This property means that the weights are not susceptible to any sort of meaningful analysis, limiting their usefulness for furthering understanding of disease. The trade-off for this lack of interpretability is usually improved performance though a greater amount of data is required for effective deep learning compared to algorithms with only one layer.

Pitfalls in Machine Learning

Different Performance Metrics for Different Questions (and Data)

Crucially, performance must be evaluated on "held-out" data, testing how generalizable weights are to data unseen during training. Ideally, this test set would be collected independently of the training set since differences can arise in data collected at different sites. Datasets can also be randomly split into training and test sets (e.g., 80/20 split), ideally with a separate validation set depending on the size. The question of how to measure performance is not necessarily straightforward. In classification tasks, there are multiple metrics that can be used to judge effectiveness, and the choice of which to maximize often depends on the question at hand. Metrics are calculated by comparing the prediction for each individual in the test set to the ground-truth label, which can then be categorized as a true-positive (TP), false-positive (FP), true-negative (TN), or false-negative (FN), depicted in the confusion matrix seen in Fig. 17.1.

A few key, common performance metrics (i.e., measures) to estimate the accuracy of ML include:

(i) Sensitivity (also termed recall)—the true-positive rate, given by [TP/(TP + FN)]
(ii) Specificity—the true-negative rate, given by [TN/(TN + FP)]
(iii) Overall accuracy, calculated as the total percentage of true-positives and true-negatives, i.e., all correct test set results
(iv) Precision—the number of instances in the test set labeled positive which are indeed positive, given by [TP/(TP + FP)]
(v) F1, the harmonic mean of precision and recall, a useful indication of the balance between the two

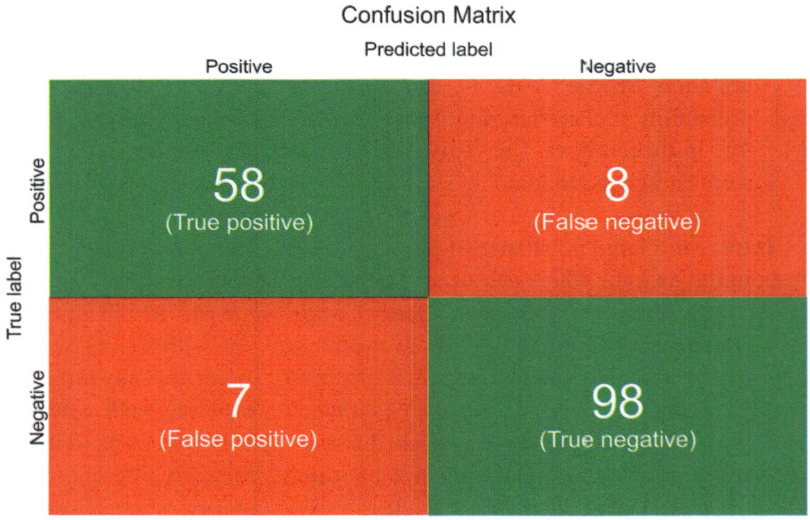

Fig. 17.1 Confusion matrix showing predicted labels against true labels, with true positives and true negatives in green and false positives and false negatives in red. *Note:* Results of classification task using a toy dataset

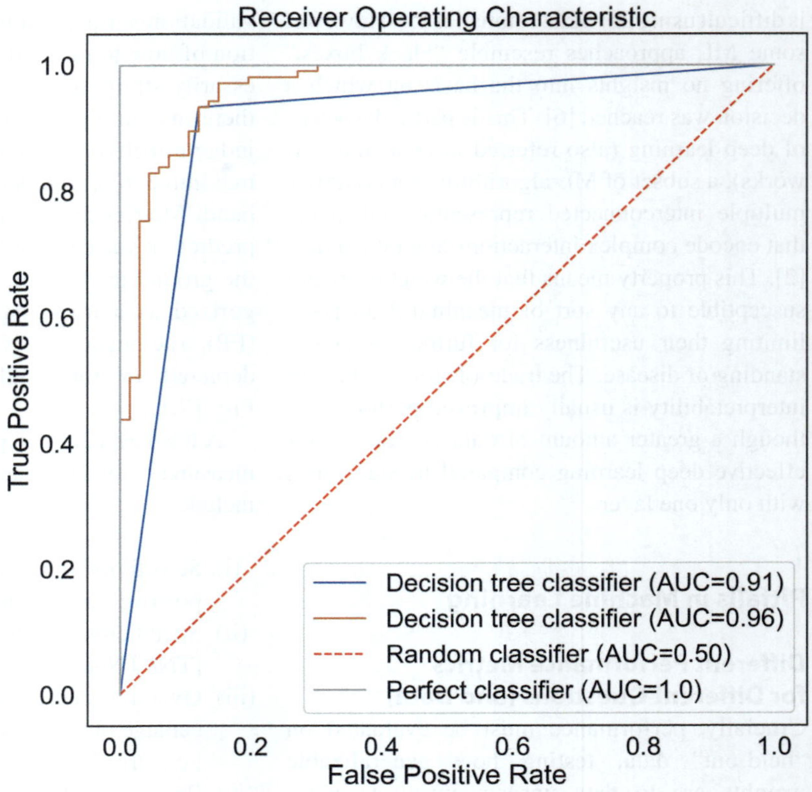

Fig. 17.2 Receiver Operating Characteristic showing performance of two classifiers, perfect and random classification. *Note:* AUC = area under the curve. For the same toy data results as seen in Fig. 17.1

(vi) ROC-AUC—the area under the curve (AUC) of the receiver operating characteristic (ROC), a result of sensitivity and specificity plotted at different thresholds. Often reported more simply as the AUC, this single number between zero and one represents classifier performance where 0.5 indicates chance level (Fig. 17.2). An intuitive interpretation of the AUC is that it is the probability a classifier would score a positive instance above a negative one, if both were chosen at random.

If there is a large imbalance of cases and controls in the dataset, which can occur particularly when a disease is rare, then use of generic accuracy to measure performance becomes meaningless. One useful metric in this scenario is balanced accuracy, which decreases if accuracy is inflated only due to superior performance on the over-represented class, otherwise it remains the same [7]. The AUC also remains robust to class imbalance since it reflects sensitivity and specificity, regardless of class distribution.

If the cost of mislabeling a false-negative or false-positive is not equal, then either sensitivity or specificity can be maximized. For example, two real-world applications of ML in the field of neurodegeneration are (i) identification of patients with a disease who may be suitable for trials of novel therapies, and (ii) widespread screening in the community, to identify individuals with an increased risk of the disease who could undergo further tests. In the first application, the cost of a false-positive is high, since if we include people in the trial who do not actually have the disease, a drug being tested will fail and the person will have been exposed to a novel therapy without any potential benefit. In this case, we want to maximize specificity. In the second example, both a false-positive and false-negative will have costs to the screened individual though they are different in kind, and—absent the availability of any disease treatment—to be told you have an untreatable and life-changing disease when you do not have would be infinitely worse than being falsely reassured for a year or two, or possibly longer.

Cross-Validation

Due to the nature and costs involved in clinical data collection, datasets available are often small. In these cases, instead of relying on one split of data, cross-validation can be used. Data is split into a number of subsets, usually 10, called "folds," and each fold used for either training or testing of the algorithm over the same number of iterations (Fig. 17.3). The final model performance is evaluated as an average across all permutations of the data. Stone [8] has shown that cross-validation can ensure a more robust estimate of performance than a single train/test split, and each instance can be used to both train and test the data though never within the same fold, as this would lead to "leakage" of unseen test set information. Also to prevent leakage, preprocessing steps such as normalization—an important transform that enables direct comparison of features regardless of scale—should be conducted within each fold. Other cross-validation approaches include leave-one-out cross-validation, in which an algorithm is trained on the whole dataset minus one instance, and leave-pair-out. Additionally, ideally only the features of interest would be associated with the target value, but in practice, unless a dataset is matched, other variables such as age and gender may also be overrepresented in one group, which an algorithm would then weight more heavily. To try and help balance these and other (sometimes unknown) confounds, splitting of data must be randomized.

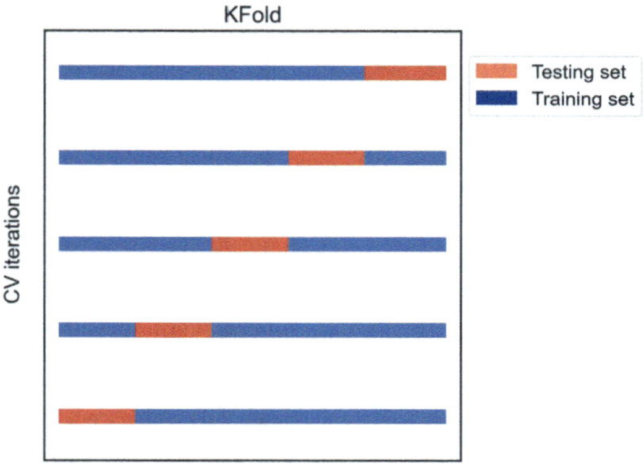

Fig. 17.3 K-fold cross-validation where $k = 5$. *Note:* The dataset is split into five sets of training and test data

Generalization

The "fit" of a model is paramount (Fig. 17.4). Underfitting leads to poor performance on both the training and test sets, which can occur if a model is too simple to explain variance in the target outcome. Conversely, if a model overfits then performance will be good on the training set, but poor on the test set. In these cases, the model is

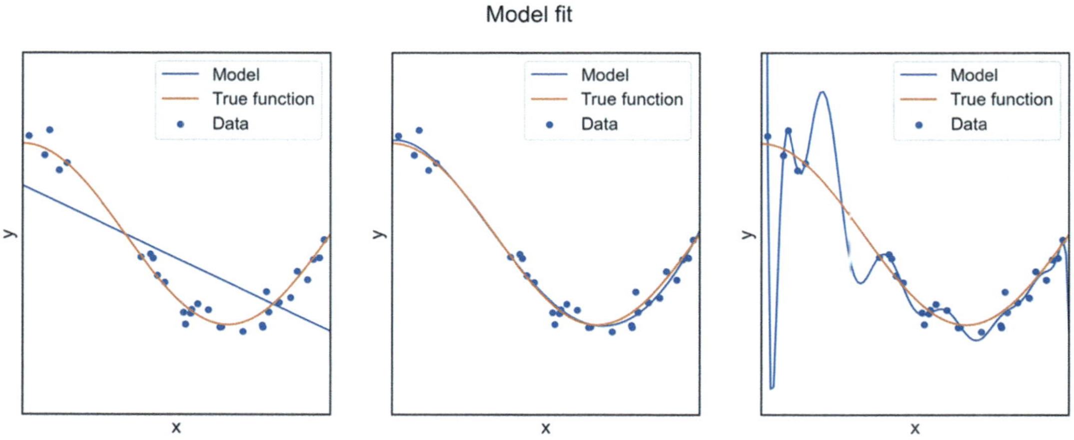

Fig. 17.4 Illustrations of model fit, visualizing underfitting, good fit, and overfitting, respectively. *Note:* All figures created using Python and scikit-learn [9, 10]

likely highly tuned to the samples in the training set, for example, if a model is too complex, and so the feature weights do not generalize well to unseen data. The type of algorithm and feature set size used will influence model fit [2].

For example, for high-dimensional data, when the number of features is close to or larger than the number of observations (i.e., $X \geq y$), they can suffer from the "curse of dimensionality," as noise and redundancy of features increases with the number of features. Dimensionality reduction and feature selection steps can be added to the algorithm to help reduce overfitting and improve speed and performance.

Natural Language Processing for Analysis of Spoken Discourse

Natural Language Processing (NLP) is an area of research and application in which computational approaches are used to model natural human language, informed by multiple schools including psychology, linguistics, engineering, and artificial intelligence [11]. Techniques and tools, seen everywhere from translation to home devices, can be used in research, assessment, and remote monitoring of patients, the need for which was heightened during the recent pandemic. Text can be preprocessed and a multitude of features spanning different linguistic domains automatically computed at speed and low cost, a process which will be described next.

Key Preprocessing Steps

Transcription

To analyze properties of discourse, as opposed to pure acoustic features of a sample, it must be available in transcribed form. During or after transcription, only speech pertaining to the individual of interest can be retained, excluding for example a conversational partner, unless such additional information is necessary for computation of features. Traditionally transcription has been done manually, which is labor intensive, costly, and open to human error. In the case where more than one transcriber works on a dataset, it is possible to compute the level of agreement between them, for example, calculating the Levenshtein similarity on a subset of overlapping transcripts [12]; see [13] for an example.

One core goal of NLP is accurate automatic speech recognition (ASR), which can be found in many mobile applications. While a lower cost and much less time-intensive option, accuracy of the technology remains, at the time of writing, problematic, particularly for populations experiencing dysarthria or highly disordered speech. Additionally, neologisms, which are likely to be of interest clinically, may be automatically corrected by the software. Once speech has been adequately transcribed, a key step in analysis is tokenization.

Tokenization

Tokenization is the process of automatically segmenting individual sentences and words into smaller, meaningful tokens. For example, *hasn't* is segmented into *has* and *n't*, and *he'll* into *he* and *'ll*. As such, punctuation and the surrounding context are key; while most periods in a string likely represent a sentence boundary, the ones in *Ph.D.* do not [14]. Tokenizing approaches include regular-expression-based rules, and ML approaches, such as the "PunktSentenceTokenizer," part of the open-source Python library Natural Language Toolkit (NLTK) [15], trained to detect sentence boundaries using the 4.5 million word Penn Treebank Corpus [16].

Part-of-Speech (POS) Tagging

Following tokenization each token can be automatically "tagged" with a label indicating its usage in the speech sample. As with tokenizing, context is important since a word can have multiple tags depending on its usage, for example, the word *match* can function as a noun in the string "a boxing match," or verb in "the jacket and trousers don't match." In fact, up to 20% of words in the English language can have multiple tags, and given the frequency with which they occur, it is estimated that 55–67% of words in a text would be ambiguous without context [14]. In other words, assigning correct tags is non-trivial.

A common set of tags to use is the Penn Treebank, which includes 45 different tags according to grammatical use such as verbs (e.g., "drink"), and subtypes such as past verbs ("drank") and gerunds ("drinking").

As with tokenization, different approaches can be applied. The ML-based NLTK "PerceptronTagger" was trained to predict tags for tokens in the Wall Street Journal corpus and assigns tags to new data based on probability given features of each token, with an accuracy of up to 97% [17]. Thus, tagging provides useful information not just about single words, but also those surrounding them.

Lemmatization

Lemmatization is a technique for normalizing text which maps a word to its lemma or base form, free from inflection. For example, the lemma of "Thought," "Thinking," and "Thinks" is "Think." Lemmas are always words found in the dictionary, unlike a word's stem. Automatic lemmatization relies not only on word meaning, but its POS tag, and as such lemmas reflect the meaning of a content word in its given context [14].

Parsing

Parsing is the process of deconstructing a sentence according to its structure and the relationships between words, governed by the rules of a language. In the most common approach, grammar rules are used to determine the syntactic structure of a sentence, resulting in a parse tree made up of clauses, sub-clauses, and their syntactic relationships, which can be visualized and analyzed using different techniques to assess complexity.

Computation of Features

Vocabulary

As with the first attempts at summarizing Shakespeare's writing, analysis of a person's vocabulary—i.e., the specific words they use—can reveal a great deal. Comparison to expected norms for the language of interest, or how an individual's vocabulary changes over time, can give insights into overall cognition and mental state. Vocabulary is measured under the "bag-of-words" assumption, in which the order of production of words is disregarded, and only their individual lexical and grammatical properties assessed [14]. An important distinction is between content and function words, also referred to as open and closed class, respectively, since new content words can be added to the group, unlike function words which rarely increase in number. Content words provide meaning to language, such as nouns, verbs, and adjectives, while function words act as the linguistic scaffold, providing structure irrespective of content, such as conjunctions and determiners.

One approach to analyzing vocabulary is calculating the type-token ratio (TTR), in which the number of unique content words in a sample (types) are compared to the total number of words used (tokens). This can be problematic when samples are of different lengths, a limitation somewhat mitigated by different approaches such as the Moving-Average Type Token Ratio (MATTR), calculated over a sliding window, Brunet's Index, and Honore's statistic [18, 19].

Lexical and Psycholinguistic Properties of Discourse

Content words have inherent psycholinguistic properties. These phenomena, associated with word use in the lexicon, can indicate lexical sophistication and include the frequency, imageability, concreteness, age-of-acquisition, and familiarity of a word. Some are estimated through human ratings, such as imageability (how easy is it to conjure an image of a word in your mind?), concreteness (can we easily see, hear, feel, smell, or touch it, or is it more abstract?), and familiarity (how often do we come across the word?). Others, such as the frequency of a word, are estimated through reference to large corpora, such as the British National Corpus, a collection of 100 million words of spoken and written language, or the SUBTLEXus corpus, a collection of subtitles from film and television [20].

When analyzing psycholinguistics, words should be lemmatized (see above); otherwise, the usage of a word in a sample could be underestimated. Other caveats are that different properties are interrelated, for example "table" occurs at high frequency, is acquired at an early age and is concrete, so researchers must take care if aiming to analyze one distinct property. Furthermore, values change with fashions in word usage, particularly for word frequency, and low frequency words are typically underrepresented in corpora [21].

Syntactic Complexity

Approaches that utilize a syntactic parse tree to analyze complexity include the mean length of sentences and clauses [22], and more complex methods such as Yngve or Frazier scoring, which calculate the depth of a tree to capture information about subordinate clauses (the presence of which would indicate greater complexity). The Yngve method assigns a score to each branch in the parse tree, starting at zero and increasing from right to left, before calculating a score for each word in the tree by summing the branches "stacked" on it. Summary metrics such as the mean score per word indicate the complexity of the sample [23]. The Frazier method traces a path from each word, applying a series of stopping criteria, and summing scores along the path for each branch [24].

Word Embeddings

Word embeddings are N-dimensional vector representations of words embedded in a semantic space. The space is built using word co-occurrences in a large corpus to capture meaning, the core idea is captured by Firth who observed that "You shall know a word by the company it keeps" [25]. The mathematical properties of embeddings, highlighted in a common example in which the vectors for *king - man + woman = queen*, can be useful for calculating the "average" meaning of a sentence. The pioneering approach to build embeddings, latent semantic analysis (LSA), derives vector dimensions from the fact that (i) particular groups of words tend to occur together (or not) across contexts, and (ii) there are associations between words that appear in contexts that are similar in meaning [26]. For example, the words "clinician" and "physician" will have vectors close together, since they occur in the same kinds of document with other similar words, and are semantically similar.

Neural approaches build embeddings by training a language model on local windows of text, predicting either a word given its context (continuous bag-of-words model) or context given a target word (skip-gram model). The weights assigned to features during training then represent the word embedding. The first approach of this type, word2vec, offers three-million pre-trained embeddings for words and phrases, each of 300 dimensions, built using the Google News dataset [27]. Other neural approaches include BERT (Bidirectional Encoder Representations from Transformer), which achieved state-of-the-art performance on NLP tasks when released [28], and more contemporary, computationally expensive language models such as GPT-3. A few caveats for word embeddings is that words should be lemmatized, which could otherwise impact results [29], and that homonyms and homographs (words with multiple meanings for the same spelling) have only one embedding. As such, the embedding for "pen" is a representation of all possible meanings, including a writing instrument and to enclose an animal, likely weighted according to the frequency of use.

Coherence and Cohesion

Semantic coherence - that is, how well a theme or series of themes is maintained - is an inherent property of discourse that can improve the ability of a listener to follow along [30]. Coherence can be studied at the local level, such as between adjacent sentences, or globally, analyzing maintenance of a theme across a whole sample of discourse. Cohesion is an objective property of individual words, and cohesive devices, such as anaphora—words which refer back to a preceding clause—can improve the coherence of speech [31].

Word Embeddings for Analysis of Coherence

Since word embeddings convey semantic information, they can be used to measure coherence using distance metrics. A common approach is to calculate the cosine of the angle between two vectors (or average vectors) to determine the degree to which they are pointing in the same direction [32]. The word movers distance can also be calculated, finding the minimum cumulative distance required to move between all embeddings in one document (or sentence) to another [33]. This approach obviates the necessity to first average the vectors in a sentence or window, and so may retain more information [13]. Metrics can also be calculated over sliding windows to investigate fine-grained local coherence, and to disregard sentence boundaries, which may be unreliable in the transcription if an individual's ability to construct sentences is impaired.

Entropy and Perplexity

Entropy stems from information theory and was first applied to language by the American mathematician Claude Shannon [34]. Entropy is a measure of the degree of information inherent in each variable in a sequence, such as characters in a string, which in turn affects the predictability and complexity of the sequence. For example, in the sentence "The king married the q..." the unseen variable is undoubtedly a "u". Given this 100% probability, revealing the character does not reduce prior uncertainty of the string. The next character provides more information: the sequence could continue '*-een*, but other endings are possible (if less likely), such as "*-antum physicist*." Entropy therefore depends not just on the likelihood of co-occurrence of individual letters and words, but on higher order considerations such as grammatical correctness and context, making it impossible to quantify with precision. In practice, however, there are ways of estimating predictability for each character in a string, allowing the average Shannon entropy of a text to be found. A sequence with high entropy can be regarded as more unpredictable and complex, while low entropy values imply that a text is predictable, repetitive, and/or of low complexity.

Perplexity is closely related to entropy and is a measure of how accurately the distribution of *n*-grams (words, word-pairs, word-triplets, etc.) in a text predicts the next, unseen, word. Often used to measure the performance of a language model, better performing models, which predict the next word with high probability of being correct, will have lower perplexity [35].

Sentiment

One application of NLP is to quantify the sentiment of words and pieces of text, which can be used, for example, in classification algorithms to automatically identify positive or negative user reviews. These approaches have been utilized in clinical research, such as for detecting signs of depression and neurodegenerative disorders based on social media posts [36, 37].

Discourse Categories and Associated Features

Categorization of discourse can depend on the field of study, but here the focus is on the approach of Dipper and Pritchard [38], who describe many of the discourse tasks adopted in research settings. Expository discourse is produced when a person talks about their own experience, such as major life events or their experiences of an illness. Narrative discourse is the process of telling a story, and may be particularly useful in the study of features of coherence, since a series of ideas must be organized and expressed to maintain a consistent theme [39]. Descriptive discourse, such as describing a scene, has been well-studied in neurogenic populations since stimuli can be standardized. This can be particularly useful for analysis of vocabulary since responses can be compared to established lists of lexical items referenced by neurotypical speakers [40]. A common scene is the Cookie Theft description task, from the Boston Diagnostic Aphasia Examination (BDAE) [41]; see Chap. 6 for details on the TalkBank project which includes the DementiaBank, a large collection of picture descriptions [42]. The type of discourse may impact classification results and important features, and is therefore an important consideration when assessing disordered speech [13].

Bringing it all Together—Some Examples from the Literature

In this chapter, the focus is on Alzheimer's disease to highlight some interesting and novel approaches using the techniques described here, much of which are "disease-agnostic." Seminal work on classifying Alzheimer's disease based on speech demonstrated the power of combining multiple linguistic features with feature selection approaches to obtain optimal performance [43]. While most studies use supervised learning techniques to classify homogeneous datasets, an unsupervised clustering approach step prior to classification was found to distinguish dementia from depression in an aggregated "noisy" dataset of speech from individuals with one or other of these diagnoses, an important task given that symptoms can overlap [44].

Ablimit and colleagues [45] used a number of interesting techniques to analyze speech in Alzheimer's disease. Calculating consecutive cosine distances between different types of features at 1-min segments throughout interview transcripts, they showed that the variation in features within speaker samples was different. An oversampling approach was then used to overcome class imbalance in the dataset, and a deep neural network architecture compared to a baseline classification algorithm, with improved performance. Saliency maps, an approach adopted from image classification to decode important pixels in classification, were used to investigate important features, overcoming the "black box" limitation [45]. Other approaches to interpreting deep learning models are reviewed by Räuker et al. [46].

Finally, the 2020 Alzheimer's Dementia Recognition through Spontaneous Speech (ADReSS) Challenge made strides in furthering ML-based speech analysis in Alzheimer's disease. Researchers taking part had access to the same dataset, with a portion held back for testing, for either classification or regression models (predicting cognitive scores). Shared tasks such as this ensure that different methodologies are directly comparable across studies [47].

Do it Yourself—Tools for Computation and Analysis of Features

There are many freely available "no-code," user-friendly tools to get started on computation of features—all you need is some transcribed speech or text you want to analyze. The Word Embedding Analysis website from the University of Colorado Boulder enables document comparison based on word embeddings of different types [48], and the suite of automatic linguistic analysis tools, mainly developed by Kyle and Crossley, can be used to compute many different variables, including lexical sophistication, cohesion, and syntactic complexity [49]. The Lexical Complexity Analyzer (LCA) and L2 Syntactic Complexity Analyzer (L2SCA) compute variables stemming from the language development literature, and offer both a web-based application programming interface (API) and command-line interface for more control over analyses [22]. Linguistic Inquiry and Word Count (LIWC), while (at the time of writing) not freely available, also offers an easy-to-use API for calculation of many features of vocabulary and sentiment, scoring words according to annotated dictionaries to reflect psychological states [50]. It is important for users to understand what is going on "under the hood"—that is, exactly how the tool generates values given samples of discourse as input, and what each value represents. This can also help in spotting bugs, erroneous values, and guide important data cleaning decisions such as how to deal with missing data.

Python is an open-source coding language with numerous libraries that can be used to load discourse in different formats and carry out preprocessing and analysis [9]. NLTK, mentioned above, has many built-in functions that ensure steps such as tokenization can be completed for thousands of speech samples with a few lines of code, and the spaCy and gensim libraries can be used to work with word embeddings in particular [15, 51, 52]. This offers greater flexibility than no-code tools when working with discourse samples and can improve understanding of features, with intermediate outputs in steps of computation available for inspection.

For ML, the Python library sci-kit learn is available [10], with excellent documentation to guide users and built-in functions for dimensionality reduction, cross-fold validation and more, and other libraries can be used to visualize results. There is a wealth of online training available for those who have the opportunity to learn to code using tools such as Python or other languages (see "Resources" Section). It will likely pay dividends in the form of increased understanding of processes and enable greater sharing among the community of analysis pipelines, aiding in reproducibility. The Waikato Environment for Knowledge Analysis (WEKA) also provides a no-code, open-source option for ML [53].

Current Issues in Clinical Translation of Computational Approaches to Speech Analysis

The progress in computation which has enabled application of computational approaches to study speech has solved many issues that once faced the field, improving the speed, cost, and breadth of feature extraction. However, a number of factors now make clinical translation of algorithms challenging. Issues with generalizability can arise from multiple sources, including a lack of diversity across research volunteers (often fitting the "WEIRD" description—white, educated, industrialized, rich, and democratic [54]); pathological heterogeneity in clinical populations, such as Alzheimer's disease; the presence of comorbidities; and differences in the distribution of true positives and true negatives, for example, a lower prevalence of disease than that seen in training [55]. Moreover, language-specific factors such as regional accent and slang usage may impact performance even between different hospitals. Research using multisite and multilingual datasets has so far provided grounds for optimism [56, 57] and attempts at addressing the lack of diversity in datasets are being made at a high level [58].

A lack of trust in ML, from clinicians and patients, can also limit adoption of new tools. This is linked to model complexity and interpretability since opaque models are difficult to understand, making it challenging to explain results to patients. Conversely, trust can be improved by using transparent algorithms with greater "explainability" [59–61], and by reporting an algorithm's confidence in its decision [62]. In view of the fact that algorithms which underserve less-well represented communities will not foster trust, these issues are undoubtedly linked.

Major Takeaways

1. ML techniques can be used to "mine" high-dimensional sets of features from language to find those associated with a disease state.
2. ML models can be evaluated using different performance metrics, and it is important to understand how these are calculated to ensure effective analysis of a dataset.
3. There are myriad features that can be computed from a speech sample, providing information about different linguistic domains—which of these are of interest will depend on the question at hand.
4. There are some brilliant open-source ML and NLP tools, as well as resources to learn to use them, but users should take care to understand how features are calculated when using "off-the-shelf" tools.
5. It is important to be aware of wider issues regarding how research using ML techniques, and speech, can impact society.

Appendix: Additional Resources

Online Resources

Knowing at least some Python is usually a prerequisite to hands-on NLP analyses. All of these resources are freely available.

1. Machine learning
   (a) Machine Learning 101 from Jason Mayes. Covers what's in this chapter, with great examples, and more depth: https://docs.google.com/presentation/d/1kSuQyW5DTnkVaZEjGYCkfOxvzCqGEFzWBy4e9Uedd9k/edit#slide=id.g28f0b1f244_0_105
   (b) UC Boulder Applied Machine Learning lecture slides (2018). Provides a great summary of ML algorithms and concepts, with equations: https://cmci.colorado.edu/classes/INFO-4604/
   (c) Blog series by Jason Brownlee, explaining ML concepts and tools in an accessible way, with code: https://machinelearningmastery.com/
   (d) Sci-kit learn library user guide: https://scikit-learn.org/stable/user_guide.html
2. Learning Python
   (a) Modules of the Montreal Brainhack school (updated annually) which include videos, exercises, and links to further resources. See the Introduction to Python for data analysis and Writing scripts in Python modules, as well as machine learning basics. If you are new to Python, you can also follow the relevant parts of the Installation module: https://school--brainhack.github.io/modules/
   (b) Python docs tutorials: https://docs.python.org/3/tutorial/index.html
   (c) Tutorial on Jupyter notebooks, a powerful resource for interactive coding: https://www.dataquest.io/blog/jupyter-notebook-tutorial/
   (d) Beware of relying on notebooks for all tasks; they are a great "sand box," but see these slides by Joel Grus to understand their limitations (also presented in the Writing scripts in python module of the Brainhack school linked above): https://docs.google.com/presentation/d/1n2RlMdmv1p25Xy5thJUhkKGvjtV-dkAIsUXP-AL4ffI/edit#slide=id.g362da58057_0_1
3. Natural language processing
   (a) Speech and Language Processing 2023 book draft by Jarafsky & Martin, with slides for some chapters: https://web.stanford.edu/~jurafsky/slp3/
   (b) Berkley course (2021) slides and readings, an accessible overview of many NLP topics covered in this chapter, and more: https://people.ischool.berkeley.edu/~dbamman/info256.html
   (c) Fast AI course (2019), including YouTube videos which can function as stand-alone videos, and accompanying code on Github. It covers ethics, and topics beyond this chapter in-depth, including neural network approaches: https://www.fast.ai/posts/2019-07-08-fastai-nlp.html

References

1. Garrard P, Maloney LM, Hodges JR, Patterson K. The effects of very early Alzheimer's disease on the characteristics of writing by a renowned author. Brain. 2005 Feb;128(Pt 2):250–60.
2. Raschka S, Mirjalili V. Python machine learning: machine learning and deep learning with python, scikit-learn, and TensorFlow 2. Packt Publishing Ltd; 2019. 772 p.
3. Petti U, Baker S, Korhonen A. A systematic literature review of automatic Alzheimer's disease detection from speech and language. J Am Med Inform Assoc. 2020;27(11):1784–97.
4. Salvatore C, Castiglioni I. A wrapped multi-label classifier for the automatic diagnosis and prognosis of Alzheimer's disease. J Neurosci Methods. 2018;302:58–65.
5. Ridgway GR, Lehmann M, Barnes J, Rohrer JD, Warren JD, Crutch SJ, et al. Early-onset Alzheimer disease clinical variants: multivariate analyses of cortical thickness. Neurology. 2012;79(1):80–4.
6. Jarrold W, Peintner B, Wilkins D, Vergryi D, Richey C, Gorno-Tempini ML, et al. Aided diagnosis of dementia type through computer-based analysis of spontaneous speech. In: Proceedings of the workshop on computational linguistics and clinical psychology: from linguistic signal to clinical reality. Baltimore, MD: Association for Computational Linguistics; 2014. p. 27–37.
7. Brodersen KH, Ong CS, Stephan KE, Buhmann JM. The balanced accuracy and its posterior distribution. In: 2010 20th International Conference on Pattern Recognition; 2010. pp. 3121–4.
8. Stone M. Cross-validatory choice and assessment of statistical predictions. J R Stat Soc. 1974;36(2):111–33.
9. Python Software Foundation [Internet]. Python.org. [cited 2023 Feb 19]. https://www.python.org/

10. Pedregosa F, Varoquaux G, Gramfort A, Michel V, Thirion B, Grisel O, Blondel M, Prettenhofer P, Weiss R, Dubourg V, Vanderplas J. Scikit-learn: machine learning in python. J Mach Learn Res. 2011;12:2825–30.
11. Chowdhury GG. Natural language processing. Annu Rev Inf Sci Technol. 2005;37(1):51–89.
12. Navarro G. A guided tour to approximate string matching. ACM Comput Surv. 2001;33(1):31–88.
13. Clarke N, Barrick TR, Garrard P. A comparison of connected speech tasks for detecting early Alzheimer's disease and mild cognitive impairment using natural language processing and machine learning. Front Comput Sci. 2021;3:634360.
14. Jurafsky D, Martin JH. Speech and language processing [Internet]. [cited 2023 Feb 19]. https://web.stanford.edu/~jurafsky/slp3/
15. Bird S, Klein E, Loper E. Natural language processing with python: analyzing text with the natural language toolkit. O'Reilly Media, Inc; 2009. 504 p.
16. Marcus M, Santorini B, Marcinkiewicz MA. Building a large annotated corpus of English: the Penn treebank. 1993 [cited 2023 Feb 19]. https://repository.upenn.edu/cis_reports/237/
17. Manning CD. Part-of-speech tagging from 97% to 100%: is it time for some linguistics? In: Computational linguistics and intelligent text processing. Springer Berlin Heidelberg; 2011. p. 171–89.
18. Covington MA, McFall JD. Cutting the Gordian Knot: The Moving-Average Type–Token Ratio (MATTR). J Quant Linguist. 2010;17(2):94–100.
19. Hess CW, Sefton KM, Landry RG. Sample size and type-token ratios for oral language of preschool children. J Speech Hear Res. 1986;29(1):129–34.
20. Brysbaert M, New B. Moving beyond Kucera and Francis: a critical evaluation of current word frequency norms and the introduction of a new and improved word frequency measure for American English. Behav Res Methods. 2009;41(4):977–90.
21. Garrard P. Cognitive archaeology: uses, methods, and results. J Neurolinguistics. 2009;22(3):250–65.
22. Lu X. Automatic analysis of syntactic complexity in second language writing. Int J Corpus Linguist. 2010;15(4):474–96.
23. Yngve VH. A model and an hypothesis for language structure. Proc Am Philos Soc. 1960;104(5):444–66.
24. Dowty DR, Karttunen L, Zwicky AM. Studies in natural language processing: natural language parsing: psychological, computational, and theoretical perspectives: psychological, computational, and theoretical perspectives. Dowty DR, Karttunen L, Zwicky AM, editors. Cambridge, England: Cambridge University Press; 2005. 428 p.
25. Firth J. A synopsis of linguistic theory, 1930-1955. Stud Linguist Anal. 1957:10–32.
26. Landauer TK, Foltz PW, Laham D. An introduction to latent semantic analysis. Discourse Process. 1998;25(2–3):259–84.
27. Mikolov T, Chen K, Corrado G, Dean J. Efficient estimation of word representations in vector space. arXiv preprint arXiv:1301.3781. 2013 Jan 16.
28. Devlin J, Chang MW, Lee K, Toutanova K. BERT: pre-training of deep bidirectional transformers for language understanding. In: Proceedings of the 2019 conference of the north American chapter of the Association for Computational Linguistics: human language technologies, volume 1 (long and short papers). Minneapolis, Minnesota: Association for Computational Linguistics; 2019. pp. 4171–86.
29. Iter D, Yoon J, Jurafsky D. Automatic detection of incoherent speech for diagnosing schizophrenia. In: Proceedings of the fifth workshop on computational linguistics and clinical psychology: from keyboard to clinic. New Orleans, LA: Association for Computational Linguistics; 2018. pp. 136–46.
30. Graesser AC, McNamara DS, Louwerse MM, Cai Z. Coh-metrix: analysis of text on cohesion and language. Behav Res Methods Instrum Comput. 2004;36(2):193–202.
31. de Beaugrande R, Dressler W. Introduction to text linguistics. Rocky Mt Rev Lang Lit. 1981;37(1/2):103.
32. Han J, Kamber M, Pei J. Data mining: concepts and techniques. Choice. 2012;49(06) 49–3305 – 49–3305.
33. Kusner M, Sun Y, Kolkin N, Weinberger K. From word embeddings to document distances. In International conference on machine learning 2015 Jun 1, pp. 957–966. PMLR.
34. Shannon CE. Prediction and entropy of printed English. Bell Syst Tech J. 1951;30(1):50–64.
35. Wankerl S, Noeth E, Evert S. An analysis of perplexity to reveal the effects of Alzheimer's disease on language. In: Speech communication; 12 ITG Symposium. ieeexplore.ieee.org; 2016. pp. 1–5.
36. Tao X, Zhou X, Zhang J, Yong J. Sentiment analysis for depression detection on social networks. In Advanced data mining and applications: 12th international conference, ADMA 2016, Gold Coast, QLD, Australia, December 12–15, 2016, Proceedings 12 2016, pp. 807–810). Springer International Publishing.
37. Wang X, Zhang C, Ji Y, Sun L, Wu L, Bao Z. A depression detection model based on sentiment analysis in micro-blog social network. In Trends and Applications in Knowledge Discovery and Data Mining: PAKDD 2013 International workshops: DMApps, DANTH, QIMIE, BDM, CDA, CloudSD, Gold Coast, QLD, Australia, April 14–17, 2013, revised selected papers 17 2013, pp. 201–213). Springer Berlin Heidelberg.
38. Dipper LT, Pritchard M. Discourse: assessment and therapy. In: Fernandes FDM, editor. Advances in speech-language pathology. London: InTech; 2017.
39. Glosser G, Deser T. Patterns of discourse production among neurological patients with fluent language disorders. Brain Lang. 1991;40(1):67–88.
40. Berube S, Nonnemacher J, Demsky C, Glenn S, Saxena S, Wright A, et al. Stealing cookies in the

twenty-first century: measures of spoken narrative in healthy versus speakers with aphasia. Am J Speech Lang Pathol. 2019;28(1S):321–9.
41. Goodglass H, Kaplan E. The assessment of aphasia and related disorders. Philadelphia: Lea & Febiger; 1983.
42. MacWhinney B. Understanding spoken language through TalkBank. Behav Res Methods. 2019;51(4):1919–27.
43. Fraser KC, Meltzer JA, Rudzicz F. Linguistic features identify Alzheimer's disease in narrative speech. J Alzheimers Dis. 2016;49(2):407–22.
44. Ehghaghi M, Rudzicz F, Novikova J. Data-driven Approach to Differentiating between Depression and Dementia from Noisy Speech and Language Data. arXiv preprint arXiv:2210.03303. 2022 Oct 7.
45. Ablimit A, Scholz K, Schultz T. Deep learning approaches for detecting Alzheimer's dementia from conversational speech of ILSE study. Proc Interspeech. 2022;2022:3348–52.
46. Räukur T, Ho A, Casper S, Hadfield-Menell D. Toward transparent ai: A survey on interpreting the inner structures of deep neural networks. arXiv preprint arXiv:2207.13243. 2022 Jul 27.
47. Luz S, Haider F, de la Fuente S, Fromm D, MacWhinney B. Alzheimer's dementia recognition through spontaneous speech: The ADReSS challenge. arXiv preprint arXiv:2004.06833. 2020 Apr 14.
48. Word Embedding Analysis [Internet]. [cited 2023 Feb 19]. http://wordvec.colorado.edu/
49. NLP tools for the social sciences [Internet]. NLP tools for the social sciences. [cited 2023 Feb 19]. https://www.linguisticanalysistools.org/
50. Pennebaker JW, Boyd RL, Jordan K, Blackburn K. The development and psychometric properties of LIWC2015. 2015 Sep 15.
51. Honnibal M, Montani I. spaCy 2: natural language understanding with Bloom embeddings, convolutional neural networks and incremental parsing; 2017.
52. Rehurek R, Sojka P. Gensim–python framework for vector space modelling. NLP Centre, Faculty of Informatics, Masaryk University; 2011.
53. Kaufmann M. The WEKA Workbench. Online appendix for data mining: practical machine learning tools and techniques. online; 2016.
54. Henrich J, Heine SJ, Norenzayan A. The weirdest people in the world? Behav Brain Sci. 2010;33(2–3):61–83; discussion 83–135.
55. Park SH, Han K. Methodologic guide for evaluating clinical performance and effect of artificial intelligence Technology for Medical Diagnosis and Prediction. Radiology. 2018;286(3):800–9.
56. Fraser KC, Lundholm Fors K, Kokkinakis D. Multilingual word embeddings for the assessment of narrative speech in mild cognitive impairment. Comput Speech Lang. 2019;53:121–39.
57. Kalafatis C, Modarres M, Apostolou P, Marefat H, Khanbagi M, Karimi H, et al. Validity and cultural generalisability of a 5-minute AI-based, computerised cognitive assessment in mild cognitive impairment and Alzheimer's dementia. Front Psych. 2021;12:1155.
58. European Commission. On Artificial Intelligence - A European approach to excellence and trust [Internet]. 2020 [cited 2021 Feb 7]. https://ec.europa.eu/info/sites/default/files/commission-white-paper-artificial-intelligence-feb2020_en.pdf
59. Chandler C, Foltz PW, Elvevåg B. Using machine learning in psychiatry: The need to establish a framework that nurtures trustworthiness. Schizophr Bull. 2020;46(1):11–4.
60. Clarke N, Foltz P, Garrard P. How to do things with (thousands of) words: computational approaches to discourse analysis in Alzheimer's disease. Cortex. 2020;129:446–63.
61. Ostrand R, Gunstad J. Using automatic assessment of speech production to predict current and future cognitive function in older adults. J Geriatr Psychiatry Neurol. 2021;34(5):357–69.
62. El-Sappagh S, Alonso JM, Islam SMR, Sultan AM, Kwak KS. A multilayer multimodal detection and prediction model based on explainable artificial intelligence for Alzheimer's disease. Sci Rep. 2021;11(1):2660.

Natasha Clarke studied psychology at Cardiff University before completing a masters in clinical psychology and mental health at Swansea University in 2011. She trained as a psychologist and in clinical dementia research at the Research Institute for the Care of Older People, Bath, and held research positions in dementia and mental health. She was awarded her Ph.D. by St George's University of London in 2021, and then moved to the Institut universitaire de gériatrie de Montréal, where she is an Institute for Data Valorization (IVADO) Postdoctoral Fellow.

Peter Garrard qualified in Medicine at Bristol University in 1990. He trained in general medicine, specializing in neurology, and completing a Ph.D. in cognitive neuroscience during a clinical training fellowship at the University of Cambridge. He has been fully accredited in neurology since 2000. He held senior clinical academic positions at the University College London and the University of Southampton, before moving to St George's, where he is currently Professor of Neurology, in 2011.

18 Tele-Assessment of Cognition and Discourse Production

Jacky Chak Pui Choy, Ruizhi Dai, Anthony Pak-Hin Kong, and Gloria H. Y. Wong

Preview of What Is Currently Known

People living with dementia and stroke survivors have difficulties accessing community services. e-health services including tele-assessment are possible solution, although development has been slow, due to challenges such as cognitive deficits and sensory loss present in these client groups. Practice wisdom is rapidly accumulating since the COVID-19 pandemic on adapting in-person assessments into tele-assessment in these populations. A number of professional organizations, such as American Speech-Language-Hearing Association and American Psychological Association, have also provided guidance and resources on tele-assessment. While recommendations for general cognitive and language testing are summarized, specific guidelines on virtual discourse evaluation seem to be missing. Inconsistent administration and sensory impairment deserve particular attention from researchers and clinicians to ensure validity and reliability.

Objectives

(a) To review the current advances in tele-assessment in the dementia and stroke populations
(b) To illustrate, using examples of cognitive screening and discourse production measures, issues in tele-assessment in these populations
(c) To discuss the key practical considerations for telephone administration, videoconference administration, and conducting computerized tests via videoconferencing
(d) To recommend future directions of tele-assessment of cognition and discourse production in the dementia and stroke populations

J. C. P. Choy · G. H. Y. Wong (✉)
Department of Social Work and Social Administration, The University of Hong Kong, Pok Fu Lam, Hong Kong SAR
e-mail: cpchoy@hku.hk; ghywong@hku.hk

R. Dai
Department of Psychology, Guangzhou University, Guangzhou, China

Center for Brain and Cognitive Sciences, Guangzhou University, Guangzhou, China
e-mail: dairuizhi@gzhu.edu.cn

A. P.-H. Kong
Academic Unit of Human Communication, Learning, and Development, The University of Hong Kong, Pokfulam, Hong Kong SAR

Aphasia Research and Therapy (ART) Laboratory, The University of Hong Kong, Pok Fu Lam, Hong Kong SAR
e-mail: akong@hku.hk

A. P.-H. Kong (ed.), *Spoken Discourse Impairments in the Neurogenic Populations*,
https://doi.org/10.1007/978-3-031-45190-4_18

Introduction

The Needs and Challenges for Tele-Assessment

Among various brain and neurological conditions, dementia and stroke attract intense attention from researchers and practitioners for ways of improving access to care. According to the Global Dementia Observatory, currently there are 55.2 million people living with dementia (PLwD) [1], while the Global Burden of Disease (GBD) estimated 12.2 million incident stroke cases in 2019 and 101 million prevalent cases worldwide [2]. A substantial proportion of these huge populations has difficulties in accessing community services due to mobility or transportation issues [3]. Particularly during the COVID-19 pandemic, community care services for PLwD and stroke survivors are often considered "non-emergency" services, which may be suspended or maintained at a minimum level; early assessment for new/suspected cases and regular progress monitoring are compromised.

Telecare and, more specifically, tele-assessment, appear to be an attractive option to address such needs. By tele-assessment, we refer to remote assessments conducted using telephone and/or videoconferencing technology, such that the assessor can have real-time interaction with the person being assessed. This covers various platforms, including telephone, smartphones, tablet computers, and PCs, and a wide range of software and applications are considered. Tele-assessment is not new: in dementia, for example, tele-assessment via videoconferencing has been used in diagnostic interviewing [4]. As tele-assessment can reduce traveling time and related costs, their use in PLwD and stroke survivors may greatly improve service access in a cost-effective manner.

The barriers and challenges are, however, many. Apart from generic ones in the implementation of e-health services [5], such as issues about digital fraud and privacy, and infrastructure support (linked to socioeconomic disadvantages) [6], many people impacted by dementia or stroke (including their caregivers) are older people, who tend to have lower IT literacy [3]; the conditions also mean lower cognitive functioning, with limited mental capacity in some cases, and can be complicated by hearing/visual impairments, distressed behaviors, and functional impairment. These barriers possibly explain the slow development in tele-assessment in PLwD and stroke survivors, until recently.

Current Advances in Dementia and Stroke: An Overview

The COVID-19 pandemic has been identified as a turning point for e-health [7], enabling wider acceptance of videoconferencing by professionals, service users, and other stakeholders, accelerating innovations that could otherwise take decades. A "digital revolution" in dementia care has been called for [8], with widespread hope that telecare could be a game-changer [6]. Some authors proposed that telecare assuming a central role connecting services in the future [9]; in research, there is also a growing interest in online/remote study visit [10].

Under this context, knowledge and experience are rapidly accumulating, addressing many previous challenges in tele-assessment in the dementia and stroke populations. For example, the Alzheimer Society of Canada Task Force on dementia care best practices for COVID-19 has published a report on remote assessment [11]. Reviewing a range of telephone and video assessment tools for screening and specific domain assessment of cognition, function, and behavior, the Task Force noted that some of the remote tests can be reliably done, although validation and norm data are needed. They concluded that tele-assessment can be implemented for people with cognitive impairment. Some of the challenges and practice wisdom in implementing tele-assessment, particularly remote cognitive screening and language assessment, will be discussed further in this chapter.

Another recent Cochrane review compared remote and in-person telephone and video call tests similarly noted that there seems to be good agreement, in that caution is needed as remote testing is complex, and scoring and cut-offs established with in-person tests may not apply to remote delivery of the tests [12], and psychometric properties such as test-retest reliability may be lacking when tests are being moved online [13]. Some authors recommend using only tools that have evidence for psychometric equivalency for remote and in-person assessments [14]. When used in rural populations, mixed results have been reported regarding differences between in-person and tele-assessment of cognition [15]. Sources of variance introduced with tele-assessment may include inconsistent administration and impact of sensory loss on use of technology which highlighted the need to screen for sensory loss, training, and improved reporting of administrative procedures [14, 16].

The potential impacts of overcoming these teething troubles are well recognized. One obvious advantage is the possibility of routine screening in indicated populations, for example, by delivering the Montreal Cognitive Assessment (MoCA) via videoconferencing as cognitive screening in all stroke survivors [13]. Tele-assessment can be a low-cost option to allow screening at scale, which may not be feasible otherwise in practice or research [17]. If delivered using the person's own electronic device such as a smartphone, detection of early cognitive decline may be made possible through more frequent and sensitive tests that are longer in duration, with attention paid to users' experience [18]. A few cognitive screening tools, including MoCA and the Oxford Cognitive Screen-Plus (OCS-Plus), have developed protocols to enable remote screening at scale: the MoCA 5-min protocol [19] can be delivered over the phone, with psychometric properties established in many languages other than English, such as Chinese; the OCS-Plus delivered using tablet computers has established feasibility in low-resources, low-IT literacy settings [20], and guidelines for remote assessment.

Another relatively untapped potential is the use of telephone or videoconferencing tools to conduct language assessments. The abovementioned Canada Task Force report included reviews of several common language assessments, such as Boston Naming Test (BNT) and Semantic Category Fluency [11]. With these traditional language-based tests, there were initial evidence suggesting that performance is not affected by videoconference administration in older people, if technical issues (such as having a high-speed network connection) can be ensured, although there may be slight variations in some of the tests such as BNT [21]. Apart from these traditional language-based tests, tele-assessment allows easy collection of speech samples, which opens new opportunities for spoken discourse research. Speech samples collected in conversations carried out remotely via videoconferencing are rich data for in-depth analysis, such as Main Concept Analysis (MCA) [22], and advances in machine learning to identify non-invasive biomarkers for accessible, cost-effective screening [23], a priority in both practice and research [24]. Like traditional cognitive tests, attention is nevertheless needed in nuanced differences of remote versus in-person language assessment. For example, some researchers noted that despite comparable quality, the quantity/duration of speech may be lower with remote assessment, with higher rates of caregiver interference [25].

To illustrate some of the key points to note in administering tele-assessments in PLwD and stroke survivors, some direct experience and lessons learned from remote cognitive screening using MoCA 5-min protocol and OCS-Plus, as well as assessment of oral discourse production using MCA (as part of a larger project "BrainLive—Connecting Families Living with Dementia In Pandemic Situations and Beyond" conducted in Hong Kong) are shared and discussed in the next sections.

Tele-Assessment of Cognition

An Example of Telephone Administration: MoCA 5-min Protocol

Montreal Cognitive Assessment 5-minute protocol (MoCA 5-min) is a brief cognitive screening tool for telephone administration [19]. It consists of four subtests tapping on different cognitive domains, including a 5-word immediate recall (attention), a 1-min verbal fluency (executive functions/language), a 6-item time and geographical orientation (orientation), and a 5-word delayed recall and recognition (memory). Compared to its full version [26], the time for administration is shortened from 10 to 5 min on average. Several subtests such as trail making, clock drawing, and object naming that required paper-and-pencil and visual stimuli were removed. It gives an advantage for assessing individuals (for instance, stroke survivors) with difficulties in holding a pen. MoCA 5-min and MoCA are equally effective in detecting cognitive impairments. Norm-derived cut-off scores corrected for age and education were established from older adults cohort (65+) in Hong Kong [27]. Moreover, score conversions from minimental state examination (MMSE) [28] and interRAI Cognitive Performance Scale (CPS) [29], two widely adopted tools in clinical and long-term care settings, respectively, are available, which facilitated comparability of scores from different cognitive assessment tools. First developed in Hong Kong Chinese, MoCA 5-min test is culturally adapted and validated in Tanzania [30] and France [31] with good validity and reliability. Two other alternate versions of shortened MoCA suitable for telephone administration, namely the Blind version of MoCA [32] and MiniMoCA [33], are available in English.

Caregiver's Involvement for Maintaining Assessment Validity

When administering tele-assessment for people with suspected cognitive impairment, the involvement of their caregivers (usually a family member) is often crucial for scheduling the appointment, setting up the environment, and providing essential information. In our experience of administering MoCA 5-min in a community survey, caregivers were interviewed as an informant before the respondent, that is, the person living with dementia or suspected cognitive impairment. Assessors are recommended to ask caregivers to help with the following preparatory actions to maintain the validity of the assessment. First, the respondent must stay in a quiet and undisturbed environment for around 5 min. Without clear instruction, caregivers may sit next to the respondent throughout the assessment mostly because they are concerned about their relative's performance, or the respondents may feel uncomfortable talking to a stranger on the phone without their caregiver. It is therefore essential to remind the caregivers that the respondent should be alone in a quiet room before the assessment. If their home environment does not allow for such arrangement (e.g., having limited space), assessors should at least suggest the caregiver to sit apart such that s/he is out of the respondent's sight. Second, calendars, smartphones, or any cues of date should be temporarily covered or removed from the respondent's sight. This is to ensure the validity of the responses to the time orientation items. Third, the respondent's address can be obtained in advance from the caregivers, especially for the first time of contact with the respondents, such as baseline assessment in research studies or large-scale screening in public health programs. This information is necessary for scoring the items of the geographical orientation. When administering other cognitive assessments that similarly require a distraction- and cue-free environment, even via videoconferencing, these preparations with involvement of a caregiver should also be considered.

When there is no caregiver or other reliable third person available, assessors should guide the respondents to stay in an environment free of distractions in order to ensure the validity of the test. Guidelines from the MoCA test website [33] suggested that, for the time orientation items, assessors could ask respondents to close their eyes before responding; and for the geographical orientation items, assessors should tell the respondents where they are calling from (e.g., name of clinic/institution) at the beginning of the call.

An Example of Computerized Test and Videoconference Administration: OCS-Plus

Oxford Cognitive Screen-Plus (OCS-Plus) is a computerized tablet-based screening tool for assessing domain-specific cognition with detailed measures on memory and executive function [34]. It comprises ten subtests including picture naming, semantics, orientation, word memory encoding, trails, verbal recall, episodic recall, figure copy/recall, rule finding, and cancelation. And these subtests tap on different cognitive functions. The time for administration is 24 min on average. The OCS-Plus app is now downloadable at Google Play Store and Apple Appstore. Details of registration and demonstration videos of in-person administration can be found online [35].

OCS-Plus is a digital tool modified from the paper-and-pencil test Oxford Cognitive Screen (OCS), which is an aphasia- and neglect-friendly instrument sensitive to cognitive deficits in stroke survivors. OCS is characterized by its low requirement on respondent's language level [36], first developed in the UK, and translated and validated among the Dutch, Danish, Spanish, Russian, Brazilian, Italian, and Hong Kong Chinese [35]. Compared with OCS, OCS-Plus is designed to be equally inclusive, and it is currently validated with normative data from neurologically healthy aged population in the UK, Germany [34], and rural South Africa [20].

One of the major advantages of computerized test is the capability of automated data entry and scoring. At the end of an assessment session of OCS-Plus, for example, a wheel-like outcome report will be automatically generated to illustrate the performance of the respondent of each subtest compared to the age-matched normative data [35]. This visualization of assessment results allows assessors to have a quick overview of the respondent's cognitive performance. Another advantage of computerized test, in addition to standardization of administration, is the recording of a more detailed response metrics. For instance, apart from accuracy-based measures, OCS-Plus reported the respondents' processing speed for the trails subtests by taking the response time into account. Respondents' tapping errors are also automatically recorded in the cancelation subtests, allowing researchers to further explore possible visuospatial processing and memory impairments. Moreover, although the tool was administered in-person in its validation studies [20, 35], its design is highly applicable for remote assessment via videoconferencing such that the respondents can stay home or in a quiet accessible location instead of traveling to a clinic or research office.

Caregiver's Involvement for Equipment Setup and Assessment Administration

Similar to telephone administration, caregiver of the PLwD or stroke survivor usually play an important role in videoconference administration, in particular, for setting up the equipment, checking internet connectivity, and checking audio, visual, and touchscreen functions. In an ongoing remote dementia intervention pilot study, we have included OCS-Plus as one of the outcome monitoring tools and administered it via videoconferencing. A tablet computer with preinstalled OCS-Plus and a videoconference app (e.g., Zoom, Microsoft Teams), a tablet stand, an earphone, and a stylus were delivered to each respondent. For those without a stable internet connection, a prepaid data SIM card for short-term use was also provided. Before the assessment, a meeting link for videoconference was sent to the caregiver. For caregivers with lower IT literacy (usually older adults themselves), our assessors would call and guide them through how to use the tablet, to open the videoconference app, and to enter the virtual meeting room. The camera, speaker, and microphone function were checked to ensure that both the assessor and respondent sides were hearing clearly and seeing smooth image.

Next, assessors would ask caregivers to share their screen and launch the OCS-Plus app on their tablet. During the assessment, although the assessor is the main administrator who reads the instructions and determines whether a response is correct, caregivers' assistance is needed to press the appropriate buttons in order to proceed to the next step and record the responses correctly (e.g., pressing "start" before starting the next subtest (see Fig. 18.1), selecting "correct/incorrect" correspondingly in the picture naming test (see Fig. 18.2), etc.). It is therefore crucial to commu-

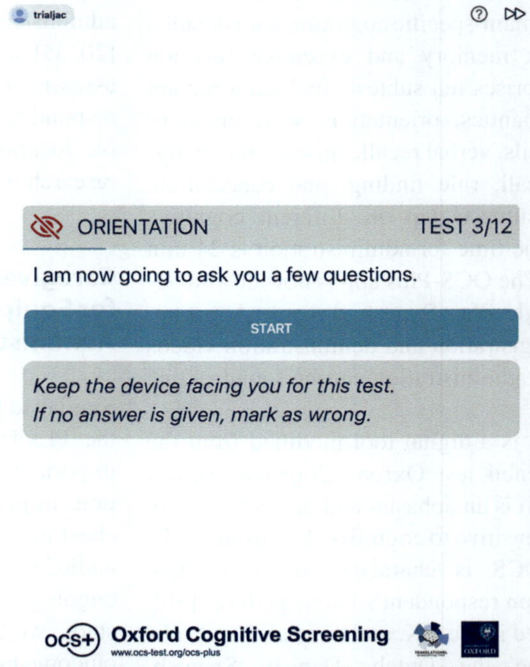

Fig. 18.1 Screenshot of OCS-Plus app: the screen before starting the orientation subtest

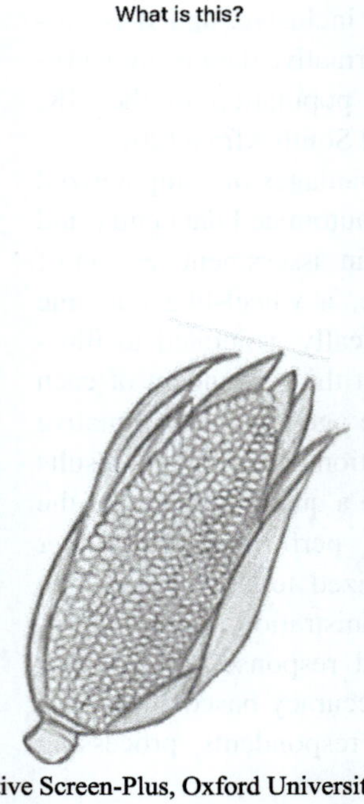

Fig. 18.2 Screenshot of OCS-Plus app: an item of the picture naming subtest

nicate with caregivers clearly about their assistive role such that they would follow the assessor's instruction and not interfere with the respondents' response during the administration. These caregiver's assistance would not, and should not, affect the respondent's performance. If an interference occurs, the assessor should take a note and redo the corresponding subtest afterwards.

Considerations for Improving Audio Quality: Speakerphone or Earphone?

Before and during the administration, extra attention should be given to the hearing, visual, and tactile difficulties either arising from respondent's sensory impairment, device limitations, or both. For respondents with hearing or visual impairments, assessors should check with the caregivers and suggest the respondents to wear hearing or visual aids if necessary and available. For audio output, we suggest using the built-in speaker of the tablet such that both the respondent and caregiver can hear the assessor, especially for OCS-Plus which requires caregiver's assistance throughout the videoconference administration. If respondents found it difficult to hear the instructions, even after adjusting the volume, using the earphone might help improve voice clarity. To keep the caregiver involved, the respondent and caregiver would need to share the earphone by using one earpiece each. However, it was noted that some older adults were quite resistant to the use of earphone as it made them feel uncomfortable.

For brief telephone assessments like MoCA 5-min that does not require caregiver's involvement during the test administration, we suggest respondents to use the phone in a traditional handheld mode such that they could have an independent conversation without interference as if they were in a private room with the assessor. The use of speakerphone or earphone is only recommended when it helps to improve the voice clarity or when respondents are unable to hold a phone (e.g., owing to physical disability).

Considerations for Reliable Touchscreen Input: Fingertips or Stylus?

For touchscreen input, as the cohort of participants in our project had lower levels of education in general and some were not familiar with holding a pen, our default mode of administration was to instruct the respondents to touch the screen with their fingertips to avoid errors or delays due to unfamiliar use of a stylus. However, in line with the findings of earlier studies on older adults' use of touch screen, it was observed that older adults often experienced touch recognition errors due to dry or wrinkled fingertips [37], or even "unregistered touch" causing frustration and confusion [38] during the test administration. If these touchscreen difficulties were observed during the assessment preparation or administration, assessors should suggest the respondents to use a stylus and allow them to practice using it for actions such as tapping on icons, swiping to the next screen, and drawing on a whiteboard (if available in the videoconference platform).

Maintaining Virtual Face-to-Face Interaction: Suggestions for Handling Disabled Camera During Screen Sharing

Allowing a virtual face-to-face contact is undoubtedly a major advantage of videoconference administration over telephone administration. However, it was noticed that for some videoconference platforms and/or models of tablets, when the screen sharing function is activated, the tablet camera will turn off and there are no floating windows showing the camera view of the others. This issue occurred when we administered OCS-Plus remotely with respondents who were using an Android tablet and Zoom for videoconferencing. Although the assessment could still be administered and completed under sole verbal communication, it is not an ideal setup as seeing each other would promote better engagement of the respondents in the task and enable the assessor to notice the non-verbal gestures, facial expressions, and physical surroundings of the respondents. Caregivers were guided to update the app, and if the issue persisted, they were asked to connect a second device with a camera (e.g., a smart phone) such that the assessor can see the respondents.

Tele-Assessment of Discourse Production

An Example of Videoconference Administration: Adapting MCA

Main Concept Analysis (MCA) is an assessment tool for oral discourse production that uses a sequential picture description task to elicit language samples, followed by a discourse analysis with reference to a rule-based system that focuses on the presence, accuracy, and completeness of targeted main concepts [39]. Respondents are presented with four sets of sequential pictures depicting a story (e.g., cooking in a kitchen, buying ice-cream) and asked to describe the happenings in each story. Administration and scoring could be completed in 20 minutes for most cases. MCA is a sensitive tool for distinguishing speakers with and without aphasia [22], and PLwD from persons with non-fluent aphasia and healthy control [40]. First developed in Cantonese [22], it is also adapted and validated in English [41], Mandarin [42], Japanese [43], Korean [44], Dutch [45], and Spanish [46]. A detailed manual was published [39] for guiding standardized administration, scoring, and interpretation. Though MCA was administered in-person during its development and validation, it is suitable for videoconference administration with appropriate adaptations. Moreover, with the recording function of the videoconferencing tool, it becomes more convenient to audio- or videotape the assessment session as the assessors do not need to prepare and set up a separate recorder.

Considerations for Replicating Procedures of In-person Administration: Preparation and Presentation of Digital Materials

Proper presentation of the stimuli is fundamental to a valid assessment, either for in-person or remote administration. In an ongoing investigation of remote dementia intervention, discourse production has been included as a secondary outcome through the administration of MCA via videoconferencing. More specifically, the screen sharing function was utilized to present the MCA sequential pictures depicting a story to the respondents. As suggested by the original in-person administration guideline, assessors first introduced the task by showing all four pictures of a story, then presented each picture and pointed to its target main concept before the respondents started their description. To follow this procedure as closely as possible, five digital image files with high resolution were prepared: the first one showing all four pictures horizontally in the correct order, and the other four corresponding to each of the sequential picture set. When presenting the first image, as the size of the image seen by the respondent was limited by the screen size, the assessor might need to enlarge the image and slowly scrolled from the left to the right as if the pictures were glanced horizontally in an in-person administration. In addition, the laser pointer tool of the videoconference platform was used during the administration to replicate the finger pointing procedure of in-person administration. If the assessor was not able to prepare digital image of the pictures, an alternative approach is to present the pictures in front of the camera and to physically point to the parts where the target main concepts are depicted. Nevertheless, the latter option was less desirable because it made the administration more difficult, with the need to steadily hold the stimulus, and to mark or take notes of the responses simultaneously.

Considerations for the Use of Verbal Cues: Be Aware of Time Delay and Overlapping Voices

Assessors should also be aware of the potential time delay in videoconferences, especially when using prompts or probing questions. It is common to make use of probing questions in psychological assessments if there is no response from the respondents, for instance, saying "what about here?" or "any more?" during the picture description task of MCA. Due to the potential time delay, it is suggested that assessors wait for 2–3 s longer than in in-person administration before giving verbal cues. Not only can it accommodate for the time delay in communications, but also avoid overlapping of verbal production between the assessor and respondent; this is particularly helpful in most videoconference platforms, as it can ensure only one voice input is delivered to the meeting participants and captured in the recordings.

Ethical, Equity, and Privacy Considerations for Tele-Assessment

Apart from maintaining the assessment validity, the ethical and data privacy standard that applies to in-person administration should also apply to tele-assessment [11]. It is the assessor's responsibility to well-explain and guide through the tele-assessment procedures and ensure it will not bring extra harm/discomfort to the respondents, such as distress and disorientation due to a low IT literacy. Although tele-assessment has the benefits of improving access to telecare, access to the suitable device (e.g., computer with a camera, tablet), attitudes toward telecare, and competence in internet and technology use are factors usually causing difficulties in tele-assessment among the older population [47, 48]. If the respondents, and/or their caregivers, do not have the required equipment and IT proficiency, or feel uncomfortable with telecare, assessors should consider shifting to in-person mode of administration instead. Moreover, assessors should make use of a safe device with password protection and identify a suitable and secure platform for videoconferencing. Platforms that are encrypted, user-friendly, and compatible with most commonly-used devices (e.g., Zoom, Microsoft Teams, GoToMeeting, Google Meet, Cisco Webex) are preferable. Last but not least, if the tele-assessment involves audio and/or video recording via the cloud drive of the videoconference platform, assessors should also consider the security of the cloud storage and transfer the recordings to another safe storage (e.g., local drive with data protection, intranet of a trusted institution) regularly.

Conclusion and Future Directions

Tele-assessment for cognitive screening and discourse production is fast developing in the dementia and stroke populations. Apart from being an alternative to paper-and-pencil neurocognitive tests to improve access, tele-assessments hold the potential to advance detection of cognitive impairments beyond what is possible with traditional, well-validated tests. In a recent collection of essays from international leaders by the World Dementia Council [49], for example, the possible roles of "digital biomarkers" is an area of focus. Although still in its infancy, intense research is exploring the predictive value of human–computer interactions in early detection of cognitive changes, such as reaction time in task-switching (e.g., between application) as a measure of executive function [50]. Initial evidence suggests that specifically designed tele-assessments delivered via the person's own device are feasible in older people, as valid digital biomarkers sensitivity to early cognitive changes for detecting Alzheimer's disease, as shown through their association with both paper-and-pencil tests and amyloid burden [51]. Electronic cognitive assessments also allow use of real-time analyses, such as item response theory, for automatic scoring for feedback and for improving measurement precision in the testing of true cognitive ability [52].

Likewise, speech-based digital biomarkers are gaining attention in their potential linkage with neuropsychiatric processes [53]. Especially with the rise of natural language processing and interest in spontaneous speech and automated speech analysis [54, 55], novel biomarkers could in theory be identified with research on their clinical validity for predicting diagnosis, disease progression, or treatment response [53]. The latter role could be particularly relevant in conversation-based non-pharmacological interventions, such as cognitive stimulation therapy (CST) in PLwD, with evidence of cognitive enhancement [56] theoretically linked to language use [57].

Some of the current challenges of tele-assessments in the dementia and stroke populations, such as low IT literacy and insufficient infrastructure, may become less relevant as the demographic profile changes over time. Currently, use of information and communications technology (ICT) devices such as smartphones is noted in more than half of PLwD and caregivers in high-income countries/areas [58]. In these areas, although device access and willingness to participate in remote cognitive testing were lower in PLwD compared with people with normal cognition or mild cognitive impairments, overall access and willingness is high, and with additional resources, representative participation in tele-assessments using videoconferencing seems feasible [59]. Questions remain, however, as to how scalable these tele-assessments will be as the technologies mature, especially when applied in low-resources settings. In a recent systematic review of digital biomarker technologies for the monitoring of cognition in home-based settings, most technologies were found to be "far removed from everyday life experiences" and thus not suitable for use in real-life settings with uncontrolled conditions [60]. As noted in a recent rapid review commissioned by the Department of Health and Social Care in England [61], a key feature of more promising digital technologies in dementia is the deployment or repurposing of existing commercial solutions. Tele-assessments conducted using or embedded in everyday life digital technologies, such as WhatsApp, WeChat, Zoom, or Microsoft Teams, could represent a promising area for future practice and research.

Major Takeaways

1. The COVID-19 pandemic had accelerated the development of tele-assessment, especially for vulnerable populations with limited mobility such as PLwD and stroke survivors. Recent reviews and guidelines have supported that tele-assessment has good agreement with in-person tests. While further studies on scale validation and norm data establishment are warranted, clinicians and researchers should pay attention to two major factors that might compromise the results of tele-assessment: inconsistent administration and sensory impairment.
2. Examples of tele-assessment where administration experience is accumulating with these populations include (1) MoCA 5-min protocol—a brief cognitive screening tool for telephone administration, (2) OCS-Plus—a computerized cognitive test that is highly applicable for videoconference administration, and (3) MCA—an assessment tool for oral discourse production suitable for videoconference administration after careful adaptations.
3. When administering tele-assessment of cognition and discourse production, assessors should consider the caregiver's involvement in maintaining assessment validity, setting up the equipment, and providing necessary assistance during administration. Administration procedures, such as the presentation of instructions and stimuli, should be replicated as closely to the original in-person version as possible. Microphone, speakerphone, display, camera, and touchscreen function of the respondent's device must be checked against the requirements of the tele-assessment with considerations of possible sensory impairments.
4. Ethical, equity, and data privacy standards that apply to in-person administration also apply to tele-assessment. Assessors should consider the respondents' access to the required device, attitudes toward technology, IT proficiency, and security of the device and

videoconference platform when planning for tele-assessment.

5. Tele-assessment of cognition and discourse production, instead of being simply an alternative to paper-and-pencil tests, has high potentials for advancing the development of digital biomarkers for detecting cognitive impairment, monitoring disease progression, and predicting treatment response. Future research and services concerning tele-assessment could focus on solutions for scaling up tele-assessment in low-resource regions and integrating it into everyday life digital technologies.

Acknowledgments The assessment options summarized in this chapter is part of a larger project "BrainLive—Connecting Families Living with Dementia In Pandemic Situations and Beyond" funded by the Simon K. Y. Lee Elderly Fund.

References

1. Alzheimer's Research UK. Dementia statistics hub: global prevalence. https://www.dementiastatistics.org/statistics/global-prevalence/.
2. G. B. D. Stroke Collaborators. Global, regional, and national burden of stroke and its risk factors, 1990-2019: a systematic analysis for the global burden of disease study 2019. Lancet Neurol. 2021;20(10):795–820.
3. Pike KE, Chong MS, Hume CH, Keech BJ, Konjarski M, Landolt KA, et al. Providing online memory interventions for older adults: a critical review and recommendations for development. Aust Psychol. 2018;53(5):367–76.
4. Loh PK, Donaldson M, Flicker L, Maher S, Goldswain P. Development of a telemedicine protocol for the diagnosis of Alzheimer's disease. J Telemed Telecare. 2007;13(2):90–4.
5. Manji H, Saxena S. Here's how digital tools can transform mental health care. International Telecommunication Union; 2019. https://news.itu.int/heres-how-digital-tools-can-transform-mental-health-care/.
6. Knapp M, Shehaj X, Wong G. Digital interventions for people with dementia and carers: effective, cost-effective and equitable? Neurodegener Dis Manag. 2022;12(5):215–9.
7. Wind TR, Rijkeboer M, Andersson G, Riper H. The COVID-19 pandemic: the 'black swan' for mental health care and a turning point for e-health. Internet Interv. 2020;20:100317.
8. Cuffaro L, Di Lorenzo F, Bonavita S, Tedeschi G, Leocani L, Lavorgna L. Dementia care and COVID-19 pandemic: a necessary digital revolution. Neurol Sci. 2020;41(8):1977–9.
9. Mok VCT, Pendlebury S, Wong A, Alladi S, Au L, Bath PM, et al. Tackling challenges in care of Alzheimer's disease and other dementias amid the COVID-19 pandemic, now and in the future. Alzheimers Dement. 2020;16(11):1571–81.
10. Nunnerley M, Mattek N, Kaye J, Beattie Z. Preferences of NIA Alzheimer's Disease Research Center participants regarding remote assessment during the COVID-19 pandemic. Alzheimers Dement (Amst). 2022;14(1):e12373.
11. Geddes MR, O'Connell ME, Fisk JD, Gauthier S, Camicioli R, Ismail Z, et al. Remote cognitive and behavioral assessment: report of the Alzheimer Society of Canada task force on dementia care best practices for COVID-19. Alzheimers Dement (Amst). 2020;12(1):e12111.
12. Beishon LC, Elliott E, Hietamies TM, Mc Ardle R, O'Mahony A, Elliott AR, et al. Diagnostic test accuracy of remote, multidomain cognitive assessment (telephone and video call) for dementia. Cochrane Database Syst Rev. 2022;4(4):CD013724.
13. Chapman JE, Cadilhac DA, Gardner B, Ponsford J, Bhalla R, Stolwyk RJ. Comparing face-to-face and videoconference completion of the Montreal cognitive assessment (MoCA) in community-based survivors of stroke. J Telemed Telecare. 2021;27(8):484–92.
14. O'Connell ME, Vellani S, Robertson S, O'Rourke HM, McGilton KS. Going from zero to 100 in remote dementia research: a practical guide. J Med Internet Res. 2021;23(1):e24098.
15. Sekhon H, Sekhon K, Launay C, Afililo M, Innocente N, Vahia I, et al. Telemedicine and the rural dementia population: a systematic review. Maturitas. 2021;143:105–14.
16. Hunter MB, Jenkins N, Dolan C, Pullen H, Ritchie C, Muniz-Terrera G. Reliability of telephone and videoconference methods of cognitive assessment in older adults with and without dementia. J Alzheimers Dis. 2021;81(4):1625–47.
17. Abdulrahman H, Jansen E, Hoevenaar-Blom M, van Dalen JW, van Wanrooij LL, van Bussel E, et al. Diagnostic accuracy of the telephone interview for cognitive status for the detection of dementia in primary care. Ann Fam Med. 2022;20(2):130–6.
18. Lancaster C, Koychev I, Blane J, Chinner A, Wolters L, Hinds C. Evaluating the feasibility of frequent cognitive assessment using the Mezurio smartphone app: observational and interview study in adults with elevated dementia risk. JMIR Mhealth Uhealth. 2020;8(4):e16142.
19. Wong A, Nyenhuis D, Black SE, Law LS, Lo ES, Kwan PW, et al. Montreal cognitive assessment 5-minute protocol is a brief, valid, reliable, and feasible cognitive screen for telephone administration. Stroke. 2015;46(4):1059–64.

20. Humphreys GW, Duta MD, Montana L, Demeyere N, McCrory C, Rohr J, et al. Cognitive function in low-income and low-literacy settings: validation of the tablet-based Oxford cognitive screen in the health and aging in Africa: a longitudinal study of an INDEPTH community in South Africa (HAALSI). J Gerontol B Psychol Sci Soc Sci. 2017;72(1):38–50.
21. Brearly TW, Shura RD, Martindale SL, Lazowski RA, Luxton DD, Shenal BV, et al. Neuropsychological test administration by videoconference: a systematic review and meta-analysis. Neuropsychol Rev. 2017;27(2):174–86.
22. Kong AP-H. The use of main concept analysis to measure discourse production in Cantonese-speaking persons with aphasia: a preliminary report. J Commun Disord. 2009;42(6):442–64.
23. Fristed E, Skirrow C, Meszaros M, Lenain R, Meepegama U, Cappa S, et al. A remote speech-based AI system to screen for early Alzheimer's disease via smartphones. Alzheimers Dement (Amst). 2022;14(1):e12366.
24. Gregory S, Linz N, Konig A, Langel K, Pullen H, Luz S, et al. Remote data collection speech analysis and prediction of the identification of Alzheimer's disease biomarkers in people at risk for Alzheimer's disease dementia: the speech on the phone assessment (SPeAk) prospective observational study protocol. BMJ Open. 2022;12(3):e052250.
25. Robin J, Novikova J, Sirotkin S, Yancheva M, Kaufman LD, Simpson W. Quality comparison of remote vs. in-person digital speech assessment for dementia. Alzheimers Dement. 2020;16(S5):e046971.
26. Nasreddine ZS, Phillips NA, Bédirian V, Charbonneau S, Whitehead V, Collin I, et al. The Montreal cognitive assessment, MoCA: a brief screening tool for mild cognitive impairment. J Am Geriatr Soc. 2005;53(4):695–9.
27. Wong A, Law LS, Liu W, Wang Z, Lo ES, Lau A, et al. Montreal cognitive assessment: one cutoff never fits all. Stroke. 2015;46(12):3547–50.
28. Wong A, Black SE, Yiu SY, Au LW, Lau AY, Soo YO, et al. Converting MMSE to MoCA and MoCA 5-minute protocol in an educationally heterogeneous sample with stroke or transient ischemic attack. Int J Geriatr Psychiatry. 2018;33(5):729–34.
29. Andersson B, Luo H, Wong GH, Lum TY. Linking the scores of the Montreal cognitive assessment 5-min and the interRAI cognitive performance scale in older adults with mild physical or cognitive impairment. Front Psychiatry. 2021;12:705188.
30. Masika GM, Yu DS, Li PW, Wong A, Lin RS. Psychometrics and diagnostic properties of the Montreal cognitive assessment 5-min protocol in screening for mild cognitive impairment and dementia among older adults in Tanzania: a validation study. Int J Older People Nursing. 2021;16(1):e12348.
31. Dujardin K, Duhem S, Guerouaou N, Djelad S, Drumez E, Duhamel A, et al. Validation in French of the Montreal cognitive assessment 5-minute, a brief cognitive screening test for phone administration. Rev Neurol. 2021;177(8):972–9.
32. Pendlebury ST, Welch SJ, Cuthbertson FC, Mariz J, Mehta Z, Rothwell PM. Telephone assessment of cognition after transient ischemic attack and stroke: modified telephone interview of cognitive status and telephone Montreal cognitive assessment versus face-to-face Montreal cognitive assessment and neuropsychological battery. Stroke. 2013;44(1):227–9.
33. Nasreddine Z. MoCA cognitive assessment. Canada: MoCA Test; 2022. https://www.mocatest.org/.
34. Demeyere N, Haupt M, Webb SS, Strobel L, Milosevich ET, Moore MJ, et al. Introducing the tablet-based Oxford cognitive screen-plus (OCS-plus) as an assessment tool for subtle cognitive impairments. Sci Rep. 2021;11(1):8000.
35. Demeyere N, Duta MD, Webb SS, Humphreys GW, Riddoch J. Oxford cognitive screening. Oxford: University of Oxford; 2022. https://www.ocs-test.org/
36. Demeyere N, Riddoch MJ, Slavkova ED, Bickerton W-L, Humphreys GW. The Oxford cognitive screen (OCS): validation of a stroke-specific short cognitive screening tool. Psychol Assess. 2015;27(3):883.
37. Burkhard M, Koch M, editors. Evaluating touchscreen interfaces of tablet computers for elderly people. Mensch and computer workshop band; 2012.
38. Harada S, Sato D, Takagi H, Asakawa C, editors. Characteristics of elderly user behavior on mobile multi-touch devices. IFIP conference on human-computer interaction; Springer. 2013.
39. Kong P-H. Main concept analysis (MCA) for oral discourse production. Shanghai: Commercial Press (HK); 2016.
40. Kong AP-H, Whiteside J, Bargmann P. The main concept analysis: validation and sensitivity in differentiating discourse produced by unimpaired English speakers from individuals with aphasia and dementia of Alzheimer type. Logoped Phoniatr Vocol. 2016;41(3):129–41.
41. Kong AP-H, Ross A, Pettigrew C. A Main concept analysis for aphasic discourse in Irish-English speakers. J Clin Speech Lang Stud. 2012;19(1):19–43.
42. Kong APH, Yeh CC. A Taiwanese Mandarin Main Concept Analysis (TM-MCA) for quantification of aphasic oral discourse. Int J Lang Commun Disord. 2015;50(5):580–92.
43. Yazu H, Kong AP-H, Yoshihata H, Okubo K. Adaptation and validation of the main concept analysis of spoken discourse by native Japanese adults. Clin Linguist Phon. 2022;36(1):17–33.
44. Kong AP-H, Kong AP-H. Main concept analysis for acquired deficits of spoken narratives: preliminary data on inter-rater agreement and potential application to the Korean-speaking population. Clin Arch Commun Disord. 2018;3(1):14–21.
45. Criel Y, Deleu M, De Groote E, Bockstael A, Kong AP-H, De Letter M. The Dutch main concept analysis: translation and establishment of normative data. Am J Speech Lang Pathol. 2021;30(4):1750–66.

46. Kong APH. Dialectally-sensitive norms of the Spanish version of main concept analysis (Span-MCA) for quantifying neurogenically impaired spoken discourse. Rev Invest Logoped. 2021;11(2):5.
47. Smith A. Older adults and technology use. 2014.
48. Chaet D, Clearfield R, Sabin JE, Skimming K. Ethical practice in telehealth and telemedicine. J Gen Intern Med. 2017;32(10):1136–40.
49. World Dementia Council. Global dialogue on technology: reflections. London; 2021.
50. Kourtis LC, Regele OB, Wright JM, Jones GB. Digital biomarkers for Alzheimer's disease: the mobile/ wearable devices opportunity. NPJ Digit Med. 2019;2:9.
51. Papp KV, Rentz DM, Buckley RF, Schneider OR, Hsieh S, Soberanes D, et al. Associations between remote cognitive testing on an individual's own digital device and amyloid burden on neuroimaging in clinically normal older adults: results from Boston Remote Assessment for Neurocognitive Health (BRANCH). Alzheimers Dement. 2021;17(S6):e056209.
52. Luo H, Andersson B, Tang JYM, Wong GHY. Applying item response theory analysis to the Montreal cognitive assessment in a low-education older population. Assessment. 2020;27(7):1416–28.
53. Robin J, Harrison JE, Kaufman LD, Rudzicz F, Simpson W, Yancheva M. Evaluation of speech-based digital biomarkers: review and recommendations. Digit Biomark. 2020;4(3):99–108.
54. Yeung A, Iaboni A, Rochon E, Lavoie M, Santiago C, Yancheva M, et al. Correlating natural language processing and automated speech analysis with clinician assessment to quantify speech-language changes in mild cognitive impairment and Alzheimer's dementia. Alzheimers Res Ther. 2021;13(1):109.
55. Lindsay H, Troger J, Konig A. Language impairment in Alzheimer's disease-robust and explainable evidence for AD-related deterioration of spontaneous speech through multilingual machine learning. Front Aging Neurosci. 2021;13:642033.
56. Woods B, Aguirre E, Spector AE, Orrell M. Cognitive stimulation to improve cognitive functioning in people with dementia. Cochrane Database Syst Rev. 2012;(2):CD005562.
57. Spector A, Orrell M, Woods B. Cognitive stimulation therapy (CST): effects on different areas of cognitive function for people with dementia. Int J Geriatr Psychiatry. 2010;25(12):1253–8.
58. Guzman-Parra J, Barnestein-Fonseca P, Guerrero-Pertinez G, Anderberg P, Jimenez-Fernandez L, Valero-Moreno E, et al. Attitudes and use of information and communication technologies in older adults with mild cognitive impairment or early stages of dementia and their caregivers: cross-sectional study. J Med Internet Res. 2020;22(6):e17253.
59. Jacobs DM, Peavy GM, Banks SJ, Gigliotti C, Little EA, Salmon DP. A survey of smartphone and interactive video technology use by participants in Alzheimer's disease research: implications for remote cognitive assessment. Alzheimers Dement (Amst). 2021;13(1):e12188.
60. Piau A, Wild K, Mattek N, Kaye J. Current state of digital biomarker technologies for real-life, home-based monitoring of cognitive function for mild cognitive impairment to mild Alzheimer disease and implications for clinical care: systematic review. J Med Internet Res. 2019;21(8):e12785.
61. Knapp M, Shehaj X, Wong G, Hall A, Hanratty B, Robinson L, et al. Digital technology to support people living with dementia and carers. London: NIHR Older People and Frailty Policy Research Unit; 2022. Contract No.: PR-PRU-1217-21502.

Additional Resources

Articles

Bilder RM, Postal KS, Barisa M, et al. Inter organizational practice committee recommendations/guidance for teleneuropsychology in response to the COVID-19 pandemic†. Arch Clin Neuropsychol. 2020;35(6):647–59. https://doi.org/10.1093/arclin/acaa046.

Rini JF, Tsoy E, Peet B, et al. Feasibility and acceptability of a multidisciplinary academic telemedicine system for memory care in response to COVID-19. Neurol Clin Pract. 2022;12(6):e199–209. https://doi.org/10.1212/CPJ.0000000000200099.

Online Resources

American Psychological Association. Guidance on psychological tele-assessment during the COVID-19 crisis. 2020. https://www.apaservices.org/practice/reimbursement/health-codes/testing/tele-assessment-covid-19

American Speech-Language-Hearing Association. Telepractice. (Practice Portal). n.d. www.asha.org/Practice-Portal/Professional-Issues/Telepractice/. Accessed 8 Jan 2023.

Jacky C. P. Choy is a research assistant professor in the Department of Social Work and Social Administration at The University of Hong Kong. With a multidisciplinary background of psychology, psychological medicine, and social work, he is an applied social scientist interested in promoting the well-being of family caregivers and older population with care needs as well as shared family caregiving among multiple members. He has recently been involved in research projects concerning tele-assessment and remote non-pharmacological intervention for people living with dementia, and professional training on cognitive stimulation therapy in collaboration with University College London.

Ruizhi Dai is a lecturer in the Department of Psychology, Faculty of Education at Guangzhou University, China. With a background in cognitive psychology, Dr. Dai studies spatial cognition, metacognition, working memory, and how cognitive functions change with healthy aging and as a result of dementia. Her research interests also include non-pharmacological interventions and cognitive assessments for people living with dementia. As a co-Principal Investigator or a co-Investigator, Dr. Dai has participated in multiple research projects funded by the University Grants Committee of Hong Kong, The University of Hong Kong, and other private foundations.

Anthony Pak-Hin Kong is a fellow of the American Speech-Language-Hearing Association (ASHA) and Academy of Aphasia. Trained as a speech-language pathologist, his research interests include stroke-induced aphasia, discourse analyses, and neurogenic communication disorders in multilingual speakers. His research has received continuous funding from the National Institutes of Health, the Hong Kong Government, National Natural Science Foundation of China, and multiple (inter)national universities and private foundations. As a world-renowned scholar in communication sciences and disorders, he serves and served as Consultant/Advisor to provide research, clinical, and/or professional consultations to many (inter)national agencies, such as Aphasia United, Project BRIDGE (Building Research Initiatives by Developing Group Effort, USA), the Hong Kong Hospital Authority, and the Hong Kong Society for Rehabilitation. Dr. Kong is the current Founding Editor-in-Chief of Cogent Gerontology (Taylor & Francis).

Gloria H. Y. Wong is a director of the MSocSc (Mental Health) programme at The University of Hong Kong. Her research and teaching aims to improve mental health in society through scientific methods, focusing on dementia, psychosis, and preventive mental health. Her work has received funding from government and key philanthropies with a total budget of approximately HK$218 million. These include clinical research that has reached over 20,000 people, including the adaptation of evidence-based non-pharmacological interventions such as Cognitive Stimulation Therapy (CST) for remote delivery during COVID. These works have led to the publication of over 100 international journal articles. She advises local and international services and knowledge exchange bodies, including Hong Kong Alzheimer's Disease Association, and the Dementia Training Academy (https://www.ucldementiatrainingacademy.org/), a University College London—Peking University—The University of Hong Kong partnership.

Part III

Evidenced-Based Training Strategies, Interventions, and Innovative Technology to Improve Neurogenic Disordered Discourse

Interventions Targeting Spoken Discourse in Aphasia

19

Lucy Dipper, Marcella Carragher, and Anne Whitworth

Preview of What Is Currently Known

Discourse assessment and treatment is not a routine part of clinical practice internationally [1, 2]. Beyond the challenges of collecting, transcribing, and analyzing a clinical discourse sample, surveys of clinicians highlight an uncertainty among clinicians as to how to implement the findings of discourse analysis for the purposes of therapy [3]. The evidence-base for the efficacy and effectiveness of discourse treatment is also both relatively small and heterogeneous. A recent systematic review of discourse interventions [4] identified 25 papers, reporting on 127 participants. The papers highlighted a lack of consensus as to what constitutes discourse treatment, along with a wide range of therapeutic activities that targeted the different components and levels of language, and used a variety of treatment approaches, all features that characterize an emerging field of both research and practice.

Objectives

(a) To guide clinicians and intervention researchers to better understand the nature and role of discourse when selecting treatment approaches to meet individuals' daily communication needs
(b) To outline the various theoretical bases that have been used to study and treat discourse
(c) To explain the linguistic framework underpinning multi-level discourse treatments and highlight the role of cognitive processes when language is used at the discourse level
(d) To summarize the discourse treatment evidence base to date, and deconstruct three key example interventions, to highlight their core components and hypothesized active ingredients
(e) To provide a framework to assist in guiding clinicians and researchers to identify and plan treatment activities that map to specific discourse treatment goals

Discourse Therapies for People Living with Aphasia: Introduction

The ultimate objective of aphasia therapy has always been to facilitate the best communication possible to enable people living with aphasia to successfully participate in life. This goal is present across the varying communication profiles of individuals with aphasia and across the different

L. Dipper (✉)
Department of Language and Communication Science, School of Health and Psychological Sciences, City University of London, London, United Kingdom
e-mail: l.t.dipper@city.ac.uk

M. Carragher
Aphasia Centre of Research Excellence, La Trobe University, Melbourne, VIC, Australia
e-mail: M.Carragher@latrobe.edu.au

A. Whitworth
School of Health Sciences, University of Tasmania, Hobart, TAS, Australia
e-mail: Anne.Whitworth@utas.edu.au

A. P.-H. Kong (ed.), *Spoken Discourse Impairments in the Neurogenic Populations*,
https://doi.org/10.1007/978-3-031-45190-4_19

philosophical approaches adopted by treating clinicians and researchers. Designing and implementing therapies that lead to lasting and meaningful change in daily activities are, however, challenging. A growing trend in aphasia intervention is addressing this, with a focus on designing multi-level language interventions that meet these challenges in daily communication. This trend includes focusing on both monologic and dialogic discourse as treatment targets and contexts; strengthening psychometric robustness of outcome measures; and including individuals with lived experience in both the design and evaluation of discourse therapies.

Key Philosophies and Terminology

Early aphasia discourse interventions were heavily influenced by the findings of Ulatowska and colleagues [5, 6] where speakers with aphasia were reported as presenting with reduced complexity, amount of output, and clarity in narrative discourse but, overall, speakers were not considered to differ qualitatively from healthy controls. In the four decades since, discourse in aphasia has been approached by researchers in numerous different ways, with current therapy models and methodologies reflecting a wide range of philosophical underpinnings. Figure 19.1 [7] outlines the wide range of domains from which researchers have drawn to guide intervention of functional communication, and where discourse is frequently situated. In relation to intervention, each of these domains has guided the goals of intervention, the active ingredients embedded within the treatment, and how success of treatment has been defined and measured.

The term "discourse" is a broad and inclusive term which encompasses a range of discourse types, or "genres." These genres differ in relation to the linguistic, cognitive, and social demands placed on the speaker—see Fig. 19.2 [8]. Discourse genres can be differentiated by the elicitation method used (e.g., picture description vs. role play), the behavior of focus (e.g., products such as words and sentences vs. process such as how a couple repair a miscommunication), and

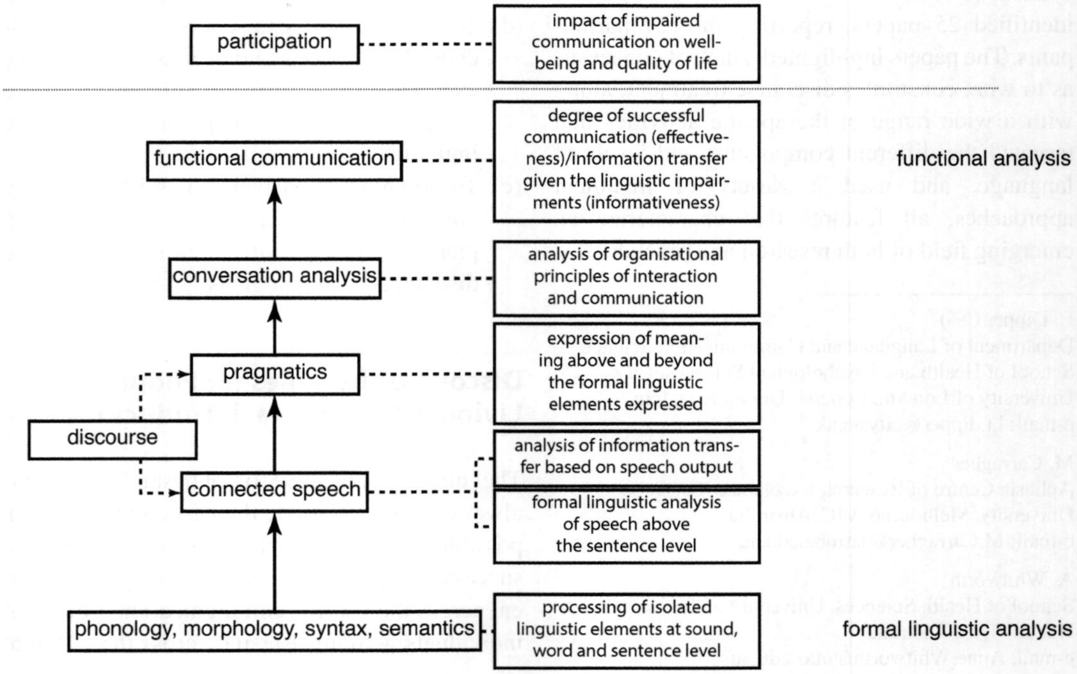

Fig. 19.1 Domains underpinning intervention for functional communication in aphasia [7]

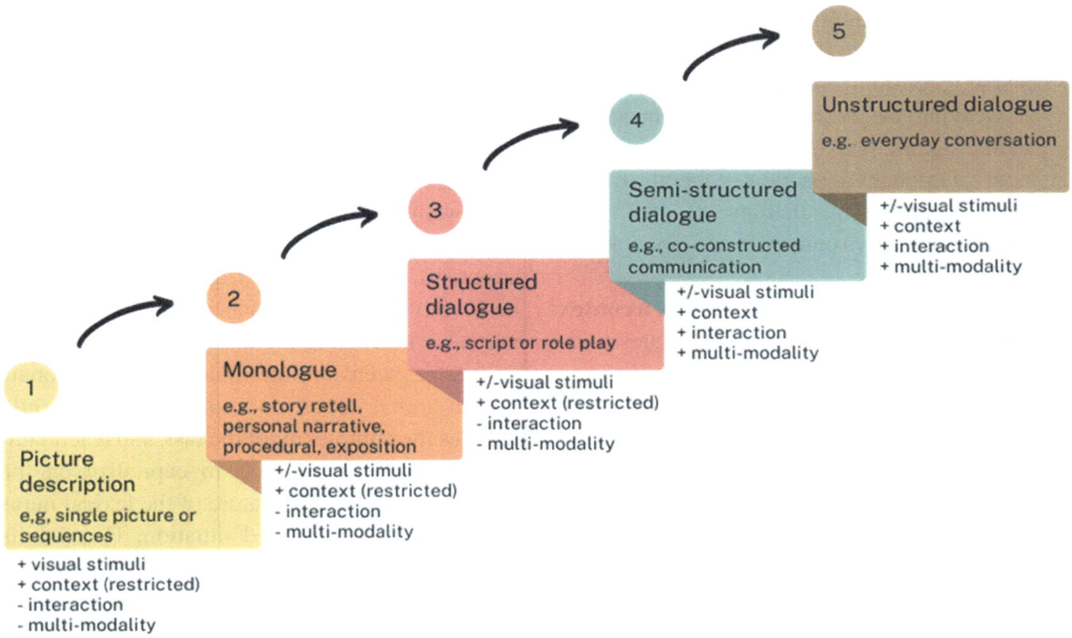

Fig. 19.2 Discourse genres (from Carragher et al., under review)

elements of complexity (e.g., availability of context, multimodal communication, and interaction [9]. Within the clinical setting, certain genres have traditionally enabled greater manipulation and control over assessment tasks and therapy targets and have therefore assumed a greater presence, such as picture description and monologues. Increasingly, researchers are interested in designing interventions that target different types of dialogue and which may be implemented within clinical settings (e.g., [10]).

The rich and varied theoretical bases that have been used to study and treat discourse give rise to a number of operational distinctions that the clinician needs to consider when deciding a course for treatment. Some of these key decisions are outlined below:

- **Structural vs. functional approaches:** Armstrong, in her seminal review of discourse in aphasia [11], suggested that there are two key philosophical perspectives. The first is the structuralist perspective which has a focus on *microstructure*, including the words, phrases, and sentences that make up discourse (e.g., [12, 13]). The second is the functionalist perspective which focuses on the construction and organizing of meaning within discourse, such that the *macrostructure* of the discourse is viewed as a semantic, organizational unit [14, 15].
- **Product vs. process**: Discourse is often conceptualized as a *product*, that is, a linguistic unit above the sentence level (e.g., [12, 13]). In contrast, in daily communication, discourse is likely to be conceptualized as a complex *process* that emerges from interaction between two or more speakers [16].
- **Monologue vs. dialogue**: Discourse interventions can include either or both monologues and dialogues [17]. This dichotomy may also be conceptualized by considering the inherent demands of in vacuo vs. in situ language [9]. In vacuo encompasses language samples that are outside of an interactional context and is a useful context for focusing on linguistic functions such as word retrieval or creating syntactic constructions. In contrast, language in situ refers to language samples from face-to-face dyadic interaction which typically include

multimodal communication and the availability of context [18, 19]. Moving along the discourse spectrum from monologue to dialogue, or weaving the two together within a treatment program, is likely to be a necessary treatment component to promote generalization of skills targeted in therapy to the more naturalistic environment of spontaneous communication.

- **Discourse therapy vs. discourse as a context for therapy**: A final distinction relates to the goal of therapy. Broadly, discourse interventions may be viewed as falling within two categories, i.e., those that actively target and seek to improve discourse structure or organization, and even the rules involved in discourse, and those that use discourse as a context for practicing microstructure targets with the intention of increasing generalization. Examples of the former include Interactive Storytelling Therapy [20], NARNIA (a Novel Approach to Real-life Communication: Narrative Intervention in Aphasia [21], and LUNA (Language Underpins Narrative in Aphasia [22] and are explored further below. In contrast, the latter category uses discourse as a context to practice and embed microlinguistic skills such as word finding, without explicit therapeutic focus on discourse structure or organization. An exemplar of this approach is seen in Rose and Douglas' study [23] where they targeted single words and combined these in a procedural discourse task to elicit words within treated categories, for example, describing "going to the zoo" to elicit "animals." Gains were recorded in both the retrieval of the treated words in isolation along with an increased number of nouns in discourse. Discourse was, therefore, used as a context for treatment to facilitate generalization rather than to specifically target discourse structure itself. This chapter will focus on the former interventions that focus on discourse organization and structure as the goal for improvement.

While our understanding of the philosophies underpinning discourse interventions may be facilitated using these dichotomous terms, increasingly the approaches are being more flexibly blended together. For example, current interventions (e.g., Interactive Storytelling Therapy, NARNIA, LUNA) explicitly target and integrate both micro- and macrostructure for therapeutic improvement. This blending of approaches suggests that traditional dichotomies, such as the structural vs. functionalist distinction, may now be overly simplistic. Intervention approaches may also involve an initial focus on monologues with later extension into dialogue. The rationale for an initial focus on monologue frequently reduces the complexity of the task and teach/consolidate rules, as well as to capitalize on the shared and predictable nature of the lexical items and topics in a controlled situation. These skills may then be embedded within a dialogic therapy context, in order to specifically target new skills and use strategies in a context where there are increased social and cognitive demands. In their review of the theoretical and methodological challenges within discourse production, Linnik and colleagues [24] reinforced, among other constructs, the importance of integrating micro- and macro structure, highlighting the relationship between linguistic competence and successful communication. This bringing together of different knowledges around discourse into integrated and comprehensive therapeutic approaches offering a logical and promising way forward to enhance communication.

Why Discourse Therapy Matters

People with lived experience of aphasia, and key stakeholders such as health professionals, have consistently indicated that assessing and treating communication difficulties is a key priority in rehabilitation [25, 26], and there is much evidence that is testimony to successful approaches that improve communication. The vast majority of aphasia therapy has targeted language impairments, with a particular focus on those components that are categorized as microstructure, e.g., improving word knowledge and access [27, 28], and the comprehension and production of sentence structure [29, 30]. While relatively consistent gains have been seen on items targeted in therapy, these gains have frequently not been maintained and the amount of transfer or generalization to untreated words and sentences, and to such daily contexts as conversation, has been far more variable and in many instances negligible [31–36]. Understanding our lack of success in generalizing to those daily contexts where communication disability is experienced by people with aphasia has resulted in a resurgence of interest in the discourse level of communication and, subsequently, discourse level therapies. A focus on discourse may provide both new theoretical insights into how generalization is best likely to be facilitated and maintained and, importantly, how we can work effectively with people with aphasia to maximize communication gains.

What Do We Know About Discourse Treatment?

Despite discourse underpinning everyday communication, it is not a routine feature in clinical practice internationally [1, 2]. A survey of UK speech-and-language therapists (n = 211) indicated that only 30% of respondents routinely analyzed discourse [3]. Beyond the challenges of collecting, transcribing, and analyzing a discourse sample, the survey data indicated an uncertainty among clinicians regarding how to implement the findings of discourse analysis for the purposes of therapy. This lack of routine assessment of discourse coincides with a low incidence of discourse level interventions both in clinical practice and in literature. A UK survey (n = 50) and related focus group (n = 6) investigated clinical implementation of intervention for one particular type of discourse, conversation therapy [37]. Findings indicated that, while conversation was a frequent target of therapy, clinical interventions often differed from published protocols, for example, by combining different treatment approaches, such that conversation therapies were variable in their implementation. Further, the authors found that clinicians felt more pressure to justify targeting conversation in therapy compared to, for example, microstructure [37].

The low clinical implementation of discourse interventions is perhaps unsurprising given that they are necessarily complex in nature [38] and a lack of consensus on the essential features, or critical ingredients, of this type of intervention [4]. Within discourse intervention, therapeutic targets may range from words to sentences to discourse, may focus on a single or multiple levels, and may or may not include the communication partner [39]. Importantly, if the clinical goal is to improve spoken discourse, evidence suggests that the discourse level should be explicit in the intervention (e.g., [21]).

While still relatively new to everyday clinical practice, the evidence base regarding the efficacy and effectiveness of discourse treatment is growing. A recent systematic review [4] found 25 papers, reporting on 127 participants, that *explicitly* reported on treatment of discourse in aphasia. Analysis of these studies revealed significant heterogeneity in treatment approaches to discourse, even within this small field. As Armstrong [11] noted, one of the reasons for this is likely related to the variety of perspectives taken in the literature. Contemporary approaches variably target the linguistic impairment (words and sentences) within a spoken discourse, macrostructural issues such as topic maintenance or story grammar, the cognitive processes involved in discourse planning, and/or more functional perspectives such as the overall communicative success of the discourse. A wide range of therapeutic activities have been reported aimed at different levels of language, with treatment approaches delivered across both individual and group settings, sometimes combining both. This heterogeneity in perspectives has resulted in a lack of consensus about what constitutes discourse treatment. In an emerging field, it is both important and appropriate to trial various treatment approaches and designs, with this variety in philosophies and approaches both illustrating not just the complexity of intervening in discourse but also that it is a strength in progressing our understanding.

While empirically appropriate, an obstacle arising from this heterogeneity is that it can be viewed as providing sparse guidance for clinicians and researchers, and that it fails to provide the impetus to move the field forward in consensus. A more productive approach may be to acknowledge the multifaceted nature of discourse, sitting as it does at the interface of language and cognition, consisting of multiple layers of processing, and comprised of multiple levels of language. The most effective discourse level interventions are likely to be complex, theoretically driven programs with solid foundations in metalinguistics and metacognitive skills.

Why Complexity?

Of the 25 discourse treatment studies reviewed by Dipper and colleagues [4], five described treatment targeting words in discourse, five targeted sentences in discourse, and two focused on discourse macrostructure only. While there were eight studies with treatment activities directed at multiple linguistic levels, only three of these studies targeted all three key levels of language (i.e., words, sentences, and discourse macrostructure). Arguably, the evidence base reporting truly *complex* interventions for discourse production is constrained to a very small number of studies. Despite these limitations, there are clear indicators that discourse treatment is beneficial. In this review, the most frequent benefit reported in the studies was improvement in word production in discourse, a finding reported in 88% of the studies; these included treatment activities with a range of targets. Changes in sentence production and discourse macrostructure were both less frequently assessed and less frequently reported. Moreover, changes in sentence production and discourse macrostructure were reported only when treatment activities explicitly targeted them.

To explore this idea further, the following sections will focus specifically on some of the studies in the evidence base that illustrate intentional targeting. Beginning with those aimed primarily at discourse macrostructure, two studies are of interest [15, 20] and involve five participants in total. Both studies reported gains in word production *and* in discourse macrostructure. The three studies describing multi-level treatments [21, 40, 41] involved 28 participants. Treatment was evaluated at multiple linguistic levels; each reported significant and maintained gains (on at least some of the assessed parameters) in word production and sentence production in discourse; discourse macrostructure was assessed in two of the studies [21, 40] and also showed significant gains.

These studies do demonstrate that, in contrast to therapies aimed specifically at improving word production (be it at the single word level or in a discourse context), therapies that also target sentence production and macrostructure in discourse do attend to two principles. First, they involve explicit, or direct, instruction in the rules and processes around sentences and macrostructure. Second, where the aim is to achieve gains in lexical access, sentence production, and macrostructure in discourse, it is important that the therapy target each of these in discourse tasks. In a later section, the mechanisms through which early evidence is proposed to occur in these complex multi-level discourse interventions will be illustrated.

Why Theory?

As highlighted earlier, one explanation for the heterogeneity in the discourse treatment evidence base relates to theory. There is scarcity in the use of a theoretical rationale for the treatments reported and, where theoretical frameworks are used, there is no dominant framework. Best practice in designing all complex interventions, including discourse treatments, is to develop them systematically, using both the best available evidence *and* theory [38]. In particular, complex treatments require a theoretical rationale linked to components of intervention in order to explain the expected mechanisms of change [38]. Only three of the 25 studies in the review by Dipper and colleagues [4] explicitly mentioned a theoretical framework for discourse macrostructure [20, 21, 40], and these authors drew on varied sources ([42] for cohesion; [14, 43, 44] for story grammar).

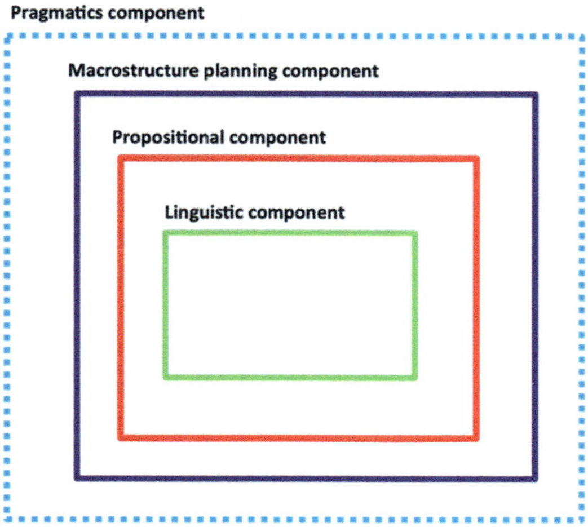

Fig. 19.3 The LUNA framework for spoken discourse [45]

While there is an evident lack of theoretical consensus in the discourse treatment evidence base, there is no lack of available theoretical frameworks. There are numerous theoretical perspectives available arising, in particular, from linguistic theory (including cognitive linguistics, psycholinguistics, sociolinguistics, and pragmatics). Dipper and colleagues [45] offered a *unified* theoretical framework based on a review of these—see Fig. 19.3.

Discourse production is described in this framework consisting of four core components: linguistic, propositional, macrostructure planning, and pragmatics. In planning a discourse, the *pragmatics* component drives decisions in relation to environmental, interpersonal, and interactional factors, all of which influence language formality and the degree to which shared knowledge can be assumed. This component takes into account the developing linguistic context and the interactional purpose of the discourse. The *macrostructure planning* component creates an organizational frame for the discourse which is likely to both draw on familiar templates and require online structural decisions. The *propositional* component is a prelinguistic organizational component that packages the discourse for linguistic processing, involving decisions about perspective, information selection/rejection, and information sequencing. The final *linguistic* component translates information into language (syntactic form, lexicalization, phonological assembly, articulation). Each of these components has the potential to influence another, with feedback occurring both "'upwards" and "downwards" between components through revisions and reshaping as the discourse is created. A word or sentence production difficulty in the linguistic component, for example, could initiate the restructuring of information in the propositional component and/or in terms of the macrostructure, which would in turn need to be picked up by the pragmatic processing.

Cognitive skills are relevant to all of these components. Executive functions, in particular, are drawn on when linguistic components become situated in propositional decisions and macrostructure planning. Perspective-taking, planning and prioritization, attention, inhibition and self-monitoring, and overall organization of thoughts all underpin the preparation of discourse. Memory (specifically episodic, prospective, and working memory) also plays a key role. Although cognition underpins many language tasks, with language being viewed by many as a cognitive process in itself, this intersection of language and cognition is particularly evident when the increased task demands of discourse processing are present.

Why Metalinguistics and Metacognition?

Being able to understand the concepts involved in language and cognition are important in discourse therapies, both underpinning the client's learning and driving the clinician's delivery. For clients to manipulate their language, they need a vocabulary to do this and, to manipulate their thinking, they equally need to understand what is involved. Much of our evidence to date is drawn from the sentence processing literature. While improvement in sentence production can occur without a person developing metalinguistic knowledge of sentences during the therapy process (see [46], for an example), this does tend to be the exception. Gaining an understanding of the roles played by words in sentences and explicitly mapping these to the sentence frame have produced consistent evidence of increased verb use and generalization to sentence production (e.g., [47–49]), even when the deficit is solely in creating the sentence frame, or predicate argument structure (also referred to as verb argument structure) [50]. The rule-based nature of mapping lexical items to sentences and being able to manipulate these rules at a metalinguistic level is viewed as playing a key role in the effectiveness of these therapies. The rules involved in discourse are likely to be even more integral to success, taking in both metalinguistics and metacognition. A metalinguistic awareness of discourse structure, frequently drawing on Stein and Glenn's story grammar [44], complements a knowledge of words and sentence structure. The increased demands on cognitive skills, discussed above, require a metacognitive awareness to be developed, including such aspects as planning, listener perspective, and evaluating how organized a discourse sample is. The clinician also plays a critical role in facilitating the client's awareness in multi-level therapies, as promoting strategy use, frequently involving direct instruction [51], draws on explicit use of metacognitive principles.

What Do We Know About How Discourse Treatment Works?

All therapeutic approaches need to be understood in relation to their aims and how each is hypothesized to achieve their unique aims. Discourse level therapies are no exception. The Rehabilitation Treatment Specification System (RTSS) was devised for rehabilitation more generally as a unified framework to allow for the systematic characterization of individual treatments [52] and has been applied to aphasia treatment [53]. Treatment theory is at the center of the framework: a tripartite structure (namely targets, ingredients, mechanisms of action) is used to describe the essential components that underpin the theory of a specific treatment. The RTSS specifies:

> *what the clinician does (ingredients) to elicit a change in a specific behaviour (target) and how that change is driven by an intrinsic mechanism (mechanism of action)* [53]. p. 577

In this way, the RTSS promotes a theory-driven specification of existing treatments, a considered approach to any modifications to these existing treatments, and a framework for future treatment developments.

Here, the RTSS is applied to discourse level therapies, to deconstruct the components within these complex interventions, and to increase transparency regarding the active ingredients within these interventions. Given the scarcity of discourse therapies and of multi-level interventions [4], three contrasting interventions are chosen to highlight how the RTSS can elucidate the components of discourse therapies. Each intervention will be summarized before the details are outlined in Table 19.1.

Interactive storytelling therapy [20] targets semi-structured dialogue and includes both the speaker with aphasia as well as their significant other. Embedded within the intervention is an acknowledgment of the multifaceted and collaborative nature of communication. Communication success is contextualized within a storytelling paradigm due to (1) the importance and prevalence of storytelling in daily life and (2) the experimental opportunities afforded by storytelling, that is, shared storytelling overlaps with some aspects of conversation but, crucially, can be benchmarked against externally set criteria which is useful for defining and quantifying "success." Interactive storytelling therapy is a complex intervention [38] in that it includes a number of actors (the individual with aphasia, the communication partner, and the couple), a number of interacting treatment targets (micro- and macrolinguistic behaviors as well as behaviors relating to the communication partner) with tailoring to the individual with aphasia and their partner. The goal of improving dialogic communication is operationalized through improving linguistic and metacognitive aspects relating to the individual with aphasia, how the communication partner receives and responds to communicative attempts and breakdown, and how the couple can reflect

Table 19.1 Illustrating how discourse level therapies are mapped against the RTSS

RTSS components	Intervention
Interactive storytelling therapy [20]	
Aim i.e., *the broad goal of the treatment*	To improve the couple's success in sharing new information in the context of storytelling
Target i.e., *a measurable behavior that is expected to improve as a result of the treatment*	• Improve the person with aphasia's storytelling from a multi-level perspective (story structure, selection of content with the partner in mind, improved argument structure, use of multimodal communication) • Optimize the interactional environment by improving the partner's competency as a communication partner
Ingredients i.e., *what the clinician does to affect change*	*Stimuli*: video clips that were funny or surprising, with minimal or no spoken language *Cues*: modeling (e.g., agent-verb construction, gesture, or a repair strategy), prompting, stepped withdrawal of support, visual record of the story *Intensity*: once weekly sessions lasting 1.5 h, over 6 weeks (total: 9 h/6 weeks) *Methods*: video feedback and self-reflection; goal-setting; story construction practice
Mechanism of action i.e., *the hypothesized reason as to why the treatment works*	For people with aphasia: • Individually tailored goals • Segment the story into a beginning, middle and end; specify the main referent (story grammar) • Consider the communication partner's needs in deciding which details to include or omit (selectivity and thinking for speaking) • Augment argument structure, e.g., agent-verb or agent-adjective structures either verbally or through verbal + multimodal resources • Increase communication success by using multimodal communication including drawing, gesture, writing • Use of a visual record of the story crafted by the person with aphasia, to aid short-term memory and decision-making For the communication partner: • Individually-tailored goals • Identify the cause of a breakdown in understanding (conversation coaching) • Discussing and trialing options for repairing breakdown (conversation coaching) For the couple: • View the video stimulus together to see the "answer" • Video feedback of the couple's shared storytelling (self-reflection, metacognitive skills)
NARNIA [21]	
Aim i.e., *the broader goal of the treatment*	To improve the content, structure, and organization of spoken discourse to optimize everyday communication and reduce the impact of language difficulties in daily life
Target i.e., *a measurable behavior that is expected to improve as a result of the treatment*	Within a range of monologic discourse genres (narratives, personal recounts, procedures, and opinions), aim to: • Increase frequency (both specificity and diversity) of verb, noun, and adjective retrieval in novel monologues • Increase use of sentences with complete verb argument structure (1, 2, and 3 argument structures and complex embedded sentences) in novel monologues • Increase the macrostructure of novel monologues across all four genres, including story grammar elements and use of cohesive ties • Increase efficiency and informativeness of novel monologues

(continued)

Table 19.1 (continued)

RTSS components	Intervention
Ingredients i.e., *what the clinician does to affect change*	The clinician ensures: • Integration of multiple language levels (words, sentences, macrostructure) into the planning and production of each discourse sample • An interactive approach with errorless learning • Lexical items driven by topic and interest; not predetermined by clinician • Explicit instruction of individualized lexical strategies where appropriate/needed • Retrieval of nouns, verbs, and adjectives to increase access to syntactic structures and semantic associations • Explicit instruction of sentence frameworks • Explicit instruction of discourse frameworks (organizational maps) for each of the four discourse genres • Explicit instruction of the role of planning, organizing, and monitoring of discourse • Visual mind maps of discourse frameworks used and can be faded out • Personal topics • Audio recording to promote self-monitoring Evidence to date: 20 × 1-h sessions (has been delivered over 4 weeks [massed practice] and over 10 weeks [distributed practice]. Home practice and carer involvement depending on person/context. Can be delivered by telepractice
Mechanism of action i.e., *the hypothesized reason as to why the treatment works*	Cognitive processing (explicit learning): • Event level processing to identify action, verb, and nouns to create explicit sentence frameworks • Metalinguistic awareness and practice of errorless and individualized lexical strategies • Metalinguistic awareness of the structure of sentence frameworks • Metalinguistic and metacognitive awareness of the organizational frameworks of a range of discourse genres • Self-evaluation of all word, sentence, and discourse elements, and overall coherence and cohesion, following each discourse production Reactivation (explicit to implicit learning): • Repeated practice of the organizational frameworks of a range of discourse genres • Enhanced salience and specificity to enhance access and linguistic connectivity
LUNA [22]	
Aim i.e., *the broader goal of the treatment*	To improve the telling of personal stories through word, sentence, and discourse macrostructure level activities. These activities aim to improve the content, structure, and organization of spoken discourse to optimize everyday communication
Target i.e., *a measurable behavior that is expected to improve as a result of the treatment*	To improve language at multiple linguistics levels: • At the *word* level, to increase use of relevant words, and the diversity of words • At the *sentence* level, to increase use of sentences with complete verb argument structure, and complex sentences with more complex structures (e.g. with two linked clauses) • At *macrostructure* level, to improve the overall structure of the story, including increased use of story grammar elements and improved coherence

Table 19.1 (continued)

RTSS components	Intervention
Ingredients i.e., *what the clinician does to affect change*	• Following a treatment handbook, the clinician and client work their way through 10 weeks of activities, each an hour long. In addition, there is another hour per week to practice the activities with a student clinician (or assistant) and challenge tasks to be completed by the client outside of the treatment sessions • The first session is on goal setting; the next 3 weeks involve word-level activities; the next 3, sentence-level activities; and the final 3, macrostructure activities • In each set of activities, the clinician provides a structure for the activity such as a semantic feature analysis chart, a color-coded sentence structure template, or a macrostructure framework. The clinician models and cues targets and also provides feedback or correction • Personalized goals and treatment targets through personally chosen story
Mechanism of action i.e., *the hypothesized reason as to why the treatment works*	• Working on individual linguistic levels (words, sentences, macrostructure) • Activities provide metalinguistic information at each linguistic level • Emphasizing the semantics of words in the story • Increasing awareness and use of core features of sentence structure • Targeting a range of sentence structures • Reflecting on reference chain use and structure, and its impact on cohesion • Segmenting the story into beginning, middle and end to work on the appropriate language for each section • Metacognitive use of treatment activities or framework as strategies to support storytelling

and learn from trialing new communicative methods in a safe space.

NARNIA (a Novel Approach to Real-life communication: Narrative Intervention in Aphasia) [21] is a structured multi-level language therapy, delivered using a natural interactive approach. Drawing on robust evidence-based therapies for improving microstructure (words and sentences), the protocol explicitly builds from microstructure to increase awareness and organization of a range of monologic genres (i.e., telling stories, giving opinions, explaining procedures, recounting events). Salient, personalized topics are introduced using a mind-mapping approach where diagrams are used to retrieve and then link ideas, events, and words in a way that leads to the organization and planning of thoughts. A focus on planning, organizing, sequencing, and monitoring ideas underpins the combining of language with cognitive skills, all skills required at the discourse level. The combination of "thinking" for "speaking" in everyday contexts is pivotal to the transfer of gains to communication outside the clinical setting.

LUNA (Language Underpins Narrative in Aphasia) is a clinical package for evaluating and treating personal narratives. LUNA was developed through a systematic process in which the research team reviewed the evidence base [4], surveyed clinicians [3], and codesigned the content of the package itself with clinicians and people with aphasia [54]. In LUNA, discourse is treated at word, sentence, and discourse macrostructure levels, using a personal narrative told by the individual. A key feature of LUNA is the use of personal narratives to generate treatment targets, thereby personalizing treatment as well as supporting salience and motivation. LUNA integrates familiar treatments—semantic feature analysis (SFA), mapping therapy, and story grammar—to provide flexible metalinguistic tools for improving people's confidence and ability to express themselves through narrative.

These three interventions conceptualize discourse and operationalize treatment in different ways. Table 19.1 draws out the underlying components of each, highlighting similarities and differences between the interventions.

How Can Clinicians Use This Information?

Given the inherent complexities within discourse interventions and the diversity of underlying theories, unsurprisingly there remains a persistent challenge of implementing these treatments within clinical practice. While this chapter has specifically focused on discourse therapies, it must be acknowledged that challenges also exist in several steps *before* therapy is offered. That is, there are a number of decisions to be made relating to what type of discourse sample to collect, which measures to use to analyze the sample, skill, and time needed to transcribe and analyze the sample, as well as skill and confidence to translate the assessment findings into a treatment program. These issues deserve detailed consideration but are not the subject of the current chapter. Here, the focus is on guiding clinicians to apply their knowledge of discourse as well as their knowledge of the individual with aphasia to decide on a treatment approach that fits with the individual's discourse goals.

All discourse level therapy should begin by careful identification of the specific goals of the individual and their close others living with aphasia. Figure 19.4 provides some examples of areas of focus in discourse, to show how a goal-setting framework including discourse context and mechanism of action might be used to guide clinical decision-making.

As Fig. 19.4 highlights, and consistent with many other interventions, overarching goals frequently need to be broken down into a number of smaller goals in order to be implemented in therapy and then built upon as therapy progresses. This figure illustrates some of the complexity in working with discourse, where almost no stone is left unturned. In collaboration with the client, and armed with a sound understanding of the components of discourse and how they interact with each other, the clinician is empowered to either gradually move through different arms of Fig. 19.4, or simultaneously incorporates several arms of the figure in a single treatment activity. A linguistically oriented treatment (such as improved sentence structure), for example, could be progressively embedded into a range of discourse targets (picture description, story monologues, conversation) within increasingly complex, interactive settings (1:1 with clinician, 1:1 with alternative practice partner, small groups). A 360-degree view of discourse, as set out in Fig. 19.4, is recommended to ensure that, first, an analysis of the components of discourse

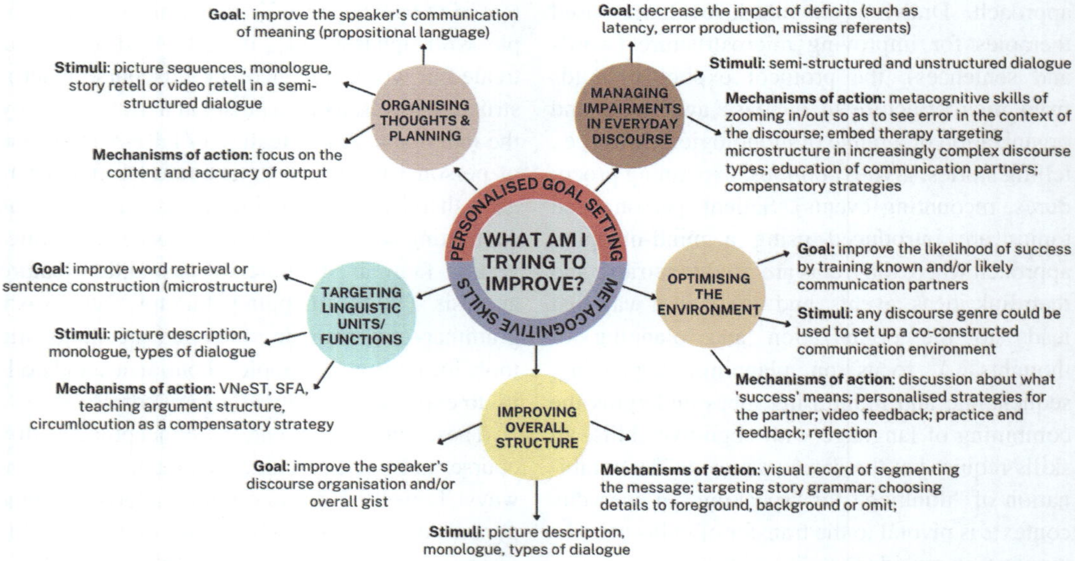

Fig. 19.4 Selected discourse treatment goals and associated treatment activities

is undertaken and targeted, and second, opportunities to combine the components into a multi-level approach are considered.

Conclusions

This chapter sought to provide an overview of developments in discourse interventions in aphasia, contextualizing these both within the historical literature in this field and the many theoretical frameworks in which discourse has been studied. We have aimed to challenge the clinician to view discourse therapy as separate to the notion of discourse being simply a *context* for therapy. We have also aimed to highlight that discourse therapy can be a combination of all the language levels that, as clinicians and researchers, we regularly target in intervention. The very nature of discourse requires us to go beyond individual linguistic structures (words and sentences). The increased complexity of different situations demanding different genres, conversational partners having unique perspectives, and the increased load in planning, inhibiting, monitoring, and generally organizing thought prior to production, all come into play. With discourse drawing on language and cognition in equal measure, intervention clearly requires innovative approaches. These approaches, however, are frequently underpinned by existing theoretical frameworks used in therapy and, as shown in this chapter, often combine approaches used routinely in clinical practice in novel and systematic ways.

Three contemporary discourse approaches have been presented. Each of these approaches is multi-level, aiming explicitly to integrate different levels of language, e.g., words, sentences, and/or macrostructure, into a single approach to improve spoken discourse. Such approaches inherently recognize that many people with aphasia have difficulty at multiple levels. Each of these approaches also acknowledges the importance of daily interaction and the desire to speak using coherent and meaningful discourse. From a learning perspective, the critical ingredients of metalinguistic and metacognitive awareness combine with the repeated exposure of practice to provide promising signs of generalized language gains, and gains that outweigh those from interventions that do not actively facilitate improved discourse. Discourse intervention involves an inherently nosier and more challenging therapeutic environment than, for example, picture naming or sentence construction, but persistence in understanding the aims, the critical ingredients, and the mechanisms through which change occurs is proposed here to be critical to more effective interventions that will impact daily communication.

Major Takeaways

1. If clinicians want to see improvement in discourse, intervention needs to target discourse.
2. If clinicians want to see change in a particular discourse genre, there is a need to direct the treatment there, informed by theory and tailored to the client's goals.
3. Multi-level therapies recognize the integrated nature of language and language breakdown.
4. These approaches do not need to be difficult or complex; they can comprise existing and familiar therapies but systematically integrate these across levels.
5. Where interventions are multi-level, there is promising evidence of greater generalization across levels that we have seen before—this is in direct contrast to seeking generalization within levels, and in expecting generalization to spontaneously occur (which it sometimes does but is best planned for).
6. As discourse is cognitively more demanding, intervention should recognize the role of cognitive processes and explicitly integrate these into therapy.
7. Metalinguistic and metacognitive strategies are likely to be key mechanisms through which discourse level interventions are effective.

References

1. Rose M, Ferguson A, Power E, Togher L, Worrall L. Aphasia rehabilitation in Australia: current practices, challenges and future directions. Int J Speech Lang Pathol. 2014;16(2):169–80.
2. Dutta M, Stark B, Murray L, Fromm D, Ramage A, Harmon T. Current practices in spoken discourse analysis in aphasia. EasyChair. 2021.
3. Cruice M, Botting N, Marshall J, Boyle M, Hersh D, Pritchard M, Dipper L. UK speech and language therapists' views and reported practices of discourse analysis in aphasia rehabilitation. Int J Lang Commun Disord. 2020;55(3):416–42.
4. Dipper L, Marshall J, Boyle M, Botting N, Hersh D, Pritchard M, Cruice M. Treatment for improving discourse in aphasia: a systematic review and synthesis of the evidence base. Aphasiology. 2021;35(9):1125–67.
5. Ulatowska HK, North AJ, Macaluso-Haynes S. Production of narrative and procedural discourse in aphasia. Brain Lang. 1981;13(2):345–71.
6. Ulatowska HK, Freedman-Stern R, Doyel AW, Macaluso-Haynes S, North AJ. Production of narrative discourse in aphasia. Brain Lang. 1983;19(2):317–34.
7. Doedens W. Situated language use in post-stroke aphasia: a systematic exploration of functional communication. 2020, University of Reading, unpublished thesis.
8. Carragher M, Mok Z, Steel G, Conroy P, Pettigrove K, Rose ML, Togher L. Towards efficient, ecological assessment of interaction: a scoping review of co-constructed communication. Int J Lang Commun Disord. 2023;58(2):482–515.
9. Clark HH. Anchoring utterances. Topics Cogn Sci. 2021;13:329–50.
10. Hall Z, Elbourne E, Togher L, Carragher M. Co-constructed communication therapy for individuals with acquired brain injury: a systematic review. Int J Lang Commun Disord. 2023.
11. Armstrong E. Aphasic discourse analysis: the story so far. Aphasiology. 2000;14:875–92.
12. Harris Z. Language and information. New York: Columbia University Press; 1988.
13. Schwartz MF, Saffran EM, Bloch DE, Dell GS. Disordered speech production in aphasic and normal speakers. Brain Lang. 1994;47:52–88.
14. Labov W. Language in the inner city: studies in the black English vernacular. Philadelphia: University of Pennsylvania Press; 1972.
15. Osiejuk E. Discourse exercises in aphasia therapy: a case study. Aphasiology. 1991;5(4–5):443–6.
16. Hengst JA, Sherrill MJ. Augmenting communicative environments for people with acquired neurogenic disorders: exploring situated discourse analysis. Top Lang Disord. 2021;41(1):27–46.
17. Armstrong E, Ciccone N, Godecke E, Kok B. Monologues and dialogues in aphasia: some initial comparisons. Aphasiology. 2011;25(11):1347–71.
18. Clark HH. Using language. Cambridge: Cambridge University Press; 1996.
19. Doedens W, Meteyard L. What is functional communication? A theoretical framework for real-world communication applied to aphasia rehabilitation. Neuropsychol Rev. 2022;32:937. https://doi.org/10.1007/s11065-021-09531-2.
20. Carragher M, Sage K, Conroy P. Preliminary analysis from a novel treatment targeting the exchange of new information within storytelling for people with non-fluent aphasia and their partners. Aphasiology. 2015;29(11):1383–408.
21. Whitworth A, Leitao S, Cartwright J, Webster J, Hankey GJ, Zach J, Howard D, Wolz V. NARNIA: a new twist to an old tale. A pilot RCT to evaluate a multilevel approach to improving discourse in aphasia. Aphasiology. 2015;29(11):1345–82.
22. Dipper, Botting, Boyle, Hersh, Marshall, Cruice, in press. PloS One.
23. Rose M, Douglas J. Treating a semantic word production deficit in aphasia with verbal and gesture methods. Aphasiology. 2008;22(1):20–41.
24. Linnik A, Bastiaanse R, Höhle B. Discourse production in aphasia: a current review of theoretical and methodological challenges. Aphasiology. 2016;30(7):765–800.
25. Stroke Association UK. Shaping stroke research to rebuild lives: the stroke priority setting partnership results for investment. 2021. https://www.stroke.org.uk/sites/default/files/research/stroke_priority_setting_partnership_full_report.pdf
26. Wallace SJ, Worrall L, Rose T, Le Dorze G, Cruice M, Isaksen J, Kong AP, Simmons-Mackie N, Scarinci N, Gauvreau CA. Which outcomes are most important to people with aphasia and their families? An international nominal group technique study framed within the ICF. Disabil Rehabil. 2017;39(14):1364–79.
27. Wisenburn B, Mahoney K. A meta-analysis of word-finding treatments for aphasia. Aphasiology. 2009;23(11):1338–52.
28. Hickin J, Cruice M, Dipper L. A systematically conducted scoping review of the evidence and fidelity of treatments for verb deficits in aphasia: verb-in-isolation treatments. Am J Speech Lang Pathol. 2020;29(1S):530–59.
29. Webster J, Whitworth A. Treating verbs in aphasia: exploring the impact of therapy at the single word and sentence levels. Int J Lang Commun Disord. 2012;47(6):619–36.
30. Hickin J, Cruice M, Dipper L. A systematically conducted scoping review of the evidence and fidelity of treatments for verb and sentence deficits in aphasia: sentence treatments. Am J Speech Lang Pathol. 2022;31(1):431–62.

31. Brady MC, Kelly H, Godwin J, Enderby P, Campbell P. Speech and language therapy for aphasia following stroke. Cochrane Database Syst Rev. 2016;2016(6):CD000425.
32. Best W, Grassly J, Greenwood A, Herbert R, Hickin J, Howard D. A controlled study of changes in conversation following aphasia therapy for anomia. Disabil Rehabil. 2011;33(3):229–42.
33. Carragher M, Conroy P, Sage K, Wilkinson R. Can impairment-focused therapy change the everyday conversations of people with aphasia? A review of the literature and future directions. Aphasiology. 2012;26(7):895–916.
34. Boyle M, Akersb CM, Cavanaugh R, Hula WD, Swiderskic AM, Elman RJ. Changes in discourse informativeness and efficiency following communication-based group treatment for chronic aphasia. Aphasiology. 2022. [Epub ahead of print].
35. Conroy P, Sage K, Ralph ML. Improved vocabulary production after naming therapy in aphasia: can gains in picture naming generalise to connected speech? Int J Lang Commun Disord. 2009;44(6):1036–62.
36. Hickin J, Cruice M, Dipper L. A feasibility study of a novel computer-based treatment for sentence production deficits in aphasia, delivered by a combination of clinician-led and self-managed treatment sessions. Aphasiology. 2022;37:1623. https://doi.org/10.1080/02687038.2022.2116928.
37. Sirman N, Beeke S, Cruice M. Professionals' perspectives on delivering conversation therapy in clinical practice. Aphasiology. 2017;31:465–94.
38. Craig P, Dieppe P, Macintyre S, Michie S, Nazareth I, Petticrew M. Developing and evaluating complex interventions: the new Medical Research Council guidance. BMJ. 2008;337(7676):a1655.
39. Webster J, Whitworth A, Morris J. Is it time to stop "fishing"? A review of generalisation following aphasia intervention. Aphasiology. 2015;29(11):1240–64.
40. Whitworth A. Using narrative as a bridge: linking language processing models with real-life communication. Semin Speech Lang. 2010;31(1):64–75.
41. Hoover EL, Caplan D, Waters G, Budson A. Effects of impairment-based individual and socially oriented group therapies on verb production in aphasia. Aphasiology. 2015;29(7):781–98.
42. Halliday MA, Hasan R. Cohesion in English. Routledge; 1976.
43. Rumelhart DE. Notes on a schema for stories. In: Representation and understanding. Morgan Kaufmann. 1975. pp. 211–236.
44. Stein NL, Glenn C. An analysis of story comprehension in elementary school children. In: Freedle RO, editor. New directions in discourse processing. Norwood: Ablex Publishing; 1979.
45. Dipper L, Marshall J, Boyle M, Hersh D, Botting N, Cruice M. Creating a theoretical framework to underpin discourse assessment and intervention in aphasia. Brain Sci. 2021;11(2):183.
46. Webster J, Gordon B. Contrasting therapy effects for verb and sentence processing difficulties: a discussion of what worked and why. Aphasiology. 2009;23(10):1231–51.
47. Fink RB, Martin N, Schwartz MF, Saffron EM, Myers JL. Facilitation of verb retrieval skills in aphasia: a comparison of two approaches. 1993:263–275.
48. Webster J, Morris J, Franklin S. Effects of therapy targeted at verb retrieval and the realisation of the predicate argument structure: a case study. Aphasiology. 2005;19(8):748–64.
49. Wambaugh JL, Ferguson M. Application of semantic feature analysis to retrieval of action names in aphasia. J Rehabil Res Dev. 2007;44(3):381.
50. Whitworth A, Webster J, Howard D. Argument structure deficit in aphasia: it's not all about verbs. Aphasiology. 2015;29(12):1426–47.
51. Ehlhardt L, Kennedy M. Instructional techniques in cognitive rehabilitation: a preliminary report. Semin Speech Lang. 2005;26(4):268–79. 2005 by Thieme Medical Publishers, New York.
52. Hart T, Dijkers MP, Whyte J, Turkstra LS, Zanca JM, Packel A, Van Stan JH, Ferraro M, Chen C. A theory-driven system for the specification of rehabilitation treatments. Arch Phys Med Rehabil. 2019;100(1):172–80.
53. Fridriksson F, Basilakos A, Boyle M, Cherney LR, DeDe G, Gordon JK, Harnish SM, Hoover EL, Hula WD, Hunting Pompon R, Phillip Johnson L, Kiran S, Murray LL, Rose ML, Obermeyer J, Salis C, Walker GM, Martin N. Demystifying the complexity of aphasia treatment: application of the rehabilitation treatment specification system. Arch Phys Med Rehabil. 2022;103:574–80.
54. Cruice M, Aujla S, Bannister J, Botting N, Boyle M, Charles N, Dhaliwal V, Grobler S, Hersh D, Marshall J, Morris S, Pritchard M, Scarth L, Talbot R, Dipper L. Creating a novel approach to discourse treatment through coproduction with people with aphasia and speech and language therapists. Aphasiology. 2022;36:1159–81.

Lucy Dipper is a linguist working in the field of Speech and Language Therapy, exploring the best ways to assess and remediate communication disorders. Prof. Dipper works with the language needed for communication in everyday life, such as storytelling and other forms of discourse; and creating feasible methods for clinicians to do so too. She joined City, University of London in 2000, and previously worked at University College London. She studied Linguistics at Sussex University and then undertook both her Masters and PhD in Clinical Linguistics at University College London.

Marcella Carragher qualified as a speech and language therapist in Northern Ireland and worked for a number of years with adults with acquired communication and swallowing disorders. Her clinical experience shaped her research interests regarding maximizing the generalization of behaviors targeted in therapy to everyday life. Her current line of work focuses on strengthening the evidence base around the validity and reliability of measures of semi-structured dialogues. Dr. Carragher is a Lead Postdoctoral Research Fellow within the NHMRC-funded Centre of Research Excellence in Aphasia Recovery and Rehabilitation at La Trobe University, Melbourne, Australia. Dr. Carragher is Deputy Treasurer for Aphasia Victoria, a consumer-advocacy group for people with aphasia.

Anne Whitworth is a clinician, researcher, and educator in the field of Speech Pathology at the University of Tasmania. Passionate about understanding communication disorders in acquired neurological disorders, Prof. Whitworth's research over 30 years has focused on developing effective evidence-based assessments and interventions for people with aphasia and dementia, and enhancing research capacity within speech-language pathology. Before joining the University of Tasmania in 2022, Anne led, taught, and researched at Curtin University and Newcastle University, UK; and had previously held clinical and managerial roles in a variety of health settings in Australia and the UK.

Neuromodulation of Impaired Spoken Discourse

20

Mehdi Bakhtiar, Maria Teresa Carthery-Goulart, and Anthony Pak-Hin Kong

Preview of What Is Currently Known

Over the recent decades, the application of safe and non-invasive brain stimulation methods for enhancement of human behaviors has received a great deal of attention by the researchers and clinicians around the world. The accumulating evidence suggests that the application of these methods will be promising as an add-on effect of behavioral training for aphasia. The majority of studies that used the neuromodulation methods in aphasia have focused on decontextualized word production such as picture naming. However, there is relatively less attention toward the effects that these methods can provide to functional communication such as discourse production. Nevertheless, the existing research is promising and suggests that neuromodulation combined with discourse production training may provide more impactful language recovery in people with aphasia.

Objectives

(a) To introduce the neuromodulation methods as an add-on treatment approach
(b) To explore the application of the neuromodulation for enhancement of language recovery in aphasia
(c) To explore the application of neuromodulation for impaired discourse production in aphasia
(d) To understand the key factors that influence the effects of non-invasive brain stimulation in functional communication in aphasia
(e) To suggest future directions on application of neuromodulation methods for impaired discourse production in aphasia

Background

Aphasia is an acquired language disorder due to brain damage, which involves different language domains resulting in difficulties using linguistic

M. Bakhtiar (✉)
Speech and Neuromodulation Laboratory, Faculty of Education, The University of Hong Kong, Hong Kong, Hong Kong SAR

Academic Unit of Human Communication, Learning, and Development, The University of Hong Kong, Pokfulam, Hong Kong SAR
e-mail: mbakht@hku.hk

M. T. Carthery-Goulart
Center for Mathematics, Cognition and Computing, Federal University of ABC, Santo André, Brazil

Cognitive and Behavioral Neurology Unit (GNCC), University of São Paulo, São Paulo, Brazil

A. P.-H. Kong
Aphasia Research and Therapy (ART) Laboratory, The University of Hong Kong, Hong Kong, Hong Kong SAR

Academic Unit of Human Communication, Learning, and Development, The University of Hong Kong, Pokfulam, Hong Kong SAR
e-mail: akong@hku.hk

A. P.-H. Kong (ed.), *Spoken Discourse Impairments in the Neurogenic Populations*,
https://doi.org/10.1007/978-3-031-45190-4_20

symbols across different modalities, i.e., listening, reading, speaking, and writing [1], across different performance levels ranging from words, phrases, sentences, to narrative discourse. The diagnosis of aphasia encompasses the exclusion of any other sensory, motor, psychiatric, and primary cognitive deficits, though they accompany aphasia frequently. These deficits have a multifactorial impact on people's communication, participation in daily living, independence, economic status, and quality of life [2]. Furthermore, with population aging, the incidence of neurodegenerative syndromes has increased all over the world. Some of these diseases affect the language network in the brain resulting in progressive aphasia syndromes. There is still no effective pharmacological treatment to address the underlying neuropathological conditions in people with aphasia (PWA). Speech-and-language therapy services are mainly used to improve the speech and language functions and reduce communication disabilities in PWA [3, 4]. However, the overall treatment progress is generally slow or minimal in this population especially among the chronic or progressive aphasia. Some studies have suggested that a minimum of 100 h of intensive behavioral therapy is necessary for significant improvement in communication skills of PWA [4], which imposes extensive financial burdens and efforts on families and healthcare professionals.

Neuromodulation Methods

One of the commonly used neuromodulation methods is Transcranial Magnetic Stimulation (TMS), which uses non-invasive magnetic fields to stimulate the neural cells. TMS can be delivered in single/paired pulses or in repetitive pulses. Single-pulse TMS is used to determine the Resting Motor Threshold (RMT) and has short-term effects [5]. Repetitive TMS (rTMS) effects can last for variable times beyond the period of stimulation [5, 6]. Low-frequency stimulation (<1 Hz) tends to inhibit neural activity, and high-frequency stimulation (>5 Hz) tends to induce excitatory effects specifically under the area of stimulation. rTMS has been extensively used for treatment of patients with different psychiatric or neurogenic disorders such as depression, motor disorders, and aphasia.

Another commonly used neuromodulation method is Transcranial Direct Current Stimulation (tDCS), which can provide two types of current stimulation, i.e., anodal (+) and cathodal (−) stimulation. Unlike TMS, tDCS alone cannot directly induce action potentiation in the neural cells. The anodal tDCS depolarizes the resting membrane potential of neurons, which allows for more spontaneous cell firing and subsequently increases the neural excitability, whereas the cathodal tDCS hyperpolarizes the resting membrane potential of neurons and consequently decreases the excitability of the regional neurons [7]. Figure 20.1 illustrates an example of polarity-specific changes in motor cortex excitability following tDCS stimulation. tDCS effects can last for variable periods (hours to months) depending on the stimulation protocol [5].

Despite the growing number of studies employing these techniques in PWA, there is no agreement about which technique is best suited to enhance the effects of speech and language interventions. tDCS is more affordable, portable and has a better placebo (sham) condition, whereas TMS can reach target areas more precisely (more focused stimulation) and has better temporal resolution [5]. In addition, although both techniques are very safe, tDCS has a neglectable risk of inducing seizures even when applied to perilesional areas in the affected hemisphere [8, 9]. Furthermore, with the introduction of high-definition tDCS systems, its spatial definition has considerably improved [10].

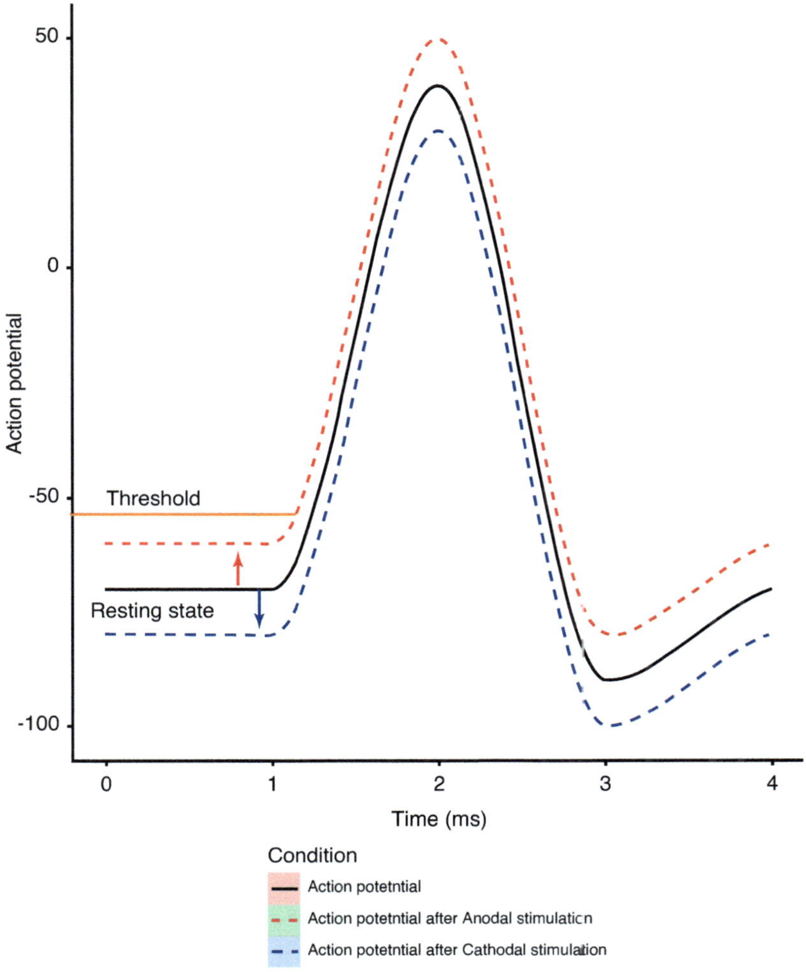

Fig. 20.1 An example of polarity-specific changes in motor cortex excitability (demonstrated by action potential) following tDCS stimulation

Neuromodulation and Language Recovery in Aphasia

It has been shown that the human brain is able to reorganize the activations of the neuronal networks in order to achieve the optimal recovery in PWA. Neuroimaging studies have suggested that spontaneous recovery is accompanied by the activation and reorganization of different brain regions [11]. There are at least two competing theories regarding the neural reorganization of language recovery in PWA [12]. Studies based on motor recovery after stroke have led some [13, 14] to postulate that the occurrence of a lesion in the left hemisphere (LH) diminishes the natural transcallosal inhibition from the dominant LH over the contralateral cortex and subsequently fails to suppress the maladaptive behaviors generated from the non-dominant right hemisphere (RH), which in turn interferes with the normal functions of LH (interhemispheric inhibition theory). This theory proposes that the neural activity of the LH regions needs to be stimulated while the neural activity in the RH regions needs to be inhibited in order to restore interhemispheric balance following a stroke. The other hypothesis, i.e., the laterality-shift hypothesis offers an alternative assumption regarding the role of RH following the LH stroke and supports the view that language function is shifted to the

RH regions that are homologous to LH areas premorbidly involved in defected language functions [15, 16]. According to the assumption of this hypothesis, the excitatory stimulation of the neural activities in RH regions might help to enhance its contribution in language recovery.

Neural reorganization is also affected by the characteristics of brain injury including etiology, location, and severity, along with age of onset and other factors associated with the concept of reserve (i.e., education, occupation, and diet). These factors are discussed to influence the neuroplasticity and severity of behavioral dysfunction in response to brain injury [17, 18]. In addition, access to the medical treatment for the brain injury and speech-and-language therapy services for communication deficits play a major role in aphasia recovery. The goals of speech-and-language therapy must be aligned to those factors and may target reactivation, substitution, or compensation of dysfunction. Neuromodulation has the potential of enhancing the effects of aphasia treatment by four mechanisms:

1. Facilitating the reactivation of the dysfunctional language network in the LH
2. Facilitating intra-hemispheric compensation by modulating the activity of unaffected areas, especially perilesional tissue
3. Reducing maladaptive plasticity due to decreased transcallosal inhibition from the LH, which results in overactivation of homotopic areas in the RH and, consequently inhibition of the LH cortex
4. Facilitating interhemispheric compensation (laterality-shift hypothesis)

The first three mechanisms are more suited to patients with less severe damage to the LH and can be achieved by increasing cortical excitability in the LH, reducing cortical excitability in the RH, or using these two types of neuromodulations simultaneously [19]. On the other hand, according to the laterality-shift hypothesis, regions of the RH need to be stimulated (instead of being inhibited). Some studies have suggested that this protocol might be more beneficial for the chronic patients with severe or extensive lesions in the LH [17, 20].

It is notable that the majority of the earlier studies that used the neuromodulation methods in aphasia treatment have focused on the decontextualized word production skills such as object or action naming. Although many of these studies suggested superior effects of neuromodulation (combined with behavioral training) compared to the behavioral training alone, the treatment outcomes are more likely limited to treated items and less commonly generalized to the functional communication. Therefore, it is quite important to develop treatment methods that are more functional and/or naturalistic such as discourse production to enhance functional communication across different contextual situations for PWA. In the upcoming sections, studies that have focused on the application of neuromodulation methods on impaired word production will first be reviewed. This is followed by more recent studies that extended to impaired discourse production.

Neuromodulation for Impaired Word Production

Naming and word-finding difficulties, which are commonly observed among different subtypes of aphasia, may critically affect functional communication. For this reason, numerous behavioral intervention protocols have targeted naming therapy. Focusing on the word-level production, the researchers can achieve a more rigorous control of the psycholinguistic properties of treated and untreated stimuli and offer a more precise quantification of the outcome measures by using a more controlled task or setting (e.g., picture naming). However, solely focusing on treatment of the word-level production in the format of picture naming has less frequently shown any benefits beyond the small sets of the treated items or toward an improvement in the meaningful functional communication [21, 22]. In this section, brief discussion and comparison of studies that used the most popular neuromodulation methods, i.e., TMS and tDCS, for treating impaired word production in PWA will be given.

Neuromodulation for Impaired Word Production in PWA

Many TMS studies in aphasia predominantly followed the assumptions put forward by the interhemispheric inhibition theory and applied low-frequency rTMS to the RH regions including the inferior frontal gyrus (homologous to Broca's area) to reduce the transcallosal inhibition and consequently facilitate the functional recovery of the language network in the LH through reactivation or intra-hemispheric compensation [5, 23–25]. This protocol has been replicated in multiple studies and suggested as an effective treatment for chronic post-stroke non-fluent aphasia [23] when coupled with speech-and-language therapy [26]. For instance, Naeser et al. [24] applied low-frequency rTMS (1 Hz, 1200 pulses, for 20 min) to the anterior portion of the homologous Broca's area in RH in four chronic non-fluent PWA. They reported better accuracy or speed of picture naming, along with improvements in elicited propositional speech for two patients (increased phrase length in the description of the Cookie Theft Picture of BDAE). Rubi-Fessen et al. [27] also investigated the add-on benefits of low frequency rTMS (1 Hz, for 20 min) over the right IFG with 10 sessions of language intervention focusing on word-retrieval. Thirty patients with subacute aphasia participated in this randomized, sham-controlled, double-blinded study. The study revealed significantly higher improvements in picture naming, and word and sentence comprehension for patients receiving TMS stimulation compared to sham. Despite the positive treatment outcomes reported across these studies, one debated concern is about the extent to which the outcomes are accompanied by the clinically relevant gains [23] such as improvements in basic communication and quality of life [28].

There are relatively limited studies that applied excitatory rTMS over the LH to balance the aberrant interhemispheric activation following the stroke in PWA. Dammekens et al. [29] applied excitatory rTMS (10 Hz, 2000 pulses) over the left IFG for 3 weeks (15 sessions) in a patient with aphasia and reported improvement in naming, comprehension, and repetition skills that was accompanied with reduction of neural activation in right IFG and normalization of electrophysiological patterns in the left IFG. Other studies that applied excitatory rTMS (intermittent theta-burst) over the left IFG (Broca's area) reported improved semantic verbal fluency among eight chronic PWA [30], and also improved performance across naming and speaking tasks among 13 non-fluent chronic PWA [31].

The studies discussed above indicated that inhibitory rTMS over the RH and excitatory rTMS over the LH can enhance the effects of word-retrieval training and lead to improvements on language expression and comprehension [28, 32]. However, there are some other studies that reported no add-on effects of rTMS for chronic [33] or subacute PWA [34]. However, it is notable that despite the lack of overall effects of rTMS, Waldowski et al. [34] revealed that a subgroup of patients (i.e., patients with left frontal lesions) obtained more improvements in naming performance while receiving rTMS compared to the sham condition. These findings may point to this issue that there is an inherent heterogeneity among PWA in terms of the response to neuromodulation treatment, which requires further investigation regarding the factors that may lead some PWA to benefit more than the others from specific neuromodulation protocols.

Given the greater availability, portability, and lower invasiveness of tDCS compared to TMS, a higher number of studies employed this neuromodulation method in PWA. This has allowed for a growing number of systematic reviews and meta-analyses being conducted with the purpose of exploring the effectiveness of tDCS in combination to behavioral interventions or as a standalone treatment [21, 22, 35–38]. The tDCS studies in PWA predominately use behavioral training that include noun and verb production [38] using different stimulation protocols such as unilateral anodal and/or cathodal stimulation of the right or left hemispheres, and bilateral (bihemispheric) stimulation including the simultaneous application of the anodal stimulation over the LH and cathodal stimulation over the RH [21]. The locations of stimulation also varied among these studies, tough comparatively more studies have investigated the effects of neuromodulation of the anterior (e.g., targeting the Broca's area and/or its homotopic area in the RH) versus the posterior (targeting Wernicke's area in LH and/or homotopic regions on the RH) cortical regions. A Cochrane systematic review of randomized controlled trial studies provided evidence for effectiveness of tDCS to improve picture naming in PWA, especially noun retrieval [22]. However, the authors indicated that there is limited report of any evidence for improved functional communication among these studies and therefore further studies are required. Other reviews have also reported positive effects of tDCS on naming skills when coupled with naming interventions (for example see [21, 37]). However, the behavioral interventions that accompanied neuromodulation varied across studies, in terms of types of exercises, dosage, duration and whether they were applied synchronously with tDCS or not [37]. Although both cathodal and anodal stimulation of the LH resulted in improvement in naming performance, more studies reported benefits associated with increasing cortical excitability in perilesional areas (see [21, 39]). In studies in which tDCS was applied to the RH, increased naming gains were observed when cathodal stimulation was applied over the frontal areas, which reported to be in line with the interhemispheric inhibition hypothesis (for example see [40]).

However, there are relatively fewer studies that applied excitatory stimulation of RH in PWA to examine the compensatory role of RH in language recovery (i.e., the laterality-shift hypothesis). The extant limited studies reported some improvement in performance of the PWA in naming accuracy, sentence production, and verbal fluency [41–43]. For instance, Flöel et al. [42] investigated the effects of 1 mA anodal stimulation of the right temporal-parietal regions combined with anomia therapy and found that anodal stimulation was associated with better outcomes in picture naming compared to the sham and cathodal stimulation of the same regions in chronic PWA. In a recent preliminary study, we applied 1 mA anodal stimulation over the right IFG combined with naming therapy to enhance the naming abilities of two chronic PWA [44]. In contrast to Flöel et al. [41], the participants showed diminished naming accuracy following the anodal stimulation of the right IFG versus the sham condition, though the difference was statistically significant in one participant [44], the results were not in the favor of the laterality-shift hypothesis. One speculation for contrasting results between Flöel et al. [41] and our study [43] might be related to different target regions of stimulation as the former stimulated the posterior brain regions (right temporal-parietal regions), whereas the later stimulated the anterior brain regions (right IFG).

Neuromodulation for Impaired Word Production in PPA

Primary progressive aphasia (PPA) is a neurodegenerative disorder that is marked with primary deterioration of language skills across different domains [45]. There are three different variants of PPA including the non-fluent PPA (naPPA), semantic variant PPA (svPPA), and logopenic variant PPA (lvPPA) [45]. The literature on the use of neuromodulation in PPA is sparse compared to PWA. Furthermore, the majority of the extant studies in PPA tend to apply the excitatory stimulation of the LH based on the neuroimaging evidence that patients with PPA to a lesser extent recruit the homotopic contralateral regions to compensate the reduced language network efficiency in the LH (see [36]). Similar to the studies on post-stroke PWA, most neuromodulation studies on PPA entertained the behavioral interventions targeting the decontextualized oral and written naming abilities and measured the treatment efficacy and generalization over a limited set of stimuli [46, 47]. Therefore, a similar research gap is the lack of report on the impacts of treatments in functional communication such as discourse production among individuals with PPA.

Despite the limitations, these studies provided evidence for add-on behavioral and underlying neural changes when excitatory stimulation of the language network in LH is combined with naming therapy. For instance, Cotelli et al. [48] compared the effects of 10 sessions of computerized naming intervention combined with excitatory tDCS (2 mA, for 25 min) over the left dorsolateral prefrontal cortex (DLPFC) among 16 patients with naPPA. The greater naming improvement was reported for patients receiving anodal tDCS (compared to sham) across both treated and untreated stimuli, which was maintained for 12 weeks after the treatment. In a subsequent study, Cottelli et al. [49] evidenced that PPA individuals with greater gray matter volume in temporal regions were more responsive to treatment and pointed to the importance of early interventions to potentiate the gains in this population. Roncero et al. [50] found similar results with a group of ten PPA individuals (non-fluent, logopenic, and semantic) with hypometabolism of the left perisylvian region. The authors conducted a double-blind crossover study in which patients received either 2 mA anodal or sham tDCS over the left inferior parieto-temporal region (the junction of angular and supramarginal gyrus) combined with 10 sessions of naming therapy. The results showed that anodal stimulation resulted in greater treatment outcomes than the sham condition along with higher generalization to untreated items.

The add-on effects of tDCS have also been investigated on written naming of people with PPA. For instance, Tsapkini et al. [51, 52] conducted a series of studies applying anodal (1–2 mA) and sham tDCS over the left IFG combined with oral and written naming training for 15 sessions among individuals with different variants of PPA. The authors reported that anodal tDCS leads to higher improvement of written naming than sham in individuals with PPA-NF and PPA-L [51, 52], with no additional benefits for individuals with semantic variant of PPA [51]. These findings point to the need of devising tailored neuromodulation protocols for patients with different variants of PPA. Further investigation of their results revealed changes in connectivity measures of the left IFG which was only induced by nodal tDCS (but not sham) [53], while the higher therapeutic gains were associated with decreases in global connectivity and higher independence of the language system (i.e., enhanced segregation of the IFG). The authors proposed that behavioral interventions combined with tDCS facilitate neuroplasticity within the left IFG, whereas behavioral interventions alone (i.e., sham condition) induce compensatory mechanisms (i.e., recruitment of other areas in the LH).

Neuromodulation in Impaired Discourse Production

Neuromodulation in Impaired Discourse Production in PWA

The initial neuromodulation studies mainly used TMS for enhancement of impaired discourse production. For instance, Hamilton et al. [54] applied inhibitory rTMS over the right posterior IFG (i.e., pars triangularis, BA45) on a patient with non-fluent aphasia with marked deficits in his propositional speech over a period of 5 years after the stroke. The patient received 1200 pulses of 1 Hz rTMS for ten daily sessions. The results showed that in addition to significant improvements in naming skills, the patient improved his propositional speech, i.e., producing longer sentences with a higher number of narrative and closed class words. The single case study was followed by a similar group study conducted by Medina et al. [55] including ten non-fluent PWA. The optimal location of the stimulation was individually determined for each patient based on the results of a picture naming task conducted before and after delivering the rTMS over the six different regions in the right inferior frontal gyrus. As a result, the pars triangularis was found to be the most optimal location of stimulation for majority of the participants (9 out of 10). Accordingly, the patients received rTMS treatment including 1200 pulses of 1 Hz rTMS for ten sessions over the 2 weeks. The performance on Cookie Theft description was measured three times at the baseline and 2 months after treatment. The results showed marked improvement in discourse productivity for the patients in the rTMS group (but not in the sham group) as indicated by increased number of narrative words (e.g., open-class and close-class words and the total number of verbs and nouns, and unique nouns). Since the measures of discourse fluency (such as sentence complexity, grammatical accuracy, or lexical selection) were not improved significantly, the authors attributed the marked improvements in discourse production to the enhanced lexico-semantic access while inhibiting the right IFG. These studies showed that inhibition of right IFG has a facilitatory role in aphasia recovery, which was in line with interhemispheric inhibition theory. However, the role of each hemisphere in neural reorganization and functional recovery still needs clarification. While the predominant approach in neuromodulation studies involves restoring balance of cortical excitability by inhibiting the RH, recent studies have explored a more individualized approach by investigating the brain areas that are associated with functional compensation using neuroimaging methods such as fMRI [19, 31]. These studies report that in some cases, the enhancement of the RH activation is associated with positive recovery. For instance, Ohara et al. [31] combined high-frequency rTMS (10 Hz, 2400 pulses) with ten sessions of language (i.e., naming, reading, repetition) and practical communication training (i.e., conversation therapy) among fluent and non-fluent PWA. Using fMRI, the authors investigated the areas related to compensation for speech production for each patient during a shadowing task (repeating words and sentences, reproducing as much as possible the speech production patterns of the model). The non-fluent patients received high-frequency rTMS in the left IFG, whereas the fluent patients received rTMS over the right or left STG. All patients exhibited long-term improvement in production skills (speaking, naming, and shadowing) after treatment, showing that personalized high-frequency rTMS was effective when applied to the right or left hemispheres across fluent and non-fluent PWA.

The tDCS has been more commonly used in the studies that applied neuromodulation methods for impaired discourse production in PWA. For instance, Marangolo et al. [56] using a sham-control crossover study design examined the application of 1 mA anodal stimulation over five sessions combined with intensive language therapy (i.e., naming the actions displayed by video clips). It was shown that tDCS stimulation resulted in an increase in verb naming up to one month after the treatment for 7 PWA. This effect was greater when the anodal stimulation was applied over the Broca's area in the LH than the Wernicke's area and also the sham condition. In the follow-up studies, the same group of researchers [57, 58] used the same tDCS protocol over the ten sessions combined by conversation therapy for each condition (i.e., anodal tDCS of the Broca' area, anodal stimulation of the Wernicke's area, and sham stimulation) to enhance the impaired discourse production in PWA. The findings were in line with their previous study as they found that PWA who received anodal tDCS over the Broca's area showed significantly better performance than the other two groups in terms of the number of content units, verbs, and sentences [57] and also significant improvement in the cohesion of speech marked with increasing the number of endophoric references (e.g., pronouns, conjunction, eclipses, and repetition) [58]. Furthermore, it was reported that the treatment outcomes were observed at one-month follow-up after the treatment and generalized to the untreated items (i.e., the video clips or pictures that were not used in conversation therapy) [57]. The effects were more pronounced for the anodal stimulation of the Broca's area than other conditions [58]. Furthermore, they conducted another study using different tDCS parameters that applied 2 mA bi-hemispheric stimulation with the anode placed on the ipsilateral lesion on the LH and the cathode placed on the contralateral lesion in the right IFG [59]. The location of stimulation was individually determined according to the location and extent of the brain lesion. The participants were randomly assigned to the sham or tDCS conditions, and then crossed over to the opposite treatment condition with 14 days of intersession interval. The tDCS stimulation was combined with intensive conversation/pragmatic therapy in which the patient and SLP exchanged information about some cartoon stories. The results showed that the tDCS stimulation improved the patient's performance in picture description (in terms of the correct use of words and SVO structure), verb naming, and picture naming. The observed effects were significantly higher in the active tDCS than the sham tDCS, and it was also observed at one-week follow-up. On the contrary, a recent study that applied a similar tDCS protocol [60] reported the lack of significant improvement in spontaneous speech following 2 mA bi-hemispheric stimulation of IFG compared to the sham condition. However, one major issue with this study is the lack of consistent, combined language training protocol across different participants.

It is notable that other groups of researchers have also applied tDCS for impaired discourse production. For instance, Galletta and Vogel-Eyny [61] reported a single case study of a participant with anomic aphasia while applying the anodal tDCS over the Broca's area combined with behavioral language therapy. Unlike many previous studies that mainly focus on decontextualized lexical training (such as picture naming), they emphasized the lexical retrieval training, which was embedded in the sentence production and focused conversation around a specific topic. The results showed that verb production (but not noun production) within the untrained sentence probes was significantly improved after anodal tDCS (+56% improvement), but not following the sham condition. Matar et al. [62] also conducted a preliminary tDCS study in six PWA and showed that anodal tDCS over left IFG combined with verb network strengthening treatment provided better treatment outcomes (i.e., the larger effect size) than sham condition in discourse production as measured by picture and procedure description, storytelling from the memory, and functional communication index. On the contrary, Aguiar et al. [63] find comparable effect among the tDCS and sham in improving the verb naming and sentence production. However, considering the higher baseline performance in sham group, the authors reported that larger treatment effect is observed among tDCS group. It is also notable the neuroimaging studies that applied anodal tDCS combined with conversation therapy reported that though tDCS can render improvement in language production, the treatment benefits are smaller for PWA with lesions in basal ganglia, insula, and superior and inferior longitudinal fasciculi [64]. Therefore, given that the treatment outcomes might be limited by the location and extent of the lesion, future studies might devise individualized neuromodulation protocol to maximize the treatment effects for impaired discourse.

In sum, the above studies suggested that neuromodulation techniques can facilitate language production of chronic PWA in a more meaningful and functional manner, when combined with a language training task such as discourse production or conversation therapy that is beyond the decontextualized word production (see Table 20.1 for more details). It is notable that the majority of these studies included the neuromodulation protocols that use excitatory stimulation over the LH regions especially the left Broca's area, or inhibition of the RH homologue regions. The studies mainly support the interhemispheric inhibition hypothesis. However, due to lack of studies that applied excitatory stimulation of the RH for enhancing the overall language and discourse production in aphasia, the arguments from the laterality-shift hypothesis remained unchallenged.

Neuromodulation in Impaired Discourse Production in PPA

The neuromodulation methods have been commonly used as an intervention strategy to enhance language skills or slow down the rate of language deterioration across different variants of PPA. As discussed, the main focus of the many studies was to enhance word production as measured by object and/or action naming tasks [48, 49, 66, 67]. Gervits et al. [65] applied tDCS to improve language skills of six PPA including four lvPPA and two naPPA. They used a unique tDCS montage that would allow an extensively large region of language network in the LH to be stimulated (see Table 20.1). They placed anodal electrode over the left frontotemporal area and cathodal

Table 20.1 Studies that applied neuromodulation for impaired discourse production in aphasia

Authors (year)	Target groups (sample size)	Neuromodulation	Location	Sessions	Task combined with neuromodulation	Outcome measures	Results
Hamilton et al. (2010) [54]	NF aphasia (1)	rTMS (1200 pulses; frequency 1 Hz; 70 mm diameter figure-of-eight coil; 10 min)	6 sites of right IFG: (1) motor cortex (2) pars opercularis (3) dorsal posterior pars triangularis (4) dorsal anterior pars triangularis (5) anterior pars opercularis (6) pars orbitalis	10 sessions	N/A	Cookie theft picture description, noun and verb naming, WAB	Significant improvements in naming skills and propositional speech where patients produced longer sentences with higher number of narrative and closed class words
Medina et al. (2012) [55]	NF aphasia (10)	rTMS (1200 pulses; frequency 1 Hz; 70 mm diameter figure-of-eight coil; 10 min)	Right pars triangularis for 9 participants; right pars orbitalis for 1 participant	10 sessions	N/A	Cookie theft picture description	Marked improvement in discourse productivity only in rTMS group as indicated by increased narrative words (e.g., open-class and close-class words, and the total number of verbs and nouns, and unique nouns)

Ohara et al. (2021) [32]	Aphasia (20)	rTMS (2400 pulses; frequency 10 Hz; 70 mm diameter figure-of-eight coil; 12 min)	Location adjusted based on fMRI results: left (13 patients) right IFG (1 patient) right STG (6 patients)	10 sessions (120 min during the 2 week hospitalization period) + 1–4 sessions per month after discharge)	Speech promotion (word-naming, word-reading, word and sentence shadowing, explanation of 4-panel cartoon, definitions, facial and oral movements, phonological exercises) + Practical communication exercises (Conversation training + Promoting Aphasics' Communication Effectiveness therapy (PACE) + self-training	Short-term assessment: SLTA naming, shadowing and revised token test of the Japanese version of WAB Long-term assessment: SLTA total score, Supplementary tests for SLTA (naming, auditory and reading comprehension, writing), shadowing and revised token test of the Japanese version of WAB	Short-term assessment (pre vs. post treatment): significant improvement of STLA naming and shadowing. Significant improvement in the shadowing task in the rTMS to LH; no significant difference in the rTMS to the RH. Significant improvement in shadowing for the fluent aphasia group and in naming for the non-fluent aphasia group Long-term (pre-treatment vs 3-month after treatment): all patients presented significant improvement in SLTA total score, auditory and reading comprehension, speaking and writing. Significant difference in STLA total score and speaking was noted in the rTMS to the LH and a significant difference in STLA total score and reading in the rTMS to the RH. STLA total score, auditory comprehension and speaking improved significantly both in the fluent group and the non-fluent group

(continued)

Table 20.1 (continued)

Authors (year)	Target groups (sample size)	Neuromodulation	Location	Sessions	Task combined with neuromodulation	Outcome measures	Results
Marangolo et al. (2013) [56]	NF aphasia (7)	tDCS (1 mA; 20 min; a pair of surface-soaked sponge electrodes (5 × 7 cm))	Anodic: Broca's area, Wernicke area	5 sessions	Action naming in video clips	Verb naming	Improvement in verb naming performance up to one month after the therapy
Marangolo et al. (2013) [57]	NF aphasia (12)	A tDCS (1 mA; 20 min; a pair of surface-soaked sponge electrodes (5 × 7 cm))	Anodic: Broca's area, Wernicke's area	10 sessions	Elicitation of conversation related to videoclips	The number of C-units, verbs, and sentences in conversation	Significant improvement in performing the number of content units, verbs, and sentences
Marangolo et al. (2014) [58]	NF aphasia (8)	A tDCS (1 mA; 2 min; a pair of surface-soaked sponge electrodes (5 × 7 cm))	Anodic: Broca's area, Wernicke's area	10 sessions	Elicitation of conversation related to videoclips	Number of endophoric references	Improvement of cohesion of speech by increasing the number of endophoric references (e.g., pronouns, conjunctions, eclipses, and repetition) while describing videos related to the daily situations
Marangolo et al. (2014) [59]	NF aphasia (7)	A tDCS (2 mA; 20 min; a pair of surface-soaked sponge electrodes (5 × 7 cm))	Anodic: ipsilesional IFG Cathodic: contralesional IFG	10 sessions	Pragmatic language training (cartoon stories)	Picture description, verb and noun naming	Improvement in picture description, verb naming, and picture naming

Aguiar et al. (2015) [63]	Aphasia (9)	tDCS (1 mA; 20 min; two 35 cm^2 electrodes)	Location adjusted based on MRI results: Anodic: Broca's area Cathodic: right hemisphere homologous of Broca's area (3 participants) Anodic: anterior and superior to Broca's area Cathodic: the homologous area in the right hemisphere (2 participants) Anodic: left superior and middle frontal gyri right homologous of Broca's area (3 participants) Anodic: posterior middle and superior temporal gyri Cathodic: a symmetrical position over the RH (1 participant)	10 sessions	ACTION treatment (Italian adaptation)	Sentence completion (finite (with three tenses) and non-finite verb production) and sentence construction (SVO)	Improvements in both measures (i.e., sentence completion and constructions)
Campana et al. (2015) [64]	NF aphasia (20)	A tDCS (2 mA; 20 min; a pair of surface soaked sponge electrodes (5 cm × 7 cm))	Anodic: ipsilesional frontal gyrus Cathodic: contralateral frontopolar cortex	10 sessions	Conversational therapy	Picture description, noun and verb naming	Improvement in all three outcome measures
Galletta and Vogel-Eyny (2015) [61]	Fluent anomic aphasia (1)	A tDCS (1 mA; 20 min; two 35 cm^2 (5 cm × 7 cm) saline-soaked sponges (Soterix Medical 1 × 1 device))	Anodic: Broca's area Cathodic: contralateral supraorbital area	10 sessions	Focused discourse (Conversation) + Sentence production training	Sentence probes with untrained set of embedded nouns and verbs	Verb production (but not noun production) within the untrained sentence probes was significantly improved

(continued)

Table 20.1 (continued)

Authors (year)	Target groups (sample size)	Neuromodulation	Location	Sessions	Task combined with neuromodulation	Outcome measures	Results
Gervits et al. (2016) [65]	PPA (6)	tDCS (1.5 mA; 20 min; 5 × 5 cm saline-soaked pads secured by a rubber strap)	Anodic: left frontotemporal region Cathodic: left occipitoparietal region	10 sessions	Narration of the wordless children's books	Speech rate in words per minute (WPM), mean length of utterance (MLU)	Continuous advancement in linguistic aptitudes (i.e., speech production and grammatical comprehension)
McConathey et al. (2017) [66]	PPA (15)	tDCS (1.5 mA; 20 min; 5 × 5 cm saline-soaked pads secured by a rubber strap)	Anodic: left prefrontal region Cathodic: left occipital region	10 sessions	Narration of the wordless children's books	Sentence repetition test, grammatical comprehension (Penn-TROG), semantic processing: Boston naming test (BNT) and pyramids and palm trees (PPT), category fluency tests	Individuals (with nfvPPA or lvPPA) who have poorer baseline performance exhibited greater tDCS-related improvements in global language performance, grammatical comprehension and semantic processing. Individuals with better baseline performance demonstrated a subtle tDCS-related effects in the speech repetition task only
Hosseini et al. (2019) [67]	PPA (6)	tDCS (1.5 mA; 20 min; 5 × 5 cm electrodes)	Anodic: left prefrontal regions Cathodic: left occipital region	10 sessions	Narration of the wordless children's books	Category fluency test, test of reception of grammar (TROG), pyramids and palm trees (PPT), Boston naming test (BNT)	Reduced difficulties in verbal fluency, particularly for lvPPA and naPPA patients, with tDCS-related benefits on semantic processing

Guillouët et al. (2020) [60]	Aphasia (10)	tDCS (2 mA; 20 min; a pair of surface-soaked sponge's electrodes (5 × 7 cm))	Anodic: IFG Cathodic: contralesional IFG	15 sessions	Speech-and-language therapy	Number of different nouns employed amid the HDAE subtest question "Describe your job" and verbal fluency tests	No statistically significant improvement
Matar et al. (2022) [62]	Aphasia (6)	A tDCS (2 mA; 20 min; two (5 × 7 cm) saline-soaked sponges)	Anodic: left IFG Cathodic: contralateral supraorbital ridge	6 sessions	Verb network strengthening treatment	Picture description, Procedure description, Storytelling from memory, Verb retrieval (verb type token ratio), functional communication index	Significant improvement in picture and procedure description, storytelling from memory and functional communication index

NF Non-Fluent, *PPA* Primary Progressive Aphasia, *WAB* Western Aphasia Battery, *SLTA* Standard Language Test of Aphasia, *IFG* Inferior Frontal Gyrus, *LH/RH* Left Hemisphere/Right Hemisphere electrode over the left occipitoparietal area. The tDCS stimulation was combined with a behavioral task in which the participants had to produce narrative speech according to a wordless picture story book. The outcome measures include several language tasks such as picture naming, semantic categorization, grammatical comprehension, and speech elicitation based on Cookie Theft picture. The participants showed improvements across different language tasks. More particularly, there was a marked increase in speech elicitation task in terms of the increase in mean length of utterances (MLU), which maintained for 3 months after the treatment.

Conclusion and Future Directions

Despite the essential role of discourse production for everyday communication [68], the majority of speech and language interventions in PWA and PPA have focused on enhancing naming abilities, which may not typically result in enhancement of functional communication [21, 22]. Not surprisingly, this chapter has summarized and discussed that only few studies have employed neuromodulation combined with conversation training or behavioral training that are designed to treat the main components of discourse production, i.e., length, informativeness, morphosyntactic structure, and global coherence and cohesion. It has been reported that different microlinguistic (e.g., informativeness, morphosyntactic aspects) and macrolinguistic (e.g., discourse structure) components of discourse production may concomitantly or even selectively be affected in PWA. This may suggest that the future neuromodulation studies may adopt behavioral training protocols that target different aspects of discourse production along with sensitive outcome measures to achieve optimal results in PWA [68]. Overall, the research studies that have been reviewed here collectively suggest that coupling neuromodulation methods with discourse production training or conversation therapy can lead to more functionally meaningful effects than decontextualized word-level training and that the effects can generalize to different linguistic domains/levels such as lexical retrieval, verbal fluency, and grammatical accuracy (see Table 20.1 for more details).

Although different locations of stimulation have been used across studies (see Table 20.1), anodal stimulation of left IFG seems to have contributed to enhancement of language recovery more effectively, particularly in discourse production, which would be more in line with interhemispheric inhibition theory. The evidence suggests that this protocol facilitates lexical retrieval for oral discourse production by balancing LH cortical excitability [55]. However, other underlying mechanisms of recovery (e.g., potential contribution of the RH in improvement of discourse production) demand further investigation. One future direction would be to examine whether the excitatory stimulation of various regions in the RH can lead to enhanced discourse production and functional communication especially among PWA with more extensive lesions on the LH. Further studies may also explore the effects of bilateral versus unilateral brain stimulation protocols on discourse production in PWA [60, 69]. It is also notable that an individualized neuromodulation according to the location and extent of the brain lesion might be more fruitful in gaining the meaningful behavioral outcomes. Perhaps, this would suggest different treatment parameters such as the polarity (anodal versus cathodal stimulation), intensity (e.g., 1 vs. 2 mA), location of the simulation, and the number of treatment sessions, in addition to language training protocol, could be customized according to the patient's pathological conditions. Lastly, future studies may also consider including participants with different types of aphasia in their treatment protocol. Since the existing neuromodulation studies have mainly focused on discourse production in non-fluent aphasia, it remains unknown whether or how neuromodulation treatments can improve the functional communication of people with fluent aphasia. These questions open new avenues for research in neuromodulation in order to achieve better functional recovery for PWA.

Major Takeaways

1. Application of neuromodulation methods can enhance the effects of behavioral training on language recovery in aphasia.
2. Application of inhibitory stimulation of the right hemisphere has been used as the most common protocol to restore the aberrant interhemispheric activation and impaired language skills in chronic patients with post-stroke aphasia.
3. Application of excitatory stimulation of the left hemisphere has been used as the most common protocol to restore impaired language skills in patients with PPA.
4. Individualized treatment based on underlying neuropathological conditions enhances the effects of neuromodulation on language recovery.
5. Neuromodulation treatments, when combined with the discourse production training compared to the decontextualized word production, will provide greater treatment outcomes across various language and functional communication skills.

References

1. McNeil MR, Pratt SR. Defining aphasia: some theoretical and clinical implications of operating from a formal definition. Aphasiology. 2001;15:901–11.
2. Cruice M, Hill R, Worrall L, Hickson L. Conceptualising quality of life for older people with aphasia. Aphasiology. 2009;24:327–47.
3. Basso A. How intensive/prolonged should an intensive/prolonged treatment be? Aphasiology. 2005;19:975–84.
4. Bhogal SK, Teasell R, Speechley M. Intensity of aphasia therapy, impact on recovery. Stroke. 2003;34:987–92.
5. Breining BL, Sebastian R. Neuromodulation in post-stroke aphasia treatment. Curr Phys Med Rehabil Rep. 2020;8:44–56.
6. Georgiou AM, Lada E, Kambanaros M. Evaluating the quality of conduct of systematic reviews on the application of transcranial magnetic stimulation (TMS) for aphasia rehabilitation post-stroke. Aphasiology. 2020;34:540–56.
7. Nitsche MA, Paulus W. Excitability changes induced in the human motor cortex by weak transcranial direct current stimulation. J Physiol. 2000;527:633–9.
8. Lerner AJ, Wassermann EM, Tamir DI. Seizures from transcranial magnetic stimulation 2012–2016: results of a survey of active laboratories and clinics. Clin Neurophysiol. 2019;130:1409–16.
9. Antal A, Alekseichuk I, Bikson M, et al. Low intensity transcranial electric stimulation: safety, ethical, legal regulatory and application guidelines. Clin Neurophysiol. 2017;128:1774–809.
10. Edwards D, Cortes M, Datta A, Minhas P, Wassermann EM, Bikson M. Physiological and modeling evidence for focal transcranial electrical brain stimulation in humans: a basis for high-definition tDCS. Neuroimage. 2013;74:266–75.
11. Fridriksson J, Richardson JD, Fillmore P, Cai B. Left hemisphere plasticity and aphasia recovery. Neuroimage. 2012;60:854–63.
12. Hamilton RH, Chrysikou EG, Coslett B. Mechanisms of aphasia recovery after stroke and the role of noninvasive brain stimulation. Brain Lang. 2011;118:40–50.
13. Murase N, Duque J, Mazzocchio R, Cohen LG. Influence of interhemispheric interactions on motor function in chronic stroke. Ann Neurol. 2004;55:400–9.
14. Takeuchi N, Oouchida Y, Izumi S-I. Motor control and neural plasticity through interhemispheric interactions. Neural Plast. 2012;2012:1–13.
15. Blank SC, Bird H, Turkheimer F, Wise RJ. Speech production after stroke: the role of the right pars opercularis. Ann Neurol. 2003;54:310–20.
16. Geranmayeh F, Brownsett SLE, Wise RJS. Task-induced brain activity in aphasic stroke patients: what is driving recovery? Brain. 2014;137:2632–48.
17. Thiel A, Hartmann A, Rubi-Fessen I, Anglade C, Kracht L, Weiduschat N, Kessler J, Rommel T, Heiss W-D. Effects of noninvasive brain stimulation on language networks and recovery in early poststroke aphasia. Stroke. 2013;44:2240–6.
18. Cappa SF. Spontaneous recovery of aphasia. In: Stemmer W, editor. Handbook of the neuroscience of language. London: Academic; 2008. p. 389–94.
19. Cappa SF. The neural basis of aphasia rehabilitation: evidence from neuroimaging and neurostimulation. Neuropsychol Rehabil. 2011;21:742–54.
20. Chieffo R, Ferrari F, Battista P, et al. Excitatory deep transcranial magnetic stimulation with H-coil over the right homologous Broca's region improves naming in chronic post-stroke aphasia. Neurorehabil Neural Repair. 2014;28:291–8.
21. Sandars M, Cloutman L, Woollams AM. Taking sides: an integrative review of the impact of laterality and polarity on efficacy of therapeutic transcranial direct current stimulation for anomia in chronic poststroke aphasia. Neural Plast. 2016;2016:8428256.
22. Elsner B, Kugler J, Pohl M, Mehrholz J. Transcranial direct current stimulation (tDCS) for improving aphasia in adults with aphasia after stroke. Cochrane Database Syst Rev. 2019;5:1–93.
23. Lefaucheur J-P, Aleman A, Baeken C, et al. Evidence-based guidelines on the therapeutic use of repetitive

transcranial magnetic stimulation (rTMS): an update (2014–2018). Clin Neurophysiol. 2020;131:474–528.
24. Naeser MA, Martin PI, Nicholas M, Baker EH, Seekins H, Kobayashi M, Theoret H, Fregni F, Maria-Tormos J, Kurland J. Improved picture naming in chronic aphasia after TMS to part of right Broca's area: an open-protocol study. Brain Lang. 2005;93:95–105.
25. Dionísio A, Duarte IC, Patrício M, Castelo-Branco M. The use of repetitive transcranial magnetic stimulation for stroke rehabilitation: a systematic review. J Stroke Cerebrovasc Dis. 2018;27:1–31.
26. Wang C-P, Hsieh C-Y, Tsai P-Y, Wang C-T, Lin F-G, Chan R-C. Efficacy of synchronous verbal training during repetitive transcranial magnetic stimulation in patients with chronic aphasia. Stroke. 2014;45:3656–62.
27. Rubi-Fessen I, Hartmann A, Huber W, Fimm B, Rommel T, Thiel A, Heiss W-D. Add-on effects of repetitive transcranial magnetic stimulation on subacute aphasia therapy: enhanced improvement of functional communication and basic linguistic skills. A randomized controlled study. Arch Phys Med Rehabil. 2015;96:1935–1944.e2.
28. Mendoza JA, Silva FA, Pachón MY, Rueda LC, Romero LAL, Pérez M. Repetitive transcranial magnetic stimulation in aphasia and communication impairment in post-stroke: systematic review of literature. J Neurol Transl Neurosci. 2016;4:1070.
29. Dammekens E, Vanneste S, Ost J, Ridder DD. Neural correlates of high frequency repetitive transcranial magnetic stimulation improvement in post-stroke non-fluent aphasia: a case study. Neurocase. 2014;20:1–9.
30. Szaflarski JP, Vannest J, Wu SW, DiFrancesco MW, Banks C, Gilbert DL. Excitatory repetitive transcranial magnetic stimulation induces improvements in chronic post-stroke aphasia. Med Sci Monit Int Med J Exp Clin Res. 2011;17:CR132–9.
31. Ohara K, Kuriyama C, Hada T, Suzuki S, Nakayama Y, Abo M. A pilot study verifying the effectiveness of high-frequency repetitive transcranial magnetic stimulation in combination with intensive speech-language-hearing therapy in patients with chronic aphasia. Neurorehabilitation. 2021;49:459–67.
32. Kapoor A. Repetitive transcranial magnetic stimulation therapy for post-stroke non-fluent aphasia: a critical review. Top Stroke Rehabil. 2017;24:547–53.
33. Heikkinen PH, Pulvermüller F, Mäkelä JP, Ilmoniemi RJ, Lioumis P, Kujala T, Manninen R-L, Ahvenainen A, Klippi A. Combining rTMS with intensive language-action therapy in chronic aphasia: a randomized controlled trial. Front Neurosci. 2019;12:1036.
34. Waldowski K, Seniów J, Leśniak M, Iwański S, Członkowska A. Effect of low-frequency repetitive transcranial magnetic stimulation on naming abilities in early-stroke aphasic patients: a prospective, randomized, double-blind sham-controlled study. ScientificWorldJournal. 2012;2012:518568.
35. Cichon N, Wlodarczyk L, Saluk-Bijak J, Bijak M, Redlicka J, Gorniak L, Miller E. Novel advances to post-stroke aphasia pharmacology and rehabilitation. J Clin Med. 2021;10:3778.
36. Norise C, Hamilton RH. Non-invasive brain stimulation in the treatment of post-stroke and neurodegenerative aphasia: parallels, differences, and lessons learned. Front Hum Neurosci. 2017;10:675.
37. ALHarbi MF, Armijo-Olivo S, Kim ES. Transcranial direct current stimulation (tDCS) to improve naming ability in post-stroke aphasia: a critical review. Behav Brain Res. 2017;332:7–15.
38. Galletta EE, Conner P, Vogel-Eyny A, Marangolo P. Use of tDCS in aphasia rehabilitation: a systematic review of the behavioral interventions implemented with noninvasive brain stimulation for language recovery. Am J Speech Lang Pathol. 2016;25:S854–67.
39. Baker JM, Rorden C, Fridriksson J. Using transcranial direct-current stimulation to treat stroke patients with aphasia. Stroke. 2010;41:1229–36.
40. Rosso C, Perlbarg V, Valabregue R, et al. Broca's area damage is necessary but not sufficient to induce after-effects of cathodal tDCS on the unaffected hemisphere in post-stroke aphasia. Brain Stimul. 2014;7:627–35.
41. Cipollari S, Veniero D, Razzano C, Caltagirone C, Koch G, Marangolo P. Combining TMS-EEG with transcranial direct current stimulation language treatment in aphasia. Expert Rev Neurother. 2015;15:833–45.
42. Flöel A, Meinzer M, Kirstein R, Nijhof S, Deppe M, Knecht S, Breitenstein C. Short-term anomia training and electrical brain stimulation. Stroke. 2011;42:2065–7.
43. Vines BW, Norton AC, Schlaug G. Non-invasive brain stimulation enhances the effects of melodic intonation therapy. Front Psychol. 2011;2:230.
44. Cheung C, Bakhtiar M, Kong APH. The inhibitory effect of anodal HD-tDCS over right inferior frontal gyrus on naming accuracy in people with aphasia. In Montreal: Academy of Aphasia 56th Annual Meeting; 2018. (Frontiers in Human Neuroscience; vol. 12).
45. Gorno-Tempini ML, Hillis AE, Weintraub S, et al. Classification of primary progressive aphasia and its variants. Neurology. 2011;76:1006–14.
46. Cotelli M, Manenti R, Ferrari C, Gobbi E, Macis A, Cappa SF. Effectiveness of language training and non-invasive brain stimulation on oral and written naming performance in primary progressive aphasia: a meta-analysis and systematic review. Neurosci Biobehav Rev. 2020;108:498–525.
47. Nissim NR, Moberg PJ, Hamilton RH. Efficacy of noninvasive brain stimulation (tDCS or TMS) paired with language therapy in the treatment of primary progressive aphasia: an exploratory meta-analysis. Brain Sci. 2020;10:597.
48. Cotelli M, Manenti R, Petesi M, Brambilla M, Cosseddu M, Zanetti O, Miniussi C, Padovani A, Borroni B. Treatment of primary progressive aphasias by transcranial direct current stimulation combined with language training. J Alzheimers Dis. 2014;39:799–808.

49. Cotelli M, Manenti R, Paternicò D, et al. Grey matter density predicts the improvement of naming abilities after tDCS intervention in Agrammatic variant of primary progressive aphasia. Brain Topogr. 2016;29:738–51.
50. Roncero C, Kniefel H, Service E, Thiel A, Probst S, Chertkow H. Inferior parietal transcranial direct current stimulation with training improves cognition in anomic Alzheimer's disease and frontotemporal dementia. Alzheimers Dement (N Y). 2017;3:247–53.
51. Tsapkini K, Webster KT, Ficek BN, Desmond JE, Onyike CU, Rapp B, Frangakis CE, Hillis AE. Electrical brain stimulation in different variants of primary progressive aphasia: a randomized clinical trial. Alzheimers Dement (N Y). 2018;4:461–72.
52. Tsapkini K, Frangakis C, Gomez Y, Davis C, Hillis AE. Augmentation of spelling therapy with transcranial direct current stimulation in primary progressive aphasia: preliminary results and challenges. Aphasiology. 2014;28:1112–30.
53. Tao Y, Ficek B, Wang Z, Rapp B, Tsapkini K. Selective functional network changes following tDCS-augmented language treatment in primary progressive aphasia. Front Aging Neurosci. 2021;13:681043.
54. Hamilton RH, Sanders L, Benson J, Faseyitan O, Norise C, Naeser M, Martin P, Coslett HB. Stimulating conversation: enhancement of elicited propositional speech in a patient with chronic non-fluent aphasia following transcranial magnetic stimulation. Brain Lang. 2010;113:45–50.
55. Medina J, Norise C, Faseyitan O, Coslett HB, Turkeltaub PE, Hamilton RH. Finding the right words: transcranial magnetic stimulation improves discourse productivity in non-fluent aphasia after stroke. Aphasiology. 2012;26:1153–68.
56. Marangolo P, Fiori V, Paola MD, Cipollari S, Razzano C, Oliveri M, Caltagirone C. Differential involvement of the left frontal and temporal regions in verb naming: a tDCS treatment study. Restor Neurol Neurosci. 2013;31:63–72.
57. Marangolo P, Fiori V, Calpagnano MA, Campana S, Razzano C, Caltagirone C, Marini A. tDCS over the left inferior frontal cortex improves speech production in aphasia. Front Hum Neurosci. 2013;7:539.
58. Marangolo P, Fiori V, Campana S, Calpagnano MA, Razzano C, Caltagirone C, Marini A. Something to talk about: enhancement of linguistic cohesion through tdCS in chronic non fluent aphasia. Neuropsychologia. 2014;53:246–56.
59. Marangolo P, Fiori V, Gelfo F, Shofany J, Razzano C, Caltagirone C, Angelucci F. Bihemispheric tDCS enhances language recovery but does not alter BDNF levels in chronic aphasic patients. Restor Neurol Neurosci. 2014;32:367–79.
60. Guillouët E, Cogné M, Saverot E, et al. Impact of combined transcranial direct current stimulation and speech-language therapy on spontaneous speech in aphasia: a randomized controlled double-blind study. J Int Neuropsychcol Soc. 2020;26:7–18.
61. Galletta EE, Vogel-Eyny A. Translational treatment of aphasia combining neuromodulation and behavioral intervention for lexical retrieval: implications from a single case study. Front Hum Neurosci. 2015;9:447.
62. Matar SJ, Newton C, Sorinola IO, Pavlou M. Transcranial direct-current stimulation as an adjunct to verb network strengthening treatment in post-stroke chronic aphasia: a double-blinded randomized feasibility study. Front Neurol. 2022;13:722402.
63. de Aguiar V, Bastiaanse R, Capasso R, Gandolfi M, Smania N, Rossi G, Miceli G. Can tDCS enhance item-specific effects and generalization after linguistically motivated aphasia therapy for verbs? Front Behav Neurosci. 2015;9:190.
64. Campana S, Caltagirone C, Marangolo P. Combining voxel-based lesion-symptom mapping (VLSM) with A-tDCS language treatment: predicting outcome of recovery in nonfluent chronic aphasia. Brain Stimul. 2015;8:769–76.
65. Gervits F, Ash S, Coslett HB, Rascovsky K, Grossman M, Hamilton R. Transcranial direct current stimulation for the treatment of primary progressive aphasia: an open-label pilot study. Brain Lang. 2016;162:35–41.
66. McConathey EM, White NC, Gervits F, Ash S, Coslett HB, Grossman M, Hamilton RH. Baseline performance predicts tDCS-mediated improvements in language symptoms in primary progressive aphasia. Front Hum Neurosci. 2017;11:347.
67. Hosseini M, McConathey EM, Ungrady M, Grossman M, Coslett HB, Hamilton RH. Proceedings #10: transcranial direct current stimulation mediates improvements in verbal fluency for patients with primary progressive aphasia. Brain Stimul. 2019;12:e69–71.
68. Dipper LT, Pritchard M. Discourse: assessment and therapy. In: Fernandes FDM, editor. Advances in speech-language pathology London: IntechOpen; 2017. p. 4–23.
69. Marangolo P, Fiori V, Cipollari S, Campana S, Razzano C, Paola MD, Koch G, Caltagirone C. Bihemispheric stimulation over left and right inferior frontal region enhances recovery from apraxia of speech in chronic aphasia. Eur J Neurosci. 2013;38:3370–7.

Mehdi Bakhtiar is an assistant professor and the director of the Speech and Neuromodulation Laboratory (https://www.snlab.hku.hk) in the Faculty of Education, at The University of Hong Kong (HKU). He obtained his MSc in Speech Therapy from Tehran University of Medical Sciences and his PhD in Cognitive Neuroscience of Language from HKU. His research interests include application of behavioural and neuromodulation methods for understanding, assessment and treatment of individuals with the fluency disorders as well as neurogenic communication disorders.

Maria Teresa Carthery-Goulart is a Lecturer and Researcher in Faculty of Education, The University of Hong Kong. She is an Associate Professor at the Center for Mathematics, Cognition and Computing, Federal University of ABC and a Researcher at the Cognitive and Behavioral Neurology Unit, Department of Neurology in the University of São Paulo. She is a speech and language therapist graduated from the Faculty of Medicine, University of São Paulo. She obtained her MSc. in Psychology in the area of Neurosciences and Behavior from the Institute of Psychology, University of São Paulo and her PhD in Sciences in the area of Neurology from the Faculty of Medicine, University of São Paulo. She has been Visiting Scientist at the Medical Research Council - Cognition and Brain Sciences Unit, Cambridge (2007–2008). She has studies in Cognitive Neuroscience of Language, Neuropsychology, Psycholinguistics, and Neurolinguistics.

Anthony Pak-Hin Kong is a fellow of the American Speech-Language-Hearing Association (ASHA) and Academy of Aphasia. Trained as a speech-language pathologist, his research interests include stroke-induced aphasia, discourse analyses, and neurogenic communication disorders in multilingual speakers. His research has received continuous funding from the National Institutes of Health, the Hong Kong Government, National Natural Science Foundation of China, and multiple (inter)national universities and private foundations. As a world-renowned scholar in communication sciences and disorders, he serves and served as Consultant/Advisor to provide research, clinical, and/or professional consultations to many (inter)national agencies, such as Aphasia United, Project BRIDGE (Building Research Initiatives by Developing Group Effort, USA), the Hong Kong Hospital Authority, and the Hong Kong Society for Rehabilitation. Dr. Kong is the current Founding Editor-in-Chief of Cogent Gerontology (Taylor & Francis).

21 FOQUSAphasia: An Initiative to Facilitate Research of Spoken Discourse in Aphasia and Its Translation into Improved Evidence-based Practice for Discourse Treatment

Manaswita Dutta, Laura L. Murray, Brielle C. Stark, and Lucy Bryant

Preview of What Is Currently Known

Accurate evaluation of language is paramount to diagnosing aphasia and to designing and implementing effective aphasia interventions. Recently, there has been growing empirical and clinical interest in spoken discourse analysis: It is considered an important tool for describing aphasia and documenting treatment outcomes. The evaluation of spoken discourse is preferred by many given its ability to provide a realistic reflection of how an individual functions in everyday communication situations and contexts. However, presently, incorporating discourse analysis into aphasia research and clinical practice has been hampered by methodological limitations (such as abundance of discourse outcome measures, poor psychometrics) and barriers including lack of time, and limited resources and training. The FOQUSAphasia working group was created to address the current state of spoken discourse in research and clinical settings, with the goal of improving its evidence base and clinical utility to yield meaningful functional outcomes for individuals with aphasia and related clinical populations.

Objectives

(a) To explain the importance of targeting spoken discourse in aphasia and related acquired language disorders
(b) To provide the rationale for creating the FOQUSAphasia working group
(c) To describe goals and deliverables of FOQUSAphasia in terms of research, collaboration, and clinical implementation of spoken discourse analysis
(d) To summarize ways to get involved in FOQUSAphasia

M. Dutta
Department of Speech and Hearing Sciences, Portland State University, Portland, OR, USA
e-mail: mdutta@pdx.edu

L. L. Murray (✉)
School of Communication Sciences and Disorders, Western University, London, ON, Canada
e-mail: lmurra57@uwo.ca

B. C. Stark
Department of Speech, Language and Hearing Sciences, Indiana University Bloomington, Bloomington, IN, USA
e-mail: bcstark@iu.edu

L. Bryant
Graduate School of Health, University of Technology Sydney, Sydney, Australia
e-mail: Lucy.Bryant@uts.edu.au

A. P.-H. Kong (ed.), *Spoken Discourse Impairments in the Neurogenic Populations*,
https://doi.org/10.1007/978-3-031-45190-4_21

Current State of Spoken Discourse Analysis in Aphasia Assessment and Treatment

Discourse (or language beyond single words, sentences, or utterances that is used for a specific purpose) is integral to an individual's everyday social and vocational communication. Impairments in discourse can significantly affect one's psychosocial well-being and quality of life [1–5]. In recent years, the analysis of spoken discourse (or connected speech) has been gaining widespread empirical and clinical attention in the assessment and rehabilitation of aphasia [6–8] and other acquired language disorders including dementia [9, 10], primary progressive aphasia [11], and cognitive-communication disorders due to traumatic brain injury [12, 13]. Spoken discourse analysis has been increasingly used in language assessment, and the measurement of language treatment outcomes as it (a) enables the concurrent examination of language structure and its use and (b) is more naturalistic than isolated language measures such as confrontational naming, verbal fluency, or repetition tasks [12, 14, 15].

Spoken discourse samples can be collected using monologue or interactional tasks such as picture description, narratives (e.g., storytelling, personal recounts), procedural descriptions, or unstructured or structured conversations with familiar or unfamiliar communication partners. The elicited language samples can be evaluated at the structural level (i.e., microlinguistic [e.g., lexical, semantic, syntactic aspects]), global level (i.e., macrolinguistic [e.g., organization, informational content]), or both to gain a comprehensive understanding of how language production can be affected across different linguistic levels [15–18]. Researchers and clinicians across the globe therefore widely acknowledge the ecological validity of and see value in pursuing spoken discourse analysis to improve our understanding of communication abilities and rehabilitation outcomes for individuals with aphasia and other acquired language disorders.

Despite frequent use of spoken discourse analysis and increased recognition of its merit in understanding and managing aphasia and related language disorders, there remains notable inconsistency and a lack of standardization in implementing and reporting spoken discourse procedures and outcomes [8, 19]. First, fundamentally, there is a lack of consensus over the definition of discourse. For instance, discourse has been traditionally described from *structural* (i.e., language use "beyond the boundaries of isolated sentences" p. 300 [20]), *cognitivist* ("a set of utterances aimed at conveying a message among interlocutors … [it] may be the most elaborative linguistic activity" p.302 [2]), or *functional* (i.e., language beyond a single simple clause that is used for specific purposes [1]) viewpoints. Further, professionals involved in discourse analysis vary in their definition preferences and some individuals adopt other descriptions of discourse [21, 22]. There are also variable definitions for describing specific discourse characteristics such as fluency [23]. These definitional inconsistencies are likely a reflection of, as researchers have argued, discourse's inherent variability across individuals that makes it difficult to measure [16]. Consequently, there are contrasting conceptions among clinicians and researchers regarding spoken language tasks that constitute as assessing language at the discourse level [8, 24]. For example, whereas single picture description is most commonly used to assess discourse-level production [8], other professionals may rely on conversational analysis to tap into interactional aspects of language.

Second, there is notable heterogeneity among research studies related to the procedures undertaken for spoken discourse analysis [22, 25, 26]. To illustrate, variations are noted throughout the discourse analysis process: from setting the criteria to segment utterances produced during a discourse task (e.g., T-units versus C-units) to establishing consistency of procedures (e.g., whereas some researchers undertake determining reliability of discourse measures, others do not report this information in their studies). A further challenge is that many studies fail to clearly report discourse analysis procedures making across-study comparisons difficult. For example, although it is common for researchers to document the stimuli used to elicit the discourse sample and to describe the discourse outcomes derived, they may not mention other methodological details imperative for study replication and reproducibility of findings as well as comparison of discourse outcomes across studies [19]. Essential details that are inconsistently reported include participant characteristics (particularly providing characteristics of both members in a conversational dyad versus describing the participant with aphasia only), personnel involved (e.g., experienced speech-language pathologists [SLPs], undergraduate research assistants), training procedures for collecting and analyzing discourse samples, and tools (e.g., recording instruments and analysis metric) used in the transcription, coding, analysis, and interpretation processes [8, 25].

Third, the extant literature has varied widely in terms of the outcome measures used to assess discourse-level language functioning [26]. Currently, across studies, there are a multitude of spoken discourse variables yet insufficient data establishing the psychometric properties of these outcome measures [27]. With the contemporary increase in discourse research, studies often introduce new outcome measures and analysis methods but fail to provide access to the assessment tools, report information related to the validity and reliability of these measures, or describe the rationale for choosing them [8, 25]. In cases where such analyses have been reported, a variety of statistical procedures have been used. Researchers may use percent agreement, simple linear correlations, or intraclass correlation coefficient (ICC) to report reliability metrics. It is important to establish the psychometric quality of discourse measures to determine their stability across time and raters: If the discourse measures used in research studies (and in turn clinical practice) are inherently unstable, then this could lead to flawed conclusions regarding discourse characteristics as well as treatment-related changes in discourse [19]. Further, at present, there are nominal normative data, even for commonly used discourse measures (e.g., lexical diversity, coherence). For instance, to evaluate conversational discourse characteristics of persons with aphasia, it would be important to determine what percentage of utterances produced by typical speakers are grammatically correct during a conversation with a close communication partner to make effective comparisons. Additionally, even though some normative data exist across research labs, free and easy access to this information is limited, with some exceptions (e.g., an open-access repository on discourse reliability data from Stark et al., available online at https://osf.io/4zcpn/). Critically, it is important to consider that it may be challenging to establish normative information for discourse data given the high variability in language productions among individuals in concert with the diversity of spoken discourse genres and outcome measures.

There are also prominent differences in practice patterns related to spoken discourse analysis when research and clinical settings are compared. Spoken discourse analysis is more commonly used by researchers than clinicians given the increased number of barriers experienced in clinical settings including lack of time, training, and availability of resources [8, 24, 28]. Thus, although clinicians value the use of discourse analysis in aphasia diagnosis and rehabilitation, their "buy-in" to use discourse analysis more routinely in their clinical practice remains limited and must be addressed in research with the goal of providing reasonable solutions and improving clinical utility and confidence.

Altogether, the persistent issues related to the vast heterogeneity in study findings and lack of standardization of discourse evaluation and reporting procedures in combination with studies involving relatively small sample sizes limit generalization and replication of research findings and have currently precluded the inclusion of spoken discourse in the set of core aphasia outcomes [19, 29]. Importantly, these challenges are currently constraining the use of spoken discourse analysis in clinical settings [8]. At present, there are limited solutions regarding how clinicians can best implement discourse analysis in practice. These limitations pose significant challenges to scientific progress and clinical translation.

Thus, there is an urgent need to improve the ways in which spoken discourse analysis is being utilized in aphasia assessment and treatment research so that it can be implemented more reliably and consistently, which in turn will improve replication and meta-analyses of study findings. With better standardization of procedures, meaningful comparisons can be made across aphasia research studies regarding language abilities and treatment outcomes. This standardization will also yield stronger tools, which can facilitate use of existing and development of additional aphasia treatments targeting discourse. With improvements in research endeavors, we expect more constructive solutions and best practices for clinical use of discourse analysis.

Fostering the Quality of Spoken Discourse in Aphasia (FOQUSAphasia)

Overview and Goals

Fostering the **Qu**ality of **S**poken Discourse in **Aphasia** (FOQUSAphasia; www.foqusaphasia.com) is an international working group that aims to improve the state of spoken discourse research and evidence in aphasia and acquired language disorders in general [19]. The working group was initially created following a round table discussion at the Clinical Aphasiology Conference in Whitefish, Montana in 2019. The working group has grown significantly since then and currently consists of an international group of researchers and clinicians who are interested in spoken discourse work in a range of neurological populations with acquired language disorders.

The goal of FOQUSAphasia is to improve the methodological rigor and standardize the procedures related to spoken discourse analysis in research. More specifically, it aims to establish the psychometric quality of and normative data for existing and commonly used discourse analysis measures to improve their validity and reliability and enhance confidence in their interpretation for both aphasia diagnostic and treatment outcome purposes. The ultimate objective of the working group is improving the research surrounding spoken discourse analysis practices for aphasia and related language disorders so they can be used frequently, efficiently, and affordably in clinical practice. FOQUSAphasia also aims to improve networking opportunities and access to spoken discourse information.

Structure of the Working Group

FOQUSAphasia has a dynamic structure that has evolved with the needs of the working group and the field. At the time of this book chapter, it includes a steering committee and task forces to serve different initiatives (see Fig. 21.1). The steering committee comprises a team of experts who oversee the creation and work of the various task forces and interface with the stakeholders to direct and ensure timely progress of the working group initiatives. The steering committee members are selected via nomination and voting by all members across the different task forces. In addition, there are two task forces within FOQUSAphasia at present, each of which serves specific initiatives: (1) the *Best Practices* and (2) *Methodology and Data Quality* task forces. Interested individuals can self-select and join a task force of interest. Each task force is supervised by a leadership team, the members of which are elected by members at large serving in the respective task forces. The leadership team directs progress of initiatives within each task force. The working group plans to change the current structure dynamically in the future and envisions (a) the creation of more task forces with more initiatives, (b) facilitation of fruitful collaborations via writing groups, and (c) interactive events based on the needs of researchers, clinicians, other stakeholder groups (e.g., individuals living with acquired language disorders), and the field at large.

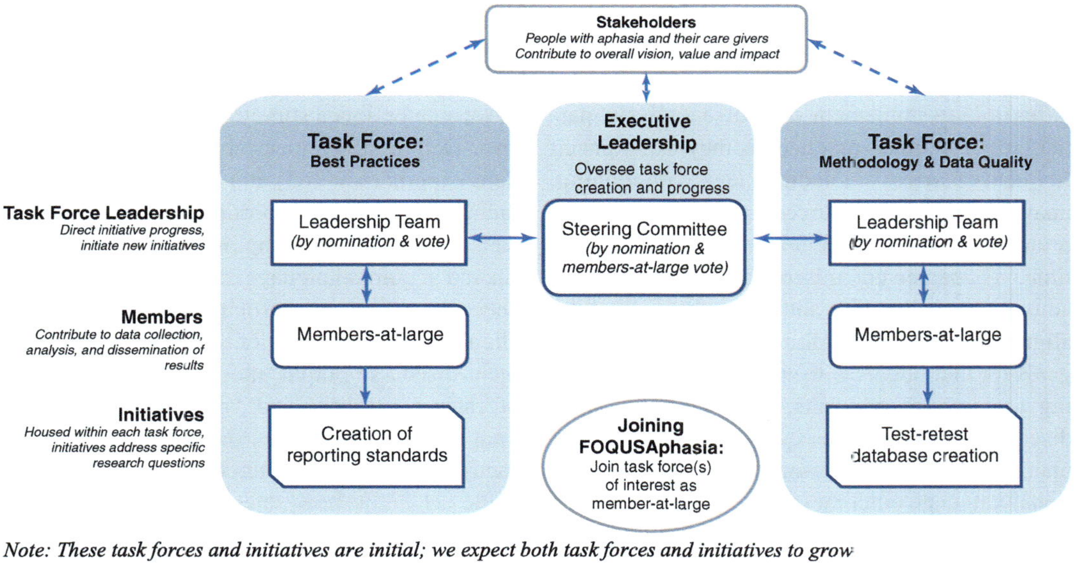

Fig. 21.1 Structure and hierarchy of the FOQUSAphasia working group. *Note:* These task forces and initiatives are initial; we expect both task forces and initiatives to grow

FOQUSAphasia Task Forces and Deliverables

Best Practices Task Force

This task force aims to establish best practice standards for the analysis and reporting of spoken discourse in studies involving individuals with aphasia and other acquired language disorders. The goal of the task force's initial initiative is to create reporting standards and ensure that all studies on spoken discourse in aphasia and other acquired language disorders consistently and transparently report information pertaining to data collection, analysis, and interpretation, thus allowing replicability across studies, improving reproducibility of findings, and facilitating synthesis (e.g., meta-analyses) of this literature.

As part of the *Best Practices* task force, a mixed-methods survey study was completed to identify current practices of SLPs and researchers globally regarding acquiring, analyzing, and reporting spoken discourse in aphasia [8]. Respondents (total n = 189) from different geographic regions, and a broad range of backgrounds and experiences (e.g., work settings, years working in aphasia, professional degrees) participated in the study. Survey findings showed that over 70% of the respondents frequently used spoken discourse analysis to describe aphasia symptoms and over 50% used it as an aphasia treatment outcome measure. Spoken discourse samples were most commonly collected using stimuli and procedures from standardized aphasia assessments (e.g., describing the Cookie Theft Picture from the Boston Diagnostic Aphasia Examination) [30]. There was significant heterogeneity in the discourse analysis procedures used across respondents and settings (e.g., elicitation tasks, whether language samples were or were not recorded, recording instruments, analysis software, outcome measures). Further, when discourse analysis practices in research and clinical settings were compared, results showed that researchers collected more samples and more frequently recorded, transcribed, and coded spoken discourse data than clinicians. Interestingly, most respondents transcribed discourse samples in real time and relied on perceptual and clinical judgment-based analysis; fewer respondents reported using sophisticated computerized tools to analyze language outcomes. Several respondents acknowledged the lack of normative data and supported the need for psychometric information of discourse measures. Qualitative findings indicated that many respondents found it unfeasible to implement discourse analysis, particularly in clinical practice, as they experienced frequent barriers including lack of training, unavailability of resources to apply discourse protocols, and the predominant concern, limited time. A perceived misconception was noted among some clinicians and researchers about the alignment of spoken discourse and functional goals for individuals with aphasia; that is, according to many respondents, the incorporation of discourse in aphasia assessment and treatment planning may not necessarily yield better functional language outcomes. In terms of research, it was perceived that discourse data were not relevant for research questions or essential for peer-reviewed publications. These misconceptions regarding discourse stem from a lack of knowledge about discourse and its clinical and empirical utility. The survey identified several ongoing challenges in the field related to spoken discourse analysis and was critical in informing future lines of research. For instance, there remains a critical need to standardize discourse analysis procedures, given the significant variability in the implementation of discourse analysis procedures across both clinical and research settings. A dearth of research regarding normative data for the vast majority of spoken discourse measures and, more critically, their psychometric properties currently confound the interpretation of these measures. Relatedly, existing psychometric and normative data for spoken discourse outcomes along with results from future research in this area should be consolidated into a single platform that can be readily available for clinicians and researchers. Furthermore, research efforts need to focus on developing time-efficient methods such as automated discourse analysis that (a) increase accuracy and replicability and (b) rely less on training and expertise to foster more frequent use of spoken discourse analysis in clinical settings. Finally, there is limited information regarding spoken discourse analysis protocols for linguistically and culturally diverse populations: Most developed spoken discourse protocols and normative data apply to English-speaking individuals living in high-income countries [31, 32].

Following the practice trends identified from the aforementioned survey, Stark et al. conducted an e-Delphi study to establish consensus from field experts ($n = 165$) and propose initial minimum standards for reporting spoken discourse data in research involving individuals with aphasia and acquired language disorders [22]. Several "necessary" (e.g., participant characteristics, elicitation task description, criteria used to segment discourse output into utterances, reporting of rater reliability) and "recommended" (e.g., total words in a sample, data analysis software used) items were identified for reporting (see Table 21.1 for how "necessary" and "recommended" were defined; https://osf.io/y48n9/). This research has provided an initial reporting framework for future spoken discourse studies to utilize, and if adopted, has the potential to improve the quality of the evidence published and to facilitate meaningful comparisons across studies.

Methodology and Data Quality Task Force

This task force focuses on improving the quality and psychometrics of spoken discourse outcomes. The initial initiatives of this task force have been to evaluate the stability of commonly used spoken discourse measures and create a test-retest database of samples and outcome measures with established psychometric and normative data. The goal of this task force is to offer investigators across multiple research sites opportunities to collaborate, test important hypotheses, and measure discourse by leveraging big data (e.g., AphasiaBank). Importantly, the goal is to make these data freely available to those interested in spoken discourse via open science platforms (e.g., OSF; https://osf.io/).

As an example, several members of the *Methodology and Data Quality* task force (Dalton et al.) recently collaborated with other researchers in a study designed to examine certain psychometric properties of an automated discourse analysis tool [33]. More specifically, spoken discourse samples from 49 individuals with aphasia

Table. 21.1 Best Practice necessary and recommended items for reporting on spoken discourse

Category	Reporting item	Necessary	Recommended
Information about the discourse sample	• Define "discourse"	☐	
	• Define "utterance" (or other unit, e.g., turn unit)	☐	
	• Number of words in sample		☐
Information about how the discourse sample was collected	• Describe elicitation task	☐	
	• *Exact instructions used to elicit discourse sample*[a]	☐	
Information about the persons included in the collection of the discourse sample	• Demographic information about primary speaker [the person whose discourse is of interest]	☐	
	• Information about the primary speaker's neurological condition	☐	
Methodology and rater agreement	• Inter-rater reliability for each analyzed variable/measure	☐	
	• Reliability statistics used	☐	
	• Details on the number (percentage) of files used for determining reliability/agreement	☐	
	• Reliability (point to point agreement) for transcription (orthographic or other)		☐
Analysis	• Type of transcription (e.g., orthographic, phonetic)	☐	
	• Detailed description of any perceptual rating scale used, including providing a copy of the scale if not previously published	☐	
	• Details of the annotation system, formal (e.g., CHAT) or informal (created by the clinician/examiner)	☐	
	• *Whether transcription was verbatim* (e.g., *including all behaviors such as fillers) or whether information was excluded in the transcription process*[a]	☐	
	• Details of any software used for transcribing/ annotating/generating data (e.g., SALT, CLAN, ELAN)		☐
	• Completeness of transcription (full, partial, transcribing errors only)	☐	
	• Who/what transcribed the sample (by a human, by a machine/software, hybrid human and software)		☐
Information about the individual discourse variables/behaviors reported	• What is being used as primary outcome measure(s) (e.g., linguistic information, speech information, etc.)	☐	
	• Theoretical rationale for selecting variable/behavior/outcome measure(s)		☐
	• Operational definition for each variable/behavior/ outcome(s)	☐	

Note: Original source of this table is Stark et al. [22], which involved an e-Delphi protocol including three rounds of expert scoring and analysis. Necessary reporting items are those noted as "highly" or "extremely" necessary by >70% participants in Round 3 or those that were not carried forward from Round 1 rated "highly" or "extremely" necessary by >70% of participants completing all three rounds. Recommended are those noted as "highly" or "extremely" necessary by >65% in Round 2 (or by participants completing all three rounds in Round 1), but which did not reach "highly" or "extremely" necessary by >70% participants in Round 3

[a]Items that should have been brought forward from a prior round due to high consensus rating, but which erroneously were not

and 48 age-, education-, and gender-matched typically aging adults were analyzed manually (using a checklist) as well as in an automated format using CORELEX, a component of the freely available computerized language analysis (CLAN) program (https://dali.talkbank.org/clan/). Both the manual and automatic scoring focused on quantifying use of core vocabulary or lexicon within the samples. The samples were collected by asking participants to tell a story about a picture or set of pictures and to describe a procedure (i.e., five AphasiaBank protocol discourse tasks); as part of the AphasiaBank data set, all samples had been previously transcribed by the individuals who contributed the samples to the data set or by AphasiaBank personnel. A comparison of results from the two analysis methods yielded excellent inter-method reliability for all discourse tasks and both participant groups (i.e., all ICCs ≥0.977). Notably, use of the automated method significantly reduced discourse analysis time for both experienced and inexperienced CORELEX users; that is, hand scoring all the transcripts took approximately 29 hours longer than the automated scoring. Keeping in mind that the samples had already been transcribed (which is also time consuming), Dalton and colleagues concluded that CORELEX offered an efficient and valid approach for analyzing use of core lexical items and acknowledged the need to develop additional automated tools that could reduce the time barrier for researchers and clinicians who utilize spoken discourse analysis.

Stark and colleagues conducted a study to evaluate the stability of spoken discourse variables and the effects of attention, lifestyle, and physiological factors on reliability in 23 persons with aphasia and 24 matched healthy controls [34]. All participants were tested using the AphasiaBank discourse protocol, and language samples were analyzed for a number of microlinguistic variables (e.g., mean length of utterance, verbs/utterance, correct information units, and related measures of efficiency and informativeness). Reliability was evaluated using ICC at two time points (test–retest; 10 ± 3 days apart) and within and across raters (intra- and inter-rater). Several reliable measures were identified to assess discourse outcomes for persons with aphasia and healthy controls; however, the reliability varied across groups and tasks. For instance, whereas some discourse variables demonstrated good to excellent test-retest reliability for the aphasia group across tasks and both time points (e.g., CIU measures), reliability of these same variables was poor for healthy controls. Proportional metrics for both groups showed consistently low reliability (e.g., open/closed class words, noun/verb ratio). The authors emphasized the need to consider the group characteristics and different tasks when evaluating the reliability of discourse measures and recommended using of minimal detectable change [35] to identify clinically meaningful discourse metrics as outcomes for aphasia treatment.

Doub et al. published a technical report detailing procedures used in the aforementioned investigation with a special focus on conducting a virtual study with persons with aphasia [36]. The authors outlined essential components to run a successful virtual study and issues to consider when testing vulnerable populations, including information related to participant recruitment, consent and assessment processes using aphasia-friendly material, data storage, and quality evaluation. This study provided practical recommendations for conducting a virtual discourse study and showed 100% retention of participants and high-quality data acquisition and feasibility.

Increasing Public Knowledge about Spoken Discourse

FOQUSAphasia has offered several free interactive workshops and lectures on a wide range of topics on spoken discourse in aphasia and related acquired language disorders (accessible online via https://www.foqusaphasia.com/interactive--events). The FOQUSAphasia lecture series was developed to engage experts and encourage early career researchers to showcase their spoken discourse work. Additionally, findings from the working group's projects have been disseminated at national and international conferences. The FOQUSAphasia website provides free access to a range of discussion forums and discourse-related resources including recent publications and presentations. The working group aims to expand its membership to increase global representation and include other important stakeholders such as persons living with aphasia and their communication partners who would serve as key contributors to obtaining consensus, identifying priorities for next steps to be undertaken by the task forces, and informing the development of evidence-based tools to improve functional language outcomes.

In summary, to achieve FOQUSAphasia's goal of improving the quality of spoken discourse analysis research, the task forces within the working group, thus far, have evaluated the current practice patterns of researchers and clinicians, established a set of best practice guidelines for reporting spoken discourse information in research, and improved the feasibility of conducting discourse analysis (e.g., automated core lexicon analysis, virtual administration procedures). In addition, FOQUSAphasia has developed a number of initiatives to facilitate collaborations between and among researchers and clinicians and improve public knowledge regarding spoken discourse.

Future Directions

Although FOQUSAphasia, as a recently developed working group, has had a productive start, its work has identified a number of gaps in spoken discourse analysis research and clinical practice that require empirical attention. First, in addition to recommending adoption of the recently created best practice standards for spoken discourse analysis, FOQUSAphasia encourages researchers to make available their study protocols to ensure transparency and in turn, foster consistency and efficiency across research studies. Second, future research must focus on not only establishing the psychometric properties of and normative data for commonly used spoken discourse measures and consolidating these findings with existing data, but also making this information freely and easily available on a shared platform such as AphasiaBank (https://aphasia.talkbank.org/). Third, to improve clinical endorsement and wider adoption in aphasia clinical trials, research efforts must continue to be directed toward developing time-efficient spoken discourse analysis tools, which do not require extensive training to use (e.g., automatized transcription tools, psychometrically sound rating scales and checklists). For example, several normed checklists have been recently developed to facilitate implementation of spoken discourse analysis and promote standardization [11, 37]. Fourth, it is important to consider populations diverse in culture, language(s) used, and other demographic variables (e.g., level of education) during the development and validation of stimuli and procedures used for spoken discourse analysis. The working group aims to bring together and facilitate productive collaborations among professionals interested in spoken discourse work with a goal of advancing the evidence base and professional, speech-language pathology practice for individuals with aphasia, and other acquired language disorders and addressing the many existing gaps in this field.

Conclusion

The FOQUSAphasia working group was initiated to address the unmet needs related to spoken discourse analysis practices in aphasia and has now expanded to other acquired language disorders. In this chapter, we have outlined the background, structure, roles of members, deliverables, and our goals. The task forces as well as the initiatives within each will be shaped by the joint efforts of existing and future stakeholders including researchers, clinicians, and those living with acquired language disorders and their family members. Individuals who are interested in contributing to this work are encouraged to contact the authors of this chapter to join our efforts toward improving the state of spoken discourse analysis in research and clinical settings and fostering reproducible science in general.

Major Takeaways

1. Spoken discourse analysis is a valued tool by both researchers and clinicians when describing aphasia and related acquired language disorders as well as when monitoring the effects of interventions for these disorders.
2. There are many current barriers to using spoken discourse analysis in aphasia research and clinical practice including inadequate psychometric data of spoken discourse measures and lack of time and resources needed for transcribing and analyzing spoken discourse data.
3. FOQUSAphasia is a recently developed international working group that aims to champion the use of spoken discourse analysis for aphasia and related acquired language disorders in both research and clinical settings.
4. The FOQUSAphasia task forces have undertaken important empirical initiatives to improve the state of spoken discourse research including: (i) completing an international survey of clinicians and researchers regarding current practices and barriers to spoken discourse analysis in aphasia; (ii) creating an initial set of best practice standards for spoken discourse analysis in research; (iii) evaluating and establishing the psychometric stability of some existing discourse measures; and (iv) facilitating discussions among those interested in spoken discourse work through interactive events and collaborative efforts.
5. Significant work remains to be done to improve the state of spoken discourse analysis research that, in turn, will facilitate its use in clinical settings. In the future, researchers are urged to focus on further standardizing discourse measurement and treatment procedures, improve psychometric evidence and normative databases, facilitate educational efforts, and consider clinical barriers and diverse populations when enhancing currently available and developing new spoken discourse assessment tools.

Acknowledgments We would like to acknowledge all members of the FOQUSAphasia working group (http://www. foqusaphasia.com). The work published as a part of FOQUSAphasia is supported by funding awarded to authors Brielle C. Stark (ASHFoundation Foundation New Investigator Award) and Angela C. Roberts (National Institutes of Health/ National Institute on Deafness and Other Communication Disorders Grant 1R21DC017255-01).

References

1. Halliday MA, Matthiessen CM, Halliday M, Matthiessen C. An introduction to functional grammar. Routledge; 2014.
2. Ska B, Duong A, Joanette Y. Discourse impairments. The MIT Encyclopedia of Communication Disorders; 2004. p. 302–4.
3. Sim P, Power E, Togher L. Describing conversations between individuals with traumatic brain injury (TBI) and communication partners following communication partner training: using exchange structure analysis. Brain Inj. 2013;27(6):717–42.
4. Elbourn E, Kenny B, Power E, Togher L. Psychosocial outcomes of severe traumatic brain injury in relation to discourse recovery: a longitudinal study up to 1-year post-injury. Am J Speech Lang Pathol. 2019;28(4):1463–78.
5. Linnik A, Bastiaanse R, Höhle B. Discourse production in aphasia: a current review of theoretical and methodological challenges. Aphasiology. 2016;30(7):765–800.
6. Cruice M, Aujla S, Bannister J, Botting N, Boyle M, Charles N, Dhaliwal V, Grobler S, Hersh D, Marshall J, Morris S. Creating a novel approach to discourse treatment through coproduction with people with aphasia and speech and language therapists. Aphasiology. 2021;1-23:1159.
7. Dipper L, Marshall J, Boyle M, Hersh D, Botting N, Cruice M. Creating a theoretical framework to underpin discourse assessment and intervention in aphasia. Brain Sci. 2021;11(2):183.
8. Stark BC, Dutta M, Murray LL, Fromm D, Bryant L, Harmon TG, Ramage AE, Roberts AC. Spoken discourse assessment and analysis in aphasia: an international survey of current practices. J Speech Lang Hear Res. 2021;64(11):4366–89.
9. Antonsson M, Lundholm Fors K, Eckerström M, Kokkinakis D. Using a discourse task to explore semantic ability in persons with cognitive impairment. Front Aging Neurosci. 2021;12:607449.
10. Murray LL. Distinguishing clinical depression from early Alzheimer's disease in the elderly: can narrative analysis help? Aphasiology. 2010;24(6):928–39.

11. Dalton SG, Hubbard HI, Richardson JD. Moving toward non-transcription-based discourse analysis in stable and progressive aphasia. Semin Speech Lang. 2020;41(01):032–44.
12. Steel J, Elbourn E, Togher L. Narrative discourse intervention after traumatic brain injury: a systematic review of the literature. Top Lang Disord. 2021;41(1):47–72.
13. Marini A, Zettin M, Bencich E, Bosco FM, Galetto V. Severity effects on discourse production after TBI. J Neurolinguistics. 2017;44:91–106.
14. Mayer J, Murray L. Functional measures of naming in aphasia: word retrieval in confrontation naming versus connected speech. Aphasiology. 2003;17(5):481–97.
15. Stark BC. A comparison of three discourse elicitation methods in aphasia and age-matched adults: implications for language assessment and outcome. Am J Speech Lang Pathol. 2019;28(3):1067–83.
16. Armstrong E. Aphasic discourse analysis: the story so far. Aphasiology. 2000;14(9):875–92.
17. Richardson JD, Dalton SG, Schultz C, Harlow V, Haley K, Jacks A, Silverman M. Story grammar analysis in persons with aphasia. In: Poster presented at the American-Speech-Language-Hearing Association convention, Denver, CO; 2015.
18. Harris Wright H, Capilouto GJ. Considering a multilevel approach to understanding maintenance of global coherence in adults with aphasia. Aphasiology. 2012;26(5):656–72.
19. Stark BC, Dutta M, Murray LL, Bryant L, Fromm D, MacWhinney B, Ramage AE, Roberts A, Den Ouden DB, Brock K, McKinney-Bock K. Standardizing assessment of spoken discourse in aphasia: a working group with deliverables. Am J Speech Lang Pathol. 2021;30(1S):491–502.
20. Ulatowska HK, Olness GS. Discourse. The MIT Encyclopedia of Communication Disorders; 2004. p. 300–2.
21. Lessa I. Discursive struggles within social welfare: restaging teen motherhood. Br J Soc Work. 2006;36(2):283–98.
22. Stark BC, Bryant L, Themistocleous C, den Ouden DB, Roberts AC. Best practice guidelines for reporting spoken discourse in aphasia and neurogenic communication disorders. Aphasiology. 2022;1-24:761.
23. Clough S, Gordon JK. Fluent or nonfluent? Part a. underlying contributors to categorical classifications of fluency in aphasia. Aphasiology. 2020;34(5):515–39.
24. Bryant L, Spencer E, Ferguson A. Clinical use of linguistic discourse analysis for the assessment of language in aphasia. Aphasiology. 2017;31(10):1105–26.
25. Dietz A, Boyle M. Discourse measurement in aphasia research: have we reached the tipping point? Aphasiology. 2018;32(4):459–64.
26. Bryant L, Ferguson A, Spencer E. Linguistic analysis of discourse in aphasia: a review of the literature. Clin Linguist Phon. 2016;30(7):489–518.
27. Pritchard M, Hilari K, Cocks N, Dipper L. Reviewing the quality of discourse information measures in aphasia. Int J Lang Commun Disord. 2017;52(6):689–732.
28. Cruice M, Botting N, Marshall J, Boyle M, Hersh D, Pritchard M, Dipper L. UK speech and language therapists' views and reported practices of discourse analysis in aphasia rehabilitation. Int J Lang Commun Disord. 2020;55(3):417–42.
29. Wallace SJ, Worrall L, Rose T, Le Dorze G, Breitenstein C, Hilari K, Babbitt E, Bose A, Brady M, Cherney LR, Copland D. A core outcome set for aphasia treatment research: the ROMA consensus statement. Int J Stroke. 2019;14(2):180–5.
30. Goodglass H, Kaplan E, Weintraub S. BDAE: the Boston diagnostic aphasia examination. Philadelphia, PA: Lippincott Williams & Wilkins; 2001.
31. Goral M, Conner PS. Language disorders in multilingual and multicultural populations. Annu Rev Appl Linguist. 2013;33:128–61.
32. Beveridge ME, Bak TH. The languages of aphasia research: bias and diversity. Aphasiology. 2011;25(12):1451–68.
33. Dalton SG, Stark BC, Fromm D, Apple K, MacWhinney B, Rensch A, Rowedder M. Validation of an automated procedure for calculating core lexicon from transcripts. J Speech Lang Hear Res. 2022:1–8.
34. Stark BC, Alexander JM, Hittson A, Doub A, Igleheart M, Streander T, Jewell E. Reliability of spoken discourse in speakers with aphasia. arXiv [Preprint]; 2022. https://osf.io/b3s27
35. Boyle M. Test-retest stability of word retrieval in aphasic discourse. J Speech Lang Hear Res. 2014;57(3):966–78. https://doi.org/10.1044/2014_JSLHR-L-13-0171.
36. Doub A, Hittson A, Stark BC. Conducting a virtual study with special considerations for working with persons with aphasia. Am J Speech Lang Pathol. 2021;64(6):2038–46.
37. Richardson JD, Dalton SG. Main concepts for three different discourse tasks in a large non-clinical sample. Aphasiology. 2016;30(1):45–73.

Additional Resources

Articles

Boyle M. Choosing discourse outcome measures to assess clinical change. In Seminars in speech and language, Thieme Medical Publishers; 2020, Vol. 41(01), pp. 001–009.

Dipper L, Marshall J, Boyle M, Botting N, Hersh D, Pritchard M, Cruice M. Treatment for improving discourse in aphasia: a systematic review and synthesis of the evidence base. Aphasiology. 2021;35(9):1125–67.

Fromm D, Forbes M, Holland A, MacWhinney B. Using AphasiaBank for discourse assessment. In seminars in speech and language. Thieme Medical Publishers; 2020, Vol. 41(01), pp. 010–019.

Books/Book Chapters

Coelho C, Cherney LR, Shadden BB, editors. Discourse analysis in adults with and without communication disorders: a resource for clinicians and researchers. San Diego, CA: Plural Publishing; 2022.

Kong AP. Analysis of neurogenic disordered discourse production: theories, assessment and treatment. New York: Routledge; 2022.

Kong AP. Analysis of neurogenic disordered discourse production: from theory to practice. New York: Routledge; 2016.

Online

Fostering the Quality of Spoken Discourse in Aphasia [Internet]; n.d. https://www.foqusaphasia.com/

TalkBank [Internet]; n.d. https://www.talkbank.org/

Manaswita Dutta is an assistant professor at the Department of Speech and Hearing Sciences at Portland State University. Her research interests include understanding the nature of cognitive-linguistic changes that occur as a result of aging and neurological impairment. More specifically, her research examines the relationship between extralinguistic cognitive functions (e.g., attention, executive functioning) and language and its impact on functional communication and psychosocial outcomes of individuals with aphasia and other acquired neurogenic language disorders. Her current work focuses on measuring spoken discourse outcomes and improving clinical utility of discourse analysis tools in aphasia and bilinguals with Alzheimer's disease.

Laura L. Murray is a full professor in the School of Communication Sciences and Disorders and Associate Dean of Graduate and Postdoctoral Studies in the Faculty of Health Sciences at Western University. She is a Fellow of the American Speech-Language-Hearing Association. Her research focuses on typical aging and acquired neurogenic cognitive and communication disorders, with specific interest not only in examining how extralinguistic cognitive deficits interact with language abilities in aphasia, right hemisphere disorders, traumatic brain injury, or progressive neurological diseases, but also in developing procedures for assessing and treating both acquired language disorders and related, extralinguistic concomitant symptoms.

Brielle C. Stark is an assistant professor of Speech, Language and Hearing Sciences at Indiana University Bloomington. She was a Gates Cambridge Trust Scholar during her Ph.D. in Clinical Neurosciences at Cambridge University (UK), where she studied the efficacy and feasibility of tablet-based therapy for individuals with chronic aphasia and the behavioral and neural correlates of inner speech in this population. She completed her postdoctoral work at the University of South Carolina, specializing in understanding the neural bases of impaired language in aphasia. She is interested in language production in post-stroke aphasia, and her research evaluates behavioral characteristics (especially spoken discourse) and neural mechanisms. Additionally, she is interested in multimodal attributes of language production in aphasia, especially gesture, and in better understanding the phenomenon of inner speech in this population. Dr. Stark is a co-founder of FOQUSAphasia, a working group revolving around discourse studies in aphasia.

Lucy Bryant is a senior lecturer, early career researcher, and a Certified Practicing Speech Pathologist at the University of Technology Sydney Graduate School of Health, Sydney, Australia. Her clinical and research expertise is in assessment and intervention of functional language and communication skills for people with developmental and acquired communication disability, with a particular focus on language in use. Lucy's work also relates to the use of computer technologies to support assessment and rehabilitation of language and communication skills.

Better Conversations with Aphasia and Primary Progressive Aphasia

22

Anna Volkmer and Suzanne Beeke

Preview of What Is Currently Known
Communication is a human right. It is fundamental to our daily lives and well-being. Adults with communication difficulties are vulnerable to social isolation, deteriorating relationships, poor mental health, reduced quality of life, and exclusion from healthcare decision-making [1–6]. It is known that communication difficulties carry a high disease burden and are often the primary cause of relationship breakdown [7].

Objectives

(a) To summarize the impact of aphasia and primary progressive aphasia on everyday conversations with family and friends
(b) To explain the principles of a Better Conversations approach to intervention targeting everyday conversation skills
(c) To illustrate ways in which a Better Conversations approach can have a positive impact on everyday conversation
(d) To demonstrate the role of a healthcare professional in supporting access to Better Conversations interventions

A. Volkmer · S. Beeke (✉)
Division of Psychology and Language Sciences, University College London, London, UK
e-mail: a.volkmer.15@ucl.ac.uk; s.beeke@ucl.ac.uk

Background

Aphasia is a communication disability caused by an acquired impairment of spoken language, comprehension, reading, and writing. The most common cause of aphasia is stroke, a condition where blood supply to the brain is disrupted [8]. Approximately one-third of people who experience a stroke have aphasia. Aphasia masks competence and may affect participation and quality of life of the person with aphasia and their significant others [9].

Primary Progressive Aphasia (PPA) describes a heterogeneous group of language-led dementias associated with Alzheimer's disease and fronto-temporal dementia [10, 11]. There are three internationally recognized PPA variants—semantic (svPPA), logopenic (lvPPA), and non-fluent (nfvPPA)—each presenting with differing profiles of progressive language difficulties (See Rukesnaite et al. [11] for a full description of each variant).

Unsurprisingly, aphasia and PPA have a significant impact on conversation. This is illustrated in qualitative studies targeting individuals' experiences. For example, Wallace et al. [12] questioned people with aphasia and family members across seven countries about the most important treatment outcomes. One priority was participation in conversation. Specifically, people with aphasia want to "reduce communication breakdown…communicate independently, and to

A. P.-H. Kong (ed.), *Spoken Discourse Impairments in the Neurogenic Populations*,
https://doi.org/10.1007/978-3-031-45190-4_22

'keep up' in conversation," and to "participate in 'normal' and more complex conversations including discussions." Their family members want people with aphasia to be able to "communicate beyond the level of basic needs to… express their thoughts, wishes and emotions" (Wallace et al., [12], p. 6). In PPA, focus groups [13, 14] and case study interviews [15] have revealed how conversation topics become needs-based rather than opinion-based, and how complex group interactions cause people with PPA to lose confidence and withdraw. These issues can, in turn, cause stress and frustration for the communication partner (CP) [15]. People with PPA and their families also report that they spend time searching for guidance and therapy to improve conversations [13, 14].

Using our language skills to have a conversation is something we do every day and take completely for granted. Conversation is the way we make decisions in our lives, and it is the glue of relationships and community participation. We follow rules we are largely unaware of, that govern who talks when (turn taking), and how we fix conversational breakdowns (repair). Communication difficulties make people vulnerable to unsatisfactory conversations because of problems with (i) finding the words, phrases, and sentences to take a turn, (ii) understanding and being understood, and (iii) problems caused (however unintentionally) by a CP.

Observational methods such as conversation analysis (CA) have shed light on the impact of aphasia and PPA on conversation. Wilkinson [16] identifies two major themes across CA studies of aphasia, which also fit well with our research in PPA, namely repair and adaptation within interaction. Repair is the conversational mechanism we use to deal with problems of speaking, hearing, and understanding [17]. All aphasia and PPA types are associated with long repair sequences, that often deal with word finding difficulties [18–20]. Wilkinson [16] defines adaptation as how people with communication difficulties and their CPs use strategies or resources to take turns in a conversation despite having limited linguistic resources. One common resource for the person with a communication difficulty is gesture [16, 21] and another is enactment, using speech, prosody, facial expression, and body movements, to convey meaning [22]. CPs also adapt their interaction in positive ways, for example, collaborating to achieve repair [23] and by using behaviors that are more challenging such as test questions (whereby a CP asks a question despite knowing the answer, which may create a situation where the person with a communication difficulty is put under pressure to answer). This behavior risks exposing the limitations of a person with a communication difficulty, resulting in a loss of face [16, 21]. In summary, the conversation difficulties associated with stroke-related aphasia and PPA can lead to the experience of loss of interactional competence [16, 21] and adaption can help or hinder the situation.

Communication partner training (CPT) is an intervention that aims to maximize participation of people with communication difficulties in conversations [24]. CPT programs are designed to enhance conversational skill and confidence, employing activities that directly address conversation and "focus on changing behaviors within the context of genuine conversation" (Simmons-Mackie et al., [24], p. 512). CPT is likely to be protective of mental health, preventing the evolution of low mood into clinical depression for people with aphasia after stroke [25].

The Better Conversations Approach to CPT

Better Conversations (BC) is an approach to CPT that focuses on individualized strategies to help people with communication difficulties and their CPs have more enjoyable and successful interactions in their everyday lives. A BC approach helps people to understand how conversation works and to explore the challenges they face because of the communication difficulty. It involves working in collaboration with people with communication difficulties and their regular CPs to develop the best strategies for their conversations. We call this partnership a *conversation dyad*. There is a focus on facilitators and barriers to conversation. Both affect the flow of conversations and how enjoyable or meaningful they are. Facilitators used by people with a communication difficulty vary, but writing, gesture, and a key word to introduce a topic can all help conversations flow. For CPs, leaving space to talk, prompting writing or gesture, and offering comments instead of questions are all useful strategies. A common barrier for people with communication difficulties is word finding difficulty, and for CPs it is asking a test question. BC interventions for stroke-related aphasia and PPA have been coproduced with people with lived experience and their family members (see, for example, Volkmer et al., [14]). There are five core principles behind a BC approach:

1. DYAD: Both parties in the conversation are involved in therapy, and both work toward achieving conversation goals. Conversation involves at least two people. This may sound obvious, but the study and treatment of communication difficulties have often focused on the speech, language, and communicative behaviors of just the person with the impairment. In BC, a key principle is how people work together to create meaningful and satisfying conversations. For BC therapy to work, it needs "buy-in" from both conversation partners. It also needs the therapist to ensure that the abilities of both participants in a dyad are addressed as part of the therapy process.
2. SKILLS: BC is about identifying, reinforcing, and building on skills as well as acknowledging difficulties. Recognizing that we all have competencies in conversation, as well as areas of difficulty, is important. Many of us have more conversational skills in certain contexts than others. The effects of conversation partner familiarity and the (in)formality of the setting, for example, can play a significant role in how we use our skills. As with principle 1 above, BC is concerned with the skills of conversation partners as well as people with communication difficulties.
3. STRATEGIES: BC aims to maximize the use of conversation facilitators and minimize the impact of conversation barriers. A strategy is a conversation behavior that can be observed, understood, and developed with practice. Again, BC focuses on strategies for conversation partners as well as for people with communication difficulties.
4. OWNERSHIP: The dyad identifies their own conversation facilitators and barriers and uses this insight to choose their preferred strategies to work on. The speech-language pathologist (SLP) has a role in facilitating the process of identification but what matters here is that facilitators, barriers, and strategies belong to the dyad and are not imposed by the SLP. This ownership or investment is key to maximizing motivation for change.
5. PRACTICE: The dyad practices using their chosen strategies in conversations coached by the SLP. Practice is a central component of BC, providing the dyad with knowledge and confidence to develop strategy use in order to make meaningful and lasting change. Practice can take place within sessions as well as outside therapy during self-directed practice. What matters is that practice is recognized, supported, and discussed. It is not simply an add-on to therapy but an integral part of the BC process.

Aphasia Case Study

Here the case study of Graham and Alex (pseudonyms) whom we previously described in detail in [26] is presented and summarized. Graham was a 63-year-old retired man who had a large left middle cerebral artery infarct 5 years before he joined the BCA intervention study (reported in Best et al., [27]). Graham had severe non-fluent aphasia and moderate dyspraxia, with severe word finding difficulties. In conversation, his comprehension appeared good; however, testing revealed moderate sentence level comprehension difficulties. Graham lived with Alex, his long-term partner. Graham's aphasia was having a negative impact on their active social life.

Before therapy, Graham and Alex independently made eight 15–20 min conversation videos at home, after being trained to use a video camera. A large number of conversations were sampled because this was a research project—this is not a common clinical practice. For clinical assessment of conversation, we recommend two videos each approx. 10 min long, or three if possible. On the BC website (tinyurl.com/BetterConversationsLab), readers can find a webinar giving advice on how to make a conversation video of a client and their CP. The SLP assessed Graham's and Alex's conversations using the BC Facilitators and Barriers Observation Tool (Table 22.1).

Graham and Alex were offered eight sessions of CPT using the Better Conversation with Aphasia (BCA) program, freely available online (https://extendstore.ucl.ac.uk/product?catalog=UCLXBCA). The program was delivered once a week for 1–1.5 h in their home. Figure 22.1 gives a summary of the intervention sessions.

Table 22.1 A completed BC facilitators and barriers observation tool for Graham and Alex

Instruction: Use this tool to record the facilitators and barriers you observe when observing a conversation between a person with a communication difficulty (PWCD) and their communication partner (CP). We encourage you to observe a video recording but you can observe the dyad in real-time.

Conversation facilitators

These are behaviors that allow the conversation to work and flow. For example, the CP giving time or checking understanding, or the PWCD using writing or gesture.

Graham (PWA)

- Initiates topics of conversation.
- Gives his opinion.
- Uses multimodal strategies to take a turn—Word plus gesture, intonation, facial expression, writing.
- Uses automatic phrases and symbolic noise to convey meaning.

Alex (CP)

- Uses gossip and opinion to initiate a conversation.
- Introduces productive topics—Friends, gardening, trips away.
- Accepts dyspraxic errors without asking Graham to say the word correctly.
- Comments on what Graham says.

Conversation barriers

These are behaviors that cause conversational difficulties or reduce conversational flow. For example, the CP asking test questions (where the answer is already known), or the PWCD taking unintelligible turns or not initiating topics.

Graham (PWA)

- Dyspraxic output makes him unintelligible at times.
- Word finding difficulties affect his ability to take a turn.
- Often his turns consist only of yes/no (because of being asked lots of yes/no questions).

Alex (CP)

- Asks lots of yes/no questions and test questions which means Graham has to do a lot of answering instead of being able to introduce topics.
- Doesn't always give time for Graham to respond to questions.

Environmental facilitators and barriers to conversation

These are environmental factors that support conversation or cause difficulties. For example, background noise from a TV, seating arrangements.

- Most conversations recorded in a facilitative environment without distraction
- Sometimes Graham has a pen and paper in front of him

Source: BC facilitators and barriers observation tool (tinyurl.com/BetterConversationsLab)

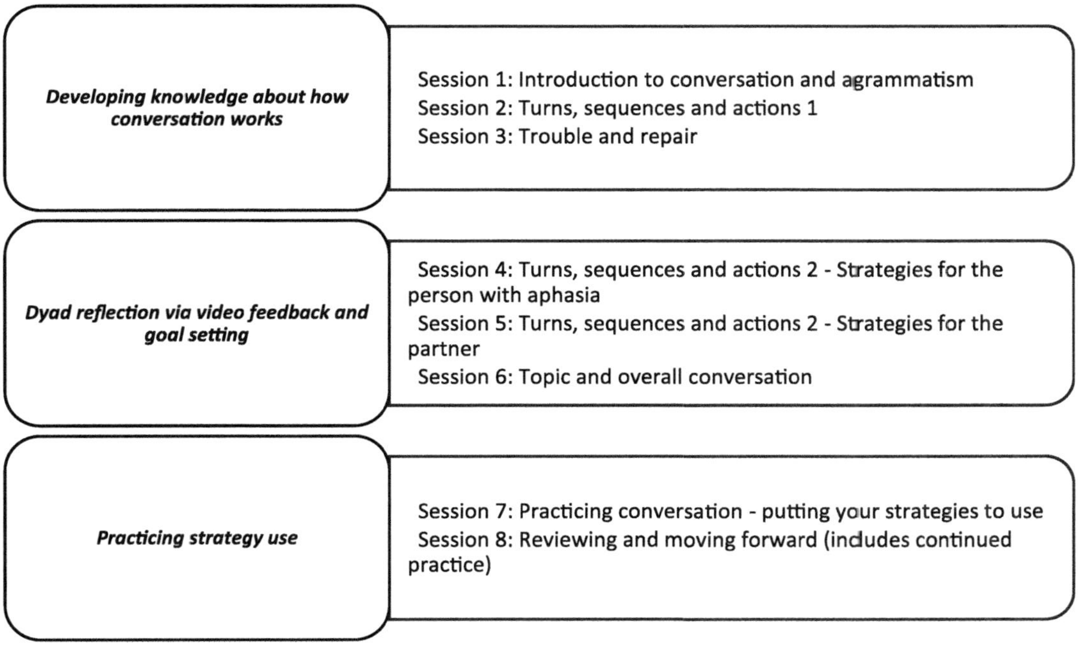

Fig. 22.1 Summary of the eight BCA intervention sessions delivered to Graham and Alex

The SLP used video feedback to help Graham and Alex reflect on their conversations and to identify for themselves the facilitators and barriers to their conversations. She prepared very short video clips (of approximately 30–90 s in duration) to show them. Some showed facilitators she had already identified: Graham initiating a topic and using multimodal strategies to take a turn, Alex commenting on Graham's turns. One video clip showed a key barrier in Alex's conversations as perceived by the SLP, the use of test questions. The SLP used two neutral questions to help Graham and Alex reflect, "what is happening here?" and (for the video clip of a barrier) "what could you have done differently?" She supported their ability to spot conversation behaviors by using handouts from the BCA online resource. After this, Graham and Alex set the following goals.

Graham chose to practice these strategies to support conversation:

1. Writing and drawing
2. Using a key word to identify a topic
3. Using mime to act out an event

Alex wanted to stop using test questions and decided to practice these strategies:

1. Letting the conversation continue (so Graham could say more)
2. Carrying on if he had understood (rather than stopping to fix an error)
3. Commenting on things that Graham said

The SLP supported Graham and Alex to practice using their strategies in conversation-based activities such as planning a holiday, and discussing a news story.

Subsequently, the Better Conversations Conversation Outcome Measure (BC-COM) was used to measure changes in post-therapy conversations. Because this was a research project, the frequency of use of their chosen facilitators and some key barriers in six conversation samples before and after therapy were tallied to account for the inherent variability across conversations. For clinical use, it is recommended to collect two or three pre-therapy samples and two post-therapy samples, all of 5 min duration. Guidance on using the BC-COM clinically can be found in

Table 22.2 A completed BC-Conversation Outcome Measure (BC-COM) sheet for Graham and Alex

Note: Conversation is inherently variable—the more samples you use the more likely you are to capture meaningful change after therapy. If possible use two or three pre-therapy samples and two post-therapy samples.		Counts in 5-min conversation samples													
		Pre-therapy samples							Post-therapy samples						
Client: Graham	**Facilitators** (expected to increase after therapy)	1	2	3	4	5	6	**Pre-therapy mean**	7	8	9	10	11	12	**Post-therapy mean**
	Writing or drawing	0	0	0	0	0	0	**0**	0	0	0	0	7	1	**1.3**
	Key word to identify topic	3	0	2	1	0	3	**1.5**	8	5	5	2	4	2	**4.3**
	Mime to act out event	0	0	0	1	0	0	**0.2**	3	3	0	0	0	0	**1**
		Pre-therapy samples							Post-therapy samples						
Conversation partner: Alex	**Facilitators** (expected to increase after therapy)	1	2	3	4	5	6	**Pre-therapy mean**	7	8	9	10	11	12	**Post-therapy mean**
	Letting conversation continue	0	0	0	0	4	7	**1.8**	2	2	1	0	5	0	**1.7**
	Carrying on if you have understood	0	2	1	3	3	3	**2**	1	3	3	2	1	0	**1.7**
	Commenting on things G says	1	1	0	4	9	12	**4.5**	3	7	5	2	5	5	**4.5**
		Pre-therapy samples							Post-therapy samples						
Conversation partner: Alex	**Barriers** (expected to decrease after therapy)	1	2	3	4	5	6	**Pre-therapy mean**	7	8	9	10	11	12	**Post-therapy mean**
	Test questions	7	1	0	10	1	16	**5.8**	2	1	0	0	2	0	**0.8**

Beeke and Bloch [26]. Table 22.2 shows a completed BC-COM sheet for Graham and Alex.

The BC-COM reveals Alex almost eradicated test questions after BCA—a pre-therapy mean of 5.8 test questions in a 5-minute conversation dropped to 0.8 after therapy. However, the three facilitators Alex chose to practice showed no change. After BCA, Graham successfully deployed his keyword strategy—a pre-therapy mean of 1.5 instances in a 5-min conversation increased to a mean of 4.3 after therapy. Graham's other two strategies, mime and writing/drawing, showed some increased use after therapy but this was variable.

PPA Case Study

Here another case study of F.F. and H.H. whom we have previously described in detail in Beeke et al. [28] is presented and summarized. F.F. is retired man with PPA and H.H., his partner. Based on a combination of brain imaging and clinical assessment F.F. was diagnosed with nfvPPA approximately 2 years prior to participating in this intervention. In line with the Gorno-Tempini et al. [29] international consensus on diagnostic criteria for nfvPPA, F.F. presented with effortful, halting (apraxic) speech and difficulties understanding syntactically complex sentences. F.F. was referred to speech and language therapy due to difficulties in his verbal output, which had become very slow. F.F. and H.H. explained that conversation had become a source of frustration for them both. This had been amplified during the COVID-19 pandemic as F.F., who worked part time and had caring responsibilities for their child, had to work from home during this time. Given the COVID-19 restrictions at the time, this intervention was delivered remotely via a video conferencing platform. Given remotely delivered interventions often fall under the broader title of telehealth we called this teleCPT.

Before starting teleCPT, F.F. and H.H were asked to make four 10-min video recordings of natural home-based conversations. In order to facilitate the transfer of these recordings, these were recorded during a video conferencing session, whereby the SLP invited F.F. and H.H. to join a video call from their home. The SLP turned their camera and microphone off and recorded the interactions. F.F. and H.H. were asked to rate whether these were representative of their everyday conversations to ensure the recordings captured something meaningful and relevant to them.

The SLP reviewed the recordings to assess their conversation, using the BC Facilitators and Barriers Observation Tool (see Table 22.3) to identify common barriers and facilitators present in the dyad's conversations.

F.F. and H.H. were then invited to attend four sessions of teleCPT using the Better Conversation with PPA (BCPPA) program. This was delivered remotely over four 1-h sessions on the video con-

Table 22.3 A completed BC facilitators and barriers observation tool for F.F. and H.H

Instruction: Use this tool to record the facilitators and barriers you observe when observing a conversation between a person with a communication difficulty (PWCD) and their communication partner (CP). We encourage you to observe a video recording but you can observe the dyad in real time.
Conversation facilitators *These are behaviors that allow the conversation to work and flow. For example, the CP giving time or checking understanding, or the PWCD using writing or gesture.* F.F. (PwPPA) • When F.F. used gestures to indicate he was still speaking (that his turn was not complete), ensured H.H. waited for him to complete his turn before embarking on her turn or another task. • Similarly, when F.F. used gestures to indicate that he was about to start a turn, this ensured H.H. waited for him to start his turn before embarking on other tasks or leaving the room. H.H. (CP) • When F.F. was unintelligible or produced an incomplete utterance and H.H. asked for clarification, F.F. was able to produce a clearer or more complete turn, allowing conversation to flow.
Conversation barriers *These are behaviors that cause conversational difficulties or reduce conversational flow. For example, the CP asking test questions (where the answer is already known), or the PWCD taking unintelligible turns or not initiating topics.* F.F. (PwPPA) • F.F. did not look to check if H.H. was present when he started speaking—meaning he often started speaking when H.H, had left the room. This often-meant H.H. was unable to hear him speaking. • F.F. took long pauses before a turn—meaning H.H. would take a turn or begin another activity. • F.F. occasionally produced unintelligible speech or incomplete utterances that were difficult for H.H. to understand. H.H. (CP) • When F.F. was unintelligible or produced an incomplete utterance, H.H. would often let these pass or respond with an unrelated comment resulting in frustration.
Environmental facilitators and barriers to conversation *These are environmental factors that support conversation or cause difficulties. For example, background noise from a TV, seating arrangements.* • F.F.'s favorite armchair was in a position which made it difficult for him to see everybody in the room. • H.H. would often be doing multiple activities at the same time. E.g., speaking to F.F. from another part of the same room where she was preparing food or arranging furniture.

Source: BC facilitators and barriers observation tool (tinyurl.com/BetterConversationsLab)

Table 22.4 Summary of the four BCPPA sessions delivered to F.F. and H.H

Session number	Focus of session
Session 1: What is conversation?	Information about how conversation works and what can go wrong was presented, discussing turn taking, questions and answers, breakdown and repair and topic maintenance. This was supported by handouts which were shared using the screen share function and then emailed afterwards. The dyad were supported to share their views on what conversation meant to them. Finally a clip of their own conversation was shown to them (an example of a positive sequence where a facilitator was used).
Session 2: Goal setting	Three further video clips were shown. The dyad were supported to use their new knowledge to identify what they felt were the potential barriers to conversational flow and what facilitated the flow. Having identified these barriers and facilitators the dyad were invited to set goals on what they wished to work on. The dyad set the following goals: For H.H. • To use more clarification questions, to deal with the barrier of not understanding F.F. and letting it pass. • To try to focus more on the conversation while not doing something else at the same time. This was identified to deal with the barrier observed on the recording whereby she undertook multiple activities while in conversation with F.F., often not in the same room as him. For F.F. • To use gesture more to indicate "I still have something to say". This was identified to deal with the barrier of long pauses in the conversation. • To check H.H. is still in the room before talking by saying her name or looking. This was identified to deal with the observed behavior whereby F.F. started talking despite H.H. not being present in the room. Having set these goals F.F. and H.H. rated them with a score, in line with goal attainment scale procedures (Turner-Stokes et al., 2009).
Session 3: Practice	F.F. and H.H. were asked to practice their goals between sessions and then discuss at the therapy session how they had managed. In this discussion, a virtual tour of the living space helped the SLP to recommend the best seating arrangement for the dyad in conversations. During this session, the couple also had another "practice" conversation, which the SLP then asked them to reflect on and evaluate in line with their goals.
Session 4: Problem solving and planning for the future	In the final session, F.F. and H.H. were provided a summary handout of the work they had undertaken to date. The SLP also provided guidance on anticipated future changes in conversation and strategies that might help, e.g., H.H. giving more time to respond as F.F.'s speech would likely become even slower. At this session F.F. and H.H. were also asked to re-visit their goals and re-rate them.

ferencing platform. Details of these intervention sessions are given in Table 22.4.

At the end of the four BCPPA sessions, H.H. and F.F. were asked to review their goals and consider if they had made any progress in these areas. As described in Beeke et al. [28], H.H. and F.F. felt that they had achieved all the goals they had set themselves. In relation to H.H.'s goal to ask more clarification questions, they both felt they had achieved this goal much more than they had anticipated. This provided a useful and tangible (and person centered) measure of progress made in therapy.

The BC Pathway—Who and When?

One of the most important aspects of the BC approach to CPT is that it is undertaken jointly with the person with a communication difficulty and a CP. It is not uncommon for clients to find it difficult to identify an available CP, or a CP who might find it most useful. Often, we start with the spouse or partner, but they might not always be the person who would benefit most from this intervention. The ideal CP might be a relative or friend who finds communication difficult. Taking time to think about the right CP can be useful, and offering the intervention to multiple people around the person, e.g., first the partner, then the adult child and friends can address conversation issues more broadly. Additionally, delivering the intervention remotely, via telehealth (teleCPT), can assist in managing time and access to the intervention [28].

Some participants might be able to identify a barrier or facilitator in their conversations immediately, others might require more guidance and practice. The BC approach has embedded a range of strategies to facilitate change including video feedback, self-reflection tasks on barriers and facilitators, joint identification of goals, and practice of strategies in sessions. In our experience, the video feedback is the most important component in this reflection process. The video recording enables people to see the impact of their communication on the other person in the conversation. By selecting brief clips (30 s to 2 min long at most), the SLP can present specific examples. One example of this might be showing a video clip of how a test question or a series of test questions makes an interaction seem like an examination instead of a conversation, another example might be presenting a video clip demonstrating how effective a gesture is in conveying meaning.

People with PPA and their families have advocated that CPT should be a standard component of a care pathway for individuals at the very start of their journey with dementia [14]. Certainly, SLPs report using CPT approaches with almost all clients with PPA. However, feedback from participants in the BCPPA pilot feasibility study indicates that people may benefit from different dosages at different times on their disease journey. Anecdotally, people with stroke-related aphasia and their families often report wishing they had received this type of intervention sooner. Based on this we would recommend BC approaches should be offered from the outset and prioritized to the same extent as impairment-based approaches.

Importantly, delivering BC may not need to be a one-off event. SLPs working with people with PPA have compared this to a dental review, highlighting that 6 month "check ups" can help monitor progression and identify new issues that arise and need to be addressed [30]. Indeed, our experience is that people with both stroke-related aphasia and progressive aphasia change over time and can benefit from brief, additional top up sessions. This can be delivered individually or in a group setting.

Remote delivery of speech and language therapy has been essential during recent years and based on our clinical experience, remote delivery of BC interventions, via video conferencing platforms, has been extremely successful. Two examples of teleCPT for PPA and PCA have been written up as case studies and demonstrate positive outcomes [28, 31]. These cases demonstrate participants achieved their goals, reported positive changes to the impact of PPA on their lives, and provided positive feedback on their experiences of remote CPT. Clinically, we have also run BC groups, with up to four dyads, on video conferencing platforms and found this to be extremely positive. Delivered over a series of eight 1-hour video conferencing sessions over 8 weeks, participants have reported positive peer learning experiences and formed ongoing relationships that have contributed to maintenance of conversation strategies [32].

To conclude, clinical experience, research, and lived experience have informed the development of both BCA and BCPPA. The BC approach to CPT is designed to address behaviors that impact on the flow of conversation. The conversation behaviors of the person with the communication difficulty and their CP are intertwined, therefore training them both is an essential component. BC provides a framework for SLPs to address these issues.

Major Takeaways

1. Aphasia and primary progressive aphasia can lead to barriers to conversation such as test questions.
2. Both the person with aphasia/primary progressive aphasia and their family member are responsible for dealing with barriers to everyday conversations. Therefore training both people in the partnership is vital.

3. The five core principles of a Better Conversations approach are DYAD, SKILLS, STRATEGIES, OWNERSHIP, and PRACTICE.
4. The clinical outcomes of a Better Conversations approach include achievement of personally relevant conversation goals and observable changes in conversation behavior.
5. A Better Conversations approach provides a framework for the speech-language pathologist to directly target change in conversation skills.

Acknowledgments We would like to thank the members of the Better Conversations lab at UCL, our wider collaborators and all the people with aphasia and PPA and their family and friends who have been part of this work.

References

1. Cruice M, Worrall L, Hickson L. Reporting on psychological well-being of older adults with chronic aphasia in the context of unaffected peers. Disabil Rehabil. 2011;33(3):219–28.
2. Hemsley B, Werninck M, Worrall L. "That really shouldn't have happened": people with aphasia and their spouses narrate adverse events in hospital. Aphasiology. 2013;27(6):706–22.
3. National Institute for Health and Care Excellence. Dementia: assessment, management and support for people living with dementia and their carers; 2018. https://www.nice.org.uk/guidance/ng97.
4. Ruggero L, Nickels L, Croot K. Quality of life in primary progressive aphasia: what do we know and what can we do next? Aphasiology. 2019;33(5):498–519.
5. Threats T. The ICF framework and third party disability: application to the spouses of persons with aphasia. Top Stroke Rehabil. 2010;17(6):451–7.
6. Victor CR, Rippon I, Nelis SM, Martyr A, Litherland R, Pickett J, Hart N, Henley J, Matthews F, Clare L, IDEAL programme team. Prevalence and determinants of loneliness in people living with dementia: findings from the IDEAL programme. Int J Geriatr Psychiatry. 2020;35(8):851–8.
7. Volkmer A, Spector A, Warren JD, Beeke S. The 'better conversations with primary progressive aphasia (BCPPA)' program for people with PPA (primary progressive aphasia): protocol for a randomised controlled pilot study. Pilot Feasibility Studies. 2018;4(1):1.
8. World Stroke Association (Viewed 2022) at https://www.world-stroke.org/
9. Berg K, Isaksen J, Wallace SJ, Cruice M, Simmons-Mackie N, Worrall L. Establishing consensus on a definition of aphasia: an e-Delphi study of international aphasia researchers. Aphasiology. 2022;36(4):385–400.
10. Marshall CR, Hardy CJ, Volkmer A, Russell LL, Bond RL, Fletcher PD, Clark CN, Mummery CJ, Schott JM, Rossor MN, Fox NC. Primary progressive aphasia: a clinical approach. J Neurol. 2018;265(6):1474–90.
11. Ruksenaite J, Volkmer A, Jiang J, Johnson J, Marshall CR, Warren JD, Hardy CJ. Primary progressive aphasia: toward a pathophysiological synthesis. Curr Neurol Neurosci Rep. 2021;21(3):1–2.
12. Wallace SJ, Worrall L, Rose T, Le Dorze G, Cruice M, Isaksen J, Kong AP, Simmons-Mackie N, Scarinci N, Gauvreau CA. Which outcomes are most important to people with aphasia and their families? An international nominal group technique study framed within the ICF. Disabil Rehabil. 2017;39(14):1364–79.
13. Loizidou M, Brotherhood E, Harding E, Crutch S, Warren JD, Hardy C, Volkmer A. 'Like going into a chocolate shop, blindfolded': what do people with primary progressive aphasia want from speech and language therapy? Int J Lang Commun Disord. 2022;58:737–55.
14. Volkmer A, Spector A, Swinburn K, Warren JD, Beeke S. Using the Medical Research Council framework and public involvement in the development of a communication partner training intervention for people with primary progressive aphasia (PPA): better conversations with PPA. BMC Geriatr. 2021;21(1):1–7.
15. Pozzebon M, Douglas J, Ames D. Facing the challenges of primary progressive aphasia: the spousal perspective. J Speech Lang Hear Res. 2018;61(9):2292–312.
16. Wilkinson R. Conversation and aphasia: advances in analysis and intervention. Aphasiology. 2015;29(3):257–68.
17. Schegloff EA. Overlapping talk and the organization of turn-taking for conversation. Lang Soc. 2000;29(1):1–63.
18. Laakso M, Klippi A. A closer look at the 'hint and guess' sequences in aphasic conversation. Aphasiology. 1999;13(4–5):345–63.
19. Taylor C, Croot K, Power E, Savage SA, Hodges JR, Togher L. Trouble and repair during conversations of people with primary progressive aphasia. Aphasiology. 2014;28(8–9):1069–91.
20. Volkmer A, Mistry S, Thompson D, Warren JD, Beeke S. Collaborative turn-construction practices of people with primary progressive aphasia and their family conversation partners. J Interact Res Commun Dis. 2023;14(3):456-485.
21. Kindell J, Keady J, Sage K, Wilkinson R. Everyday conversation in dementia: a review of the literature to inform research and practice. Int J Lang Commun Disord. 2017;52(4):392–406.
22. Kindell J, Sage K, Keady J, Wilkinson R. Adapting to conversation with semantic dementia: using enactment as a compensatory strategy in everyday social interaction. Int J Lang Commun Disord. 2013;48(5):497–507.

23. Beeke S, Beckley F, Best W, Johnson F, Edwards S, Maxim J. Extended turn construction and test question sequences in the conversations of three speakers with agrammatic aphasia. Clin Linguist Phon. 2013;27(10–11):784–804.
24. Simmons-Mackie N, Raymer A, Cherney LR. Communication partner training in aphasia: an updated systematic review. Arch Phys Med Rehabil. 2016;97(12):2202–21.
25. Baker C, Worrall L, Rose M, Hudson K, Ryan B, O'Byrne L. A systematic review of rehabilitation interventions to prevent and treat depression in post-stroke aphasia. Disabil Rehabil. 2018;40(16):1870–92.
26. Beeke S, Bloch S, editors. Better conversations with communication difficulties: a practical guide for clinicians. J&R Press Limited; 2023.
27. Best W, Maxim J, Heilemann C, Beckley F, Johnson F, Edwards SI, Howard D, Beeke S. Conversation therapy with people with aphasia and conversation partners using video feedback: a group and case series investigation of changes in interaction. Front Hum Neurosci. 2016;10:562.
28. Beeke S, Volkmer A, Farrington-Douglas C. TeleCPT: delivery of a better conversations approach to communication partner training during a global pandemic and beyond. Perspect ASHA Special Interest Groups. 2021;6(6):1776–85.
29. Gorno-Tempini ML, Hillis AE, Weintraub S, Kertesz A, Mendez M, Cappa SF, Ogar JM, Rohrer JD, Black S, Boeve BF, Manes F. Classification of primary progressive aphasia and its variants. Neurology. 2011;76(11):1006–14.
30. Volkmer A, Cartwright J, Ruggero L, Beales A, Gallée J, Grasso S, Henry M, Jokel R, Kindell J, Khayum R, Pozzebon M. Principles and philosophies for speech and language therapists working with people with primary progressive aphasia: an international expert consensus. Disabil Rehabil. 2022;45:1063–78.
31. Volkmer A, Farrington-Douglas C, Crutch S, Beeke S, Warren J, Yong K. Better conversations: a language and communication intervention for aphasia in posterior cortical atrophy. Neurocase. 2022;28(4):356–63.
32. Volkmer A, & Farrington-Douglas, keeping conversations going during the COVID-19 pandemic: communication partner training for people with TBI, Aphasia and PPA. Centre for Neurorehabilitation Symposium, Clinical Networking Event UCLH September 2020.

Additional Resources

Books

Beeke S, Bloch S, editors. Better conversations with communication difficulties: a practical guide for clinicians. J&R Press Limited; 2023.

Volkmer A, Broomfield K, editors. Seldom heard voices in service user involvement: the how and why of meaningful collaboration. J&R Press Limited; 2022.

Online Resources

BC Webpage; n.d. tinyurl.com/BetterConversationsLab

Better Conversations with Aphasia: An E-Learning Resource; n.d. https://extendstore.ucl.ac.uk/product?catalog=UCLXBCA

Anna Volkmer is an honorary consultant speech and language therapist within the cognitive disorders service at the National Hospital for Neurology and Neurosurgery, University College London Hospital. She is also employed as a lecturer and NIHR funded advanced research fellow within the Department of Language and Cognition at University College London. Anna's research focuses on developing and trialling interventions for people with primary progressive aphasia. More about her research and publications can be found on www.ucl.ac.uk/pals/people/anna-volkmer.

Suzanne Beeke is an associate professor in the Department of Language and Cognition at University College London. Her research focuses on understanding the impact of language and communication disorders on the everyday conversations of adults with acquired neurological conditions. She leads the Better Conversations lab and is lead author of Better Conversations with Aphasia, a free online training resource and therapy programme available at https://extendstore.ucl.ac.uk. More about her research and publications can be found on www.ucl.ac.uk/pals/people/suzanne-beeke.

Improving Communication with People Living with Dementia: A Socio-Cognitive Approach

23

Lenisa Brandão, Juliana Onofre de Lira, and Maria Isabel d'Ávila Freitas

Preview of What Is Currently Known
Studies on the discourse skills of people living with dementia (PWD) have been regarded as a window to the cognitive mechanisms and brain networks involved in discourse processes. Different dementia types have characteristic profiles of discourse deficits [1] which can ultimately progress [2–4]. There is a consensus that functional communication interventions involving the PWD and their communication partners should be introduced at the earliest stages of dementia [5] and that therapies should be multidisciplinary and adopt a person-centered approach (PCA), a guiding principle in dementia care centering on the fulfillment of physical, psychological, and social needs [6].

Objectives
(a) To present a socio-cognitive approach to discourse and a therapeutic person-centered approach
(b) To discuss the process of assessment and goal-setting for functional communication interventions
(c) To analyze discourse strategies for use by people living with dementia (PWD) and their communication partners
(d) To address aspects of communication that involve the dignity and well-being of PWD

L. Brandão (✉)
Department of Speech, Language and Hearing Sciences, Federal University of Santa Maria, Santa Maria, Brazil
e-mail: lenisa.brandao@ufsm.br

J. O. de Lira
Faculty of Ceilândia, University of Brasília, Brasília, Brazil
e-mail: julianalira@unb.br

M. I. d'Ávila Freitas
Department of Speech, Language and Hearing Sciences, Federal University of Santa Catarina, Florianópolis, Brazil
e-mail: maria.isabel@ufsc.br

A Socio-Cognitive Approach to Discourse

The starting point of any discourse production process is the selection of relevant information from mental models in memory. Mental models are cognitive representations of experiences, occurrences, and situations held in episodic memory [7, 8]. Both generic and specific episodic and semantic information interact in the construction of mental models. These give rise to discourse content, but discourse production also relies heavily on representations of communication situations. Therefore, besides accessing representations of events, mental representations of the communication events are regularly constructed and updated to form context models. This type of model contains information on the intentions of the language user and the purpose of the communication situation. The context model also incorporates assumptions about the listener's intentions and their episodic and semantic knowledge, as

A. P.-H. Kong (ed.), *Spoken Discourse Impairments in the Neurogenic Populations*,
https://doi.org/10.1007/978-3-031-45190-4_23

well as expected social behaviors in this context. Knowledge management is guided not only by the intentions of the language user, but also by the goals and purpose of the communication event and by the interlocutor's (presumed) knowledge [8]. An important note about the model presented is that context is a mental representation of the communication situation as constructed by the language user. In other words, it is not the social situation per se that determines the mode of expression during conversational interactions, but the subjective representation of social facts and the manner in which one represents partners in communication. This subjective and interpretive view of context ascribes an active role to language users in discourse construction and justifies the inclusion of diversity in context models.

Cognitive Skills and Communication

Alzheimer's Disease (AD) is the most frequent type of dementia. Throughout early, moderate, and severe stages of progression of AD, the structural systems of language, such as syntax, morphology, and phonology, are typically affected. On the other hand, macro-linguistic aspects of discourse production such as global coherence and informativeness are significantly impacted from the early stages of the disease [9–14]. These dissociations have provided a wealth of materials for understanding the distinct phases of discourse production, as well as their relationships with cognitive skills in the course of dementia. Difficulties accessing semantic and episodic knowledge have been shown to progressively affect discourse production among people living with dementia (PWD) [15]. Executive functioning also plays an important role in discourse production. This can be observed in AD and vascular dementia, but most particularly in the manner the behavioral variant of frontotemporal dementia affects pragmatic abilities [16, 17]. Executive functions such as planning, monitoring, organizing, selecting relevant information, while keeping track of what has been said and inhibiting irrelevant or socially inappropriate content, are important in the maintenance of discourse skills [18–20] and are often progressively affected across various dementia etiologies.

While it is valuable to elucidate the mechanisms underlying difficulties PWD face when producing discourse, after many decades, researchers and clinicians are recognizing the importance of communication skills that can remain relatively preserved throughout the different stages of dementia. Communication is a fundamental part of life, and efforts to promote the quality of life of PWD should be at the center of care decision processes. The quality of communication encompasses mainly social and interactive goals and can coexist with discourse diversity [21]. It is important to acknowledge that certain communication contexts facilitate discourse production and use of discourse strategies by PWD [22, 23]. Promoting communication roles that favor agency and the use of preserved knowledge has been shown to improve communication with PWD [24]. Studies have also shown that non-verbal comprehension and expression of emotions [25, 26], as well as complex emotion-based learning capacities [27], are preserved in dementia. Therefore, quality of life-oriented goals can guide the focus of therapeutic efforts to build emotionally meaningful, dignified, and pleasurable contexts of communication, rather than aiming exclusively at achieving standard patterns of discourse production [21, 28].

Movements advocating person-centered dementia care argue that dementia causes a change in communication, rather than a loss of the ability to communicate [29, 30]. Communication is a human need which cannot be treated as an unidirectional skill to be improved only by the PWD. Instead, it is a reciprocal and collaborative process that relies greatly on the mental representations that communication partners (CP) have about the context of communicating with a person living with dementia. This chapter presents a brief review of a sociocognitive model of discourse to highlight important aspects for the person-centered perspective of improving communication with PWD.

Communication Strategies and Diversity of Mental and Context Models

Discourse and cognitive models have increasingly adopted the idea that a difference in the discourse or cognitive performance of individuals with dementia may reflect the use of a strategy in response to a difficulty [31, 32]. In other words, some discourse features which were once considered signs of deficits of PWD are already recognized in the scientific literature as strategies enabling communication [32]. Focus on the strategic nature of discourse takes account of the active role of the speaker and the way she or he keeps communication flowing despite difficulties. Discourse strategies are learned during language development and may require more or less explicit control. Certain strategies seem to depend on the preservation of the conscious ability to monitor discourse production, being part of explicit knowledge, whereas others seem to become automated, as part of procedural or implicit knowledge [33, 34].

Planning and organizing the expression of ideas in a coherent manner heavily involves monitoring discourse production and conducting dynamic management of available knowledge [8]. Although these abilities are affected by AD, the presence of certain strategies shows that the ability to manage discourse does not vanish in the early and moderate stages of AD. At least until the stages of moderate cognitive decline of AD, the person still seems to recognize difficulties and often makes comments and inquiries to justify reduced informativeness and to obtain knowledge from the CP [32, 35–37]. Nespoulous [31] used the term "modalizers" to refer to these metadiscourse strategies, regarding them as comments and requests for help in an attempt to overcome discourse difficulties. These denote monitoring of propositional content expressed in discourse production [32, 36, 37] and are used to maintain the continuity of communication [35]. From a pragmatic perspective, the use of such strategies should be seen as a skill, not as a failure in communication [37].

The type of strategy outlined above relies greatly on the ability to monitor one's own discourse production. However, although much of discourse is constructed from deliberate access to explicit knowledge, this does not mean the speaker constructs a new mental model every time he or she is faced with a different communication situation. The greater one's repository of experiences accrued from different social situations, the more implicit or tacit the (pre)construction of a context model can become. This implies that different levels of conscious control are involved in the manner in which communication events are represented [8]. Thus, talking about familiar topics and meaningful personal events that have been told many times in conversations with well-known CP may require less effort from the discourse production system. In later stages of AD, for example, it becomes even more important to provide easily accessible life events, as well as familiar communication situations [21]. In addition, it is also vital to recognize the importance of maintaining implicit strategies, such as the ability to accept and take turns in conversations, throughout advanced stages of AD [38, 39].

Being aware of and recognizing discourse strategies are crucial roles of the CP of PWD. Communication partner responses during interactions, and their attitudes toward speakers with dementia, have a major influence on the experience of communication [21]. Reciprocity in interaction and skillful use of discourse markers is therefore important [22]. While certain discourse features may not seem like conventional expected responses, the context model of the CP of PWD must account for the use of certain atypical communication strategies. For example, the expression of what Davis, Moorek, and Peacock [40] call *frozen phrases* or *frozen-coping strategies* can be interpreted as a way that someone with AD uses to close a topic or maintain "conversational credibility" when he or she is unable to answer a question. A collaborative manner of building communication in face of a topic closure may be by summarizing the current topic, so that in turn, the closure is reconfirmed and either participant may start a new topic. A frozen-coping phrase is usually preceded by a discourse marker and a pause and occurs at the beginning of a turn. For example:

A CP's question: "What did you like doing?"
Response from the person with AD: "Just... what I was doing."

Although a typical speaker may interpret this response as evasive or vague, the answer should be perceived as a collaborative response. Replying with positive feedback may encourage the PWD to continue taking turns in conversation without losing face [38]. In certain situations, atypical strategies can be interpreted as effective signals of communication if the CP of PWD is able to let go of conventional top-down principles that usually regulate conversations. The context of communication in this case draws attention to local underlying factors important for social interaction [21].

Validating what PWD comment on and request, even when their assertions or inquiries result from confabulations or memory distortions, can be regarded as a social interaction strategy that takes into consideration the fact that their mental and context models are functioning differently. Insistence on the truth and constantly correcting a person's autobiographical memory flaws, for example, is not recommended for achieving success in communication. Instead, CP can take an approach that favors the well-being of the PWD during communication. Does it matter whether the person thinks that their CP is that friend from the old neighborhood or is the conversation enjoyment what counts the most [41]? Family, friends, and professionals who communicate with PWD may face neuropsychiatric symptoms such as agitation, aggression, hallucination, or delusions from the PWD. In these situations, is it recommendable that CP confront the person with reality? Another example is, due to memory problems, PWD often ask about or want to see a deceased relative. Instead of providing them with painful information every time this happens, CP may consider applying a common strategy called therapeutic lying [42]. Although dismissing the truth may be regarded as unethical in conventional communication situations, 66–96% of family carers and healthcare staff that communicate with PWD have admitted using this strategy to prevent distress when considered necessary [43]. However, it is very important to avoid attitudes that damage the person's right to autonomy [44]. Careless generalization of this type of strategy can contribute to depersonalizing people with dementia [45]. When asked about this strategy, people in the early stages of dementia who were interviewed by Day et al. [46] said they felt more comfortable with the idea of "small" lies. Undoubtedly, applying this strategy in later stages seems to be considered more acceptable, and the use of distraction, defined as the ability to divert attention to other matters or to shift topics, is suggested as a better alternative [47]. Recommendations that align well with the person-centered approach point to the relevance of providing non-verbal and empathic responses to the emotions expressed by PWD, rather than expressing precise verbal responses that would contain information likely to cause distress [48].

Non-verbal communication is also a powerful communication strategy when interacting with PWD. Improving communication in any way possible should be facilitated from the earliest stages of dementia, and should also be maintained in the more advanced stages. There is evidence of retained awareness of self and functional communication skills at very late stages of dementia, showing a desire and ability to communicate in people with severe dementia, even when speech is no longer present [49]. Difficulties expressing or understanding non-verbal communication are associated with the presence of neuropsychiatric symptoms, lower quality of life, and greater caregiver burden [50]. Therefore, exploring non-verbal communication is an important aspect of dementia care throughout disease progression [51]. Some authors propose that caregivers and professionals should be trained in recognizing and interpreting non-verbal signals, as well as in responding to facial expressions of positive emotions, among others. These strategies may enhance, in general, the mood of PWD, while facilitating care activities (such as bathing or other daily activities) and decreasing negative behavior (such as anger). These strategies may also lead to an improvement in eye contact and contextualized smiling, as well as in verbal communication [52–54]. Chen [55] found that home-care workers in Taiwan used strategies such as smiling, maintaining eye contact, using gentle touching, pointing with one finger to draw attention to something important in the environment, and giving instructions to squeeze hands firmly in the event of acceptance or refusal of instructions. The author also found the main non-verbal communication signals of PWD, which varied in meaning, were eye movements, turning the face to the side, looking downward, and maintaining steady eye contact. It is important to highlight that the stigma faced by PWD, especially in advanced stages, can mean that these non-verbal signals may not be interpreted as signs of intentional communication. Therefore, the way PWD are represented in CP' context models—assigning intentionality to PWD behaviors or otherwise—can determine whether communication will be established or not (Fig. 23.1).

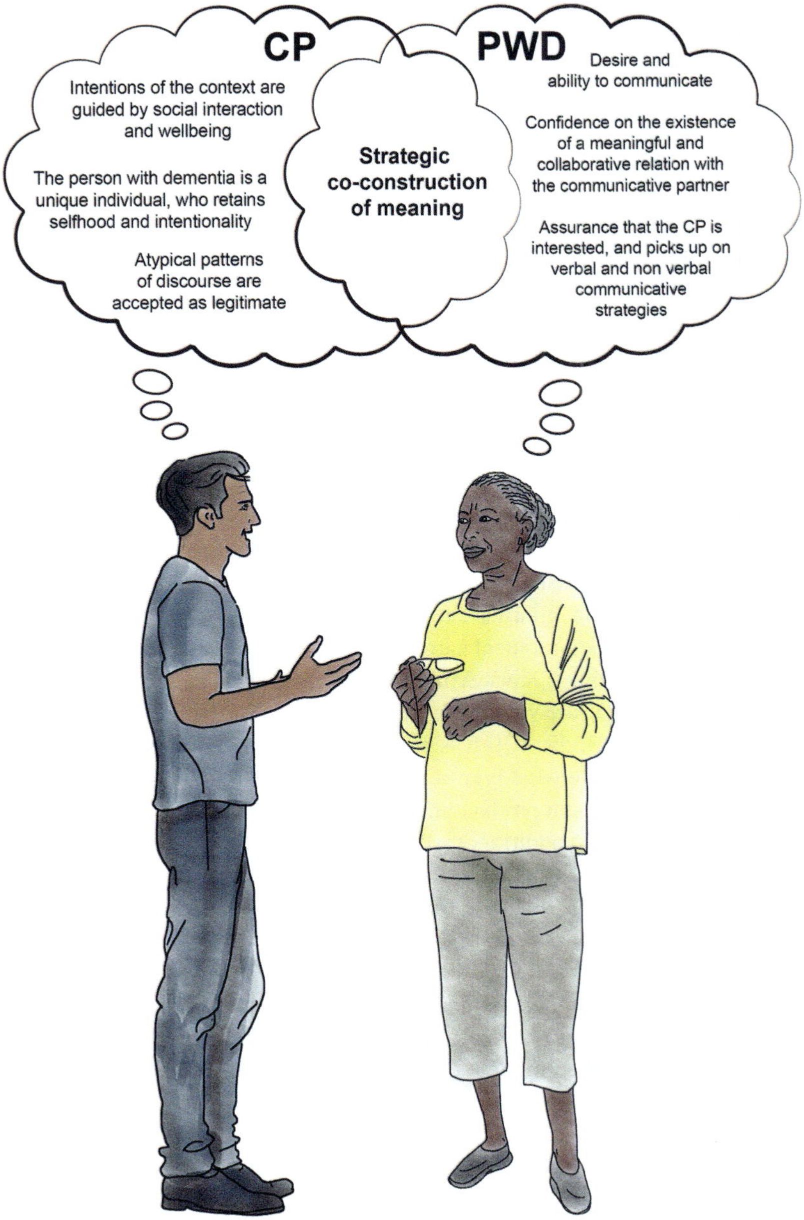

Fig. 23.1 Respect for diversity and strategic co-construction of meaning

Person-Centered Communication Care

Coherent with the socio-cognitive model for discourse and its perspective regarding communicative strategies, the person-centered approach (PCA) emphasizes that the quality of life of PWD should be at the center of therapeutic decisions [6]. According to Maki et al. [56], during the therapeutic process, communication should be assessed and facilitated from the early stages of dementia. Multidimensional aspects must be considered when setting goals, including clinical, cognitive, behavioral, motivational, functional, environmental, and social factors [56].

Before initiating intervention, PWD's ability to communicate in different situations should be assessed, independently of speech, language, or cognitive impairment. This assessment should consider the possible need for environmental modifications, use of hearing aids, time available to communicate, and the presence of behaviors that may interfere with communication abilities in ecological situations [57]. Functional activity assessment scales allow the disability caused by dementia to be quantified and qualified in terms of functioning. These instruments also facilitate therapeutic planning and family/caregiver guidance [58]. Discourse tasks, such as having a conversation about a familiar topic, eliciting storytelling or autobiographical narrative, describing pictures, or telling a story while looking at a sequence of pictures, are very useful ways of evaluating discourse [13, 59, 60]. It is recommended that therapists observe what types of prompts and cues can help the person produce informative and coherent discourse. In addition, the interaction of PWD and their CP can be analyzed with assessment tools designed to evaluate the support provided by the conversation partner and the resultant participation of the person with dementia [61]. To enhance reflective learning about communication, conversations recorded in the evaluation process can be used later to provide CP with concrete examples and insights [62].

Therapeutic goals should, wherever possible, be set through a shared decision-making process with the PWD, respecting the wishes of the person, regardless of dementia stage. Goals selected should be individualized, meaningful, practical, and relevant to the daily living of the PWD and to their CP. There are methods of assessing and facilitating joint decision-making for selecting goals and activities that can be applied to communication interventions. Eliciting issues or areas that might form the basis for intervention goal-setting in an interview may be very helpful to allow the person to be active in this process [63]. For each issue, the person being interviewed can rate the perceived importance of making changes to a certain activity, as well as their readiness to make these changes. The most important stage of setting therapeutic goals involves revisiting each activity and negotiating specific goals that conform to the SMART principles (i.e., *S*pecific, *M*easurable, *A*chievable, *R*ealistic, and *T*ime-delineated). Once a goal is set, and current performance described, possible barriers and facilitators to achieving the goal are discussed using specific prompts, with an emphasis on identifying the resources available to support the changes to be promoted [63]. Within these interviews, there is scope to elicit input from informants and, therefore, this type of interview applies to main CP. Thus, the assessment can also involve the supportive capacity of the CP in helping achieve selected goals, including those that can contribute to reducing caregiver burden.

Hickey and Bourgeois [64] highlight that therapeutic processes focused on communication should not be designed with the exclusive purpose of restoring brain function or cognition, although these aspects may naturally benefit from therapies centered on communication. The goals for communication should attempt to maintain autonomous functioning of this area, as far as possible, throughout all phases of dementia. Promoting quality of life should be a directive of the therapeutic process, and this can be achieved through participation in content-motivating meaningful activities that are contextualized for the PWD and their main CP.

Functional Communication Interventions (FCI)

Functional communication is the ability to receive or convey a message, as well as to communicate effectively and independently, in a natural environment regardless of the mode of communication [65]. Focusing on functional communication helps maintain social interactions and thus reduce social isolation, depression, caregiver burden, and improve the quality of life of PWD, family, and caregivers. Functional Communication Interventions (FCI) are based on The International Classification of Functioning, Disability and Health [66] as the theoretical-practical construct. FCI includes individuals with different language deficit profiles and levels of symptom severity and identifies optimal strategies according to the participant's communication strengths and weaknesses [67]. The main aim of this type of intervention is to maintain an optimum level of communication and social connectedness. FCI may involve direct and indirect strategies that focus on active participation of PWD in communication activities. Promoting participation in daily communication situations includes proposing environmental modifications (e.g., working with families and caregivers), raising awareness about compensatory strategies or aids that can enhance communication, and encouraging engagement in everyday tasks or situations [68]. For example, introducing the use of cooperative assistive devices, such as information prompts or memory aids provided by CP, can contribute to building meaningful conversations [69, 70]. Using visual cues, such as memory wallets or presenting pictures and short informative sentences on a screen, has been shown to augment discourse informativeness and coherence of PWD [71, 72]. Given the fact that the desire to communicate and stay connected remains relatively well preserved into the later stages of dementia [73, 74] and since communication requires joint construction of the message by CP, all participants share responsibility in the process [75]. Thus, therapeutic processes should involve both the PWD and their CP [76].

Communicating with PWD can be a highly challenging task for caregivers and family members. Therefore, CP should receive information and training on how to facilitate PWD participation and avoid creating barriers to PWD communication [77]. Feelings of guilt are often reported by CP when realizing that PWD fail to maintain expected discourse during conversations. It is important that CPs understand that PWD may have difficulties communicating when more than one person is speaking at the same time, filtering out varied verbal or environmental sounds, or recognizing unusual vocabulary and strange expressions. It may also be difficult for PWD to understand topic change signals, making it challenging for them to continue talking about newly introduced themes. The CP, as a listener, needs to be guided on how to continue communication when conventional expected communication behaviors are not manifested. In trying to manage feelings of guilt, CP may reject conversational attempts to avoid eliciting communication breakdowns of PWD. Moreover, CP may also try repeatedly to make sense of confused discourse, while taking excessive responsibility for not getting positive results from their conversational efforts. Thus, CP must understand that achieving conversation and communication are two different matters; the latter must be facilitated in any way possible (verbal or non-verbal) allowing the expression of PWD to be different from that expected in exchanges between people without dementia [78]. In this chapter, aspects of communication care for both PWD and CP are covered. However, we recommend reading Chap. 26 of this book about CP training.

Promoting Dignity for PWD in Communication Contexts

As outlined above, caregivers often perceive that communication poses different challenges at each stage of the disease, affecting the quality of their relationship with PWD [79–81]. Lack of communication between the caregiver and care receiver can lead to conflict in the relationship, social isolation, depression in one or both individuals, caregiver burden and stress, an increased risk of early institutionalization and may affect the relationship quality and well-being of caregivers and PWD [79, 82]. All these aspects may lead to PWD distress [83]. "Responsive behaviors," such as aggression, frustration, repeated questioning, and cursing, can be typically more pronounced as dementia progresses, and are frequently cited as targets of behavioral interventions designed for PWD. However, expressions of distress may also be appropriate signs of affect arising from frustration due to difficulties of both parties in communicating, misunderstandings, and negative attitudes of CP toward PWD. According to Sabat [84], negative positioning toward PWD is based on the notion that every instance of seemingly "abnormal" behavior seen in the person diagnosed is due to brain damage, and that these individuals are immune to being treated in dysfunctional ways by others. The author explained that if, for example, a person diagnosed with probable AD is treated in a way that could be humiliating and embarrassing, and reacts with anger or grief or by pulling away from others, such behaviors are viewed as symptoms of dementia instead of symptoms of dysfunctional social treatment, thereby falsely validating the original ill-conceived position of the CP.

According to van der Geugten and Goossensen [85], certain institutional environments (where PWD may spend long periods or reside) may develop daily communication routines that are undignifying. Objectivation takes place when PWD are treated as a homogeneous group. This is often the case when professionals fail to see PWD as unique individuals and do not tailor care to individual needs. Some professional communication attitudes can exacerbate objectification, such as being bossy, enforcing will, being disrespectful, not taking PWD seriously, or badly disguising maneuvers of diversion. People in general tend to negatively modify communication when interacting with people who differ cognitively [86]. The concept of "Elderspeak" refers to the patronizing way of communicating with an older person, and this can be particularly salient in communication with PWD. Oversimplified vocabulary, inappropriate use of familiar names, and overuse of tag questions have been found to increase resistiveness to care in PWD [87]. Not communicating with the PWD or talking about them in front of them also shows attitudes that ignore the relationality of the person. Shortage of time for communication also creates a general atmosphere of business that lowers the quality of relationships. Being cared for by strangers, due to a lack of continuity in caregiver staff of institutions, also promotes undignifying communication routines. Undignifying communication contexts which objectivate or stigmatize PWD make them feel worthless, meaningless, and useless. The inability of PWD to clearly communicate through language what they feel under these circumstances contributes to a lack of understanding of their suffering and wishes by the professional care providers. Therefore, it is very important to promote awareness about stigma, change perspectives about dementia, and learn to draw attention to non-verbal communication.

Dignifying communication practices ensure that PWD enjoy confirmation as unique human beings, with a name, a history, and a unique personality and identity. These practices include taking an interest in the background of the PWD, their past roles, hobbies, beliefs, and values. Keeping connection with CP that have family and friendship ties is a very important part of this process. In addition, taking part in enjoyable and identity-strengthening activities, associated with previous or present interest and formal and informal skills is also important. Engaged listening and attention to understand discourse choices that may be unexpected are crucial attitudes when talking to PWD [88]. Collaborative storytelling can also be a powerful source of well-being [89]. However, although coherence and informativeness of storytelling can be facilitated with visual prompts such as pictures and short written phrases when necessary, communication activities should not be limited to those which rely heavily on exclusive expression through oral language skills. Figure 23.2 outlines favorable and disruptive representations on context models.

Context model of communicative partner (CP) of person living with dementia (PWD) in a given communication situation (CS)									
	Purpose of communication situation	Intention of CP of PWD	Representation of PWD	Relationality expected	Communication modality expected	Conceptions about discourse diversity	How atypical forms of discourse are handled	Availability of time for interaction	Emotions that may be associated or experienced
FAVORABLE	Social interaction Collaborative storytelling Shared embodied activities Daily care and activities of daily living that can be done in collaboration	To engage in exchange and co-management of topics centered on past and present interests, skills and values of PWD To share feelings of connection and wellbeing	Unique person who has a singular history, knowledge and personality and whose wishes, tastes and decisions must be considered Individual who has his/her own personal way of dealing with dementia	Personalization Horizontality and interdependency are valued, interaction is oriented toward building reciprocity, accessibility and engagement	Multimodal channels of expression, including eye contact, touch, vocal, facial and bodily gestures which may or may not be accompanied by speech	Strategic person-centered view	Validation, collaboration, attention to understand unexpected expression; help in maintaining and shifting themes; attention to local and bottom-up signals of cooperation	Enough time is given for both parties to take turns; Time is available for longer pauses, repetitions, hesitations and modalizers	Empathy, comfort and acceptance Feelings of belonging to network that shares similar context models Constructive coping of emotions related to facing the cognitive changes of PWD
DISRUPTIVE	To achieve practical goal that does not require interaction To demand independence in discourse production To conduct activities which are not contextualized and meaningful	To direct and impose continuation of topics not centered on interests of PWD	Subject suffering from a disease, lack of selfhood, intentionality; Subject represents homogeneous group	Objectivation Verticality (power and status positioning of CP) and independence in communication are valued; interaction is oriented by one's individual goals; talking about and not with the person	Interaction is established only if oral language is present	Impairment-based view	Frequent interruptions, does not let go of top-down standard discourse patterns, language and memory flaws are corrected, insistence on the truth, and generalized use of therapeutic lying.	Shortage of time, manifesting as busyness and avoidance; Unease with different response rhythms	Burden, frustration and guilt; Excessive self-demand and responsibility; Feeling poorly supported by other CPs of the PWD

Fig. 23.2 Favorable and disruptive context models

Communicating through bodily gestures and facial expression can be a great source of joy for PWD. Dignifying care practices incorporate the use of all senses and imagination to facilitate interaction with others [85]. For example, taking a short walk out in nature, while holding hands with someone with whom there is a meaningful connection, can be a shared bodily experience that communicates without words. According to Kontos [90], the existence of selfhood does not depend solely on cognitive monitoring abilities. Self must be understood as being enacted in the actual movements of the body. Embodied activities that are meaningful for the person, and that rely on implicit memory, can be embedded in daily communication routines, such as knitting or saying a prayer together. Embodied communication activities can also be practiced in groups through art, which is a failure-free social activity that does not require participants to communicate using strict conversational rules [91]. Engaging in dancing or sharing emotions with clown visitors are also examples of practicing embodied communication activities [92, 93]. Intergenerational programs often entail interactive activities such as painting or drawing, listening or making music, and singing [94]. By interacting with PWD, children, teenagers, and young adults can learn about dementia and positive attitudes toward PWD, improving their social skills and increasing self-confidence [95]. Breakfast club, a structured multi-modality group social intervention, is another suggested approach to involve PWD in a functional and interesting way, which may increase involvement with residual communication strengths [96]. These programs can also be an excellent way of promoting inclusion of PWD in society and of changing perspectives about dementia. All these possible actions described above foster the concept of dementia-friendly communities, or places, where PWD can be respected, supported, and actively involved to contribute as much as possible [97, 98]. This can lead to effective social inclusion and is interdependent on public awareness education, reduction of stigma, and inclusive environmental design [99, 100]. This view is facilitated within a "culture of care," where all members of the community, not only relatives or caregivers of PWD, have a sense of reciprocity and caring for each other [96, 101].

Major Takeaways

1. This chapter provided a brief introduction to a socio-cognitive model of discourse which is coherent with person-centered perspectives on improving communication with PWD.
2. Emphasis was placed on functional aspects of communication, considering its different channels and the diverse ways in which communication can manifest. The presented perspectives highlighted therapeutic processes which focus on promoting joint decisions respecting the wishes of PWD and their CP in planning communication interventions.
3. The approach presented also raises awareness of preserved communication skills of PWD and strategies that can be used by PWD and their CP to enhance communication.
4. Finally, the promotion of dignity and well-being in communication contexts was addressed, considering the need for raising awareness on the importance of maintaining personhood when interacting with PWD. At a time when dissemination of the idea of dementia-friendly communities is increasing awareness on the relevance of promoting a better life for PWD and their families, it is crucial that therapeutic perspectives embrace the goal of combating stigma and empowering PWD to participate in communication situations.

Acknowledgments The authors would like to pay their special regard to the Global Brain Health Institute for the support on promoting academic work that can contribute to building inclusive societies for people living with dementia. The authors also express their respect and appreciation to the broad interdisciplinary work and teachings of Teun Adrianus van Dijk, for the long-lasting positive impact of his socio-cognitive approach to discourse on research applied to the discourse of people living with dementia. In addition, the authors thank Caroline Jagoe for her comments on the content of this chapter.

References

1. El-Wahsh S, Monroe P, Kumfor F, Ballard K. Communication interventions for people with dementia and their communication partners. Dementia Rehabil. 2021:35–56.
2. Ash S, Moore P, Vesely L, Grossman M. The decline of narrative discourse in Alzheimer's disease. Brain Lang. 2007;1(103):181–2.
3. Henry JD, Phillips LH, Von Hippel C. A meta-analytic review of theory of mind difficulties in behavioural-variant frontotemporal dementia. Neuropsychologia. 2014;56:53–62.
4. Woodward M. Aspects of communication in Alzheimer's disease: clinical features and treatment options. Int Psychogeriatr. 2013;25(6):877–85.
5. Royal College of Speech & Language Therapists. Speech and language therapy provision for people with dementia; 2014.
6. Manthorpe J, Samsi K. Person-centered dementia care: current perspectives. Clin Interv Aging. 2016;11:1733.
7. Johnson-Laird PN. Mental models: towards a cognitive science of language, inference, and consciousness. Harvard University Press; 1983.
8. Van Dijk TA. Discourse and context: a socio-cognitive approach. Cambridge University Press Cambridge; 2008.
9. Feyereisen P, Berrewaerts J, Hupet M. Pragmatic skills in the early stages of Alzheimer's disease: an analysis by means of a referential communication task. Int J Lang Commun Disord. 2007;42(1):1–17.
10. Glosser G, Deser T. Patterns of discourse production among neurological patients with fluent language disorders. Brain Lang. 1991;40(1):67–88.
11. Ripich DN, Terrell BY. Patterns of discourse cohesion and coherence in Alzheimer's disease. J Speech Hear Disord. 1988;53(1):8.
12. de Lira JO, Ortiz KZ, Campanha AC, Bertolucci PHF, Minett TSC. Microlinguistic aspects of the oral narrative in patients with Alzheimer's disease. Int Psychogeriatr. 2011;23(3):404.
13. de Lira JO, Minett TSC, Bertolucci PHF, Ortiz KZ. Evaluation of macrolinguistic aspects of the oral discourse in patients with Alzheimer's disease. Int Psychogeriatr. 2019;31(9):1343–53.
14. Kim BS, Kim YB, Kim H. Discourse measures to differentiate between mild cognitive impairment and healthy aging. Front Aging Neurosci. 2019;11:221.
15. Laine M, Laakso M, Vuorinen E, Rinne J. Coherence and informativeness of discourse in two dementia types. J Neurolinguistics. 1998;11(1):79–87.
16. Ash S, Moore P, Antani S, McCawley G, Work M, Grossman M. Trying to tell a tale: discourse impairments in progressive aphasia and frontotemporal dementia. Neurology. 2006;66(9):1405–13.
17. Chapman SB, Bonte FJ, Wong SBC, Zientz JN, Hynan LS, Harris TS, et al. Convergence of con-

nected language and SPECT in variants of frontotemporal lobar degeneration. Alzheimer Dis Assoc Disord. 2005;19(4):202–13.
18. McDonald S. Pragmatic language skills after closed head injury: ability to meet the informational needs of the listener. Brain Lang. 1993;44(1):28–46.
19. McDonald S, Pearce S. Clinical insights into pragmatic theory: frontal lobe deficits and sarcasm. Brain Lang. 1996;53(1):81–104.
20. McDonald S, Pearce S. Requests that overcome listener reluctance: impairment associated with executive dysfunction in brain injury. Brain Lang. 1998;61(1):88–104.
21. Matsumoto Y. Pragmatics of understanding: centrality of the local: cases from Japanese discourse and Alzheimer's interaction. Contrast Pragmat. 2020;2(1):24–51.
22. Davis B. Alzheimer talk, text and context: enhancing communication. Springer; 2005.
23. Ramanathan V. Alzheimer discourse: some sociolinguistic dimensions. Routledge; 2013.
24. Dijkstra K, Bourgeois M, Youmans G, Hancock A. Implications of an advice-giving and teacher role on language production in adults with dementia. Gerontologist. 2006;46(3):357–66.
25. Magai C, Cohen C, Gomberg D, Malatesta C, Culver C. Emotional expression during mid-to late-stage dementia. Int Psychogeriatr. 1996;8(3):383–95.
26. Luzzi S, Piccirilli M, Provinciali L. Perception of emotions on happy/sad chimeric faces in Alzheimer disease: relationship with cognitive functions. Alzheimer Dis Assoc Disord. 2007;21(2):130–5.
27. Evans-Roberts CE, Turnbull OH. Remembering relationships: preserved emotion-based learning in Alzheimer's disease. Exp Aging Res. 2010;37(1):1–16.
28. Astell AJ, Ellis MP. The social function of imitation in severe dementia. Infant Child Dev. 2006;15(3):311–9.
29. Benson S, Kitwood TM. The new culture of dementia care. Hawker; 1995.
30. Kitwood TM. Dementia reconsidered: the person comes first. Open University Press; 1997.
31. Nespoulous J-L. De deux comportements verbaux de base: référentiel et modalisateur. De leur dissociation dans le discours aphasique. Cahiers de psychologie; 1980.
32. Ripich DN, Vertes D, Whitehouse P, Fulton S, Ekelman B. Turn-taking and speech act patterns in the discourse of senile dementia of the Alzheimer's type patients. Brain Lang. 1991;40(3):330–43.
33. Van Dijk TA, Kintsch W. Strategies of discourse comprehension. Academic Press New York; 1983.
34. Van Dijk TA, Kintsch W. A caminho de um modelo estratégico de processamento do discurso. Van Dijk, Teun A Cognição, discurso e interação São Paulo: Contexto 1992:9–35.
35. Asp E, Song X, Rockwood K. Self-referential tags in the discourse of people with Alzheimer's disease. Brain Lang. 2006;97(1):41–52.
36. Bayles KA. Communication in dementia. The aging brain: Communication in the elderly; 1985, pp. 110–34.
37. Duong A, Tardif A, Ska B. Discourse about discourse: what is it and how does it progress in Alzheimer's disease? Brain Cogn. 2003;53(2):177–80.
38. Green NL, Davis B, editors. Dialogue generation in an assistive conversation skills training system for caregivers of persons with Alzheimer's disease. American Association for Artificial Intelligence; 2003.
39. Brandão L, Parente MAMP, Peña-Casanova J. Estratégias comunicativas de pessoas com doença de Alzheimer. Psicologia: reflexão e crítica. 2010;23:308–16.
40. Davis B, Moore L, Peacock J. Frozen phrases as requests for topic management: effect and affect in recipient design by a speaker of Alzheimer's discourse. NWAV2000. Michigan State University; 2000.
41. Santo Pietro MJC, Ostuni E. Successful communication with persons with Alzheimer's disease: an inservice manual. Butterworth-Heinemann Medical; 2003.
42. James IA, Wood-Mitchell AJ, Waterworth AM, Mackenzie LE, Cunningham J. Lying to people with dementia: developing ethical guidelines for care settings. Int J Geriatr Psychiatry. 2006;21(8):800–1.
43. James I, Powell I, Smith T, Fairbairn A. Lying to residents: can the truth sometimes be unhelpful for people with dementia. Psychol Special Interest Group Older People (PSIGE) Newsletter. 2003;82:26–8.
44. Muller-Hergl C. Distress does not justify lying. J Dementia Care. 2007;15(4):10.
45. Mitchell G, Agnelli J. Person-centered care for people with dementia: Kitwood reconsidered. Nurs Stand (2014+). 2015;30(7):46.
46. Day AM, James IA, Meyer TD, Lee DR. Do people with dementia find lies and deception in dementia care acceptable? Aging Ment Health. 2011;15(7):822–9.
47. Hertogh CM, The BAM Miesen BM, Eefsting JA. Truth telling and truthfulness in the care for patients with advanced dementia: an ethnographic study in Dutch nursing homes. Soc Sci Med. 2004;59(8):1685–93.
48. Feil N. Validation therapy. Geriatr Nurs. 1992;13(3):129–33.
49. Ellis MP. Maintaining personhood and self-image in dementia: an exploration of collaborative communication. [Doctoral dissertation], University of St Andrews, 2009.
50. Khan Z, Da Silva MV, Nunez KM, Kalafatis C, Nowicki S, Walker Z, et al. Investigating the effects of impairment in non-verbal communication on neuropsychiatric symptoms and quality of life of people living with dementia. Alzheimer's Dementia. 2021;7(1):e12172.
51. Machiels M, Metzelthin SF, Hamers JP, Zwakhalen SM. Interventions to improve communication

between people with dementia and nursing staff during daily nursing care: a systematic review. Int J Nurs Stud. 2017;66:37–46.
52. Magai C, Cohen CI, Gomberg D. Impact of training dementia caregivers in sensitivity to nonverbal emotion signals. Int Psychogeriatr. 2002;14(1):25–38.
53. van der Weert JC, van Dulmen AM, Spreeuwenberg PM, Ribbe MW, Bensing JM. Effects of snoezelen, integrated in 24 h dementia care, on nurse–patient communication during morning care. Patient Educ Couns. 2005;58(3):312–26.
54. Haberstroh J, Neumeyer K, Schmitz B, Pantel J. Development and evaluation of a training program for nursing home professionals to improve communication in dementia care. Zeitschrift fur Gerontologie und Geriatrie. 2008;42(2):108–16.
55. Chen C-H. Long-term home care communication with dementia elders in Taiwan: a focus on nonverbal communication strategies; 2021.
56. Maki Y, Sakurai T, Okochi J, Yamaguchi H, Toba K. Rehabilitation to live better with dementia. Geriatr Gerontol Int. 2018;18(11):1529–36.
57. de Carvalho IAM, Bahia VS, Mansur LL. Functional communication ability in frontotemporal lobar degeneration and Alzheimer's disease. Dement Neuropsychol. 2008;2(1):31–6.
58. Frattali C, Thompson C, Holland A, Wohl C, Ferketic M. ASHA functional assessment of communication skills for adults (FACS). Rockville, MD: American Speech-Language-Hearing Association; 1995.
59. Mueller KD, Hermann B, Mecollari J, Turkstra LS. Connected speech and language in mild cognitive impairment and Alzheimer's disease: a review of picture description tasks. J Clin Exp Neuropsychol. 2018;40(9):917–39.
60. Toledo CM, Aluísio SM, Dos Santos LB, Brucki SMD, Trés ES, de Oliveira MO, et al. Analysis of macrolinguistic aspects of narratives from individuals with Alzheimer's disease, mild cognitive impairment, and no cognitive impairment. Alzheimer's Dementia. 2018;10:31–40.
61. Mok Z, Steel G, Russell C, Conway E. Measuring the interactions of people with dementia and their conversation partners: a preliminary adaption of the Kagan measures of support and participation in conversation. Aging Ment Health. 2021;25(1):13–21.
62. O'Rourke DJ, Lobchuk MM, Thompson GN, Lengyel C. Video feedback: a novel application to enhance person-centered dementia communication. Int J Nurs Pract. 2020;26(4):e12820.
63. Clare L, Hindle JV, Jones IR, Thom JM, Nelis SM, Hounsome B, et al. The AgeWell study of behavior change to promote health and wellbeing in later life: study protocol for a randomized controlled trial. Trials. 2012;13(1):1–9.
64. Hickey E, Bourgeois MS. Dementia: person-centered assessment and intervention. Routledge; 2017.
65. American Speech-Language-Hearing Association. Report of the advisory panel to ASHA's functional communication measures reports. Rockville MD: American Speech-Language-Hearing Association; 1990.
66. World Health Organization. IFC: International Classification of Functioning, Disability and Health; 2001.
67. Rogalski EJ, Saxon M, McKenna H, Wieneke C, Rademaker A, Corden ME, et al. Communication bridge: a pilot feasibility study of internet-based speech–language therapy for individuals with progressive aphasia. Alzheimer's Dementia. 2016;2(4):213–21.
68. Volkmer A, Spector A, Meitanis V, Warren JD, Beeke S. Effects of functional communication interventions for people with primary progressive aphasia and their caregivers: a systematic review. Aging Ment Health. 2020;24(9):1381–93.
69. Bourgeois MS. Effects of memory aids on the dyadic conversations of individuals with dementia. J Appl Behav Anal. 1993;26(1):77–87.
70. Brandão L, Castelló FG, van Dijk TA, Parente MAMP, Peña-Casanova J. Cognition and discourse production in Alzheimer's disease: using informative prompts. Psychol Neurosci. 2009;2(2):147–55.
71. Lanzi A, Burshnic V, Bourgeois MS. Person-centered memory and communication strategies for adults with dementia. Top Lang Disord. 2017;37(4):361–74.
72. Brandão L, Monção AM, Andersson R, Holmqvist K. Discourse intervention strategies in Alzheimer's disease: eye-tracking and the effect of visual cues in conversation. Dementia Neuropsychol. 2014;8:278–84.
73. Chapman S, Ulatowska H. The nature of language disruption in dementia: is it aphasia. Texas J Audiol Speech Pathol. 1992;17:3–9.
74. Hamilton HE. Conversations with an Alzheimer's patient : an interactional sociolinguistic study. Cambridge, UK; New York, NY: Cambridge University Press; 1994. xii, 184 p.
75. Ferguson A. Maximizing communication effectiveness. Pragmatics in speech and language pathology studies in clinical applications. Amsterdam/Philadelphia: John Benjamins; 2000. p. 53–88.
76. Wong SB, Anand R, Chapman SB, Rackley A, Zientz J. When nouns and verbs degrade: facilitating communication in semantic dementia. Aphasiology. 2009;23(2):286–301.
77. O'Rourke A, Power E, O'Halloran R, Rietdijk R. Common and distinct components of communication partner training programmes in stroke, traumatic brain injury and dementia. Int J Lang Commun Disord. 2018;53(6):1150–68.
78. Eaves L. Strategies to increase communication with dementia patients. Northern Speech Services, Inc; 2008.
79. Orange JB, Colton-Hudson A. Enhancing communication in dementia of the Alzheimer's type. Top Geriatr Rehabil. 1998;14(2):56–75.
80. Hendryx-Bedalov PM. Effects of caregiver communication on the outcomes of requests in spouses with dementia of the Alzheimer type. Int J Aging Hum Dev. 1999;49(2):127–48.
81. Small JA, Geldart K, Gutman G. Communication between individuals with dementia and their caregivers during activities of daily living. Am J Alzheimers Dis Other Dement. 2000;15(5):291–302.

82. Steeman E, Abraham IL, Godderis J. Risk profiles for institutionalization in a cohort of elderly people with dementia or depression. Arch Psychiatr Nurs. 1997;11(6):295–303.
83. Savundranayagam MY, Hummert ML, Montgomery RJ. Investigating the effects of communication problems on caregiver burden. J Gerontol Ser B Psychol Sci Soc Sci. 2005;60(1):S48–55.
84. Sabat SR. A bio-psycho-social approach to dementia. Excellence in dementia care: research into practice; 2008, pp. 70–84.
85. van der Geugten W, Goossensen A. Dignifying and undignifying aspects of care for people with dementia: a narrative review. Scand J Caring Sci. 2020;34(4):818–38.
86. Giles H, Coupland N, Coupland I. 1. Accommodation theory: communication, context, and. Contexts of accommodation: developments in applied sociolinguistics; 1991, p. 1.
87. Williams KN, Herman R, Gajewski B, Wilson K. Elderspeak communication: impact on dementia care. Am J Alzheimers Dis Other Dement. 2009;24(1):11–20.
88. Learned WWH. Conclusion: keeping the conversation going. Learning from the talk of persons with dementia: a practical guide to interaction and interactional research; 2020, p. 243.
89. Hydén L-C. Storytelling in dementia: collaboration and common ground. Living with dementia. London: Palgrave; 2017. p. 116–34.
90. Kontos PC. Embodied selfhood: an ethnographic exploration of Alzheimer's disease: thinking about dementia. Rutgers University Press; 2006. p. 195–217.
91. Lazar A, Cornejo R, Edasis C, Piper AM, editors. Designing for the third hand: empowering older adults with cognitive impairment through creating and sharing. Proceedings of the 2016 ACM Conference on Designing Interactive Systems; 2016.
92. Kontos P, Miller K-L, Mitchell GJ, Stirling-Twist J. Presence redefined: The reciprocal nature of engagement between elder-clowns and persons with dementia. Dementia. 2017;16(1):46–66.
93. Kontos P, Grigorovich A, Kosurko A, Bar RJ, Herron RV, Menec VH, et al. Dancing with dementia: exploring the embodied dimensions of creativity and social engagement. The Gerontologist. 2021;61(5):714–23.
94. Galbraith B, Larkin H, Moorhouse A, Oomen T. Intergenerational programs for persons with dementia: a scoping review. J Gerontol Soc Work. 2015;58(4):357–78.
95. Baker JR, Goodenough B, Jeon Y-H, Bryden C, Hutchinson K, Low L-F. The Kids4Dementia education program is effective in improving children's attitudes towards dementia. Dementia. 2019;18(5):1777–89.
96. Pietro MJS, Boczko F. The breakfast Club: results of a study examining the effectiveness of a multi-modality group communication treatment. Am J Alzheimers Dis. 1998;13(3):146–58.
97. Alzheimer's Disease International. Dementia friendly communities: key principles internet. Alzheimer's Disease International; 2016. https://www.alzint.org/u/dfc-principles.pdf
98. Wu SM, Huang HL, Chiu YC, Tang LY, Yang PS, Hsu JL, et al. Dementia-friendly community indicators from the perspectives of people living with dementia and dementia-family caregivers. J Adv Nurs. 2019;75(11):2878–89.
99. Hung L. Creating dementia friendly community for social inclusion: a scoping review: developing topics. Alzheimers Dement. 2020;16:e047147.
100. de Vugt M, Dröes R-M. Social health in dementia. Towards a positive dementia discourse. Taylor & Francis; 2017. p. 1–3.
101. Wiersma EC, Denton A. From social network to safety net: dementia-friendly communities in rural northern Ontario. Dementia. 2016;15(1):51–68.

Lenisa Brandão is an associate professor in Department of Speech, Language and Hearing Sciences at Federal University of Santa Maria, Brazil. Dr. Brandão is a Speech-Language Pathologist and received her PhD in Federal University of Rio Grande do Sul. Her postdoctoral research was conducted on discourse and dementia at Lund University (Sweden) and Universidade Nova de Lisboa (Portugal). She is a Life Long Atlantic Fellow for Equity in Brain Health and currently investigates art-based therapeutic approaches. The Alzheimer's Society has awarded her with the Pilot Awards for Global Brain Health Leaders for a study on the therapeutic effects of clowning.

Juliana Onofre de Lira is an Adjunt Professor of Faculty of Ceilândia of University of Brasília, Brazil. Dr. de Lira is a Speech-Language Pathologist and received her PhD from Federal University of São Paulo. Her doctorate and postdoctoral research was on discourse and dementia. She is a member of the Brazilian Society of Speech, Language and Hearing Pathology (SBFa), former vice-coordinator of the Department of Language (2020-2022) and vice-coordinator of Oral and Written Language Committee for the Adult and Elderly of this institution (2023–2025).

Maria Isabel d'Ávila Freitas is an associate professor in Department of Speech, Language and Hearing Sciences at Federal University of Santa Catarina, Brazil. Dr. Freitas is a Speech-Language Pathologist and received her PhD from University of São Paulo. Her doctorate and postdoctoral research on dementia was carried out in Behavioral and Cognitive Neurology Unit Hospital das Clinicas, University of São Paulo. She is a member of the Brazilian Society of Speech, Language and Hearing Pathology (SBFa) and former coordinator of the Oral and Written Language Committee for the Adult and Elderly of this institution (2017–2022).

24 Communication Treatment Approaches to Improve Discourse Production in Traumatic Brain Injury

Leanne Togher, Elise Elbourn, and Joanne Steel

Preview of What Is Currently Known
Historically, there has been a lack of empirical evidence around communication approaches for discourse production. Innovations in understanding core principles of rehabilitation for traumatic brain injury (TBI) have helped to address traditional intervention challenges with the TBI population such as engagement, motivation, and generalization. Furthermore, advances in the conceptualization of discourse have led to the development of treatments that target the nuanced interactional and social elements that commonly breakdown in discourse after TBI. Challenges remain for the clinician seeking direction for diverse clinical caseloads with TBI, and while the number of reported treatments has increased, these may appear heterogeneous due to the range of techniques, methods, and targets reported in discourse treatment literature [1]. However, recent theoretical advances, such as the Rehabilitation Treatment Specification System, are being used to identify key components of successful social communication treatments from published studies. This information, combined with existing international recommendations for best practice [2], can guide speech-language pathologists (SLPs) in their decision-making for discourse-level interventions after TBI.

Objectives
(a) To summarize key theoretical approaches and clinical guidelines with respect to communication treatment approaches that aim to improve discourse production in traumatic brain injury (TBI)
(b) To establish an understanding of how to use goal attainment scaling to facilitate goal setting
(c) To explain communication partner training approaches and their evidence
(d) To explain group-based social skills training programs and their evidence
(e) To describe a range of treatment approaches that will meet specific patient goals (e.g., return-to-work)
(f) To promote identification of key components of existing evidence-based treatments to apply to individual cases

Background

Discourse production occurs naturally in everyday conversations yet requires a complex integration of skills to execute effectively. A traumatic

L. Togher (✉) · E. Elbourn
Department of Speech Pathology, The University of Sydney, Sydney, Australia
e-mail: leanne.togher@sydney.edu.au; elise.elbourn@sydney.edu.au

J. Steel
School of Health Sciences (Speech Pathology), The University of Newcastle, Callaghan, Australia
e-mail: Joanne.steel@newcastle.edu.au

A. P.-H. Kong (ed.), *Spoken Discourse Impairments in the Neurogenic Populations*,
https://doi.org/10.1007/978-3-031-45190-4_24

brain injury (TBI) can impact everyday conversations when a person's underlying cognitive impairments disrupt their discourse production [3]. Features of impaired discourse production can include difficulties with initiation and maintenance of topics, providing insufficient or excessive detail [4, 5] or failing to respond to the needs of the communication partners with whom they are conversing [6]. Such difficulties can detrimentally impact on the success of interpersonal relationships, career or study aspirations, and participation in social engagements [7]. Communication treatment approaches aim to mitigate these detrimental impacts by targeting the unique difficulties that arise following TBI.

A prerequisite for treatment success is comprehensive assessment and targeted goal setting. It is important to gain multiple perspectives on communication changes after injury, including from the person with TBI, family, health professionals, and employers to determine priorities for treatment [8]. These opinions need to be integrated with measures of performance both in standard tests of neuropsychological and psychosocial functioning, but also non-standardized discourse evaluation to establish direction for treatment [9]. The clinician additionally needs to evaluate factors influencing communication performance such as communication partners, the external environment, fatigue, or personal characteristics to appropriately guide treatment decisions [8].

Theoretical Models and Principles Context-based Interventions

Treatment programs which focus on improving the discourse of people with TBI vary widely, which makes comparison difficult. It can also be problematic to identify which aspect(s) of a treatment program are contributing to changes that may be occurring because of the treatment. Frameworks which describe treatment components have been developed to address these issues, including the Rehabilitation Treatment Specification System (RTSS) [10], the Template for Intervention Description and Replication (TIDieR) [11], and the Intervention TAXonomy (ITAX) [12]. The RTSS describes treatment according to the ingredients or the actions undertaken by the clinician toward the patient and/or the speaking environment, the mechanisms of action that are proposed to be underpinning the improvement, and the targets of the intervention. For example, Meulenbroek and colleagues [13] described treatment targets and ingredients for social communication treatments in TBI, concluding that common targets comprised changed skilled behaviors in natural contexts through systematic instruction with practice, role play, peer group interactions, and education. Mechanisms of action were not well described in current treatment studies, suggesting that more work is required in this domain of enquiry [13].

Using the TIDier framework to describe treatments which aim to improve the spoken discourse of people with TBI is becoming more commonplace (e.g., [14, 15]). The TiDieR checklist assesses the reporting quality of interventions and is designed to improve reporting of results, interpretation, and scientific reproducibility [11]. The TiDieR checklist consists of 12 items: Name, Rationale, Materials, Procedure, Provider, Mode-of-Delivery, Setting, Dosage, Tailoring, Modifications, How-Well-Planned, and How-Well-Actual. This checklist has proved to be beneficial in describing treatments which aim to improve spoken discourse in people with TBI. For example, in a study of project-based intervention for people with TBI [14], the TIDieR was used to describe the features of the program (also see Section "Project-based Treatments" below). The "why" of project-based treatment comprised six essential elements, including (i) that there was a project or tangible end product, (ii) intervention was group based, (iii) that it included individualized communication-based goals, (iv) communication partners were involved which helped to maintain treatment goals, (v) acknowledgment and support were provided in relation to the participant's cognitive abilities, and (vi) considerations and planning were undertaken to address impaired awareness. The impact of this improved reporting of key features of treatment such as the "why" will guide clinicians in their delivery of patient-centered, goal-directed treatment, which is a key recommendation of the INternational panel of experts in COGnitive rehabilitation (INCOG) guidelines [2].

The ITAX is a classification system used to identify and describe the key features of interventions, comprising the delivery characteristics (such as the mode of treatment, materials, location), and the content and goals of intervention (including treatment content strategies and mechanisms of action). For example, the ITAX was used to describe communication partner training (CPT) programs for TBI, aphasia, and dementia, to reveal common features of CPT programs across diagnoses [16]. The common features of CPT included the delivery characteristics whereby all treatments were in face to face, group, or individual contexts, but there was wide variation noted in the duration of CPT programs (from 1 to 35 h). Categories of information that were common to all programs included, for example, negative behaviors to avoid and the explicit purpose of the program being stated for participants. The most common skill building techniques included the use of videos, discussions, and trainer demonstrations. Remarkably, of the 96 strategies identified to train partners, only three were common to all CPT programs, including teaching the use of short simple sentences, giving one piece of information at a time, and giving time to respond.

These three classification systems offer clinicians and researchers valuable information regarding the specific characteristics that are critical to discourse treatment success for people with TBI. This vital information, combined with models of communication and social cognition following TBI [17–19], provides guidance for which treatment is suitable for which patient, and how it should be conducted and measured.

Measuring Treatment Outcomes

Establishing the effect or outcome of a treatment is the primary determinant of treatment success. The person-centered treatments outlined in this chapter necessitate outcome measures that can capture individualized progress. Goal attainment scaling (GAS) has emerged as a leading evidence-based approach to evaluating treatment outcomes in TBI [20]. GAS uses a standard method of scoring that has been shown to demonstrate clinically important change. The individualized system involves use of a five-point scale that provides objective documentation of patient progress on personally relevant, meaningful goals. A long-term goal is established as the baseline level of achievement (0). A rating of −1 or −2 reflects below expected or well below expected level of attainment, respectively, while a +1 or +2 rating indicates above expected or well above expected achievement. The scale has also been adapted for people with TBI so that it ranges from 1 to 5, to enhance a feeling of success [21]. The goals are developed in collaboration with the patient and other stakeholders. The GAS format enables clear illustration of goal attainment in a manner that is accessible to the patient, family, funding bodies, and the multidisciplinary team. GAS scoring is also useful for measuring progress in groups, as different individualized goals can be scaled and aggregated to determine general group progress [22]. An example of GAS for the case example (Section "Case Report: Treatment of Discourse Production Following TBI") is illustrated below:

Goal attainment scaling (GAS)	Example
+2	Jason contributes 50% of spoken output in conversations in varied communication contexts.
+1	Jason contributes 50% of spoken output in 80% of conversations with Sharon at home.
0	Jason contributes 50% of spoken output in a 10-min conversation with Sharon at home.
−1	Jason contributes 70% of spoken output in a 5-min conversation with Sharon at home.
−2	Jason contributes 80% of spoken output in a 5-min structured conversation with Sharon at home.

Communication Partner Training (CPT) Interventions

Communication partner training is an evidence-based approach to addressing the environment in which a person with TBI communicates. It is based on the premise that a positive, facilitative communication partner will provide linguistic, social, emotional, and cognitive support to enable the person with TBI optimal communication opportunities. Training programs have been developed and successfully trialed, including a 10-week face-to-face program comprising individual and group therapy sessions (with a total dose of 35 hours) [23] and a 10-week program which was delivered via videoconference 90 min per week during individual sessions (total dose of 15 hours) [24]. A third program called *interact-ABI-lity* is a self-directed and freely available 2 hour online module for any person who wishes to learn how to communicate effectively with a person with acquired brain injury with aphasia, dysarthria, and/or cognitive communication disorders (https://abi-communication-lab.sydney.edu.au/courses/interact-abi-lity/).

In all programs, the emphasis is on training communication partners to learn how to ask questions that will elicit new information, opinions, and feelings, rather than test the person's knowledge or memory, to offer background information to support a person's memory and executive functioning when introducing and maintaining topics (i.e., cognitive supports) and to approach their conversation with the person with TBI with a positive, interested attitude (i.e., emotional supports). This approach to intervention has been described in two systematic reviews, with recommendations that larger clinical trials are needed [25, 26] and has been recommended as best practice in international cognitive rehabilitation guidelines [2].

Social Communication Interventions

Several group-based and individualized intervention approaches to treat social skills and social communication have been described in research literature. These have some common components, including explicitly targeting self-awareness and self-monitoring ability, usually incorporating video or audio feedback, role play, and instruction on linguistic components of successful interactions.

Group Interactive Social Skills Treatment (GIST) [27–29] is a manualized program that targets social communication ability. The program, developed by a speech-language pathologist (SLP) and social worker, is a structured cognitive-behavioral therapy targeting the cognitive, communicative, and emotional impairments that are impacting the person's social competence. The treatment, which can be co-facilitated by social work or psychology, consists of 13 group sessions: starting with a group orientation session followed by twelve 1.5-h weekly modules and set homework tasks. Content includes conversation management, learning to recognize different communicative styles (aggressive, passive, and assertive), understanding boundaries, conflict resolution, and workplace-based communication and incorporates video self-review. Outcome measures used with GIST include the La Trobe Communication Questionnaire (LCQ) (self-report) [30], and the Profile of Pragmatic Impairment in Communication [31], the GAS and other measures including the Satisfaction with Life Scale (SWLS) [32], and the Craig Handicap Assessment and Reporting Technique Short Form (Social Integration and Occupation subscales) [33]. GIST has a focus on increasing the person's self-awareness of communication and includes training in metalinguistic/metacognitive strategies, patient-centered goal setting, and training in non-verbal behavior within a hierarchical training structure. GIST incorporates a contextualized approach with the opportunities for functional practice of learned skills in the group setting. There have been two randomized controlled trials using this program [28, 29], with good maintenance of gains in social skills reported at follow-up.

From a different perspective, the Communication-specific Coping Intervention (CommCope-I) is a treatment program that teaches the person with TBI and their communication partner to identify communication breakdowns and train communication-specific coping strategies for functional use [34, 35]. Rather than focusing on the impairment, this treatment targets the development of productive strategies the person with TBI may already be using in their interactions. CommCope-I is a hierarchical program, comprising 12 hours of intervention (2 sessions/week over 6 weeks with 6 individual sessions and 6 with communication partner(s) in the community). The program works through increasing self-awareness, in this case, by improving insight into behaviors that are leading to unsuccessful interactions. The three key components include: *facilitating self-awareness*, *developing skill* (in personally relevant coping strategies), and *evaluating performance*. Development of personally relevant coping strategies might incorporate creation of scripts, use of personally relevant imagery, role play, rehearsal, and video feedback for self-evaluation. To date, the CommCope-I has been reported in two single-case experimental design studies (A–B–A design with follow-up) [34, 35]. Gains in social communication were made for some of the participants, including reduction in psychological distress; and these gains were mostly maintained longer term. Communication-based outcome measures reported with this approach included the LCQ and The Discourse Coping Scale – Clinician Rating (DCS–CR), and The Communication-specific Coping Scale – research version (CommSpeCS), both of which were developed by the authors of CommCope-I to measure the target coping strategies.

Improving Natural Social Interaction: Group reHabilitation after Traumatic Brain Injury (INSIGHT) is another manualized group-based program that can be delivered face-to-face or online [21]. INSIGHT provides an authentic contextualized and natural context to support individualized social communication goals [21]. Patients engage in 2-hour sessions over 8 weeks which incorporate treatment ingredients of environment modification, strategies, guidance, practice, instruction, role play, feedback, modeling, education, cueing, and prompting [21]. Significant improvements in GAS scores were observed when the program was delivered virtually with a group of six participants with mild-severe TBI [21]. Interestingly, this program was delivered effectively by student clinicians [21].

Another treatment approach using Metacognitive Strategy Training (MST) to target discourse-level communication is IMPACT (Intervention for Metacognition and Social Participation: an Acquired Cognitive-communication Disorder Treatment) [36–38]. This is a manualized program, developed by SLPs and occupational therapists. IMPACT is a goal-directed therapy that targets metacognitive skills ("thinking about thinking") during meaningful activities for the person with TBI. Similar to the CommCope-I program, IMPACT targets increasing awareness of the person's performance through an individualized goal setting process using the GAS, contextualized delivery, and MST. The theory underpinning IMPACT is that metacognitive strategies (i.e., learning skills to reflect on and evaluate one's own cognitive performance) can be explicitly taught, resulting in the person having increased control over unwanted communication behaviors. IMPACT is a 6-week intervention program, with individual sessions twice weekly and one group session per week, with homework tasks also assigned. The person with TBI learns to identify and use compensatory strategies to address areas of cognitive difficulty. Specific targets reported in studies using IMPACT include receptive and pragmatic skills [36, 38] and self-awareness more specifically [37]. IMPACT has been successfully implemented with adults with TBI to target executive function, receptive language ability, and self-awareness. The program has been reported in cohort studies with adults with moderate and severe TBI. Outcome measures reported in use with the IMPACT program include the GAS [39], Self-Awareness of Deficits Interview (SADI) [40], and the LCQ [30].

Cognitive pragmatic treatment [41–43] is a group-based, manualized social communication/pragmatics program based on cognitive behavior therapy, targeting linguistic and non-linguistic social abilities, pragmatics, social appropriateness, theory of mind, and narratives among other areas. The treatment was developed by psychologists and has been reported in published studies as being delivered by psychologists, although authors state the program could be delivered by SLPs if trained. Cognitive pragmatic treatment is a 12-week program of 24 1-hour sessions, conducted in small groups of five to six participants. The sessions target various aspects of interaction, with one session focused on narrative discourse production specifically. As with other group treatment programs, the intervention begins by working on improving awareness of both the individual's communication difficulties and of aspects of successful interactions generally. However, the treatment has a focus on metalinguistic awareness rather than MST. Cognitive pragmatic treatment has been reported in four cohort studies, including people with severe [41, 42, 44] or moderate to severe TBI [43]. These studies found that cognitive pragmatic treatment improved some aspects of social communication (mainly pragmatics) and narrative discourse, with maintenance of these gains 3 months post-treatment. Cognitive pragmatic treatment has also been reported in use with people with other clinical diagnoses, such as adolescents with autism spectrum disorder [45] and adults with schizophrenia [46].

Narrative-Based Interventions

A few studies have reported on interventions aimed at improving monologic discourse after TBI, including story grammar [47] and, more broadly, narratives [48, 49]. Although these studies, with small sample sizes of one or two participants, have reported gains on some measures for treated narratives following intervention, there has been mixed results for effect generalization and/or maintenance. Not all have consistently incorporated contextualized, personally relevant materials in therapy, which is now recommended practice [2]. Key therapy components for improving narratives include MST and metalinguistics (i.e., training in the structure and elements of narrative), within a structured and hierarchical approach. One such treatment reported in the literature is NARNIA (Novel Approach to Real-life communication: Narrative Intervention in Aphasia). This is a 6-week manualized program, delivered individually face-to-face in 25 sessions of 45–60 min. NARNIA is a hierarchical, scaffolded treatment using visual cues, direct instruction, and errorless learning in individual sessions with the person with TBI. The protocol is based on traditional learning theory using a metacognitive and metalinguistic approach. While targeting narratives, the program includes other genres, including recounts, procedures, and expositions. Spoken discourse tasks are supported by videos, picture sequences, or picture scenes depending on the genre targeted. The NARNIA program has been reported with some success in studies treating adults with different acquired communication diagnoses, including in a single-case study of a patient with mild TBI [49], as well as post-stroke aphasia and primary progressive aphasia [50].

Discourse Processing Treatment (DPT) [48] is another therapy aimed at improving the person's spoken narratives with both metacognitive and metalinguistic strategies. This is a non-manualized treatment comprising 16 individual 1-hour treatment sessions with four sessions/week. Narrative stimuli include sequential wordless cartoons, with therapy resources including comprehension questions and a six-category story guide like those used in story grammar analysis (see [51]). The treatment includes structured comprehension cues, audio recording, self-evaluation, prompting, and scaffolding, with cues gradually being withdrawn. DPT is based on theory that knowledge of discourse schemas is an essential prerequisite to understanding and producing a narrative. In other words, one must be able to understand the story topic and identify salient information to retell a logical version of that story to others. Therefore, DPT teaches the client the typical structure of stories and provides hierarchically based strategies for improving production skills. DPT has been reported in two single-case design studies [52] with participants making small to moderate increase on completeness and informativeness measures of narrative discourse, which were maintained at follow-up 1 month after completion of therapy.

Cannizzaro and Coelho targeted production of story grammar elements in a case study with a person with severe TBI [47] through two treatment conditions: a story retelling condition that required the participant to retell a story from film strips and a story generation condition where the participant was presented with pictures and was required to generate a story. The treatment comprised 20 1-hour sessions (3×/week, over 6 weeks). In the narrative retell condition, the participant was guided through a series of five training steps to facilitate story episode identification, with the gradual fading of prompts. The intervention for the story generation component also involved a guided stepped training process, working toward generating multiple complete episodes for the narrative. Evidence for story grammar is currently based on one single-case study, where therapy gains were not maintained at follow-up. It is suggested that in future studies, the inclusion of contextualized, personally relevant training materials and functional practice should be considered to promote maintenance and generalization of skills gained in therapy.

Other Interventions

Social Cognition Treatments

Reading a smile is a manualized program that targets emotion perception [53], which is a critical skill required to effectively engage in interactive discourse. The program is delivered face-to-face in individual sessions with a health professional, and dosage is 25 hours across 8 weeks [53]. *Reading a smile* draws upon established principles of remediation and follows a hierarchical structure, beginning with interpretation of emotion in conventional social contexts and working toward making social inferences using situational cues. The program employs techniques such as errorless learning, self-instruction training, rehearsal, positive reinforcement, feedback, and cumulative review [53]. *Reading a smile* was evaluated in a randomized control trial, including 12 participants with severe, chronic TBI and was found to facilitate improvements in judging emotions in naturalistic formats and making social inferences [53].

SIFT IT is another social cognition treatment program that is structured around Sensing social cues, Interpreting filters, considering Feelings, interpreting Thoughts and Intentions and Trying the response (*SIFT IT*). SIFT IT is a 14-week group-based treatment with 90-minute sessions administered by a health professional [54]. *SIFT IT* targets processes such as emotion perception, and detecting hints and sarcasm, which are important for participation in interactive discourse. Participants work toward personally relevant and meaningful goals and complete five modules covering perception of social cognitive cues, interpretation of perceived social cues, and translation into socially adaptive behavior [54]. In a small group evaluation where the program was delivered face-to-face with two participants with severe TBI, *SIFT IT* was identified as acceptable and gains were reported with generalization and self-awareness of social cognition [54]. Future research with a randomized control trial is required to establish stronger efficacy for this promising intervention [54].

Project-based Treatments

Project-based treatment refers to a communication-focused intervention whereby participants work collaboratively in a group on a project with a tangible and meaningful end product [55]. Participants work toward individualized communication goals while engaging in the project. The manualized program is administered by a SLP and is delivered as a 20-hour program over 6 weeks [55]. Elements of the program include the discussion of facilitative conversational strategies, self-reflection on goals, compensatory memory supports, simplified goal planning framework, visual scaffolds, and implementation of project roles [55]. Initial efficacy with a face-to-face program was evaluated with 21 individuals with chronic acquired brain injury (ABI) and was identified as feasible, with high acceptability and noted improvements identified with GAS

[55] and quality of life. Recent adaption was explored in a telehealth context across the UK and USA concluding that project-based interventions showed potential for improving communication and engagement in meaningful social activities [56].

Another form of project-based treatment is advocacy-based project treatment where participants work collaboratively in a small group with the aim of developing an educational presentation for health professionals [57]. Drawing upon their experiences of brain injury, participants are encouraged to generate narratives that focus on successes following their injury. The treatment targets cognitive-communication impairments and identity formation [57]. Advocacy-based treatment is conducted online over 10 sessions of 1.5 hours duration delivered by a SLP [57]. Preliminary qualitative evidence from a study of 10 individuals with chronic ABI indicates potential to improve perceived clarity and conciseness in spoken discourse as well as positive influences on sense of self [57]. Further research is required to establish stronger efficacy for this intervention.

Vocational Treatments

The Work Related Communication Training (WoRC) program is a vocational program that uses computer-based social skills training to enhance spoken discourse in the workplace [58]. WoRC is based on sociolinguistic theory and speech act performance. The simulated work program is conducted face-to-face and includes 4 modules of 1.5-hours duration [58]. WoRC embeds role play, didactic training, and immediate feedback strategies. The training targets politeness markers or "words that work" that are essential to cooperative interactions in workplace settings. WoRC was evaluated in an initial trial with eight adults with chronic TBI and identified social communication impairment [58]. The program was effective in increasing use of politeness markers and improving perceived social communication skills [58]. WoRC also has an identified cost-benefit, with a 50.2% reduction in treatment costs and is usable and acceptable by participants [58]. Further research on larger samples is required.

Case Report: Treatment of Discourse Production Following TBI

Case History and Diagnostic Information

Jason is a 36-year-old male who sustained a severe TBI as the result of a workplace accident where he fell from a building during his work as a carpenter. On admission to hospital, Jason had a Glasgow Coma Scale score of 5, and his period of post-traumatic amnesia extended for 28 days, indicating an extremely severe traumatic brain injury. MRI investigations revealed generalized edema, with a right temporal subdural hematoma and right frontotemporal extradural hematoma and cerebral contusions. He had an extraventricular drain and intracranial pressure monitor inserted. At the time of his accident, Jason was married with three children and operated his own building business. Jason's wife, Sharon, his friends, and workmates were actively involved in his rehabilitation.

Jason was diagnosed with a moderate to severe cognitive-communication disorder. This was based on observations of communication during videotaped conversations with his wife, Sharon, as well as other non-standardized and standardized assessment measures. Jason's communication was characterized by word finding difficulties, rapid changes of topic, difficulty thinking of what to say, flat affect, difficulty responding to the emotions of others with an apparent failure in understanding if his conversational partner was sad or distressed, difficulty following group conversations, reduced frustration tolerance (with a tendency to lose his temper when fatigued), and his conversations were often difficult to follow due to disorganized topic development. He was also noted to be egocentric in his topic choices (i.e., talking about himself) and he rarely asked questions.

During the observed conversation, it was noted that Jason was slow to introduce topics, asked very few questions of Sharon, and failed to develop and continue topics that Sharon started. Sharon was observed to ask Jason testing questions (e.g., "Can you remember where we went last weekend?") and corrected him when he made word finding errors. She did the majority of the talking during the conversation and did not appear to give Jason time to formulate his contributions. Jason was administered the La Trobe Communication Questionnaire (LCQ) (self-report form), and Sharon completed the LCQ other form. This test comprises 30 questions which are based on Grice's conversational maxims [59] as well as communication behaviors known to be problematic following TBI. Questions (such as "When you talk to others do you have difficulty following group conversations?") are scored using a 4-point scale ranging from 1 (never) to 4 (always). Total scores on the LCQ range from 30 to 120, where 30 indicates there are no perceived communication difficulties and 120 indicates frequent communication problems. Jason scored 90 on the LCQ and his wife's score was 80, which indicates they both perceived that his communication had changed because of his injury. For example, they both reported that he often went over and over the same ground in conversations, often switched to a different topic of conversation too quickly, sometimes needed a long time to think before answering the other person and often had difficulty thinking of things to keep the conversation going. This assessment reflected the descriptions Jason and Sharon gave during the case history regarding his difficulties conversing with family, friends, and workmates. Two standardized tests were administered including The Awareness of Social Inferencing Test (TASIT) [60] and the Functional Assessment of Verbal Reasoning and Executive Strategies (FAVRES) [61]. Jason had severe difficulties with social cognition including the ability to comprehend negative emotions or differentiate lies from sarcasm with a score in the lowest fifth percentile on the TASIT. On the FAVRES, his results indicated poor verbal reasoning and executive strategies with extremely slow completion of tasks (less than the first percentile).

Clinical Management Plan

A combination of conversational treatment, communication partner training, and communication related to return-to-work approaches were employed with Jason, Sharon, and his family. Refer to Table 24.1 for suggested treatment programs and goals to address Jason's cognitive-communication disorder.

Table 24.1 Treatments for discourse following TBI

Treatment goal	Method
1. ***Improve interactional discourse skills*** • Improve initiation and maintenance of conversational topics • Improve question asking skills • Work with Jason to determine how he would like to be perceived by others in conversational interactions (e.g., respected, businessman, mate, appear calm and collected)	• Use Goal Attainment Scaling (GAS) to develop conversational goals for Jason which are focused on meaningful, personally relevant situations • Use video feedback, rating scales of conversational performance to improve self-monitoring and self-regulation, e.g., **WSTC**: **W**hat am I doing? What's the best **S**trategy? **T**ry it. **C**heck it out? • Develop a range of topics that Jason is interested in and provide him with structure • Work with Jason to develop a range of question asking strategies and using active listening techniques (such as formulating a question based on what his communication partner has just said) • Explore how Jason can use his language skills to present the image of himself he is aiming for, using Ylvisaker's metaphor/self-identity training [65] and Ownsworth's self-identity training (in collaboration with a psychologist) [66]

(continued)

Table 24.1 (continued)

Treatment goal	Method
2. ***Communication partner training—*** *Maximizing communicative success across a range of communication environments* • Introduce Jason and Sharon to a communication partner training group where they both attend together with the goal of improving their conversations	• Sharon's goals are as follows: – To approach her interactions with Jason in a positive and supportive way – To avoid correcting Jason in a punitive manner – To avoid pointing out his word finding difficulties – To use a balance of questions and comments – To help support the organization of Jason's conversation by using cognitive and communication supports – To give him time to formulate his answers and to provide information rather than using testing questions • Jason's goals are as follows: – To start conversations with Sharon and keep them going – To have a more equal share in the conversation – To share information about what he is thinking and feeling – To minimize the effects of his word finding problems by describing the target word. • Work with both Jason and Sharon to determine which speaking situations are important to them and practice their conversational strategies in those conversations
3. ***Facilitate cognitive-communication skills to enable return-to-work and social activities*** • Enhancing opportunities for participation across social and vocational contexts • Improve Jason's ability to recount stories in a coherent manner • Providing information to family/friends/work colleagues about the nature of Jason's communicative disability and strategies they can use to enhance his communication	• Provide education and training to Jason's family, friends, and workmates which provide a description of why he is having difficulty with his communication; strategies they can use to help him have positive interactions, such as introducing topics which are of interest to him • Practice working on Jason's narrative skills, by helping him recount his brain injury story in a coherent, organized way, by targeting story grammar elements to ensure that his story is complete and logically structured • Arrange for social activities in quiet environments and limit the number of people attending social events initially to assist with his slowed information processing and difficulty communicating in complex environments • Structure return-to-work activities in a way that Jason's workday is scheduled to allow for breaks, use cognitive supports, such as the notes and calendar functions on his smart phone to remind him of appointments through the day • Practice scripted conversations, such as typical conversations at the start of the day, and conversations that would occur over lunch breaks to give Jason practice formulating some everyday conversational routines and questions (e.g., so how are things going with you? How was your weekend?)

Future Directions for Discourse Intervention

Innovative discourse interventions and refinements to existing programs are continuing to be developed. Notably, advances in digital health may offer new directions for treatment with recent scoping identifying the need for treatment in virtual reality [62], self-directed communication partner training [63], and social media safety [64].

With reference to the intervention approaches summarized and discussed in this chapter, there is a current need for discourse treatments with a focus on the following areas:

(i) Treatments designed for people with mild TBI in addition to existing studies with a return-to-work focus.
(ii) Treatment for monologic discourse, in addition to conversation therapy/communication partner training.
(iii) Clearer indicators on ideal therapy dosage across all domains of discourse intervention.
(iv) Indicators for timing for commencing discourse therapy, particularly in the early stages after injury. Typically, this is when the person with TBI has most access to services, however, most studies report on participants at least 6 months post-TBI.

Major Takeaways

1. Goal attainment scaling (GAS) offers an individualized approach to measuring goal achievement for discourse production goals.
2. Interventions targeting emotion perception and social cognition may support engagement in interactional discourse.
3. Project-based interventions may support achievement of discourse goals and improvements in quality of life within meaningful social activities.
4. Success of return-to-work may be facilitated by the WoRC vocational treatment that targets discourse production in workplace interactions.
5. Social communication group treatments may be effective in improving interactive skills, providing a functional setting for practice of social communication skills.
6. Narrative discourse treatments should incorporate metalinguistics and metacognitive training, and use a structured, hierarchical approach.
7. Key therapy ingredients for spoken discourse treatment include structured skills training in contextualized, real-life settings, feedback provision, targeting of self-awareness through video or role play, and a goal-directed approach.

References

1. Steel J, Elbourn E, Togher L. Narrative discourse intervention after traumatic brain injury: a systematic review of the literature. Top Lang Disord. 2021;41(1):47–72.
2. Togher L, Douglas J, Turkstra LS, Welch-West P, Janzen S, Harnett A, et al. INCOG 2.0 guidelines for cognitive rehabilitation following traumatic brain injury, part IV: cognitive-communication and social cognition disorders. J Head Trauma Rehabil. 2023;38(1):65–82.
3. Coelho C, Grela B, Corso M, Gamble A, Feinn R. Microlinguistic deficits in the narrative discourse of adults with traumatic brain injury. Brain Inj. 2005;19(13):1139–45.
4. Barnes S, Bransby-Bell J, Gallagher-Beverley Z, Mullay J, McNeil R, Taylor C. Verbosity, traumatic brain injury, and conversation: a preliminary investigation. Aphasiology. 2021:1–24.
5. Power E, Weir S, Richardson J, Fromm D, Forbes M, MacWhinney B, et al. Patterns of narrative discourse in early recovery following severe traumatic brain injury. Brain Inj. 2020;34(1):98–109.
6. Chia AA, Power E, Kenny B, Elbourn E, McDonald S, Tate R, et al. Patterns of early conversational recovery for people with traumatic brain injury and their communication partners. Brain Inj. 2019;33(5):690–8.
7. Elbourn E, Kenny B, Power E, Togher L. Psychosocial outcomes of severe traumatic bain injury in relation to discourse recovery: a longitudinal study up to 1 year post-injury. Am J Speech Lang Pathol. 2019;28(4):1463–78.
8. Togher L, Wiseman-Hakes C, Douglas J, Stergiou-Kita M, Ponsford J, Teasell R, et al. INCOG recommendations for management of cognition following traumatic brain injury, part IV: cognitive communication. J Head Trauma Rehabil. 2014;29(4):353–68.
9. Sohlberg MM, MacDonald S, Byom L, Iwashita H, Lemoncello R, Meulenbroek P, et al. Social communication following traumatic brain injury part I: state-of-the-art review of assessment tools. Int J Speech Lang Pathol. 2019;21(2):115–27.
10. Hart T, Tsaousides T, Zanca JM, Whyte J, Packel A, Ferraro M, et al. Toward a theory-driven classification of rehabilitation treatments. Arch Phys Med Rehabil. 2014;95(1 Suppl):S33–44.e2.
11. Hoffmann TC, Glasziou PP, Boutron I, Milne R, Perera R, Moher D, et al. Better reporting of interventions: template for intervention description and replication (TIDieR) checklist and guide. BMJ. 2014;348:g1687.

12. Schulz R, Czaja SJ, McKay JR, Ory MG, Belle SH. Intervention taxonomy (ITAX): describing essential features of interventions. Am J Health Behav. 2010;34(6):811–21.
13. Meulenbroek P, Ness B, Lemoncello R, Byom L, MacDonald S, O'Neil-Pirozzi TM, et al. Social communication following traumatic brain injury part 2: identifying effective treatment ingredients. Int J Speech Lang Pathol. 2019;21(2):128–42.
14. Behn N, Marshall J, Togher L, Cruice M. Reporting on novel complex intervention development for adults with social communication impairments after acquired brain injury. Disabil Rehabil. 2021;43(6):805–14.
15. Howell S, Beeke S, Pring T, Varley R. Measuring outcomes of a peer-led social communication skills intervention for adults with acquired brain injury: a pilot investigation. Neuropsychol Rehabil. 2021;31(7):1069–90.
16. O'Rourke A, Power E, O'Halloran R, Rietdijk R. Common and distinct components of communication partner training programmes in stroke, traumatic brain injury and dementia. Int J Lang Commun Disord. 2018;53(6):1150–68.
17. Cassel A, McDonald S, Kelly M, Togher L. Learning from the minds of others: a review of social cognition treatments and their relevance to traumatic brain injury. Neuropsychol Rehabil. 2019;29(1):22–55.
18. Keegan LC, Hoepner JK, Togher L, Kennedy M. Clinically applicable sociolinguistic assessment for cognitive-communication disorders. Am J Speech Lang Pathol. 2022:1–11.
19. MacDonald S. Introducing the model of cognitive-communication competence: a model to guide evidence-based communication interventions after brain injury. Brain Inj. 2017;31(13–14):1760–80.
20. Behn N, Marshall J, Togher L, Cruice M. Setting and achieving individualized social communication goals for people with acquired brain injury (ABI) within a group treatment. Int J Lang Commun Disord. 2019;54(5):828–40.
21. Keegan LC, Reilley K, Stover M, Togher L. Virtual INSIGHT: improving natural social interaction: group reHabilitation after traumatic brain injury. Int J Lang Commun Disord. 2022;1–11.
22. Turner-Stokes L, Williams H, Johnson J. Goal attainment scaling: does it provide added value as a person-centred measure for evaluation of outcome in neurorehabilitation following acquired brain injury? J Rehabil Med. 2009;41(7):528–35.
23. Togher L, McDonald S, Tate R, Power E, Rietdijk R. Training communication partners of people with severe traumatic brain injury improves everyday conversations: a multicenter single blind clinical trial. J Rehabil Med. 2013;45:637–45.
24. Rietdijk R, Power E, Attard M, Heard R, Togher L. Improved conversation outcomes after social communication skills training for people with traumatic brain injury and their communication partners: a clinical trial investigating in-person and telehealth delivery. J Speech Lang Hear Res (Online). 2020;63(2):615–32.
25. Behn N, Francis J, Togher L, Hatch E, Moss B, Hilari K. Description and effectiveness of communication partner training in TBI: a systematic review. J Head Trauma Rehabil. 2021;36:56.
26. Wiseman-Hakes C, Ryu H, Lightfoot D, Kukreja G, Colantonio A, Matheson FI. Examining the efficacy of communication partner training for improving communication interactions and outcomes for individuals with traumatic brain injury: a systematic review. Arch Rehabil Res Clin Transl. 2020;2(1):100036.
27. Braden C, Hawley L, Newman J, Morey C, Gerber D, Harrison-Felix C. Social communication skills group treatment: a feasibility study for persons with traumatic brain injury and comorbid conditions. Brain Inj. 2010;24(11):1298–310.
28. Harrison-Felix C, Newman JK, Hawley L, Morey C, Ketchum JM, Walker WC, et al. Social competence treatment after traumatic brain injury: a multicenter, randomized controlled trial of interactive group treatment versus noninteractive treatment. Arch Phys Med Rehabil. 2018;99(11):2131–42.
29. Dahlberg CA, Cusick CP, Hawley LA, Newman JK, Morey CE, Harrison-Felix CL, et al. Treatment efficacy of social communication skills training after traumatic brain injury: a randomized treatment and deferred treatment controlled trial. Arch Phys Med Rehabil. 2007;88(12):1561–73.
30. Douglas JM, O'Flaherty CA, Snow PC. Measuring perception of communicative ability: the development and evaluation of the La Trobe Communication Questionnaire. Aphasiology. 2000;14(3):251–68.
31. Linscott RJ, Knight RG, Godfrey HP. The profile of functional impairment in communication (PFIC): a measure of communication impairment for clinical use. Brain Inj. 1996;10(6):397–412.
32. Diener E, Emmons RA, Larsen RJ, Griffin S. The satisfaction with life scale. J Pers Assess. 1985;49(1):71–5.
33. Whiteneck GG, Charlifue SW, Gerhart KA, Overholser JD, Richardson GN. Quantifying handicap: a new measure of long-term rehabilitation outcomes. Arch Phys Med Rehabil. 1992;73:519–26.
34. Douglas JM, Knox L, De Maio C, Bridge H. Improving communication-specific coping after traumatic brain injury: evaluation of a new treatment using single-case experimental design. Brain Impairment. 2014;15(3):190–201.
35. Douglas JM, Knox L, De Maio C, Bridge H, Drummond M, Whiteoak J. Effectiveness of communication-specific coping intervention for adults with traumatic brain injury: preliminary results. Neuropsychol Rehabil. 2019;29(1):73–91.
36. Copley A, Smith K, Savill K, Finch E. Does metacognitive strategy instruction improve impaired receptive cognitive-communication skills following acquired brain injury? Brain Inj. 2015;29(11):1309–16.
37. Copley A, Smith C, Finch E, Fleming J, Cornwell P. Does metacognitive strategy instruction improve

impaired self-awareness in adults with cognitive-communication disorders following an acquired brain injury? Speech Lang Hear. 2022;25(2):125–37.
38. Finch E, Cornwell P, Copley A, Doig E, Fleming J. Remediation of social communication impairments following traumatic brain injury using metacognitive strategy intervention: a pilot study. Brain Inj. 2017;31(13–14):1830–9.
39. Kiresuk T, Sherman R. Goal attainment scaling: a general method for evaluating comprehensive community mental health programs. Community Ment Health J. 1968;4:443–53.
40. Fleming JM, Strong J, Ashton R. Self-awareness of deficits in adults with traumatic brain injury: how best to measure? Brain Inj. 1996;10(1):1–15.
41. Bosco FM, Parola A, Angeleri R, Galetto V, Zettin M, Gabbatore I. Improvement of communication skills after traumatic brain injury: the efficacy of the cognitive pragmatic treatment program using the communicative activities of daily living. Arch Clin Neuropsychol. 2018;33(7):875–88.
42. Gabbatore I, Sacco K, Angeleri R, Zettin M, Bara BG, Bosco FM. Cognitive pragmatic treatment: a rehabilitative program for traumatic brain injury individuals. J Head Trauma Rehabil. 2015;30(5):E14–28.
43. Parola A, Bosco FM, Gabbatore I, Galetto V, Zettin M, Marini A. The impact of the cognitive pragmatic treatment on the pragmatic and informative skills of individuals with traumatic brain injury (TBI). J Neurolinguistics. 2019;51:53–62.
44. Sacco K, Gabbatore I, Geda E, Duca S, Cauda F, Bara BG, et al. Rehabilitation of communicative abilities in patients with a history of TBI: behavioral improvements and cerebral changes in resting-state activity. Front Behav Neurosci. 2016;10
45. Gabbatore I, Longobardi C, Bosco FM. Improvement of communicative-pragmatic ability in adolescents with autism spectrum disorder: the adapted version of the cognitive pragmatic treatment. Lang Learn Dev. 2022;18(1):62–80.
46. Bosco FM, Gabbatore I, Gastaldo L, Sacco K. Communicative-pragmatic treatment in schizophrenia: a pilot study. Front Psychol. 2016;7:7.
47. Cannizzaro MS, Coelho CA. Treatment of story grammar following traumatic brain injury: a pilot study. Brain Inj. 2002;16(12):1065–73.
48. Kintz S, Hibbs V, Henderson A, Andrews M, Wright HH. Discourse-based treatment in mild traumatic brain injury. J Commun Disord. 2018;76:47–59.
49. Whitworth A, Ng N, Timms L, Power E. Exploring the viability of NARNIA with cognitive-communication difficulties: a pilot study. Semin Speech Lang. 2020;41(1):83–98.
50. Whitworth A, Cartwright J, Beales A, Leitão S, Panegyres PK, Kane R. Taking words to a new level: a preliminary investigation of discourse intervention in primary progressive aphasia. Aphasiology. 2018;32(11):1284–309.
51. Stein NL, Glenn CG. An analysis of story comprehension in elementary school children. In: Freedle RO, editor. New directions in discourse processing: Ablex.; 1979.
52. Henderson A, Roeschlein MA, Wright HH. Improving discourse following traumatic brain injury: a tale of two treatments. Semin Speech Lang. 2020;41(5):365–82.
53. Bornhofen C, McDonald S. Treating deficits in emotion perception following traumatic brain injury. Neuropsychol Rehabil. 2008;18(1):22–44.
54. Cassel A, McDonald S, Kelly M. Establishing 'proof of concept' for a social cognition group treatment program (SIFT IT) after traumatic brain injury: two case studies. Brain Inj. 2020;34(13–14):1781–93.
55. Behn N, Marshall J, Togher L, Cruice M. Feasibility and initial efficacy of project-based treatment for people with ABI. Int J Lang Commun Disord. 2019;54(3):465–78.
56. Behn N, Hoepner J, Meulenbroek P, Capo M, Hart J. Core components of project-based intervention after acquired brain injury: delivering meaningful groups online. Int J Lang Commun Disord. 2022;
57. Hoepner JK, Keegan LC. "I avoid interactions with medical professionals as much as possible now": health care experiences of individuals with traumatic brain injuries. Am J Speech Lang Pathol. 2022;32:848.
58. Meulenbroek P, Cherney LR. Computer-based workplace communication training in persons with traumatic brain injury: the work-related communication program. J Commun Disord. 2021;91:106104.
59. Grice HP. Logic and conversation. In: Cole P, Morgan JL, editors. Syntax and semantics, Vol 3, speech acts. New York: Academic Press; 1975. p. 41–58.
60. McDonald S, Flanagan S, Rollins J. The awareness of social inference test. Thames Valley Test Company: Harcourt Assessment/Psychological Corporation; 2002.
61. MacDonald S. Functional assessment of verbal reasoning and executive strategies. Guelph: Clinical Publishing; 1998.
62. Brassel S, Power E, Campbell A, Brunner M, Togher L. Recommendations for the design and implementation of virtual reality for acquired brain injury rehabilitation: systematic review. J Med Internet Res. 2021;23(7):e26344.
63. Avramovic P, Rietdijk R, Attard M, Kenny B, Power E, Togher L. Cognitive and behavioral digital health interventions for people with traumatic brain injury and their caregivers: a systematic review. J Neurotrauma. 2022;40:159.
64. Brunner M, Rietdijk R, Avramovic P, Power E, Miao M, Rushworth N, et al. Developing social-ABI-lity: an online course to support safe use of social media for connection after acquired brain injury. Am J Speech Lang Pathol. 2022:924.
65. Ylvisaker M, McPherson K, Kayes N, Pellett E. Metaphoric identity mapping: facilitating goal setting and engagement in rehabilitation after traumatic brain injury. Neuropsychol Rehabil. 2008;18(5–6):713–41.
66. Ownsworth T. Self-identity after brain injury. 1st ed. Psychology Press, Routledge; 2014.

Additional Resources

Online Resources

Goal Attainment Scaling: Free Online Resources Available from the Kings College London Website to Support GAS; n.d. https://www.kcl.ac.uk/cicelysaunders/resources#GAS

Interact-ABI-lity: Free Online Self-guided Communication Partner Training Program for ABI (Available from the ABI Communication Lab); n.d. https://abi-communication-lab.sydney.edu.au/courses/interact-abi-lity/

Social-ABI-lity: Free Online Program to support Social Media Skills and Safety After ABI (Available from the ABI Communication lab); n.d. https://abi-communication-lab.sydney.edu.au/courses/social-abi-lity/

Leanne Togher is a full Professor at The University of Sydney, Sydney, Australia. A certified speech pathologist, Leanne is internationally recognized as a leader in the field of communication disorders following acquired brain injury (ABI). As the Director of the Acquired Brain Injury Communication Lab, Leanne leads a program of clinical research which incorporates multidisciplinary sources, including neurological rehabilitation and digital health perspectives, to develop cutting edge treatment programs for people with ABI and their families. To date, Leanne has led the publication of evidence-based treatments including *TBI Express*, *TBI ConneCT,* and *interact-ABI-lity and convers-ABI-lity* which form part of the recently launched *Social Brain Toolkit*. Leanne is also the Director of speechBITE team which is based at The University of Sydney, and she leads the TBI Bank initiative with colleagues at Carnegie Mellon University.

Elise Elbourn is a senior lecturer of acquired brain injury at The University of Sydney. Elise is a certified speech pathologist with clinical interests in supporting individuals with acquired brain injury, in both private and public sectors. Elise's research aims to improve communication support for people affected by acquired brain injury by establishing an understanding of factors influencing recovery and prognosis. Elise's research focuses on discourse-level communication disorders and promoting evidence-based practice. Elise engages regularly with clinical interest groups and regularly presents her research in national and international forums.

Joanne Steel is a lecturer in acquired communication disorders at the University of Newcastle, NSW and a certified practicing speech pathologist. Joanne has a clinical and research interest in improving outcomes for adults with acquired neurogenic communication disability, particularly after traumatic brain injury. Her research focus has been on cognitive and social communication assessment and treatment across the recovery continuum, with a focus on the early stages including post-traumatic amnesia (PTA). Recommendations based on this research have been implemented in clinical practice internationally by speech pathologists working with adults in PTA.

25 Telepractice in Language and Discourse-based Interventions for Older Adults: Theoretical and Methodological Approaches

Lilian Cristine Hübner,
Maria Teresa Carthery-Goulart,
and Erica dos Santos Rodrigues

Preview of What Is Currently Known

Certain sociocultural factors and habits can aid in managing cognitive decline associated with aging. Linguistic-cognitive stimulation emerges as a promising tool to promote cognitive maintenance, enhancement, or cognitive rehabilitation. Evidence has pointed to the contribution of this type of stimulation to avoid or postpone cognitive decline in aging. Higher linguistic abilities result in more effective daily communication. The use of linguistic tasks in cognitive stimulation mobilizes several cognitive constructs; therefore, the stimulation of cognition can be fostered by the use of linguistic stimulation, mainly based on discourse tasks, a more naturalistic approach than the use of isolated words or sentences. Furthermore, there is growing evidence of the effectiveness of telepractice, which indicates that this approach needs to be further explored, due to its efficiency and convenience in self-administration. Finally, telepractice allows the provision of individualized treatment design, updated tasks, and online monitoring by the stimulation or rehabilitation program provider.

Objectives

(a) To discuss the feasibility and effectiveness of the use of telepractice to improve, maintain, or recover linguistic-cognitive abilities in healthy and atypical cognitive aging
(b) To analyze theoretical and empirical evidence on the use of language tasks with a focus on discourse to stimulate language and cognition in typical and atypical cognitive aging
(c) To analyze methodological aspects to be observed in designing and delivering telepractice with language/discourse-based tasks to healthy and neuroatypical aging populations
(d) To foster awareness of the role of cognitive training or stimulation via telepractice over modifiable risk factors associated with cognitive decline or dementia in the aging population worldwide, mainly among individuals with lower and middle-to-low SES, with an impact on public health policies

L. C. Hübner (✉)
School of Humanities in the Graduate Course of Linguistics, Pontifical Catholic University of Rio Grande do School (PUCRS), Porto Alegre, Brazil
e-mail: lilian.hubner@pucrs.br

M. T. Carthery-Goulart
Center for Mathematics, Cognition and Computing, Federal University of ABC, Santo André, Brazil

Cognitive and Behavioral Neurology Unit (GNCC), University of São Paulo, São Paulo, Brazil

Academic Unit of Human Communication, Learning, and Development, Faculty of Education, The University of Hong Kong, Pokfulam, Hong Kong SAR
e-mail: teresa.carthery@ufabc.edu.br

E. dos Santos Rodrigues
Departament of Letters, Center for Theology and Human Sciences, Pontifical Catholic University of Rio de Janeiro (PUC-Rio), Rio de Janeiro, Brazil
e-mail: ericasr@puc-rio.br

A. P.-H. Kong (ed.), *Spoken Discourse Impairments in the Neurogenic Populations*,
https://doi.org/10.1007/978-3-031-45190-4_25

Introduction

Telemedicine and telehealth have been studied since the beginning of the twentieth century (see Houston et al. [1] for a comprehensive historical review) and consist of practices that make use of information and communication technologies (ICT) to improve and maximize access to qualified healthcare beyond the in-person, face-to-face settings. Continuous advances in technology and telecommunications have made these options increasingly feasible and the focus of extensive research, especially in the last decades and particularly during the COVID-19 pandemic.

Discursive skills allow individuals to communicate and interact via oral or written modes and are the basis for social life. An effective and efficient discourse ability in terms of comprehension and processing of auditory and written information along with oral and written production is crucial in everyday functioning in any social context. Discourse is a complex linguistic unit and involves all the other sub-linguistic components, such as phonology, morphosyntax, semantics, and pragmatics. It also requires the coordination of several cognitive processes including attention, executive functions, and short and long-term memory. Therefore, it enables the study of linguistic and cognitive changes associated with typical aging as well as of symptoms that may indicate the emergence of a pathology, such as mild cognitive impairment (MCI) and dementias, among which Alzheimer's Disease (AD) is the most prominent and may contribute to 60–70% of cases [2]. Moreover, it can be used to differentiate typical older adults as a function of sociodemographic and cultural aspects [3] and represents an exciting arena to study interventions focusing on the prevention and treatment of cognitive decline, as well as in the rehabilitation of language and communication impairments due to cerebrovascular accidents (CVA). Despite its relevance in studies on language and cognition in healthy and neuroatypical populations through the lifespan, research on interventions focusing on discourse is incipient, especially regarding the literature on telehealth.

This chapter aims at providing theoretical and methodological bases on telehealth practices focusing on language and discourse directed to healthy younger and older adults and to those with language and communication impairments following CVA or diagnosed with MCI or dementia, including AD and Primary Progressive Aphasia (PPA). Firstly, the concept of telepractice, which is the term adopted for the purposes of this chapter, is introduced. Then the theoretical and empirical data from studies with healthy older adults are present in Section "Language-based Telepractice Interventions in Healthy Aging", followed by studies developed with CVA, MCI, AD, and PPA populations in Section "Language-based Telepractice Interventions in Neuroatypical Aging". Then, in Section "Methodological Guidelines on Language/Discourse-based Telepractice for Researchers and Clinicians". We discuss some general methodological aspects to guide researchers and clinicians in designing and administering discourse stimulation, training, or rehabilitation by online means.In the last section we present our final considerations and conclusions.

Telepractice Modalities: Features, Advantages, and Challenges

Telerehabilitation can be considered an umbrella term that refers to the use of information and computer technology (ICT) to provide rehabilitation and habilitation services [4]. Telerehabilitation services can be adopted in different contexts/settings—clinical, community, or home care settings, and may be applied to fulfill distinct functions/purposes, including assessment, consultation by multidisciplinary professionals, therapeutic intervention, monitoring, education, and supervision [5]. The terminology associated with telerehabilitation is quite broad, with some terms associated with a more specific usage, referring to the nature of the telerehabilitation, like "tele mental health," and others receiving a more generic scope, such as teletherapy and telehealth, which is the preferred term regardless of the discipline [1]. In this chapter, we will use the term telepractice, endorsed by the American Speech-Language-Hearing Association [4, 6] to refer to health and educational practices directed to younger and older adults for identifying, assessing, treating, and preventing linguistic and cognitive communicative deficits, conducted remotely with a range of devices (e.g., phones, smartphones, tablets, and computers) and using ICT. This definition was based on ASHA's guidelines for speech-language pathologists but, in this chapter, we will also refer to practices focusing on language and discourse delivered by other professionals in health care and education. The term will be used to refer to telehealth, teletherapy, telerehabilitation, teletraining, and telestimulation. Similar to ASHA definitions and guidelines, we will employ this term to practices delivered primarily remotely or that complement those offered in-person in different contexts and not restricted to health services, including synchronous, asynchronous, or hybrid (those that combine in-person and remote services and/or synchronous and asynchronous remote activities) (please refer to ASHA [6] for a detailed conceptualization of these terms).

Telepractice allows the intervention program providers to design and individualize therapy or stimulation tasks to be transferred to a platform for download or access by the clients or by healthy users on their mobile devices or computers. The program deliverer is enabled to remotely create, adapt, and update offline tasks and to remotely monitor individuals' performance. While telepractice offered in a synchronous way allows an on-time interaction between the therapist, researcher, or speech-language pathologist with the person engaged in the program, asynchronous telepractice is an emerging service delivery model which has the benefit of eliminating scheduling issues and ensuring efficiency and flexibility [7] . Moreover, it favors self-paced presentation, minimal transportation barriers, higher user independence, protection from virus infections, cost-effectiveness, and the provision of core components at home [8]. Although both modalities favor customized interventions, there are some challenges to implement these services to certain populations, especially older adults, including internet access, familiarity with technology, and digital literacy [5], as well as sensory conditions, since visual and hearing limitations are highly prevalent in older adults [9].

Language-based Telepractice Interventions in Healthy Aging

The growth of the aging population worldwide and the concurrent rise of dementia rates associated with advanced age have led to concerns about recovering, maintaining, and improving linguistic and other cognitive abilities. Furthermore, the concern about cognition beyond the *WEIRD* (Western, Educated, Industrialized, Rich, and Democratic) samples of populations has increasingly pointed to the necessity of considering individual differences in cognitive development, maintenance, and treatment, or on the onset of cognitive impairment, or on cases of dementia due to the influence of factors such as reading and writing habits, education [10, 11], socioeconomic status (SES) [12], general health, physical and sleep conditions, to cite some. To illustrate, Borelli et al. [13] used the public database of the Brazilian Longitudinal Study of Aging (ELSI-Brazil) to calculate the Population Attributable Fraction (PAF) for 10 risk factors: education level, hearing loss, hypertension, alcohol consumption, obesity, active smoking, depression, social isolation, physical inactivity, and diabetes. They found that the 10 preventable risk factors for dementia accounted for 50.5% of the PAF in the Brazilian population while hearing loss (14.2%), physical inactivity (11.2%), and hypertension (10.4%) accounted for the highest PAF among all the risk factors. The authors suggest that the health of the Brazilian population could be considerably improved by focusing on the modifiable risk factor of dementia.

Online initiatives to enhance linguistic and other cognitive abilities by training new abilities in the aging population have focused mainly on online courses designed for the elderly within a field called Geragogy [14], or in learning a second language in advanced age and its neural correlates [15], or still on training specific cognitive constructs, such as working memory, sometimes combined with other stimulation practices, such as transcranial magnetic stimulation (TMS) [16]. However, the administration of telepractice designed for neurotypical older adults with a focus on language is still scarce.

Myhre et al. [17] evaluated the impact of introducing communication via social media (Facebook) as an intervention to maintain or enhance cognitive function in a sample of 41 older persons: 14 participants learned how to use Facebook and were compared to an active control intervention group (online diary website, $n = 13$) and a passive control group (waiting list, $n = 14$). A significant increase in working memory (updating component of executive function) was evidenced in the Facebook group compared to no significant change in the control groups. Other cognitive functions and social support measures were not differently impacted in the intervention and control groups.

Alaimo et al. [18] overviewed the protocols used in eight studies which administered remotely controlled cognitive training with individualized feedback to healthy older adults and individuals with subjective memory complaints. Their review highlighted the efficiency of telepractices in administering cognitive interventions since most of the studies showed improvement in memory, sustained attention, working memory, executive functions, and language, together with reduced anxiety and depression symptoms, as well as in subjective memory difficulties. In the studies, linguistic components (and especially discourse) were not the focus of stimulation, but rather one of the components integrating the protocols of some of the studies.

Hubner et al. [19] designed a telepractice program under the hypothesis that stimulation and training of specific language abilities can enhance or maintain cognitive functioning in typical older adults. The pilot feasibility study was implemented in an online platform, during the COVID pandemic in 2021. General health, cognitive, and neuropsychological pre-and post-intervention assessments were performed on a total of 58 participants (88% females, mean age 69.5 (SD = 6.3)), 5–24 years of education (70% finished college or university) that completed at least 75% of the program, which consisted of 15 days of asynchronous 20-min language stimulation sessions over 3 weeks, including daily activities focusing of discourse comprehension and production. The linguistic activities did not involve teaching of encoding strategies and delayed retrieval of verbal information, as programs targeting episodic memory. Interestingly, immediately after the intervention, participants presented significantly higher scores in the following measures:

(a) Global cognition (the Brazilian version of ACE-R [20, 21]
(b) Verbal episodic memory measures (delayed recall tasks of ACE-R and BCSB [22, 23], and learning of face-name associations)
(c) Executive function, lexical-retrieval and processing speed (letter and verbs' fluency)
(d) Faster responses on language and inhibitory control tasks (auditory sentence comprehension and Stroop color-word test).

There were no changes in the scores of working memory (digit span forward and backwards) nor in other language tasks (naming, word and sentence comprehension, repetition). The results provided preliminary evidence on the impact of linguistic stimulation on cognitive functions that need confirmation in a blinded randomized control trial. The pilot study demonstrated the feasibility of telepractice in the form of linguistic-cognitive stimulation for healthy older adults. In Section "Methodological Guidelines on Language/Discourse-based Telepractice for Researchers and Clinicians", we further discuss the methodological features of this remote language training program.

Despite our still developing knowledge about the impact of textual and sociodemographic aspects in the use of discourse for cognitive assessment and for linguistic/cognitive stimulation, it is evident that discourse ability is crucial for successful engagement and interaction in everyday life functioning, and, therefore, a focus on its exploration should be central in the delivery of programs for language maintenance, improvement, and recovery.

Language-based Telepractice Interventions in Neuroatypical Aging

Online interventions have mostly been designed and implemented with neuroatypical adult and older adult populations as compared to healthy ones. In this section, we focus on studies that employed telepractice directed to language and communication difficulties following stroke, MCI, AD, and PPA.

Telepractice in Aphasia Due to CVA

Aphasia is a common symptom associated with stroke, therefore rehabilitation for recovery from this breakdown that affects linguistic and communicative performance is very often mentioned in studies on stroke, and telepractices have recently emerged as a promising method. For example, Agostini et al. [24] compared the feasibility of telerehabilitation to a face-to-face treatment of naming delivered to five chronic people with aphasia (PWA) due to a stroke. Their study used a controlled crossover design, with lists of words in picture naming tasks with progressive phonological cues, including follow-up testing. The study yielded comparable results regarding the type of treatment (online vs face-to-face), and both modalities showed an effect of time (better performance right after treatment and in the follow-up compared to baseline).

Marshal et al. [25] developed a virtual reality platform (EVA Park) for speech-language therapy. They tested its impact on communication skills, social connectedness, and feelings of social isolation in 20 PWA, in an intervention of 5 weeks (5 sessions of 1 h per week). Participants set their own goals for the treatment, including both general goals (i.e., asking questions, initiating conversation, improving word finding) and context-related goals (based on their individual experiences such as ordering food in a restaurant, making a doctor's appointment, etc.). The participants were assisted by a communication support worker to plan and select from a variety of activities those more appropriate to achieve their personal goals. The activities included naming, role-plays in suitable settings of EVA Park, and free conversation motivated by several features of the platform (e.g., news panels). The authors compared the intervention group with a waitlist control group in measures of communication skills and social isolation. Participants were satisfied with the communication opportunities provided by EVA Park and presented significant gains in functional communication (Communicative Abilities in Daily Living Test, CADL-2, [26]) in the post-treatment assessment. The authors reported gains in naming fluency and communication confidence but mentioned that these results could not necessarily be due to the intervention. Word retrieval in conversation and narrative did not change; nor did the Friendship Scale [27]. Another study tested the use of this platform (EVA Park) in telepractice with three PWA [28]. The participants received 20 h of speech therapy (4× a week over 5 weeks) aimed at improving storytelling (producing a story from novel videoclips) and two of them presented significant improvement in oral narrative discourse after the intervention.

Pitt et al. [29] described the development and preliminary results of the applicability of Telerehabilitation Group Aphasia Intervention and Networking (TeleGAIN), an online synchronous group therapy program of 12 sessions (1.5-h weekly) for PWA. TeleGain aims at improving communication-related quality of life, language functioning, and participation levels of PWA by providing opportunities for friendship-building among participants. The program was applied to four PWA and was considered feasible and acceptable by the participants. The sessions comprised conversation and formal activities (e.g., naming, word comprehension) organized around a topic. Sessions were tailored to fit the heterogeneous clinical profile of the group (aphasia type and severity) and included materials sent by the participants to the speech-language pathologist (e.g., photos) before the session. All participants had experience using computers both before and after the stroke. Three individuals evidenced significantly higher scores both on oral expression (naming and picture description) and comprehension (auditory and reading).

Another pilot randomized controlled trial testing telepractice was conducted by Øra et al. as a resource to complement speech-language therapy delivered to PWA [30] . The authors compared groups receiving the usual treatment ($n = 27$) and augmented telepractice treatment ($n = 30$), offered 1 h per day, five times per week over four consecutive weeks. The teleintervention was delivered by videoconference and aimed at enhancing functional expressive communication and combining different functional and impairment-directed activities. A client-centered approach was used with tailored activities according to the needs of the participants. The intervention included a range of activities (e.g., oral and written naming, reading sentences and text, and discussion about familiar topics) based on available specialized resources for aphasia treatments (structured exercises) and materials from the internet. The study evidenced higher gains in repetition skills and sentence production in the group exposed to telepractice plus usual care. There were comparable gains in both groups regarding naming, auditory comprehension, and functional language.

Zhou et al. [31] investigated the effects of computerized intervention for PWA combining speech-language and cognitive training on recovery, in both inpatient and discharged participants. The rationale was that improvement in non-verbal cognitive ability could drive language recovery. A total of 40 PWA were recruited for the study and four groups were defined: inpatient training group (ITG), inpatient control group (ITG), discharged training group (DTG), and discharged control group (ITG). The ITG did the training in the hospital for 14 days under on-site supervision while the DTG was submitted to remote treatment (telerehabilitation) for 30 days. The training program was adaptive at the participant level, with tasks designed with different levels of difficulty and also with the possibility of adjusting the number of stimuli. The speech-language module involved a large set of oral and written tasks and promoted training in comprehension and production abilities related to the word, sentence, and linguistic levels. The cognitive module trained attention, memory, and executive functions. The results regarding language function and communication skills, assessed, respectively, by the Western Aphasia Battery (WAB) [32] and CADL [26] showed significantly better performance of the training groups compared to the control ones. The effects of computerized training were smaller for the DTG in comparison to the ITG, even though the former received twice as long training. The study shows that combining language and cognitive training fosters aphasia recovery.

Telepractice in MCI and AD

Telepractice has increasingly been adopted for language stimulation and treatment of people with cognitive decline and dementia both in clinical and research settings.

A recent scoping review [5] analyzed the usage of telerehabilitation among older adults with MCI and cognitive frailty. They included six studies, three of them with a qualitative approach. The studies focused on conversational approaches, discussions on television-based health and social support, semi-structured interviews, or virtual cognitive health programs. Among the digital platforms, the most used were smartphones, television-based assistive integrated technology, mobile application, and videoconference. The authors concluded that telerehabilitation is useful to improve participants' quality of life and that it can be useful for delivering health care. They also suggest that social support is required to improve the adherence and effectiveness of telerehabilitation, pointing to the necessity of more studies on its feasibility and acceptability.

Yet Jelcic et al. [33] conducted a study to compare the effectiveness of a lexical-semantic stimulation (LSS) delivered in-person versus online to individuals with AD. Twenty-seven participants were allocated to three groups: face-to-face LSS (n = 10), face-to-face control intervention (n = 10), and LSS delivered via teleconference (n = 7) conducted biweekly over 6 weeks (12 sessions). LSS protocol consisted of semantic processing tasks in the word, sentence, and discourse levels (short stories). Group discussions about response choices were also stimulated to enhance verbal competencies. The results revealed that LSS offered face-to-face or via telepractice were more effective than the control intervention. Both types of stimulation resulted in a significant improvement in global cognition (as measured by the Mini-Mental State Examination). Face-to-face LSS resulted in a significant improvement of short-term memory (immediate story recall and forward digit span) and long-term memory (delayed verbal recall). On the other hand, LSS delivered as telepractice resulted in significantly higher scores on phonemic and semantic verbal fluency.

The study of Nousia et al. [34] analyzed the efficacy and feasibility of a telerehabilitation program in multidomain amnestic MCI (md-aMCI), including 30 individuals aged 60–80 years. Half of the participants received computerized cognitive training (RehaCom) and paper-pencil language training, while the other half (control group) received standard clinical care (e.g., psychotherapy or/and physiotherapy), over a period of 15 weeks (60 min/session twice a week). Their results revealed that the telerehabilitation intervention improved performance in the domains of delayed and working memory, episodic memory, confrontation naming, verbal fluency, and global cognition. They suggest that telerehabilitation is an efficient tool in improving or stabilizing cognitive decline in md-aMCI individuals.

Telepractice in PPA

Primary Progressive Aphasia (PPA) poses a complex and instigating scenario for language studies due to its differential impact on language functioning according to each of the three variants (logopenic, semantic, or non-fluent/agrammatic). In most of the cases, anomia and word-finding difficulties are the first clinical manifestations of these syndromes, impacting functional communication. For this reason, several interventions target these impairments [35].

Meyer et al. [36] evaluated the efficiency and feasibility of anomia treatment within the three subtypes of primary progressive aphasia (PPA) by adopting a telerehabilitation-based approach. Three participants, each one diagnosed with a distinct subtype of PPA, received a baseline language and cognition evaluation, followed by a phonological and an orthographic treatment over 6 months, with a post-treatment evaluation 1 month after the end of treatment. Treatment effects were examined inter- and intra-subjects and also compared to a group of PPA with the same clinical conditions but treated in a face-to-face modality. The results showed that the three participants exhibited positive treatment effects, also when compared to in-person treatment with the same subtype of PPA, and these effects were either within the expected range or even larger than expected.

Dial et al. [37] also investigated the feasibility and utility of treatment delivered via teletherapy to individuals diagnosed with PPA. The researchers used a non-randomized group comparison design to compare the feasibility and utility of speech-language treatment delivered via teletherapy related to treatment administered in person for individuals diagnosed with PPA. Ten participants with the semantic and 11 with the logopenic variant received lexical-retrieval treatment, while 10 non-fluent PPA participants received video training for speech production and fluency promotion. Telepractice was delivered for approximately half of the participants. Testing of treatment outcomes and cognitive abilities was done previously and after the program implementation, followed by testing done 3-, 6-, and 12-months post-treatment. Their study showed comparable treatment outcomes for individuals receiving teletraining versus face-to-face therapy, supporting the application of teletherapy to treat cognitive-linguistic aspects in mild-to-moderate PPA.

Rogalski et al. [38, 39] developed an intervention for PPA and their communication partners via telepractice (Communication-Bridge) which addresses communication, language and speech difficulties by providing tailored activities on the word, sentence, and discourse levels (script-training). The project consists of a comprehensive assessment before the intervention, followed by eight person-centered internet-based speech-language therapy sessions and two post-therapy evaluations. The authors analyzed the feasibility of providing online rehabilitation services, the strategies used, participants' functional gains, and the duration of the benefit. Communication functional gains and confidence levels were higher at 2 months and maintained 4 months after the intervention. The researchers raised the issue of clients' engagement and familiarity with computers in telepractice efficiency. They concluded that person-centered intervention via internet-based speech-pathology therapy is a feasible way to treat individuals with dementia and mild and/or moderate aphasia symptoms who have an engaged care partner and familiarity with a computer.

Taken together, the studies reported above and others that have been done so far including adult and older adult healthy and neuroatypical populations, ranging from stroke and cognitive decline (MCI) to neurodegenerative diseases (AD and PPA) have brought evidence on the feasibility and efficiency of language and discourse-based telepractice for cognitive-linguistic stimulation, training, and rehabilitation. In order to implement telepractice, some common methodological guidelines should be observed, as discussed in the following section.

Methodological Guidelines on Language/Discourse-based Telepractice for Researchers and Clinicians

Beyond language, spoken discourse production demands the recruitment of several cognitive domains, such as attention, executive functions, and memory (long-term episodic and semantic, and short-term and working memory). Therefore, oral discourse practice has been reliably and comprehensively used as a tool to support the assessment of cognition [3, 11], since speech connectedness (an expression currently used in studies of computational analyses of language to describe a continuous meaningful sequence of utterances or conversations in spoken language) depends on the joined mobilization of communication, language, and other cognitive abilities. Apart from its role in cognitive assessment, discourse consists on its own as an instrument of clinical intervention, as it promotes cognitive engagement and stimulation.

Furthermore, the degree of recruitment of these cognitive domains, with a possible impact on cerebral circuitry, may vary as a function of the oral discourse typology (narrative, descriptive, expository, or injunctive), genre (for example, autobiographical story or picture descriptions), or type of stimuli prompt used to generate the oral discourse (whether presented in an oral or in a written form). To illustrate, sequences of scenes have been shown to elicit more verbal material during discourse oral production than single pictures do, since the latter tend to generate descriptions or naming of the elements which integrate the picture [40], and semantic memory has shown to be important for a coherent oral narrative production of a story based on a sequence of pictures in people with AD compared to typical older adults [10].

Together with the text, genre, and mode of presentation typologies, the processing of this complex linguistic level is affected by the participants' sociodemographic characteristics, such as age, gender, and education [41], as well as by cultural aspects, such as reading and writing habits [10] and bilingualism [42]. These aspects need to be further addressed for a better understanding of their impact on oral discourse production and discourse-based interventions, both in face-to-face and online treatment and training/stimulation.

Discourse assessment and treatment can be implemented in a more ecological way as compared to the assessment and treatment at the word or sentence levels, since it demands the linguistic content to be inserted in a context, which may refer to and recruit the individual's background knowledge, thus extrapolating the content of the text itself. In fact, older persons seem to rely more than their younger counterparts on strategies related to vocabulary knowledge and on the context in discourse processing, which is hindered in the case of tasks using isolated words [43]. This ecological advantage poses some issues, though. Among the aspects to be observed when designing an online synchronous or asynchronous intervention program for discourse stimulation or treatment, one can cite aspects related to the topic of the text chosen, text genre, the type of stimulus prompt (whether text or picture), the procedures for task administration, and the procedures for data scoring and analyses.

The *choice of the text or of the picture(s) as a stimulus prompt* that will promote oral discourse production is the first decision to make in designing a task. Texts can be read aloud by the examiner in the case of synchronous assisted intervention, or audio recorded in a male/female voice for the participant to listen (synchronously or asynchronously), or still read by the participant himself (if literate) followed or not by (open or structured) comprehension questions. Alternatively, questions can be asked as a stimulus to elicit written or oral text recall, but this will demand a detailed recall or a summary of the text. There is a variety of text genres (chronicles, news, science/instructional texts, recipes, etc.), with varying levels of length, complexity, and topics. Narratives have been the types of texts more studied due to their clear propositional segmentation, normally including a setting, a complication, a resolution, and a final state. The content should not be complex for naïve readers of a specific topic, nor too simple, of common sense, or irrelevant. The length should also be observed, as well as the inclusion of illustrations, which may facilitate text comprehension and impact a subsequent retelling or comprehension activity. When it comes to the use of a picture as a prompt to generate oral discourse production, the two most commonly used are single pictures, similar to the Cookie Theft picture [44], or sequences of scenes that form a story. Some aspects to observe are the complexity of the vocabulary portrayed in the picture(s)/scene(s), the number of characters (which may impact, for example, pronouns/references use), and the number and complexity of inferences that the picture(s) may generate, which should be guided by the research questions in the case of its use as an experiment or by the intended comprehension complexity analyses in the clinics.

When designing the linguistic activities which may accompany discourse tasks (especially in telepractice), several important measures worth extra attention to adopt, such as

(a) Organizing the activities with a gradual level of difficulty
(b) Adopting gamification in designing the tasks so as to make them more enjoyable
(c) Adjusting the number of stimuli according to the severity of the clinical profile (for example, some tasks may need to be shortened for clients with low attentional span)
(d) Providing feedback on errors and allowing the user to repeat a particular item (in the case of incorrect responses) or the whole activity to enhance practice, if this procedure does not affect the aim of the research
(e) Ensuring layout adequacy for older users, considering cleanness, typos size, sound volume, and color choices in order to avoid the participant getting distracted or having difficulties in seeing the stimuli
(f) Ensuring the activities automatically adjust to the screen display, whether on a laptop, a computer, or a cellular/smartphone

The use of pictures or texts to prompt oral discourse production is an example of cued activities. Free or less-cued oral discourse production can be obtained using instructions that request, for example, the production of a procedural text (e.g., how to prepare a sandwich), an autobiographical story (e.g., the best trip in one's life), a free conversation, a (semi) structured interview, a conversation with some special topics introduced by the examiner, among other types. In any case, the instructions need to be clear, especially in the case of asynchronous protocols, when the client and other participants (e.g., caregiver) may not have immediate assistance from the examiner or health care provider.

Among the *procedures for task administration*, the time given for task resolution matters a lot when it comes to older individuals, especially in online practices. This is even more relevant in the case of adults and older adults who are not very familiar with the use of computers, and with low or no digital literacy. The fear of disappointing the examiner, of not being smart enough with regard to technology use, the lack of practice with assessment, or even a long period without completing academic-like tasks may pose emotional burdens to older participants, which may impact the results obtained. Therefore, timing adjustment and balancing the number of time-limited activities have to be considered in stimulus design and administration. For some participants, these types of tasks may be challenging, while they may be stressful for others.

Another issue regarding task administration is the observance of voice volume and pace, which have to be adequate to each participant's preferences, as well as the size of the images or texts, when used, on the device screen (computer, laptop, or smartphone). Moreover, on the participants' side, the examiner should provide constant technical support, since some technical issues may emerge during the process of telepractice.

Finally, another concern regards *the procedures for data scoring and analyses*, since the complex linguistic material produced in an oral discourse task may demand some specialization to be scored and interpreted in order to control for subjectivity. Whenever a normalized activity is adopted, it may include a scoring manual. In other cases, the criteria for assessment should be established by the clinician or researcher. The assessment of the data generated in discourse elicitation may require a special analysis method, depending on the aim of the study or clinical practice. For example, several studies have used software (such as CLAN—Computerized Language ANalysis—https://talkbank.org, Coh-Metrix—http://cohmetrix.com/, and LIWC - Linguistic Inquiry and Word Count—https://www.liwc.app/) to analyze mainly microstructural aspects of oral productions, whose content needs first to be transcribed, or graph analyses, which analyze macrostructural aspects of connected speech. It is important to state that for the sake of publishing, statistical procedures such as interrater agreement methods (for example, the Kappa interrater reliability measure) should be adopted to minimize possible subjective interpretations.

To illustrate, we present some methodological decisions taken for the implementation of our telepractice program delivered to adults and older adults in Brazil, named *AtivaMente-PalavrAtiva* Program for Linguistic-Cognitive Training, whose results were presented earlier in Section "Language-based Telepractice Interventions in Healthy Aging" [19]. The project aimed to evaluate whether a program of linguistic stimulation could induce cognitive changes in the domains of executive functions and episodic memory. The feasibility study implemented the assessment of a pre- and post-test protocol (some tasks were adapted to be administered online) to evaluate the outcomes of remote linguistic training. The sample was recruited by convenience by announcements of the project in social media linked to the four universities integrating the project, in different states in Brazil (UFABC and USP; PUCRS and PUC-Rio), reaching participants all over the country. The authors conducted synchronous meetings and video recordings explaining the research procedures approved by the Ethics Committee of the participating universities. Participants were also invited to take part in interactive talks about healthy aging (open to the public) offered as part of an outreach project to reduce social isolation in the context of the COVID-19 pandemic in Brazil in 2021. A total of 181 participants enrolled in the open talks. Of those, 74 signed the informed consent to participate in the assessments and intervention phase and 58 completed all phases of the study. During recruitment, participants were invited to fill out two forms online, one with the consent to participate in the study and another to give rights of image and voice use, and they got access to Moodle to learn how to use it and to practice tasks similar to those to be used in the study so to get familiar with them. The program included synchronous and asynchronous activities (hybrid). The synchronous activities consisted of three components:

(a) Education in health and cognition in aging (open talks)—sessions in which the participants engaged in interactive zoom sessions with specialists approaching different topics (sleep, nutrition, voice care, mental health, cognitive reserve), and these meetings were recorded so that participants could watch them again or at any time
(b) Chat and individual support: each participant was assigned a tutor for interactions via WhatsApp. No formal script for those interactions was provided but the topics typically included help to assess the system, motivational contact by the tutor, and information about the availability of new activities. There was also a WhatsApp group for all participants (optional) for general information and interaction to promote more engagement to the program
(c) Pre- and post-intervention assessments

On the other hand, the asynchronous activities consisted of linguistic-cognitive intervention with exercises implemented on Moodle for 15 days, including one or two tasks at the word level (tackling semantic knowledge and lexical access), one at the sentence level (dealing with syntactic complex structures like passives, relative sentences, WH-questions, syntactically ambiguous sentences), and one at the discourse level. On average participants took about 20 min to undertake the activities daily. The exercises were uploaded daily and they could do them at their preferred time and location, one or more times. The exercises provided automatic feedback and also offered the participant opportunities to evaluate the complexity and enjoyability of the activities. The participants referred to having enjoyed participating in the study and reported an increase in self-confidence after joining a challenging project which demanded technical ability and cognitive stimulation, especially for those who were not very familiar with computers and who had been away from formal education for years. They also reported that their participation in the project motivated them to engage in other online cognitive activities to keep on challenging themselves.

Final Words

The growth of the older population worldwide raises concerns about the emergence of neurodegenerative diseases associated with aging. Modifiable aspects that impact the maintenance and treatment of cognitive decline, including cognitive-linguistic stimulation, appear as an alternative to this situation and could be on the agenda of public health policies. Telepractice—an umbrella word here referring to telestimulation, teletraining, and telerehabilitation—has emerged as a promising way to allow researchers and health practitioners to establish synchronous, asynchronous, or hybrid (combining digital and in-person) interaction with research participants, or clients to deliver cognitive-linguistic interventions. Other clinical populations, including stroke survivors, have also benefited from telepractices, as discussed in this chapter. Online practices have several advantages as compared to face-to-face interactions, such as flexible time scheduling, customized intervention, and remote monitoring of individuals' performance, in line with the trend of providing clients with higher autonomy and self-engagement in treatment development. One of the biggest challenges, though, is to adapt tests, batteries, and tasks to the digital environment, which may pose restrictions to the researcher and clinician, for example, in reducing observation of the client or participant's moves and whole-body response. Furthermore, another limitation to its implementation concerns the reduced access to the internet by people with low socioeconomic and/or education levels, mainly in under- developing and developing countries. Finally, technological adaptations have to be developed for successful delivery to account for sensory impairment, mainly visual and hearing impairment, which is highly prevalent in older adults; moreover, successful telepractice may require the support of care partners to navigate technologies [9].

Despite these challenges, tele language stimulation and treatment, mainly focusing on discourse—this rich and ecological linguistic and communicative resource—has been shown as a feasible and efficient tool to promote not only linguistic but also general cognitive maintenance, enhancement, and rehabilitation. Future studies should further investigate the transfer of the learned strategies to everyday life, and methodological aspects, such as the most efficient types of discourse tasks, the amount and frequency of exposure, as well as the neural correlates of stimulation and treatment in healthy and neuroatypical aging.

Major Takeaways

1. Telepractice of linguistic abilities, including discourse comprehension and production has been shown to have similar effects as face-to-face, in-person interventions.
2. Studies demonstrated a positive impact of telepractice focusing on language and communication in the enhancement, maintenance, and recovery of cognitive and linguistic functions, which should impact social policies concerned with growing aging worldwide.
3. Internet-based rehabilitation has shown effective results for language and communication rehabilitation following CVA, as well as in cognitive decline and dementia.
4. Mastering technological resources and access to good quality internet can hinder access to the benefits of online training in older populations, mainly those with low SES and education.
5. Telepractice may require the delivery of technical support by caregivers and practitioners for older adults engaged in therapeutic or research programs.
6. Future research should investigate the role of variables related to the individual level (socioeconomic and sociocultural aspects, healthy versus neuroatypical condition), as well as to the methodological level (types of text-based/oral discourse stimuli and data analyses) in the feasibility and effectiveness of telepractices.
7. Randomized controlled trials as well as studies on the neural correlates of changes associated with telepractice to typical and neuroatypical aging populations are needed.

Acknowledgments The authors thank the following institutions for financial support for research development: CAPES (Coordination of Superior Level Staff Improvement); L.C.H.: Chamada MCTIC/CNPq Universal #4524362508342994—28/2018; Programa de Internacionalização da Pós-Graduação no RS—Edital FAPERGS #012/2013, and grants as productivity researcher at CNPq (National Council for Scientific and Technological Development). MTCG: ProEC—UFABC; Edital: CNPq/MCTI/FNDCT N° 18/2021-B, number: [407022/2021-0].

References

1. Houston KT, Flemming AM, Brown KJ, Weinberg TR, Nafe JM. History, definitions, and overview of telepractice models. In: Houston KT, editor. Telepractice in speech-language pathology. 1st ed. Plural Publishing, Incorporated; 2014. p. 14–27.
2. World Health Organization (WHO); 2022. https://www.who.int/news-room/fact-sheets/detail/dementia. Accessed Jan 2023.World Health Organization.
3. Malcorra BLC, Mota NB, Weissheimer J, Schilling LP, Wilson MA, Hübner LC. Reading and writing habits compensate for aging effects in speech connectedness. NPJ Sci Learn. 2022;7(1):13.
4. Richmond T, Peterson C, Cason J, Billings M, Terrell EA, Lee ACW, et al. American Telemedicine Association's principles for delivering telerehabilitation services. Int J Telerehabil. 2017;9(2):63–8.
5. Md Fadzil NH, Shahar S, Rajikan R, Singh DKA, Mat Ludin AF, Subramaniam P, et al. A scoping review for usage of telerehabilitation among older adults with mild cognitive impairment or cognitive frailty. Int J Environ Res Public Health. 2022;19(7):4000.
6. American Speech-Language-Hearing Association (ASHA). Telepractice. (Practice Portal); n.d. www.asha.org/Practice-Portal/Professional-Issues/Telepractice/. Accessed Jan 2023.
7. Hill AJ, Breslin HM. Refining an asynchronous telerehabilitation platform for speech-language pathology: engaging end-users in the process. Front Hum Neurosci. 2016;10
8. Rabanifar N, Abdi K. Barriers and challenges of implementing telerehabilitation: a systematic review. Iran Rehabil J. 2021;19(2):121–8.
9. Yi JS, Pittman CA, Price CL, Nieman CL, Oh ES. Telemedicine and dementia care: a systematic

review of barriers and facilitators. J Am Med Dir Assoc. 2021;22(7):1396–1402.e18.
10. Malcorra BLC, Wilson MA, Schilling LP, Hübner LC. Lower education and reading and writing habits are associated with poorer oral discourse production in typical adults and older adults. Front Psychol. 2022;13
11. Malcorra BLC, Mota NB, Weissheimer J, Schilling LP, Wilson MA, Hübner LC. Low speech connectedness in Alzheimer's disease is associated with poorer semantic memory performance. J Alzheimers Dis. 2021;82(3):905–12.
12. Nitrini R, Barbosa MT, Dozzi Brucki SM, Yassuda MS, Caramelli P. Current trends and challenges on dementia management and research in Latin America. J Glob Health. 2020;10(1):010362.
13. Borelli WV, Leotti VB, Strelow MZ, Chaves MLF, Castilhos RM. Preventable risk factors of dementia: population attributable fractions in a Brazilian population-based study. Lancet Region Health Am. 2022;11:100256.
14. Bulbul A, Gunaydin S, Odabasi H. Embracing older adults in online learning. Turkish Online J Educ Technol TOJET. 2022;21(1):55–67.
15. Legault J, Fang SY, Lan YJ, Li P. Structural brain changes as a function of second language vocabulary training: effects of learning context. Brain Cogn. 2019;134:90–102.
16. Assecondi S, Hu R, Kroeker J, Eskes G, Shapiro K. Older adults with lower working memory capacity benefit from transcranial direct current stimulation when combined with working memory training: a preliminary study. Front Aging Neurosci. 2022;14
17. Myhre JW, Mehl MR, Glisky EL. Cognitive benefits of online social networking for healthy older adults. J Gerontol B Psychol Sci Soc Sci. 2017;72(5):752–60.
18. Alaimo C, Campana E, Stoppelli MR, Gobbi E, Baglio F, Rossetto F, et al. Cognitive tele-enhancement in healthy older adults and subjects with subjective memory complaints: a review. Front Neurol. 2021;12
19. Hubner LC, Rodrigues ES, Carthery-Goulart MT. A linguagem no envelhecimento: o impacto de fatores individuais e o conceito de reserva cognitiva. In: Maia M, editor. Psicolinguística: Diversidades, Interfaces e Aplicações. 1st ed. Rio de Janeiro: Editora Contexto; 2022.
20. Carvalho VA, Caramelli P. Brazilian adaptation of the Addenbrooke's Cognitive Examination-revised (ACE-R). Dement Neuropsychol. 2007;1(2):212–6.
21. César KG, Yassuda MS, Porto FHG, Brucki SMD, Nitrini R. Addenbrooke's cognitive examination-revised: normative and accuracy data for seniors with heterogeneous educational level in Brazil. Int Psychogeriatr. 2017;29(8):1345–53.
22. Brucki SMD, Mansur LL, Carthery-Goulart MT, Nitrini R. Formal education, health literacy and mini-mental state examination | Educação formal, alfabetismo em Saúde e mini-Exame do Estado mental. Dementia e Neuropsychologia. 2011;5(1):26–30.
23. Takada LT, Caramelli P, Fichman HC, Porto CS, Bahia VS, Anghinah R, et al. Comparison between two tests of delayed recall for the diagnosis of dementia. Arq Neuropsiquiatr. 2006;64(1):35–40.
24. Agostini M, Garzon M, Benavides-Varela S, de Pellegrin S, Bencini G, Rossi G, et al. Telerehabilitation in poststroke anomia. Biomed Res Int. 2014;2014:1–6.
25. Marshall J, Booth T, Devane N, Galliers J, Greenwood H, Hilari K, et al. Evaluating the benefits of aphasia intervention delivered in virtual reality: results of a quasi-randomised study. PLoS One. 2016;11(8):e0160381.
26. Holland A. Communicative abilities in daily living: a test of functional communication for aphasic adults. Baltimore: University Park Press; 1980.
27. Hawthorne G. Measuring social isolation in older adults: development and initial validation of the friendship scale. Soc Indic Res. 2006;77(3):521–48.
28. Carragher M, Steel G, Talbot R, Devane N, Rose ML, Marshall J. Adapting therapy for a new world: storytelling therapy in EVA Park. Aphasiology. 2021;35(5):704–29.
29. Pitt R, Theodoros D, Hill AJ, Russell T. The development and feasibility of an online aphasia group intervention and networking program—TeleGAIN. Int J Speech Lang Pathol. 2019;21(1):23–36.
30. Øra HP, Kirmess M, Brady MC, Partee I, Hognestad RB, Johannessen BB, et al. The effect of augmented speech-language therapy delivered by telerehabilitation on poststroke aphasia—a pilot randomized controlled trial. Clin Rehabil. 2020;34(3):369–81.
31. Zhou Q, Lu X, Zhang Y, Sun Z, Li J, Zhu Z. Telerehabilitation combined speech-language and cognitive training effectively promoted recovery in aphasia patients. Front Psychol. 2018;9
32. Kertesz A, Poole E. The aphasia quotient: the taxonomic approach to measurement of aphasic disability. Can J Neurol Sci Journal Canadien des Sciences Neurologiques. 1974;1(1):7–16.
33. Jelcic N, Agostini M, Meneghello F, Busse C, Parise S, Galano A, et al. Feasibility and efficacy of cognitive telerehabilitation in early Alzheimer's disease: a pilot study. Clin Interv Aging. 2014;1605
34. Nousia A, Pappa E, Siokas V, Liampas I, Tsouris Z, Messinis L, et al. Evaluation of the efficacy and feasibility of a telerehabilitation program using language and cognitive exercises in multi-domain amnestic mild cognitive impairment. Arch Clin Neuropsychol. 2022:cac078. Advance online publication. https://doi.org/10.1093/arclin/acac078.
35. Carthery-Goulart MT, da Silveira AC, Machado TH, Mansur LL, Pimenta Parente MAM, Hosogi Senaha ML, et al. Nonpharmacological interventions for cognitive impairments following primary progressive aphasia: a systematic review of the literature. Dement Neuropsychol. 2013;7(1):122–31.
36. Meyer AM, Getz HR, Brennan DM, Hu TM, Friedman RB. Telerehabilitation of anomia in primary progressive aphasia. Aphasiology. 2016;30(4):483–507.

37. Dial H, Hinshelwood H, Grasso S, Hubbard HI, Gorno-Tempini ML, Henry M. Investigating the utility of teletherapy in individuals with primary progressive aphasia. Clin Interv Aging. 2019;14:453–71.
38. Rogalski EJ, Saxon M, McKenna H, Wieneke C, Rademaker A, Corden ME, et al. Communication bridge: a pilot feasibility study of internet-based speech-language therapy for individuals with progressive aphasia. Alzheimer's Dementia. 2016;2(4):213–21.
39. Rogalski E, Roberts A, Salley E, Saxon M, Fought A, Esparza M, et al. Communication partner engagement: a relevant factor for functional outcomes in speech–language therapy for aphasic dementia. J Gerontol Ser B. 2022;77(6):1017–25.
40. Lima TM, Brandão L, de Parente MA, Peña-Casanova J. Doença de alzheimer: cognição e discurso narrativo com apoio em figuras. Revista CEFAC. 2014;16(4):1168–77.
41. MacKenzie C. Adult spoken discourse: the influences of age and education. Int J Lang Commun Disord. 2000;35(2):269–85.
42. Gallo F, DeLuca V, Prystauka Y, Voits T, Rothman J, Abutalebi J. Bilingualism and aging: implications for (delaying) neurocognitive decline. Front Hum Neurosci. 2022;16
43. Kavé G, Goral M. Do age-related word retrieval difficulties appear (or disappear) in connected speech? Aging Neuropsychol Cognit. 2017;24(5):508–27.
44. Goodglass H, Kaplan E, Barresi B. Boston diagnostic aphasia examination-third edition (BDAE-3). San Antonio: Pearson; 2000.

Lilian Cristine Hübner is an Associate Professor at the School of Humanities, in the Graduate Course of Linguistics at the Pontifical Catholic University of Rio Grande do School (PUCRS) and researcher at the Institute of Geriatrics and Gerontology (IGG-PUCRS). She obtained her M.A. at the Federal University of Rio Grande do Sul (UFRGS) in the field of language acquisition and bilingualism, and her Ph.D. at the Federal University of Santa Catarina (UFSC) in language studies in aging and bilingualism in a psycho- and neurolinguistic perspective. She has conducted two post-doc trainings in the area of Speech-Pathology and Medicine, at the University of Montreal in Canada and at Sorbonne—Paris VI in France. She has been a researcher of CNPq (National Council for Scientific and Technological Development) since 2013. As a trained linguist, her main research interests are (i) language and cognition in (a) typical aging, (ii) language and cognition in bi- and multilingualism, (iii) language and cognition in cognitive decline, dementia, and following a stroke, as well as, (iv) adaptation and development of linguistic and cognitive assessment instruments in a lifespan. Her research fields comprise Neurolinguistics and Psycholinguistics, with an interface with Neuropsychology, Speech-Pathology and Education.

Erica dos Santos Rodrigues is an Associate Professor in the Department of Letters of the Center for Theology and Human Sciences at the Pontifical Catholic University of Rio de Janeiro (PUC-Rio). She has been developing research in the field of Psycholinguistics, with interfaces on Education and Neuropsychology, in the Graduate Program in Language Studies at the PUC-Rio. Dr. Rodrigues is the vice-coordinator of the Psycholinguistics and Language Acquisition Laboratory in the same institution. She obtained her M.A. and her Ph.D. in language studies, at PUC-Rio, with research on writing as a cognitive process and on subject-verb agreement errors in speech, respectively. As a psycholinguist, she has been conducting studies on (i) writing and reading processes using keystroke logging and eye-tracking tools; (ii) syntax processing in language production and comprehension; and (iii) language processing in (a)typical aging. She has been a researcher of CNPq (National Council for Scientific and Technological Development) since 2020.

Maria Teresa Carthery-Goulart is an Associate Professor at the Center for Mathematics, Cognition and Computing, Federal University of ABC and a researcher at the Cognitive and Behavioral Neurology Unit (GNCC), University of São Paulo. She is a speech and language therapist graduated from the Faculty of Medicine, University of São Paulo. She obtained her M.Sc. in Psychology in the area of Neurosciences and Behavior from the Institute of Psychology, University of São Paulo and her Ph.D. in Sciences (Neurology) from the Faculty of Medicine, University of São Paulo. She has been a Visiting Scientist at the Medical Research Council - Cognition and Brain Sciences Unit, Cambridge (2007–2008) and is currently a Lecturer in Unit of Human Communication, Learning, and Development, Faculty of Education, The University of Hong Kong. She has studies in Cognitive Neuroscience of Language, Neuropsychology, Psycholinguistics, and Neurolinguistics.

Communication Partner Training (CPT) to Improve Conversation, Communication, and Mental Health

26

Analisa Pais and Caroline Jagoe

Preview of What Is Currently Known

Communication Partner Training (CPT) focuses on the communication environment through addressing the communicative competence (of both communicators), co-construction and participation [1] in order to facilitate better interactions between the person with aphasia and those around them. CPT has consistently been recommended in best practice guidelines as a means to improve the communication of people with aphasia [2, 3]. Although CPT is most well established in relation to aphasia, research with other groups shows a wider applicability. Given that exclusion and isolation, common experiences for persons with communication disability are linked to lower well-being, CPT has the potential to enhance mental health and well-being by optimizing inclusion and engagement.

Objectives

(a) To outline the evidence for the link between conversation, mental health, and well-being, arguing that the relationship is bi-directional
(b) To define Communication Partner Training (CPT) and present the evidence related to different groups of communication partners, in particular in relation to well-being outcomes
(c) To present Communication Accommodation Theory as a framework suited to investigating the nuances of communicative adjustments that can be observed following CPT
(d) To use data from families where one person has aphasia to illustrate these communicative adjustments and the evidence for changes in well-being
(e) To discuss the potential for CPT in mental health settings

Conversation, Mental Health, and Well-being

Conversation is critical to well-being. It is "a vehicle for social participation" [4] (p. 625)—a means for making social connections, building relationships, engaging in services, and accessing information. Where communication is experienced as disrupted, well-being is almost inevitably affected. This link between communication and well-being is arguably bi-directional, that is, communication influences mental health

A. Pais
School of Health and Social Care, University of Essex, Colchester, UK
e-mail: ap21904@essex.ac.uk

C. Jagoe (✉)
Department of Clinical Speech and Language Studies, Trinity College Dublin, The University of Dublin, Dublin, Ireland

Human & Community Development, University of the Witwatersrand, Johannesburg, South Africa
e-mail: cjagoe@tcd.ie

A. P.-H. Kong (ed.), *Spoken Discourse Impairments in the Neurogenic Populations*,
https://doi.org/10.1007/978-3-031-45190-4_26

and well-being, and mental health and sense of well-being influence communication. For example, in typically communicating couples of older age, enjoyable interactions in which people feel confident and in control have been associated with higher life satisfaction [5]. Where communication is the difficulty, as is the case for people with aphasia (PWA), the psychosocial consequences of the communication disability may manifest in the form of reduced motivation, participation, and treatment outcomes [6] and may in turn impact on mental health, specifically mood [7]. Indeed, there is reason to believe that the reduction in conversation experienced by PWA is a critical mediating factor in their mental health: evidence suggests that people post stroke are far more likely to experience depression if they have aphasia, than if they have no aphasia [8]. On the other side of the communication and mental health equation, research suggests that people with mental health disorders may experience communication difficulties, particularly, although not exclusively, during periods where psychiatric symptoms are prominent (see Walsh et al. [9] for overview).

Across the different disorders of communication, aphasia is arguably the best researched with regard to psychosocial well-being. This chapter will therefore focus specifically on PWA, and the role of Communication Partner Training (CPT) in addressing communication, conversation, and mental health or well-being more generally. A summary of the evidence for CPT across different types of communication partners (CPs) will be briefly presented. Social contact is central to well-being [10], and the analysis presented in this chapter focuses predominantly on primary data from PWA and their family members. We use data from the Indian context as a deliberate attempt to broaden the cultural—linguistic and geographic representation in CPT research. Finally, implications for persons with primary diagnoses of mental health disorders will be briefly explored, acknowledging that there remain significant gaps in research on CPT and primary mental health disorders such as schizophrenia or bipolar mood disorder.

Communication Partner Training

The notion of communicative competence as a joint responsibility, with conversation as co-constructed and participatory, is at the heart of CPT. Although easily reduced to the capacity residing in an individual, communicative competence is most accurately understood as manifest in interaction, as eloquently articulated by Ferguson [11]:

> *'It is possible to extend our notion of communicative competence beyond consideration of how competence is vested in the individual, by recognizing competence as arising from the interactive relationship of communication partners as they negotiate messages.'* (p. 56).

The overarching aim of CPT therefore is to optimize the interactive relationship and thereby improve the communication between the PWA and their typically-communicating partners [12–14].

Barriers in the communication environment may manifest across various settings, from family life, to friendship, work, healthcare, retail encounters, and others. A feeling of disconnect in relation to social contact may contribute to a sense of loneliness and depression [10] and therefore addressing the communication skills and resources of the CPs across any of these domains is appropriate within CPT with outcomes reasonably expected in terms of mood in particular. For this reason, the "target"' of CPT may be any number of familiar or unfamiliar communication partners, and evidence is accumulating across the categories of CPT for family members, healthcare professionals, students/volunteers, and service employees.

The evidence published in English is dominated by a focus on family members as targets of CPT, either alone, or alongside their significant others with aphasia [15]. Mental health outcomes, in terms of mood in particular, have been considered in a subset on studies on CPT with family members or significant others. In a systematic review of the evidence, Baker et al. [16] conclude that CPT may be effective for PWA (and perhaps their significant others) in improving mood where depression is not at a clinically significant level of severity. Potentially, CPT may also play a preventative role with regard to depression, although empirical evidence in this regard is lacking.

CPT for healthcare professionals has developed in response to evidence that PWA are afforded less than ideal opportunities to participate in healthcare encounters (e.g., Brown et al. [17]) and that healthcare professionals experience challenges in provision of healthcare to this population (e.g., van Rijssen et al. [18]; Carragher et al. [19]). Addressing the healthcare workers as communication partners in CPT interventions has largely been explored in relation to nursing, medical, and other allied healthcare professionals in stroke or rehabilitation services and is typically provided in a group setting using generic or programmatic training materials comprising general background on aphasia as well as skills training. Synthesizing the existing literature on the experiences of PWA in healthcare encounters, Vallumrød and colleagues [20] argue that skilled empathic or attuned communication is necessary to uphold social dignity (and by extension, well-being). CPT in this sense has a role to play at the very root of well-being within a healthcare context—through active recognition of the dignity of each individual engaging with the service.

Access to mental health interventions, and the ability of mental health professionals to support the communication of those with aphasia, is a domain of healthcare that warrants particular consideration, given that the higher rates of depression among PWA post-stroke than in the general stroke population [21]. Early depression and mental health concerns are linked to an increased risk of depression later in the stroke journey [22, 23]. Despite the high levels of depression and anxiety in this group, those with communication disability face significant barriers in accessing mental health interventions [24], particularly the "talking therapies" that are typically available for people with depression [25]. Interventions that address mental health and well-being are so often delivered through a conversational medium. However, when the medium of communication itself is interrupted, addressing these complex, hidden psychosocial needs becomes challenging. People with communication disabilities such as aphasia are often excluded from such opportunities, risking a further impact on their health and well-being. Recent work in relation to addressing psychological outcomes for PWA has focused on adapting mental health interventions for this population (e.g., Northcott et al. [26]) and interdisciplinary working with speech and language therapists and psychologists (e.g., Santro Pietro et al. [27]). There has been little published on CPT for mental health professionals specifically, although the potential for CPT delivered to mental health professions is under-explored but potentially powerful [28].

Research [29, 30] on CPT for volunteers, including, but not limited to, students in healthcare programs, suggests that these groups can acquire knowledge and skills that enable successful conversation and befriending. There is evidence of the benefit of student volunteers providing opportunities for successful conversation following training in CPT, acknowledging that the benefits are also experienced by the students themselves who accumulate valuable learning from the process of engaging with PWA [29]. More recently attention has been given to interventions designed to enable "peer-befriending" for people with stroke and aphasia (e.g., Hilari et al. [31]). The training for peers in such programs often involves training to be better communication partners [31–33].

CPT for service employees, such as transport workers, hospitality employees, and others, has the potential to increase community participation and inclusion. Researchers recognize that in the context of service industries, disorder-specific training imposes limitations and generic training regarding communication support is more appropriate [34] but there is a limited evidence base at present.

Taken as a whole then, research on CPT has been demonstrated to be effective in improving the knowledge and skills of various groups of communication partners, with distal outcomes being improved interactions with PWA. Specifically, individuals with aphasia want to "communicate their emotions, reduce communication breakdown and stress… participate in 'normal' and more complex conversations including discussions" [35] (p. 1369). Given the link between positive interactions and well-being, as outlined at the start of this chapter, CPT has the potential to be one intervention that promotes well-being and adjustment in stroke—factors which in themselves may prevent depression [16]. Across multiple settings and communication partners, there is the opportunity to enhance well-being and mental health outcomes through improving communication.

What makes communication "good," and what is the nature of conversations that contribute to a sense of connection and well-being? Communication Accommodation Theory (CAT) [36–38] which is discussed next provides a particularly useful framework to address this question and explore the nature of conversation and the impact of CPT.

Communication Accommodation Theory (CAT): A Framework to Explore the Communication Experience

A feature of conversation is how communication partners adjust or accommodate within the flow of the interaction. When people interact, they adjust their behavior with respect to their communication partner [39]. These adjustments are usually guided by the purpose or motivation to adjust and the skills or abilities of the communicators to adjust their own styles of communication [40]. Knowledge of the communication abilities of an interacting partner also influences the ways in which people adjust their own behavior. This adjustment in conversational behavior can be explained by CAT.

CAT suggests that people adjust their communicative behavior "in pursuit of positive personal and social identities" [39] (p. 28). Adjustment is considered to serve two distinct purposes [39, 40]. The affective function relates to the social and relational identity aspects of communication [39, 41]; and the cognitive function [39] focuses on the comprehensibility and the accessibility of the information being shared during communication and serves to attain communication efficiency [40, 41].

Adjustments in behavior are often influenced by perceptions of the speaker and can be explained by considering "personal, situational, and cultural circumstances" [41] (p. 469) that might influence an individual's perception, evaluation, and consequential attributions (e.g., personality, competence, intelligence, friendliness) of a CP [39]. These factors interact in complex ways to influence accommodation in communicative interaction. For example, an individual's desire to portray themselves as the more powerful communication partner is more likely to lead to divergence in communicative behavior [41]. However, when such differences in behavior associated with role and power differences (e.g., interviewer–interviewee, doctor–patient, parent–child interactions) are mutually attempted and accepted, it is considered as "complementarity" and may be perceived favorably [42]. Prior communicative experiences in communication as well as expectations [40] of how the other interactant will behave also impact adjustment in communicative behavior for both individuals and groups. For example, in interactions with PWA, the observed association between broader CP perceptions of the personality (e.g., ability to make friends, intelligence, and confidence) of PWA with their perceived non-fluency (e.g., Khvalabov [43]) might offer an explanation for the reduced skill in communication observed among untrained CPs who have been exposed to PWA [44]. It could be suggested that CP perceptions that undermine the competence of PWA which manifest in communicative behavior can negatively impact the well-being of PWA.

Adjustment in communication involves the responsive adaptation [41] of an individual's verbal and non-verbal communicative behavior to that of an interlocutor [39]. It may take different forms and various types of adjustment have been introduced in the CAT literature as its application expanded and extended to a wide range of fields of study. Table 26.1 presents four broad categories of adjustment.

In a recent application [45] of CAT to interactions involving PWA and their primary CPs, PWA were observed to adjust their communicative behavior in the context of that of their CPs and vice versa. The observed adjustments included changes to the "medium" of communication (language, modality, or style), the use of non-verbal supports such as gestures, pointing and written

Table 26.1 Categories of adjustment

Type	Definition	Examples
Accommodation	Refers to the adjustment in communication that usually serves to improve the communicative interaction, reduce differences, and enhance the meaningfulness and effectiveness of the communication.	Conversation partner uses gestures and keywords to support the conversation with the PWA.
Nonaccommodation	Refers to the adjustment in communicative behavior that functions to increase the social distance between interlocutors or hinder effective communication	Conversation partner maintains verbal communication without any effort to support the PWAs ability to participate in conversation.
Reluctant accommodation	Refers to the adjustment in communicative behavior that occurs when an individual converges to the style of the interlocutor in consideration of the societal and hierarchical norms and not due to a personal desire for affinity.	Conversation partner attunes to the PWA's style of conversation owing to external factors such as the presence of the clinician in the room.
Avoidant communication	Refers to the adjustment in communicative behavior that occurs when an individual withdraws from participation in communication due to a prior negative experience, stereotypes, etc.	Conversation partner tries to minimize the conversation or end the conversation to avoid continually engaging in conversation.

Note: Table adapted from Pais [45]

keywords, the topic/content of the discussion, the rate of speech, and intonation. The adjustments made in each turn of the conversation influenced the adjustments made in the turns that followed and were therefore observed to impact on the participation and effectiveness of the interaction positively or negatively.

Intentional and unintentional adjustments in the conversational styles were observed as being used by both the PWA and their CPs. Both interlocutors were observed to use facilitative adjustments (including accommodation and reluctant accommodation) as well as obstructive adjustments (including nonaccommodation and avoidant communication). In addition to these categories of accommodation types described in the literature on CAT, two further types were identified in the data. These types account for adjustment that are not captured by the original categories and entail accommodation where constraints on communication are imposed by aphasia. The two additional categories proposed include *Constrained Accommodation* and *Unavoidable Nonaccommodation. Constrained Accommodation* may be perceived as "underaccommodation" by the listener. *Unavoidable Nonaccommodation* may be perceived as "nonaccommodation" or "avoidant communication" by the listener. Constrained accommodation (facilitative) and unavoidable nonaccommodation (obstructive) were adjustments observed in the conversational turns of the participants with aphasia, due to the nature of the communication difficulties/impairments.

The impact of aphasia can be observed across various types of interactions. For example, the communication consequences can directly impact the level and nature of interaction between the PWA and the friends and family. Spouses, for instance, have been reported to demonstrate increased negative communicative behaviors than positive attitudes during interactions [46]. Simmons-Mackie and Damico [47] applying principles of interaction to aphasiology suggest that the way people react to one other is based on their experiences and social constructions of interaction. For example, Pais [45] demonstrates how when untrained familiar and unfamiliar CPs view PWA as "impaired," this perception can manifest in CPs behavior during interaction and result in PWA not wanting to participate. This was sometimes seen in the form of test questions, practice tasks, negative comments as illustrated below using extracts from conversational and interview data from Pais [45].

In an interaction between a father (Chandrak) and son (Paarth) illustrated in Excerpt (1) below, instances of test questions (turn 3) and practice tasks (turns 17–98) initiated by the son are subsequently met with arguably avoidance behaviors (turn 98) by the father who has aphasia. While Chandrak initially complies with tasks (turns 3–90), following turn 98, the father was observed to respond in a manner that deviated from the task of "copywriting" initiated by the son. What was lacking throughout this conversation, however, was any instance of a clear exchange of information.

Excerpt (1)

Turn	Speaker	Utterance
3	Paarth	nin per emme? ((*points to PWA with finger*)) **what is your name?**
4	Chandrak	(unintelligible utterance) ((*looks at the CP, grasps pen and holds it to the sheet of paper*))
(…)		
17	Paarth	iDu haTu rupai ((*grasps pen and demonstrates on sheet how to write 10, looks at sheet where PWA has written*)) haTu **this is ten rupees. ten**
18	Chandrak	(unintelligible utterance) ((*grasps pen and writes, looks at sheet where CP has written*))
19	Paarth	((*clicks tongue indicating disapproval*)) vonDu ((*leans forward to look at what PWA is writing. Demonstrates writing one*)) **One.**
20	Chandrak	((*grasps pen and writes down one*))
(…)		
97	Paarth	aaru ((*points out the numeric keywords on the sheets*)) **six**
98	Chandrak	ah ((*points to written numbers*))

In interactions with PWA, unfavorable attitudes toward communication and negative perceptions of disability can also have a significant impact on participation in future interactions as well as in other daily activities. In an interview with another PWA (Chet), and his sister (Payal), see Excerpt (2), Payal describes an upsetting incident that resulted in Chet discontinuing going to his own place of work as a shopkeeper, owing to the reactions of his neighboring shopkeepers.

Excerpt (2)

Speaker	Utterance
Payal	avaru eevaga ee ((*points towards the PWA*)) hogalva, alla? (…) aaDrannu, angadi aTra hogbaekaDrae, avaru kelasaDavaru Della irTara alla? vonTara hangsTare—oo ivaru hangiDa. eevaga nodi hingaagbittu avannu maTDak avaru **Now he ((*points towards the PWA*)) doesn't go, right? (…) Even then, if you have to go near the shop, they, the workers would there be right? They laugh in some peculiar way—Ohh he used to be that way. Now look, after this has happened, he is one who doesn't speak up.**
(…)	
Payal	aDarinDanae avarigae bejara aguDu. algoTae kelasakaTrae hogalla **It is from that itself, that he has gotten upset. Because of that, now he doesn't go there for work.**

Adjustment in interaction can be reactive or proactive. The motivational processes surrounding communication, may be altered during the course of the interaction and may be based on the ongoing communicative experience [40, 48]. Negative communicative experiences can result in reduced engagement, and participation or "avoidant communication" for one or both interlocutors. For people with communication disorders, where there is a risk of communication breakdown during interaction, the impact can therefore be adverse. Spouses have also been reported to experience changes in their emotions, behavior, and reactions during interaction with their partner with aphasia [49, 50].

Adjustments to communication behavior may be repeatedly observed across interactions with specific partners or similar groups of people. While some of these adjustments may only be observed across some interactions (termed short-term adjustments), some adjustments can be maintained across multiple communicative interactions and for a longer duration (termed long-term adjustments). Where the long-term adjustments are obstructive in nature, they risk repeated negative experiences in interaction which can impact a person's well-being as well as participation in future interactions.

A common observation in interactions involving PWA is the use of test questions, test tasks, which can impact negatively on communication and interaction as illustrated earlier. PWA have been observed to often comply with these behaviors overtime (as seen in the interaction between Paarth and his father Chandrak). This shifts the dynamic from family interactions to that of a "tester" and a "testee" and can impact on the sense of self and well-being of the PWA. Application of CAT could also suggest that the increased compliance by PWA might be a manifestation of the negative psychosocial impact of such nonaccommodation during communication.

Communication experiences can therefore influence the nature of communicative behavior and the level of interaction in ongoing and future interactions. In general, in the study conducted by Pais [45], adjustments in the communicative behavior of the untrained CPs were observed to be more obstructive (nonaccommodation including underaccommodation and overaccommodation) rather than facilitative (accommodation) in nature. In terms of participation, PWA were found to make attempts to participate contribute to interactions only 50% of the time, on average, during the recorded interactions with their CPs, with support offered by the CPs only 25% to 50% of the time during the baseline conversations. Negative communication experiences can and were observed to impact on social interaction and often participation in life. Such negative experiences can risk resulting in feelings of loneliness, isolation [51], grief, anger [52], and depression [53].

There is therefore a significant risk in terms of the approaches to interaction, from the reactions of people with low levels of awareness, those who see disability as a curse, to atypical styles of interaction, and communication breakdown. These consequences can impact the experiences of PWA, causing a chain reaction. Understanding these processes, therefore, is crucial to addressing them, and to paint a picture to drive change. CAT offers a framework that has the ability to facilitate structured identification of facilitative [54] and nonaccommodative behaviors [39, 55] and suggest causal explanations for the associated self-imposed consequential communicative experiences [38]. CAT also has the unique ability to capture the way accommodation is grounded in the achievement of communication actions as they transpire in interaction [48].

Impact of CPT as Explained by Application of CAT

While the impact of CPT on communication and interaction for both trained CPs and the PWA they interact with is known: application of CAT to the interactions of PWA and their trained partners within the Indian context discussed in this chapter demonstrated changes in nature of adjustment such as reduced nonaccommodative behaviors by way of reduced maintenance of and divergence to solely verbal forms of communication, reduced nonaccommodative discourse management behavior (such as reduced interruptions, use of test questions), and increased accommodation by way of interpretability and discourse management strategies (such as the communication supports and providing more time). The change in behavior of the CPs created opportunities for their partners with aphasia to respond in turn, correct incorrect inferences made by the CP and contribute further to the ongoing topic of discussion. The improved participation of the PWA is in line with the literature which suggests that improvement in the (M)SCA (i.e., Measure of Support in Conversation for adults with Aphasia) [57] has a direct impact on the (M)PCA (i.e., Measure of Participation in conversation for adults with Aphasia) [56, 57].

The changes in adjustment observed in the data from the Indian context suggest an increased focus on the acknowledging competence. For some participants, such improvements also suggested changes to long-term negative communicative patterns and behaviors following training. There was also an apparent increase in sharing the responsibility for communicative breakdowns. For example, following CPT-In (a CPT program adapted and developed for use in the Indian context) [45], communication partners who had difficulty writing and using keywords successfully used line drawings and symbols to support PWAs expression and enhance the meaningfulness of the discourse. While regaining the ability to communicate verbally may have remained a goal for some participants, an improvement in facilitatory communicative behavior was evidenced in the follow-up conversations. The hope to regain normality in verbal communication, however, has been seen in other contexts as well, and has been associated with acceptance of the changes following the stroke including changes to communication, personality, roles, and pre-morbid identity (e.g., Wallace et al. [35]). For participants in the acute phase particularly, adopting new strategies and reduced engagement with recommended strategies might be harder [58]. Culture as an influencing factor has had limited consideration, however. For example, socio-cultural factors may have influenced the acceptance of supportive strategies observed in some follow-up interactions. For example, in follow-up conversations with Chet and Payal, a reduction in the use of taught strategies was observed in Payal's communication with reduced engagement, participation, and transaction observed in Chet's turns. This was associated with negative reactions such as laughter and taunting behavior from neighboring shopkeepers when Chet attempted to use non-verbal strategies to get his message across as discussed by them during a follow-up interview. While these challenges may not be specific to the Indian context, they may be strengthened in dyads with a strong preference for verbal language and can influence the impact of CPT and consequentially the impact on well-being.

Improvements in interaction for PWA and their trained CPs following CPT created opportunities for communication that extended beyond "yes and no" questions, and reduced "practice tasks." Participants were observed to engage in discussions about shopping, likes and dislikes, planning for festivities, participation in decision-making, and more. Increased participation of PWA in interactions in some cases also reportedly extended beyond the trained family members. During a follow-up interview post CPT-In with a father and son (Chandrak and Paarth), Excerpt (3), Paarth shared how following the training, there were observed adjustments in the communication of his father as well, which supported the ability of the family members (both trained and untrained) to understand Chandrak better.

Excerpt (3)

Speaker	Utterance
Paarth	madam firstu yaenenDa, firstu maTanadvaaga, yaaru yaena arTanae aagalilla. eevaga yaenagoTiDaaDrae, kai alli action maadsTarae, bariTarae, ((pencil grasp gesture indicates 'writing')), illayaenan TorisTarae ((lifts both hands and uses each hand to touch the other, gesture indicates 'shows with hand')), aDarinDa yella find out madabouDu. avaga, naavu Tilkondakkae easy aguTae, maTaevarannu ((points to PWA)) arTamadslikkae easy aagiDae. **Madam, at first, whenever he would speak, no one could understand anything. Now, whatever he knows, he will use hand gestures, he writes ((pencil grasp gesture indicates 'writing')), if not, whatever it is, he shows us ((lifts both hands and uses each hand to touch the other, gesture indicates 'shows with hand')), And from that, we are able to find out all of it. At that point, what we have learnt to put to use, it becomes easy. Then, it has become easy for him to make us understand.**

As reduced communication access is expected to be detrimental to QOL [47], improvements in the communication may have a positive impact on quality of life and well-being over time, however this was not clearly evidenced in the data from the Indian context and may have been associated with a range of factors not limited to the complexities associated with communication and the complex socio-cultural context.

Implications for Mental Health Contexts

Given the bi-directional relationship between communication difficulties and mental health difficulties, the focus on CPT to address well-being for people with primary disorders of communication (e.g., aphasia) represents only one side of the equation. People who have a primary diagnosis of mental health difficulties, such as schizophrenia, bipolar mood disorder, or major depression, may experience a range of difficulties with regard to communication [9]. While these difficulties have received some attention in the literature, there is limited research on how intervention is best structured.

CPT has the potential to provide a potent environmental change that respects the communication processes of the person with the mental health diagnosis, and provides both interlocutors with strategies to optimize conversation. Brophy and O'Connor [59] describe the use of communication support plans (a common tool in some fields of speech and language therapy), as a means to empower service users to actively influence the communication environment and better their opportunities for connectedness. While not CPT in a traditional sense, the communication support plan as envisaged by their practitioners lays the foundation for individualized conversations about what features of communication help or hinder connection. The communication behaviors identified by service users in relation to "what I can ask others to do different" provides a potential blueprint for CPT, or for conversations led by the service user, that in themselves can be considered as user-driven CPT. Similarly, Jagoe [60] suggests that CPT in mental health settings is likely to be best served by communication partners appraising their own communication skills from within a framework that explicitly recognizing the fallibility of human communication in general (thereby shifting the focus on breakdown away from the individual with the diagnosis and to the interactional space). CPT remains a potentially powerful and yet under-utilized intervention in mental health contexts.

Conclusion

Communication partner training, as an environmental intervention, is supported by an increasing body of evidence, mostly well established in relation to aphasia. Gaps in the evidence exist with regard to specific types of communication partners or settings. However, when taken in conjunction with evidence of the link between satisfying interactions and well-being, there is a clear argument for CPT as having the potential to influence the distal outcomes of mood and mental health more broadly. The data presented on family interactions between PWA and their family members in the Indian context demonstrates the potential of CPT to influence the nuances of how communication partners adjust their communication during interaction. Although evidence on quality of life remains unclear, it is suggested here that the use of frameworks such as CAT may play a valuable role in revealing the proximal outcome of changes in communication adjustment, with careful selection of outcome measures related to mood and well-being warranted.

Major Takeaways

1. Communication experiences can impact ongoing and future adjustment in communicative behavior for both people with aphasia (PWA) and those interacting with them.
2. Communication experiences during daily activities can impact ongoing and future participation in social activities for PWA and their family members.
3. Communication Partner Training (CPT) improves meaningful interaction between PWA and their CPs, allowing conversations surrounding feelings, emotions, and decisions and rehabilitation needs which has implications for their mental health and well-being.
4. Communication Accommodation Theory (CAT) offers structure that supports rigorous and rich analysis of conversation and the psychosocial process underlying interaction.

References

1. McVicker S, Parr S, Pound C, Duchan J. The communication partner scheme: a project to develop long-term, low-cost access to conversation for people

living with aphasia. Aphasiology. 2009;23(1):52–71. https://doi.org/10.1080/02687030701688783.
2. Power E, Thomas E, Worrall L, Rose M, Togher L, Nickels L, Hersh D, Godecke E, O'Halloran R, Lamont S, O'Connor C, Clarke K. Development and validation of Australian aphasia rehabilitation best practice statements using the RAND/UCLA appropriateness method. BMJ Open. 2015;5(7):e007641. https://doi.org/10.1136/bmjopen-2015-007641.
3. Simmons-Mackie N, Worrall L, Murray LL, Enderby P, Rose ML, Paek EJ, Klippi A, on behalf of the Aphasia United Best Practices Working Group. The top ten: best practice recommendations for aphasia. Aphasiology. 2017;31(2):131–51. https://doi.org/10.1080/02687038.2016.1180662.
4. Kagan A, Black SE, Duchan JF, Simmons-Mackie N, Square P. Training volunteers as conversation partners using "supported conversation for adults with aphasia" (SCA): a controlled trial. J Speech Lang Hear Res. 2001;44(3):624–38.
5. Nezlek JB, Richardson DS, Green LR, Schatten-Jones EC. Psychological Well-being and day-to-day social interaction among older adults. Pers Relat. 2002;9(1):57–71.
6. Haley KL, Womack JL, Harmon TG, McCulloch KL, Faldowski RA. Life activity choices by people with aphasia: repeated interviews and proxy agreement. Aphasiology. 2019;33(6):710–30. https://doi.org/10.1080/02687038.2018.1506087.
7. Baker C, Worrall L, Rose M, Ryan B. 'It was really dark': the experiences and preferences of people with aphasia to manage mood changes and depression. Aphasiology. 2020;34(1):19–46. https://doi.org/10.1080/02687038.2019.1673304.
8. Kutlubaev MA, Hackett ML. Part II: predictors of depression after stroke and impact of depression on stroke outcome: an updated systematic review of observational studies. Int J Stroke. 2014;9:1026–36. https://doi.org/10.1111/ijs.12356.
9. Walsh IP, Jagoe C, Brophy J. Language and communication in adults with mental health disorders: considerations for understanding speech and language therapy process and practice. In: Jagoe C, Walsh IP, editors. Communication and mental health disorders: developing theory, growing practice. Guildford: J&R Press Ltd; 2020. p. 53–78.
10. Palmer AD, Carder PC, White DL, Saunders G, Woo H, Graville DJ, Newsom JT. The impact of communication impairments on the social relationships of older adults: pathways to psychological Well-being. J Speech Lang Hear Res. 2019;62(1):1–21. https://doi.org/10.1044/2018_JSLHR-S-17-0495.
11. Ferguson A. Describing competence in aphasic/normal conversation. Clin Linguist Phon. 1996;10(1):55–63. https://doi.org/10.3109/02699209608985161.
12. Byng S, Duchan JF. Social model philosophies and principles: their applications to therapies for aphasia social model philosophies and principles: their applications to therapies for aphasia. Aphasiology. 2005;19(10–11):906–22. https://doi.org/10.1080/02687030544000128.
13. Simmons-Mackie N, Raymer A, Armstrong E, Holland A, Cherney LR. Partner training in aphasia: a systematic review. Arch Phys Med Rehabil. 2010;91(12):1814–37.
14. Simmons-Mackie N, Raymer A, Cherney LR. Communication partner training in aphasia: an updated systematic review. Arch Phys Med Rehabil. 2016;97:2202. https://doi.org/10.1016/j.apmr.2016.03.023.
15. Cruice M, Blom Johansson M, Isaksen J, Horton S. Reporting interventions in communication partner training: a critical review and narrative synthesis of the literature. Aphasiology. 2018;32(10):1234–65. https://doi.org/10.1080/02687038.2018.1482406.
16. Baker C, Worrall L, Rose M, Hudson K, Ryan B, O'Byrne L. A systematic review of rehabilitation interventions to prevent and treat depression in post-stroke aphasia. Disabil Rehabil. 2018;40(16):1870–92. https://doi.org/10.1080/09638288.2017.1315181.
17. Brown SE, Scobbie L, Worrall L, Brady MC. A multinational online survey of the goal setting practice of rehabilitation staff with stroke survivors with aphasia. Aphasiology. 2023;37:479. https://doi.org/10.1080/02687038.2022.2031861.
18. van Rijssen MN, Veldkamp M, Bryon E, Remijn L, Visser-Meily JMA, Gerrits E, van Ewijk L. How do healthcare professionals experience communication with people with aphasia and what content should communication partner training entail? Disabil Rehabil. 2022;44(14):3671–8. https://doi.org/10.1080/09638288.2021.1878561.
19. Carragher M, Steel G, O'Halloran R, Torabi T, Johnson H, Taylor NF, Rose M. Aphasia disrupts usual care: the stroke team's perceptions of delivering healthcare to patients with aphasia. Disabil Rehabil. 2021;43(21):3003–14. https://doi.org/10.1080/09638288.2020.1722264.
20. Vallumrød S, Johannessen A, Lyberg AM. Factors that influence social dignity in persons with aphasia in their contact with healthcare professionals: a systematic literature review of qualitative studies. Int Pract Dev J. 2020;10(2):1. https://doi.org/10.19043/ipdj.102.009.
21. Kauhanen ML, Korpelainen JT, Hiltunen P, et al. Aphasia, depression, and non-verbal cognitive impairment in ischaemic stroke. Cerebrovasc Dis. 2000;10:455–61.
22. Hilari K, Wiggins R, Roy P, Byng S, Smith S. Predictors of health-related quality of life (HRQL) in people with chronic aphasia. Aphasiology. 2003;17(4):365–81.
23. Thomas SA, Lincoln NB. Predictors of emotional distress after stroke. Stroke. 2008;39(4):1240–5.
24. Ryan B, Bohan J, Kneebone I. Help-seeking and people with aphasia who have mood problems after stroke: perspectives of speech–language pathologists. Int J Lang Commun Disord. 2019;54(5):779–93. https://doi.org/10.1111/1460-6984.12476.

25. Bullier B, Cassoudesalle H, Villain M, Cogné M, Mollo C, De Gabory I, Dehail P, Joseph PA, Sibon I, Glize B. New factors that affect quality of life in patients with aphasia. Ann Phys Rehabil Med. 2020;63(1):33–7. https://doi.org/10.1016/j.rehab.2019.06.015.
26. Northcott S, Thomas S, James K, Simpson A, Hirani S, Barnard R, Hilari K. Solution focused brief therapy in post-stroke aphasia (SOFIA): feasibility and acceptability results of a feasibility randomised waitlist controlled trial. BMJ Open. 2021;11(8):e050308. https://doi.org/10.1136/bmjopen-2021-050308.
27. Santo Pietro MJ, Marks DR, Mullen A. When words fail: providing effective psychological treatment for depression in persons with aphasia. J Clin Psychol Med Settings. 2019;26(4):483–94.
28. Sheehy A. That was really the only meaningful time that he actually had to have a genuine conversation that was all about him": reviewing a counselling service for people with acquired communication disorders following stroke: service user and team perspectives. [Thesis] Trinity College Dublin. School of Linguistic Speech & Communication Sciences; 2016.
29. Cameron A, Hudson K, Finch E, Fleming J, Lethlean J, McPhail S. 'I've got to get something out of it. And so do they': experiences of people with aphasia and university students participating in a communication partner training programme for healthcare professionals. Int J Lang Commun Disord. 2018;53(5):919–28. https://doi.org/10.1111/1460-6984.12402.
30. Moss B, Behn N, Northcott S, Monnelly K, Marshall J, Simpson A, Thomas A, McVicker S, Goldsmith K, Flood C, Hilari K. "Loneliness can also kill:" a qualitative exploration of outcomes and experiences of the SUPERB peer-befriending scheme for people with aphasia and their significant others. Disabil Rehabil. 2022;44(18):5015–24. https://doi.org/10.1080/09638288.2021.1922519.
31. Hilari K, Behn N, James K, Northcott S, Marshall J, Thomas S, Simpson A, Moss B, Flood C, McVicker S, Goldsmith K. Supporting wellbeing through peer-befriending (SUPERB) for people with aphasia: a feasibility randomised controlled trial. Clin Rehabil. 2021;35(8):1151–63. https://doi.org/10.1177/0269215521995671.
32. Corsten S, Knieriemen, M, Kurfess C, Kreiter D, Lauer N. Structural and functional studies of protein interactions in gene expression. [conference presentation] international aphasia rehabilitation conference. 12–24 June 2022, Philadelphia.
33. Behn N, Moss B, Mcvicker S, Roper A, Northcott S, Marshall J, Thomas S, Simpson A, Flood C, James K, Goldsmith K, Hilari K. SUpporting wellbeing through PEeR-befriending (SUPERB) feasibility trial: Fidelity of peer-befriending for people with aphasia. BMJ Open. 2021;11(8):e047994. https://doi.org/10.1136/bmjopen-2020-047994.
34. Tessier A, Power E, Croteau C. Paid worker and unfamiliar partner communication training: a scoping review. J Commun Disord. 2020;83:83. https://doi.org/10.1016/j.jcomdis.2019.105951.
35. Wallace SJ, Worrall L, Rose T, Le Dorze G, Cruice M, Isaksen J, Kong APH, Simmons-Mackie N, Scarinci N, Gauvreau CA. Which outcomes are most important to people with aphasia and their families? An international nominal group technique study framed within the ICF. Disabil Rehabil. 2017;39(14):1364–79. https://doi.org/10.1080/09638288.2016.1194899.
36. Jones E, Gallois C, Callan V, Barker M. STRATEGIES OF ACCOMMODATION: development of a coding system for conversational interaction. J Lang Soc Psychol. 1999;18(2):123–51. https://doi.org/10.1177/0261927x99018002001.
37. Gallois C, Ogay T, Giles H. Communication accommodation theory: a look back and a look ahead. In: Gudykunst WB, editor. Theorizing about communication and culture. Thousand Oaks: Sage; 2006. p. 121–48.
38. Giles H, Coupland N, Coupland J. Accommodation theory: communication, context and consequence. In: Giles H, Coupland J, Coupland N, editors. Contexts of accommodation. Cambridge University Press; 2010. p. 1–68.
39. Gasiorek J. Theoretical perspectives on interpersonal adjustments in language and communication. In: Giles H, editor. Communication accommodation theory: negotiating personal relationships and social identities across contexts. Cambridge University Press; 2016. p. 13–35.
40. Dragojevic M, Gasiorek J, Giles H. Accommodative strategies as core of the theory. In: Giles H, editor. Communication accommodation theory: negotiating personal relationships and social identities across contexts. Cambridge University Press; 2016. p. 36–59.
41. Tomsha L, Hernandez R. Communication accommodation theory. In: West R, Turner LH, editors. Introducing communication theory: analysis and application. 4th ed. The McGraw-Hill Companies, Inc; 2010. p. 465–82.
42. Street RL. Accommodations in medical consultations. In: Giles H, Coupland J, Coupland N, editors. Contexts of accommodation. Cambridge University Press; 2010. p. 131–56.
43. Khvalabov N. Listener judgements of fluency and perceptions of aphasia [thesis] The University of Iowa; 2019. https://ir.uiowa.edu/honors_theses/299
44. Kagan A, Simmons-Mackie N, Victor JC. The impact of exposure with no training: implications for future partner training research. J Speech Lang Hear Res. 2018;61(9):2347–52. https://doi.org/10.1044/2018_JSLHR-L-17-0413.
45. Pais AM. Communication partner training for the primary caregivers of people with aphasia in India: a multi-phase exploratory study. [Thesis] Trinity College Dublin. School of Linguistic Speech & Communication Sciences; 2022. http://hdl.handle.net/2262/98560
46. Singh P, Pauranik A. Supportive conversational strategies for persons with aphasia and their significant

others. Journal of Indian Speech Language Hearing Association. 2017;31:57–65. https://doi.org/10.4103/jisha.JISHA_13_14.
47. Simmons-Mackie N, Damico JS. Access and social inclusion in aphasia: interactional principles and applications. Aphasiology. 2007;21(1):81–97. https://doi.org/10.1080/02687030600798311.
48. Gallois C, Weatherall A, Giles H. CAT and Talk in action. In: Giles H, editor. Communication accommodation theory: negotiating personal relationships and social identities across contexts. Cambridge University Press; 2016. p. 105–22.
49. Croteau C, McMahon-Morin P, Le Dorze G, Baril G. Impact of aphasia on communication in couples. Int J Lang Commun Disord. 2020;55(4):547–57. https://doi.org/10.1111/1460-6984.12537.
50. Michallet B, Tétreault S, Le Dorze G. The consequences of severe aphasia on the spouses of aphasic people: a description of the adaptation process. Aphasiology. 2003;17(9):835–59. https://doi.org/10.1080/02687030344000238.
51. Hilari K, Northcott S, Roy P, Marshall J, Wiggins RD, Chataway J, Ames D. Psychological distress after stroke and aphasia: the first six months. Clin Rehabil. 2010;24(2):181–90. https://doi.org/10.1177/0269215509346090.
52. Sorin-Peters R. Viewing couples living with aphasia as adult learners: implications for promoting quality of life. Aphasiology. 2003;17(4):405–16. https://doi.org/10.1080/02687030244000752.
53. Morrison M. I would tell you if I could: language loss, depression, and the challenge of treating patients with aphasia. UBCMJ. 2016;8(1):42–4. https://ojs.library.ubc.ca/index.php/ubcmj/article/view/188026
54. Simmons-Mackie N. Communication partner training in aphasia: reflections on communication accommodation theory. Aphasiology. 2018;32(10):1135–44. https://doi.org/10.1080/02687038.2018.1428282.
55. Gasiorek, J. The "Dark Side" of CAT: Nonaccommodation. In Giles H (ed.), Communication accommodation theory: negotiating personal relationships and social identities across contexts. Cambridge University Press; 2016. p. 85–104.
56. Eriksson K, Hartelius L, Saldert C. On the diverse outcome of communication partner training of significant others of people with aphasia: an experimental study of six cases. Int J Lang Commun Disord. 2016;51(4):402–14. https://doi.org/10.1111/1460-6984.12216.
57. Kagan A. "Supported conversation for adults with aphasia": Methods and evaluation [Thesis] University of Toronto; 1999. https://tspace.library.utoronto.ca/bitstream/1807/12973/1/NQ45755.pdf
58. Blom Johansson M, Carlsson M, Östberg P. A multiple-case study of a family-oriented intervention practice in the early rehabilitation phase of persons with aphasia. Aphasiology. 2013;27(2):201–26. https://doi.org/10.1080/02687038.2012.744808.
59. Brophy J, O'Connor S. The role of speech and language therapy in guiding service user involvement for mental health service users with communication support needs. In: Jagoe C, Walsh IP, editors. Communication and mental health disorders: developing theory, growing practice. Guildford: J&R Press Ltd; 2020. p. 191–218.
60. Jagoe C. Developing theoretically-grounded approaches to pragmatic intervention with people with schizophrenia. In: Jagoe C, Walsh IP, editors. Communication and mental health disorders: developing theory, growing practice. Guildford: J&R Press Ltd; 2020. p. 129–50.

Analisa Pais is a lecturer in the Speech and Language Therapy Division, at the School of Health and Social Care, University of Essex. She qualified as an Audiologist and Speech Language Pathologist from Manipal University, India and completed her Ph.D. at Trinity College Dublin, Ireland. Her research relates to communication access and participation for people with aphasia with a focus on majority world contexts and applying and extending communication theory to aphasia. Analisa is a member of the Collaboration of Aphasia Trialists (CATs) Societal Impact and Re-integration Research working group (http://aphasiatrials.org) and is the lead of the CATs Facebook Dissemination group.

Caroline Jagoe is an associate professor in the Department of Clinical Speech and Language Studies, Trinity College, The University of Dublin and a Research Associate in the School of Human and Community Development, University of the Witwatersrand, South Africa. Using insights from theoretical pragmatics, she works on communication access and disability inclusion in humanitarian contexts and scenarios of extreme adversity. She is the co-editor of the recent text Communication and mental health disorders: Developing theory, growing practice and sits on the Executive Committee of the Collaboration of Aphasia Trialists (http://aphasiatrials.org).

Index

A. P.-H. Kong (ed.), *Spoken Discourse Impairments in the Neurogenic Populations*, https://doi.org/10.1007/978-3-031-45190-4

GPSR Compliance

The European Union's (EU) General Product Safety Regulation (GPSR) is a set of rules that requires consumer products to be safe and our obligations to ensure this.

If you have any concerns about our products, you can contact us on ProductSafety@springernature.com

In case Publisher is established outside the EU, the EU authorized representative is:

Springer Nature Customer Service Center GmbH
Europaplatz 3
69115 Heidelberg, Germany

Batch number: 10732807

Printed by Printforce, the Netherlands